Complement in Health and Disease

Second edition

IMMUNOLOGY AND MEDICINE SERIES

Immunology of Endocrine Diseases
Editor: A. M. McGregor

Clinical Transplantation: Current Practice and Future Prospects
Editor: G. R. D. Catto

Complement in Health and Disease
Editor: K. Whaley

Immunological Aspects of Oral Diseases
Editor: L. Ivanyi

Immunoglobulins in Health and Disease
Editor: M. A. H. French

Immunology of Malignant Diseases
Editors: D. B. Jones and D. H. Wright

Phagocytes and Disease
Editors: M. S. Klempner, B. Styrt and J. Ho

Immunology of Sexually Transmitted Diseases
Editor: D. J. M. Wright

Mast Cells, Mediators and Disease
Editors: S. T. Holgate

Immunodeficiency and Disease
Editor: A. D. B. Webster

Immunology of Pregnancy and its Disorders
Editor: C. M. M. Stern

Immunotherapy of Disease
Editor: T. J. Hamblin

Immunology of Prophylactic Immunization
Editor: A. J. Zuckerman

Immunology of Eye Disease
Editor: S. Lightman

Lymphoproliferative Diseases
Editors: D. B. Jones and D. H. Wright

Immunology of Renal Diseases
Editor: C. D. Pusey

Biochemistry of Inflammation
Editors: J. T. Whicher and S. W. Evans

Immunology of ENT Disorders
Editor: G. Scadding

Immunology of Infection
Editors: J. G. P. Sissons, J. Cohen and L. K. Borysiewicz

Immunology of HIV Infection
Editor: A. G. Bird

Immunology of Gastrointestinal Disease
Editor: T. T. MacDonald

IMMUNOLOGY
SERIES · SERIES · SERIES · SERIES · SERIES AND SERIES · SERIES · SERIES · SERIES · SERIES
MEDICINE

VOLUME 20

Complement in Health and Disease

Second edition

Edited by
K. Whaley
Department of Immunology
University of Leicester
Leicester, UK

M. Loos
Institut für Medizinische Mikrobiologie
University of Mainz
Mainz, Germany

J. M. Weiler
University of Iowa
Iowa City, Iowa, USA
Series Editor: K. Whaley

KLUWER ACADEMIC PUBLISHERS
DORDRECHT / BOSTON / LONDON

Distributors

for the United States and Canada: Kluwer Academic Publishers, PO Box 358, Accord Station, Hingham, MA 02018-0358, USA
for all other countries: Kluwer Academic Publishers Group, Distribution Center, PO Box 322, 3300 AH Dordrecht, The Netherlands

A catalogue record for this book is available from the British Library

ISBN 0-7923-8823-2

Library of Congress Cataloging in Publication Data

Complement in health and disease / edited by K. Whaley, M.Loos, J. Weiler. -- 2nd ed.
p. cm. -- (Immunology and medicine series)
Includes bibliographical references and index.
ISBN 0-7923-8823-2
1. Complement (Immunology)) I. Whaley, Keith. II. Loos, M. III. Weiler, J. IV. Series.
[DNLM: 1. Complement--immunology. 2. Complement--genetics. 3. Immune Complex Diseases--immunology. QW 680 C7374 1993]
QR185.8.C6C68 1993
616.07'9--dc20
DNLM/DLC
for Library of Congress 93-9789
CIP

Copyright

Published in the United Kingdom by Kluwer Academic Publishers, PO Box 55, Lancaster, UK.

Kluwer Academic Publishers BV incorporates the publishing programmes of D. Reidel, Martinus Nijhoff, Dr W. Junk and MTP Press.

Typeset by EXPO Holding, Malaysia

Printed and bound in Great Britain by Hartnolls Ltd, Bodmin, Cornwall

Contents

List of Contributors

D Bitter-Suermann
Institut für Medizinische Mikrobiologie
Medizinische Hochschule Hannover
Konstanty-Gutschow Strasse 8
W-3000 Hannover 61
Germany

RD Campbell
MRC Immunochemistry Unit
Department of Biochemistry
University of Oxford
Oxford OX1 3QU
UK

HR Colten
Department of Paediatrics
Washington University Medical School
400 S Kingshighway Boulevard
St Louis, MO 63110
USA

AJ Day
MRC Immunochemistry Unit
Department of Biochemistry
University of Oxford
Oxford OX1 3QU
UK

P Densen
Department of Internal Medicine
University of Iowa College of Medicine
200 Hawkins Drive
Iowa City
IA 52242-1009
USA

AW Dodds
MRC Immunochemistry Unit
Department of Biochemistry
University of Oxford
Oxford OX1 3QU
UK

MK Frank
Department of Pediatrics
Duke University Medical Center
Durham, NC 17710
USA

J Köhl
Institut für Medizinische Mikrobiologie
Medizinische Hochschule Hannover
Konstanty-Gutschow Strasse 8
W-3000 Hannover 61
Germany

SKA Law
MRC Immunochemistry Unit
Department of Biochemistry
University of Oxford
South Parks Road
Oxford OX1 3QU
UK

BP Morgan
Department of Clinical Biochemistry
University of Wales
College of Medicine
Heath Park
Cardiff CF4 4XN
UK

YC Ng
Department of Medicine
King Fahd Armed Forces Hospital
PO Box 9862
Jeddah 21159
Saudi Arabia

KBM Reid
MRC Immunochemistry Unit
Department of Biochemistry
University of Oxford
Oxford OX1 3QU
UK

FS Rosen
Department of Pediatrics
Harvard Medical School
800 Huntington Avenue
Boston, MA 02115
USA

J Schifferli
Division de Néphrologie
Départment de Médecine
Hôpital Cantonal Universitaire
CH-1211 Geneva 4
Switzerland

RC Strunk
Department of Pediatrics
Washington University Medical School
400 S Kingshighway Boulevard
St Louis, MI 63110
USA

M Tosi
Unite d´Immunogenetique
INSERM U276
Institut Pasteur
25 rue du Docteur Roux
75724 Paris Cedex 15
France

JM Weiler
Department of Internal Medicine
Iowa City VA Medical Center and
University of Iowa College of Medicine
Iowa City
IA 52242
USA

JB Weitzman
MRC Immunochemistry Unit
Department of Biochemistry
University of Oxford
South Parks Road
Oxford OX1 3QU
UK

K Whaley
Department of Immunology
University of Leicester
Leicester Royal Infirmary
Leicester LE2 7LX
UK

Preface

Since the first edition of *Complement in Health and Disease* was published in 1986, significant advances have been made. The cDNAs for all of the components and some of the receptors have been cloned and sequenced. The chromosomal localization and the structural organization of a number of these genes have now been determined. These advances are now facilitating research into the structure of the complement proteins, the nature of the complement deficiency syndromes, the regulation of complement gene expression and the role of complement in different diseases. This edition contains contributions from both basic and clinical scientists in a format which we hope will appeal to both immunologists and physicians who wish to know more about this fascinating and important host defence system.

The introductory chapter by John Weiler presents a historical background to research on the complement system and describes the biochemical events occurring during activation of the system. In Chapter 2 Alastair Dodds and Tony Day discuss the phylogeny and evolution of the complement system. The techniques of protein chemistry and molecular biology have provided powerful insights into the modular structure of complement proteins and the evolution of the complement system. The structure and organisation of the complement genes is described in Chapter 3 by Ken Reid and Duncan Campbell. This chapter describes the modular structure of the complement proteins and some of the mutations which are responsible for deficiencies of individual components. The regulation of expression of the complement genes is discussed in Chapter 4 by Harvey Colten and Bob Strunk. Although the liver is the site of synthesis of most of the plasma complement components (with the possible exceptions of properdin, factor D and C1q), most of the fluid-phase complement proteins are also synthesized by cells outwith the liver. Despite the fact that we do not know the biological significance of extrahepatic complement synthesis, the accessibility of such cells provides an invaluable tool for the investigation of complement gene expression.

The remaining chapters have a more clinical focus. In Chapter 5, Fred Rosen provides an introduction to the topic of complement deficiency drawing on his wealth of experience in this field, and Peter Denson (Chapter 6) discusses the problem of bacterial infections in complement deficient patients. Mario Tosi then describes the genetic lesions underlying C1-inhibitor deficiency (Chapter 7). New ideas on the pathogenesis and treatment of C1-inhibitor deficiency are discussed by Mike Frank in Chapter 8. To continue the theme of complement in defence against bacterial infections, Jonathan Weitzman and Alex Law (Chapter 9) discuss the role of complement receptor type III (CR3) as a phagocytic receptor. Yin Ng and Jurg Schifferli (Chapter 10) then discuss the role of complement and complement deficiency in immune complex disease. The generation of anaphylatoxins during complement activation provides a powerful stimulus to the inflammatory process. Jorg Köhl and Dieter Bitter-Suermann discuss the biological activities of anaphylatoxins, the structure of the C5a receptor and the role of anaphylatoxins in different diseases. The membrane attack complex of complement, which was for so long considered to be exclusively a cytolytic effector, is now known to be a powerful activator of different cells. Paul Morgan describes the non-cytolytic effector mechanisms of the membrane attack complex in Chapter 12 and in Chapter 13 he discusses the role of complement in neurological diseases.

We wish to thank the authors for their contributions and collaborations, and Miss Sharon Crow for her secretarial work.

December 1992

Keith Whaley, *Leicester*
Michael Loos, *Mainz*
John Weiler, *Iowa City*

1 Introduction

J. M. WEILER

The complement system consists of at least 18 serum proteins and 10 membrane proteins that interact in a complex cascade leading to a wide variety of important biological responses. There are two complement activating sequences called the classical and the alternative pathways. The classical pathway was the first to be discovered and was originally thought to be activated by the Fc portion of IgM and IgG after specific immunity develops. It is now known that the classical pathway can be activated independently of antibody in the non-immune state. The alternative pathway was discovered more recently but is older phylogenetically and was originally felt to be a more important mechanism for natural immunity because activation was thought to be entirely antibody independent. However, antigen–antibody complexes may activate the alternative pathway directly through the Fab portion of the molecule. The substances involved in antibody-independent activation of the classical pathway are usually negatively charged whereas most of those producing antibody-independent activation of the alternative pathway are polysaccharides. Both pathways lead to the cleavage of the third component (C3), the complement component with the highest serum concentration. The alternative pathway is also recognized as the amplification pathway because C3 cleavage is greatly enhanced when alternative pathway components interact. A final common terminal pathway, known as the terminal complement complex (TCC) or the membrane attack complex (MAC), can lead to lysis of cells or infecting organisms.

The existence of a complement system has been known for more than 100 years although the exact nature of its components and their complex interactions are still being studied. Indeed, many of the biological consequences of complement activation await elucidation. This book serves to define progress towards understanding the complement system and its effects on the host.

A BRIEF HISTORY OF COMPLEMENT

The complement system has a rich history, dating back to the 1880s, and includes contributions from Bordet, Ehrlich and Metchnikoff as well as a large number of more modern immunologists[1–19]. Grohmann first reported in 1884 that cell-free plasma is able to kill bacteria[20]. Nuttall, in 1888, reported that defibrinated blood lyses anthrax bacillus *in vitro* and that this capacity is lost when the blood is heated or when the blood is stored for a few days at room temperature[21]. Buchner confirmed these observations in 1889 and called the heat-labile factor in the blood 'alexin', a term that survived until well into the first half of the 20th century[22,23].

Pfeiffer and Issaeff showed, in 1894, that blood obtained from guinea pigs who have recovered from cholera infection is able to protect normal guinea pigs from cholera infection if given at the same time as the bacteria[24]. These experiments demonstrated that both fresh and heat-inactivated immune serum have the capacity to lyse bacteria *in vivo* whereas only fresh immune serum causes lysis *in vitro*. Jules Bordet then reported a series of experiments showing that the capacity of heat-inactivated immune serum to lyse bacteria *in vitro* can be restored by the addition of non-immune serum[25–27]. Thus, Bordet identified two factors in blood that cause lysis: one is heat stable and depends upon previous sensitization and the other, a heat-labile factor, is present in non-immune serum. Bordet suggested that the heat-labile factor is identical to 'alexin'. In 1899, Paul Ehrlich called the heat-stable immune factor 'amboceptor', which we now know as antibody, and the heat-labile factor 'complement', a term that remains today[28,29]. Ehrlich proposed that one end of amboceptor bound to the bacteria and the other end bound to complement, a concept that has been refined with the advent of immunochemical and molecular biological techniques (Figure 1.1).

During the early part of the 20th century, investigators found that complement consists of more than one component. Ferrata showed that serum dialysed against water can be separated into two fractions, both of which are required for complement lysis; neither the precipitate nor the supernatant alone is able to cause lysis by itself[30]. Others found that, if the precipitate (which subsequently was shown to contain C1) is added first, the activity is greater than if the supernatant is added first[31]. This suggested that amboceptor ('front-piece') first reacts with a 'mid-piece' which then reacts with an 'end-piece'. Additional experiments, performed by Ritz, Coca, and Gordon *et al.*, suggested that there are four components to the complement system named C′1 (mid-piece), C′2 (end-piece), C′3 and C′4 corresponding to the order in which these components were discovered[32–34]. It is now clear that the mid-piece and end-piece both contain additional components necessary for lysis.

In the 1940s, Pillemer's group purified the first four components of complement, allowing investigators to show that the order in which these components were discovered is not the order in which they interact; C′1 interacts first with C′4 and C′2 and then C′3 is activated[35]. The first meeting of complement researchers was held in the mid-1940s on Long Island to discuss quantitative methods for examining complement. Abraham Osler remembers this meeting as being attended by about 16–20 scientists, including Pappenheimer, Mayer and

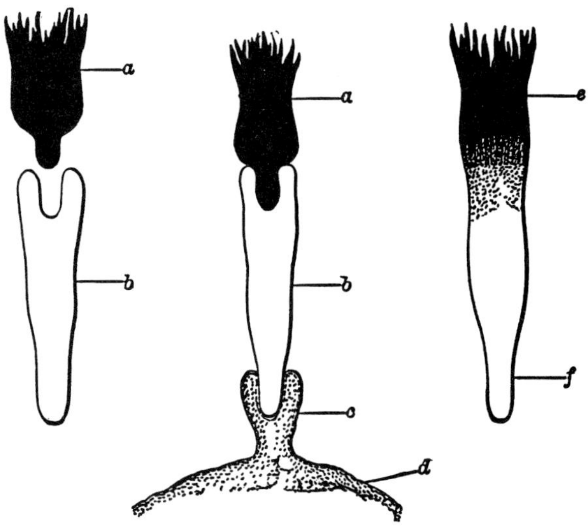

a, complement; *b*, interbody (immune body); *c*, receptor; *d*, part of a cell; *e*, toxophore group of the toxin; *f*, haptophore group.

Figure 1.1 Paul Ehrlich's view of complement as presented in his 1906 treatise *Studies on Immunity*, which was translated into English by Charles Bolduan and republished in 1917[29]

Heidelberger. No written record of this meeting exists and it appears that almost 10 years passed before the next meeting was held in 1956 at Walter Reed Army Medical Center. This second meeting is remembered by some as the 'Battle of Walter Reed' for its often confrontational nature. The modern history of complement is reflected in these meetings, symposia and workshops held over the past 30–40 years (summarized in Tables 1.1 and 1.2).

In the 1950s, Manfred Mayer developed the 'one hit theory', that only one lytic event is necessary to lyse a red blood cell[5]. Based upon this theory, it was possible to quantitate the presence of complement molecules. The assays described in *Experimental Immunochemistry*, second edition, by Elvin Kabat and Manfred Mayer, published in 1961 are still used today to measure complement functional activity[5]. Thus, it has been possible to quantitate most of the haemolytic components since the 1950s and this has allowed progress in complement to move forward at an ever increasing rate.

In the 1960s, Hans Müller-Eberhard's group at Scripps Clinic in La Jolla examined the chemical nature of the complement components and reported[58] that C3 is a major constituent of serum known as β_1C. Robert Nelson and his colleagues then reported that C′3 actually consists of six components[59]. These components were named C′3, C′5, C′6, C′7, C′8 and C′9 at the Second Complement Workshop held in 1966 in La Jolla, California[45]. Finally, in 1968 at the Third Complement Workshop, which was held in Boston, the current nomenclature was adopted in which the components are named C1, C4, C2, C3, C5, C6, C7, C8 and C9[60,61].

Table 1.1 Selected complement meetings, symposia and workshops

Date	*Location*	*Brief description*
1940s	Long Island	There were approximately 16–20 attendees. The focus of discussion was on quantitative methods.
1956	Walter Reed, Washington, DC	Described by some as the 'Battle of Walter Reed', this workshop debunked the existence of the 'properdin' pathway and may have contributed to the death of Pillemer.
1963	National Institutes of Health; Ciba Symposium; Bethesda, MD	This meeting was attended by 25 scientists and resulted in a publication that included 15 manuscripts. Organized by J. H. Humphrey and H. J. Rapp, this Ciba Symposium considered a wide range of complement topics, including primarily the biological activities associated with complement activation[6].
October, 1976	Bochum	This symposium was divided into six parts: methods and method standardization; diagnostic and prognostic usefulness of complement in determination in diseases; pathophysiology; complement and activation by drugs; genetic aspects; and a final round table discussion[12].
May 30–31, 1984	Bellagio (Como), Italy	Titled 'Clinical Aspects of Complement-mediated Diseases', this meeting was divided into nine sessions that dealt with the biological activity of complement fragments and peptides, genetic aspects of complement, and hereditary and acquired deficiencies[36].
October 29–31, 1984	Coconut Grove, FL	This was a Complement Receptor Workshop. There were 31 published abstracts that focused primarily on CR1, CR2, CR3 and CR4 as well as DAF and anaphylatoxin receptors[37].
September 3–5, 1986	Veszprem (Lake Balaton), Hungary	Titled the 'European Meeting on Complement in Human Disease', there were 83 published abstracts covering a wide variety of clinical topics[38].
September 19–22, 1988	Bari, Italy	This was the Second European Meeting on Complement in Human Disease. 100 abstracts were published. Topics included: inherited and acquired complement deficiencies; infections; mechanism of tissue damage; artificial membranes and biocompatibility; immune complexes, complement and receptors; drugs and complement; and complement analysis in the routine diagnostic workup[39].
June 27–19, 1989	Mainz, Germany	This was the Sixth Complement Genetics Workshop and Conference. There were 57 published abstracts; this workshop focused on complement polymorphisms. Previous workshops were held in Boston (1986 and 1982), Cologne (1979) and Cambridge (1977). The first workshop held in Bonn was titled 'First International Symposium on the Polymorphism of the Third Component of Human Complement'[40, 41].
September 15–17, 1990	Bratislava, CSFR	This was the Third European Meeting on Complement in Human Disease. 146 abstracts were submitted, of which 41 were from scientists from Eastern European countries. Topics included: deficiency states; complement and infections with special regard to HIV; diagnosis; tissue damage; complement in autoimmunity; biocompatibility of biomedical polymers; clinical intervention; complement and cytokines[42].

Table 1.1 (*contd*)

Date	*Location*	*Brief description*
September 21–23, 1991	Cardiff, Wales, UK	This satellite Complement in Disease Workshop was held at the University of Wales College of Medicine. 56 abstracts were published as well as eight full-length review-type manuscripts that corresponded to the talks that were given. The topics were: clinical assays and bioincompatibility; inhibitory proteins and non-lethal effects; complement and killing of pathogens; complement deficiencies; and complement in specific diseases[43].
May 1–4, 1992	Leiden, Netherlands	The Fourth Complement in Disease Workshop was held in 1992.

Table 1.2 International Complement Workshops

Workshop	*Date*	*Location*	*Number of published abstracts*	*Reference*
1	February 28–March 1, 1963	National Institutes of Health, Bethesda, MD	Summary only	(44)
2	January 17–19, 1966	LaJolla, CA	30	(45)
3	June 3–5, 1968	Harvard Medical School, Boston, MA	30	(46)
4	January 27–29, 1971	Johns Hopkins University, Baltimore, MD	39	(47)
5	February 23–25, 1973	Hotel Del Coronado, Coronado, CA	68	(48)
6	November 23–25, 1975	Sarasota, FL	101	(49)
7	November 20–22, 1977	St. Petersburg Beach, FL	137	(50)
8	October 14–16, 1979	Key Biscayne, FL	140	(51)
9	November 22–25, 1981	Key Biscayne, FL	177	(52)
10	May 25–27, 1983	Mainz, Germany	214	(53)
11	November 3–5, 1985	Key Biscayne, FL	266	(54)
12	September 18–21, 1987	Chamonix, France	320	(55)
13	September 10–15, 1989	San Diego, CA	308	(56)
14	September 15–20, 1991	Cambridge, UK	320	(57)
15	September 27–October 1, 1993	Kyoto, Japan (planned)		

During the first half of this century, it was known that a factor found in cobra venom is able to activate complement and that this activation does not proceed by classical mechanisms[62]. In the 1950s, the existence of a second pathway, called the properdin pathway for complement activation, was reported by Louis Pillemer and co-workers[63](Figure 1.2) and then disputed by Robert Nelson[64]. Pillemer's group, in 1954, described the critical elements of this second pathway, subsequently called the alternative pathway, and now recognized as older phylogenetically than the classical pathway[63]. Pillemer reported that this pathway of complement activation is important in natural immunity, a concept still considered important. His group used yeast walls (zymosan) and showed

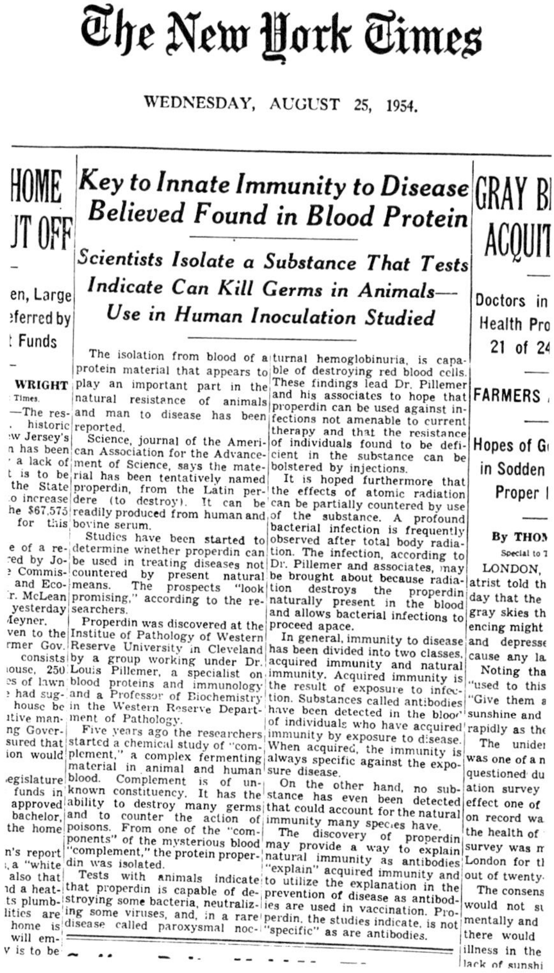

The New York Times

WEDNESDAY, AUGUST 25, 1954.

Key to Innate Immunity to Disease Believed Found in Blood Protein

Scientists Isolate a Substance That Tests Indicate Can Kill Germs in Animals— Use in Human Inoculation Studied

The isolation from blood of a protein material that appears to play an important part in the natural resistance of animals and man to disease has been reported.

Science, journal of the American Association for the Advancement of Science, says the material has been tentatively named properdin, from the Latin perdere (to destroy). It can be readily produced from human and bovine serum.

Studies have been started to determine whether properdin can be used in treating diseases not countered by present natural means. The prospects "look promising," according to the researchers.

Properdin was discovered at the Institue of Pathology of Western Reserve University in Cleveland by a group working under Dr. Louis Pillemer, a specialist on blood proteins and immunology and a Professor of Biochemistry in the Western Reserve Department of Pathology.

Five years ago the researchers started a chemical study of "complement," a complex fermenting material in animal and human blood. Complement is of unknown constituency. It has the ability to destroy many germs and to counter the action of poisons. From one of the "components" of the mysterious blood "complement," the protein properdin was isolated.

Tests with animals indicate that properdin is capable of destroying some bacteria, neutralizing some viruses, and, in a rare disease called paroxysmal nocturnal hemoglobinuria, is capable of destroying red blood cells. These findings lead Dr. Pillemer and his associates to hope that properdin can be used against infections not amenable to current therapy and that the resistance of individuals found to be deficient in the substance can be bolstered by injections.

It is hoped furthermore that the effects of atomic radiation can be partially countered by use of the substance. A profound bacterial infection is frequently observed after total body radiation. The infection, according to Dr. Pillemer and associates, may be brought about because radiation destroys the properdin naturally present in the blood and allows bacterial infections to proceed apace.

In general, immunity to disease has been divided into two classes, acquired immunity and natural immunity. Acquired immunity is the result of exposure to infection. Substances called antibodies have been detected in the blood of individuals who have acquired immunity by exposure to disease. When acquired, the immunity is always specific against the exposure disease.

On the other hand, no substance has even been detected that could account for the natural immunity many species have.

The discovery of properdin may provide a way to explain natural immunity as antibodies "explain" acquired immunity and to utilize the explanation in the prevention of disease as antibodies are used in vaccination. Properdin, the studies indicate, is not "specific" as are antibodies.

Figure 1.2 *New York Times* report on the existence of the alternative pathway of complement

that complement could be activated without the participation of classical complement proteins. This first report describes factor A (C3), factor B, factor D and properdin. Properdin binds to zymosan (PZ) and, in the presence of Mg^{2+}, causes lysis of cells. The details of this stormy period in the history of complement are recommended reading[65,66]. Pillemer's descriptions of a second pathway were confirmed in the late 1960s when the methods to purify and characterize components had improved[67,68]. Nevertheless, Nelson's rebuttal at the complement symposium held at Walter Reed Army Medical Center in 1956 appears to have been convincing and may have persuaded Pillemer to take his own life by drinking one of the complement buffers[66]. One of Pillemer's students, Irwin Lepow, continued these studies[69,70] but the existence of a second pathway remained unaccepted by most immunologists until the late 1960s when work on the alternative pathway resumed[67,68]. In short order the components of this pathway were purified and characterized as factors B and D, C3 and properdin[71–76].

Complement regulatory proteins were also discovered, including C1 esterase inhibitor[77,78], β_1H[79,80], C3b inactivator[81–84] and C4 binding protein[85,86]; these proteins are now known as C1 inhibitor (C1-INH), factor H, factor I and C4-bp, respectively. Membrane proteins were also discovered. Receptors for C3 fragments were described by several authors[87–91]: CR1, now known as CD35, binds primarily to C3b; CR2, now known as CD21, binds primarily to C3dg and to C3d; CR3, now known as CD11b/CD18, binds primarily to iC3b; and CR4, which is less well characterized. A series of glycophospholipid-anchored membrane proteins was found to have complement regulatory activity and includes membrane cofactor protein (MCP, CD46)[92,93], decay accelerating factor (DAF, CD55)[94,95], homologous restriction factor (HRF)[96,97] and CD59[98,99].

The terminal pathway of complement, also called the membrane attack complex or MAC, was studied in detail[100–106]. Perforin peptide sequences were found in the terminal components of complement[102]. Investigators argued over the nature of the lytic lesion[105,106], now believed to be caused by C5b8 complexes, which produce slow lysis, and which can interact with C9. Then, C9 molecules polymerize to form channels in the cell membrane[104–106].

Rapid strides were made in understanding the chemical nature of the components with the advent of molecular biological techniques. cDNA-derived sequences were determined for virtually all complement proteins and genomic sequences were reported for many of the complement proteins. Recent workshops have devoted large blocks of time to the molecular characterization of the complement proteins[56,57].

In parallel, investigators have developed an increased understanding of the biological role of complement[56,57,107]. Complement has been shown to be responsible for: generation of anaphylatoxins (C3a and C5a) and chemotactic factor activity (C5a), opsonization (C3b), clearance of immune complexes, regulation of B lymphocyte responses, induction of phagocytosis, regulation of monocyte migration, neutrophil and monocyte activity, cell adherence, degranulation and release of intracellular enzymes from granulocytes, production of toxic oxygen species, spreading and adherence of macrophages, neutralization of virus, and induction of leukocytosis as well as a variety of other biological activities. These topics are presented in more detail in subsequent chapters. This brief review of the history of complement provides the background to understand the complement system in the 1990s. The reader is also referred to other reviews of the history of the complement system[1–19].

The 1990s, which begins the second century of complement research, will be the time in which the biological consequences of this cascade system will be examined in even greater detail. Complement will be studied for its effect on a variety of host systems and the full biological significance of the complement system will be elucidated.

NOMENCLATURE[8,45,60,61,108]

Classical pathway components are designated with a C and a number (e. g. C1 and C3). The first four components are numbered C1, C4, C2 and C3 for historical reasons. Components of the alternative pathway are designated by letters (factors B, P and D). Activated C1 and its subcomponents have a bar over them to indicate activation (e. g. C$\bar{1}$, C$\bar{1}$r and C$\bar{1}$s). Cleavage fragments are indicated by a suffixed lower case letter (e.g. C3a and C3d are fragments of C3). Inactivated C3b is iC3b. Peptide chains of complement components are denoted with a Greek letter after the component (C5α and C5β are the alpha and beta chains of C5). C3 receptors are CR1, CR2, CR3 and CR4 and have been assigned CD designations as have other membrane proteins with complement regulatory activity (CD46, CD59).

THE COMPONENTS

Table 1.3 lists the components of the classical and alternative pathways and the membrane attack complex as well as the regulatory proteins and the membrane proteins known as of 1992. Additional complement proteins may well be added to this list, particularly membrane proteins that regulate complement activity. The proteins listed in Table 1.3 constitute about 10% of the serum proteins; the third component of complement is present in blood in the highest concentration of any of the complement proteins at about 1.5 mg/ml.

THE CLASSICAL PATHWAY: ACTIVATION (Figures 1.3 and 1.4)

The classical pathway of complement consists of a recognition protein, a macromolecule called C1, and two effector proteins, called C4 and C2. The classical pathway mediates specific immunity. Under normal circumstances, activation of C1 by immunoglobulins requires the binding of IgG of the appropriate subclass ($IgG_3 > IgG_1 > IgG_2$) or IgM to the C1q portion of C1. C1 contains one C1q (Mr 410 000), two C1r (688 amino acids, monomeric Mr 83 000) and two C1s (673 amino acids, monomeric Mr 85 000) molecules; calcium is necessary for the integrity of this macromolecular complex[109–113]. Without calcium, the subcomponents dissociate and are found as individual components[114]. The C1q subcomponent has been visualized by electron microscopy and contains six globular heads each attached to a collagen-like fibrillar stalk so that the molecule looks like a bunch of tulips[115–117] (Figure 1.3). Each of the stalks consists of three chains, designated as A (Mr 27 500), B (Mr 34 000) and C (Mr 31 600), which contain mostly glycine, lysine and proline residues[118]. Thus, the C1q subcomponent contains 18 chains, each consisting of 226 amino acids, assembled into six stalks that are linked together at the base[119]. The globular region (about 136 amino acids) has the capacity to interact with antibody[119]. The remainder of each chain is the collagen-like stalk region (about 81 amino acids) and the inner aspect of these stalks interacts with two C1r and two C1s subcomponents[120].

Table 1.3 Complement proteins, regulatory proteins and membrane receptors

A. Serum proteins

Component	*Serum Conc. (μg/ml)*	*Mr*	*Chain structure*	*Cleavage fragments*	*Biological activities*	*Chromosome*
Classical pathway						
C1q	70–300	460 000	18 (6 × 3)	—	Binds to antibody and other activators	1
C1r	34–100	83 000	1	—	Activates C1s	12
C1s	30–80	85 000	1	—	Activates C4 and C2	12
C4	350–600	204 000	3	C4a	Anaphylatoxin	6
				C4b	Binds covalently to membrane	
					Binds to C2	
				C4c		
				C4d		
C2	15–30	102 000	1	C2a	Enzymatic site of C4b2a	6
					Binds to C4	
				C2b		
Alternative pathway						
B	140–240	100 000	1	Ba	Chemotactic	6
				Bb	Enzymatic site of C3bBb	
P	20–30	56 500	4	—	Stabilizes C3bBb	X
D	1–2	24 000	1	—	Cleaves B to Ba and Bb	?
Third component						
C3	1200–1500	190 000	2	C3a	Anaphylatoxin	19
				C3b	Part of alternative pathway	
					Part of C5 convertase	
					Interacts with CR1 (CD35)	
					Solubilization of immune complexes	
					Opsonic fragment	
				C3d, C3d,g	Interacts with CR2(CD21)	
				'C3e', C3d-K	Leukoccytosis	
				C3f		

Table 1.3 (*contd*)
A. Serum proteins

Component	*Serum Conc. (μg/ml)*	*Mr*	*Chain structure C3c*	*Cleavage fragments*	*Biological activities*	*Chromosome*
Terminal pathway or membrane attack complex (MAC)						
C5	70–85	196 000	2	C5a	Anaphylatoxin, chemotaxis	9
				C5b	Formation of MAC	
C6	60–70	125 000	1	—	Part of MAC	5
C7	55–70	120 000	1	—	Part of MAC	5
C8	55–80	150 000	3	—	Part of MAC	1, 9
C9	50–160	66 000	1	—	Part of MAC	5
Control						
C1 Inhibitor (C1-INH)	180–275	105 000	1	—	Stoichiometric inhibitor of C1	11
C4 Binding protein(C4-bp)	250	550 000	7	—	Cofactor for factor I in C4b degradation; decay of C4b2a	1
Factor H	300–560	150 000	1	—	Cofactor for factor I in C3b degradation, decay of C3bBb	1
Factor I	34–50	100 000	2	—	Degrades C3b and C4b	4
Anaphylatoxin inactivator	35	310 000	—	—	Inactivates C3a and C5a to $C3a_{desarg}$ and $C5a_{desarg}$	?
S protein (vitronectin)	150–500	83 000	—	—	Controls membrane insertion of MAC	?

Table 1.3 *(contd)*

B. Receptor proteins

Membrane receptor	*Mr*	*Chain structure*	*Primary ligand(s)*	*Biological activities*	*Chromosome*	*Primary cellular location*
CR1 (CD35)	160 000–250 000	1	C3b, C4b	Immune complex transport	1	Monocytes, RBC, B cells
CR2 (CD21)	140 000	1	C3d, C3dg, iC3b	B cell regulation	1	B cells
CR3 (CD11b/CD18)	265 000	2	iC3b	Adherence	21 + ?	Monocytes, PMN, macrophages
CR4	?	1	C3dg		?	Platelets
Decay accelerating factor (DAF, CD55)	70 000	1	C4b2a, C3bBb	Decay of convertase	1	RBC, platelets B and T cells
Membrane cofactor protein (MCP, CD46)	45 000–70 000	1	C3b, C4b		?	PMN, monocytes
C3a receptor	?	?	C3a, C4a?	Mast cell degranulation	?	PMN, mast cells?
C5a receptor	45 000	1	C5a, $C5a_{desarg}$?	Mast cell degranulation		PMN, mast cells? monocytes, platelets
Homologous restriction factor (HRF)	65 000	1	C8, C9	Homologous lysis	?	RBC
CD59	19 000	1	C8, C9	Homologous lysis	?	Monocytes, RBC, T cells

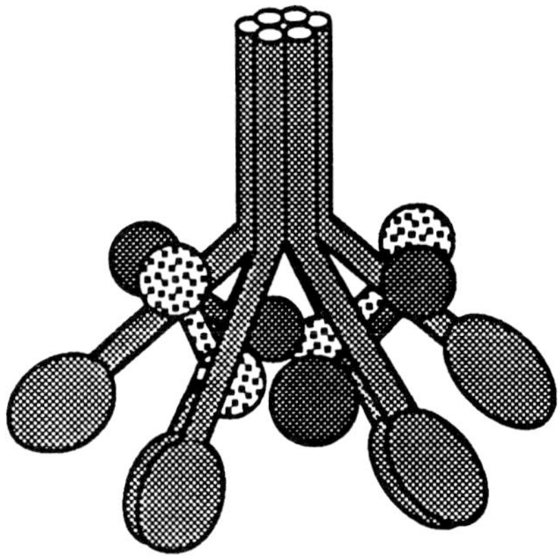

Figure 1.3 The C1 macromolecule consists of one C1q, two C1r and two C1s subcomponents. This model has been derived from electron microscopic data, demonstrating sizes and angles of these components[115–117]

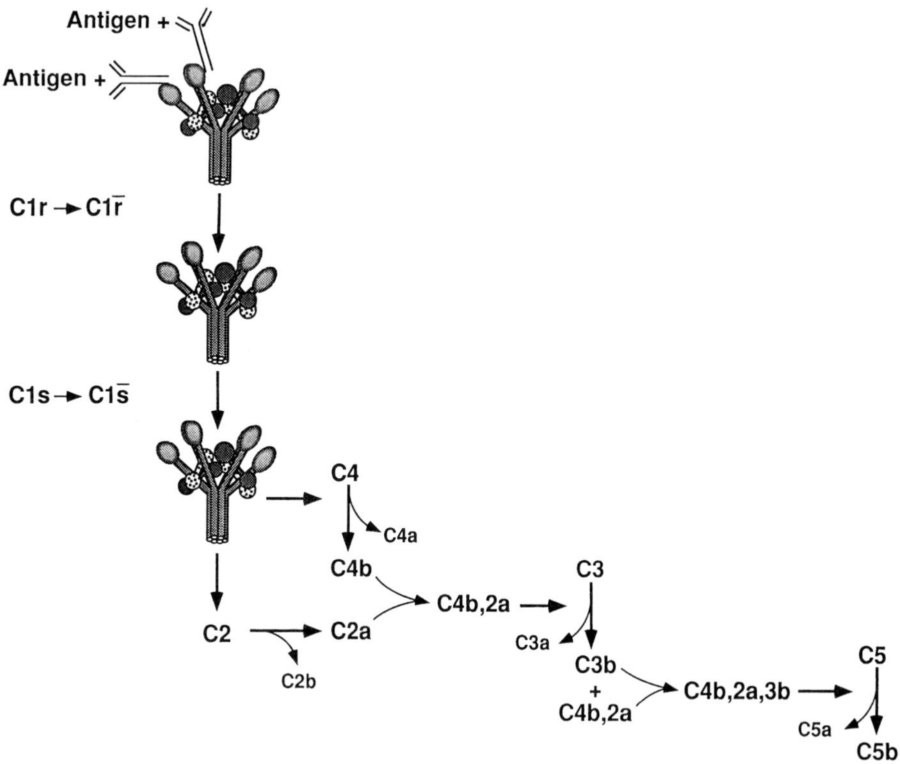

Figure 1.4 Activation of the classical pathway of complement leads to an enzyme complex capable of cleaving C3 (C4b2a, a C3 convertase) and then to an enzyme complex capable of cleaving C5 (C4b2a3b, a C5 convertase)

Activation of C1q requires the minimum binding of two of the six globular heads to the CH2 domain of the Fc region of two complement-activating IgG molecules[121]. C1 may also bind to one pentameric IgM molecule. Originally, this was thought to occur through interaction with the CH4 domain of IgM[122–124] but recent studies suggest that the interaction is with the CμH3 region[125]. Complement-activating immunoglobulin must be aggregated either physically by the formation of an antigen–antibody complex or chemically. Two IgG molecules must be properly spaced to cause activation, whereas a single pentameric IgM has the proximity built into its structure that allows activation of C1[121]. Consequently, IgM is a more efficient complement activator than is IgG.

Once immunoglobulin has bound to the globular head, the C1q molecule undergoes a change in tertiary structure that allows autocatalytic cleavage of C1r[114,126]. No fragment is released from C1r when cleavage occurs and the C1$\bar{r}$ is now able to cleave C1s to produce C1$\bar{s}$, again without release of any fragment. Cleavage fragments of C1$\bar{r}$ and C1$\bar{s}$ are held together by disulphide bonds. C1$\bar{r}$ and C1$\bar{s}$ are structurally similar, are both inhibited by diisopropyl fluorophosphate (DFP) and are classified as serine proteases[127–129]. The active enzymatic site on each of these molecules is located on the smaller of their two cleavage fragments.

C1$\bar{s}$ is also called C1 esterase and this enzyme cleaves C4, a glycoprotein of Mr 204 000 that consists of alpha (Mr 90 000), beta (Mr 80 000), and gamma (Mr 20 000) chains. Cleavage occurs near the amino terminus of the alpha chain to produce C4a anaphylatoxin, a peptide of 77 amino acids (Mr 8650), and C4b (Mr 196 000), which binds covalently to the activating particle[130–135] through a labile thiolester bond (described below for C3)[136]. C4b that does not bind remains in the fluid phase and loses its binding site. C4b also contains regions that interact with Mg^{2+}, C2, CR1 and membrane cofactor protein[137,138].

C4, unlike C3, has two genetic loci called C4A and C4B, which exist in the 'class III' major histocompatibility complex (MHC) on the sixth chromosome[139]. The resulting product is two distinct proteins that differ at only six amino acids[140–142]. Substitution of one of these amino acids, an aspartic acid for histidine, converts the functional activity of C4B to C4A and shifts C4B from having a preference for transacylation to hydroxyl to a preference for transacylation to amino nucleophiles on activating surfaces[142]. Consequently, C4B is about 4 times more active in haemolytic assays than C4A whereas C4A is more important in binding to immune complexes than C4B[139].

C1$\bar{s}$ also cleaves free C2, a glycoprotein of Mr 102 000 to produce C2a (509 amino acids, Mr 73 000) and C2b (223 amino acids, Mr 34 000)[143–146]. Although in the fluid phase this is an inefficient process, cleavage of C2 that has bound to C4b is very efficient and produces the classical pathway C3 convertase (C4b, C2a) with the release of free C2b[147,148]. C2a is the major cleavage fragment of C2 and contains the active site of the C3 convertase[149,150]. The initial binding site for C4b is located on the C2b part of the molecule and requires Mg^{2+} although, once cleaved, C2a binds to C4b independently of Mg^{2+}. C2a decays from the C4b2a complex but enzymatic activity can be regenerated if C2 and C1$\bar{s}$ are still present[5,147,148]. C4b2a cleaves the alpha chain of C3 to produce a 9 kDa fragment (C3a anaphylatoxin), leaving a major fragment, C3b, which can bind to the activating particle.

The classical pathway can also be activated independently of antibody. Heparin, a polyanionic anticoagulant, and protamine, a polycation that is used to block heparin, can form complexes that activate the classical pathway[151]. A variety of other polyanions, such as DNA, react directly with C1q to activate the classical pathway[152,153]. C reactive protein (CRP) leads to classical pathway activation without the necessity for antibody, possibly by interacting with other serum proteins or pneumococcal polysaccharides[154].

A variety of bypass pathways have also been described by multiple authors. A C1 bypass pathway was described by May and Frank in 1973 in which antibody interacts with C1, resulting in C3 cleavage by the alternative pathway without involvement of C2 and C4[155–157]. More recently, another bypass pathway was described that involves antibody, C1 and C4 but not C2 and leads to alternative pathway activation[158,159]. Finally, Masaki *et al.* described the generation of a C5 convertase in the absence of C3[160].

THE CLASSICAL PATHWAY: REGULATION

Classical pathway activation is regulated by a variety of proteins and natural processes. There are substances present in serum that appear *in vitro* to have the capacity to regulate C1q interaction with immunoglobulin[161,162]. The role of these proteins remains to be fully defined.

The early classical pathway is regulated by C1 esterase inhibitor or C1 inhibitor (C1-INH), an α_2-neuroaminoglycoprotein (Mr 105 000), which binds stoichiometrically (1:1) to C1s as well as to C1r to lead to permanent inactivation of these proteins[77,78,163–168]. C1-INH competes with natural substrates for interaction with C1r and C1s and serves as a false substrate. The active centre of C1-INH is located towards the carboxy terminal end and contains the residues -VAL-ALA-ARG(P1)-(P1′)THR-LEU-LEU-, with P1 and P1′ being the active centre. During enzyme–inhibitor interaction, C1-INH is cleaved between the P1 and P1′ residues and a covalent bond is formed between enzyme and inhibitor. In addition, the C1r:C1s:C1-INH complex (molar ratio 1:1:2) dissociates from C1 leaving C1q bound to the activating particle. Measurement of these complexes in plasma provides a useful assessment of C1 activation. C1-INH also binds stoichiometrically to plasmin, kallikrein, activated Hageman factor and coagulation factor XIa [167]. C1-INH deficiency leads to hereditary angio-oedema (also known as hereditary angioneurotic oedema or HAE) as described in Chapter 7[77,78].

The classical pathway is also regulated by C4 binding protein (C4-bp), membrane cofactor protein (MCP also known as CD46), decay accelerating factor (DAF also known as CD45), factor I and CR1 (also known as CD35) (Table 1.4). C4-bp, which contains an alpha (Mr 70 000) and beta (Mr 45 000) chain, may disassemble the C4b2a complex or may prevent C2 from binding to C4b[85,86,169–172]. C4-bp serves as a cofactor for factor I (Mr 100 000) to allow permanent inactivation of C4b[86]. MCP (Mr 45 000–70 000) does not dissociate the C4b2a complex but serves as a cofactor for factor I in the permanent inactivation of C4b[92,93,173–175]. In contrast, DAF (Mr 70 000) dissociates C4b2a but does not serve as a factor I cofactor[94,95,176–178]. CR1 (Mr about 200 000)

Table 1.4 Control of classical and alternative pathways

	Primary location	*Causes decay of*		*Factor I cofactor for*	
		C4a2a	*C3bBb*	*C4b*	*C3b*
C4 binding protein	Serum	Yes	No	Yes	No
Factor H	Serum	No	Yes	No	Yes
Decay accelerating factor	Membrane	Yes	Yes	No	No
Membrane cofactor protein	Membrane	No	No	Yes	Yes
CR1 (CD35)	Membrane	Yes	Yes	Yes	Yes

serves both to dissociate C4b2a and as a factor I cofactor in the inactivation of C4b[179]. Finally, it is important to recognize that the classical pathway convertase (C4b2a) is inherently unstable with a half-life of 3–4 minutes[5]. Thus, multiple factors serve to regulate the formation and decay of the classical pathway C3 convertase.

THE ALTERNATIVE PATHWAY: ACTIVATION (Figure 1.5)

The alternative pathway of complement consists of factors B, P and D as well as C3b and is activated by a diverse set of 'natural' substances, including yeast walls[180], bacterial cell walls[13], cobra venom factor[181] and nephritic factor[182–185]. *In vitro*, even rabbit erythrocytes are capable of causing activation by the alternative pathway of complement[186]. Thus, the alternative pathway does not require prior sensitization and therefore is a mediator of natural immunity[63].

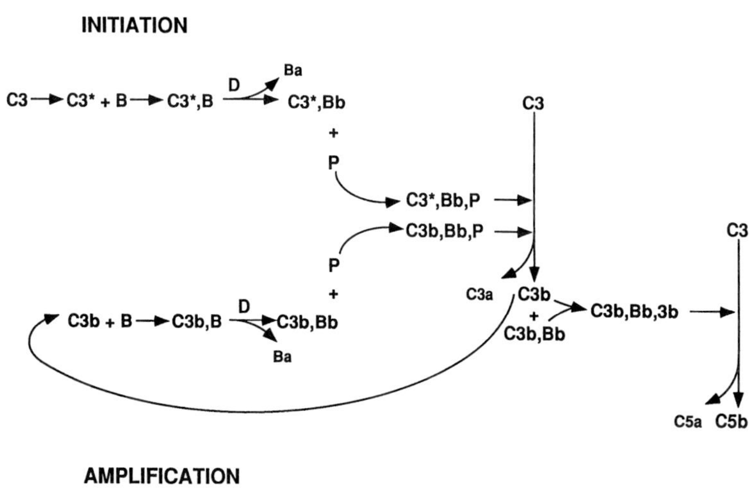

Figure 1.5 Activation of the alternative pathway of complement is an inefficient process until the amplification mechanism is recruited. C3* is C3 in which the labile thiolester bond has been cleaved. Activation of the alternative pathway leads to the formation of the alternative pathway C3 convertase (C3bBb) and then to the formation of the alternative pathway C5 convertase (C3bBb3b)

Initial activation appears to depend upon: (1) low-grade hydrolysis at the metastable binding site (the thiolester) in C3 to form a C3b-like molecule (often called $C3_{H_2O}$) that can bind factor B and form a low-efficiency fluid-phase C3 convertase ($C3_{H_2O}$,Bb); or (2) constant cleavage of small amounts of C3 into C3a and C3b. Natural cleavage of C3, although poorly understood, is thought to occur through the non-specific action of enzymes on C3 or by low-level activity of the classical pathway. C3b then serves as a substrate for factor B, a single-chain glycoprotein (739 amino acids, Mr 100 000) to produce the complex C3bB[71,75,187,188]. Factor D, a serine protease (288 amino acids, Mr 24 000) that exists in an activated form in plasma, cleaves bound factor B to Ba (Mr 35 000) and Bb (Mr 65 000) to produce C3bBb with release of Ba into the fluid phase[72,189]. Factor D has no activity on unbound factor B[73].

A glycoprotein called factor P or properdin stabilizes this C3bBb complex to retard its decay[190]. Properdin has a monomeric Mr of 56 500 and is found in plasma in multiple polymeric forms[191–195]. Trimers (P_3) and tetramers (P_4) are thought to be the most prominent forms (Mr 169 500 and 226 000); higher polymeric forms appear to be artifacts of isolation[193,194].

C3bBb and C3bBbP are the alternative pathway C3 convertases, the enzymes that cleave C3 into C3a and C3b[196,197]. Bb contains the enzymatic site for cleaving C3. The C3bBb complex requires the presence of Mg^{2+} and decays over time, dependent upon temperature. The alternative pathway is also an amplification pathway because one C3bBb or C3bBbP complex may cleave many C3 molecules. Amplification also occurs at other steps in the complement pathways, such as when C$1\overline{s}$ is produced and when C4b2a is formed. Each of these enzymes may cleave many substrate molecules leading to rapid complement activation. Consequently, amplification is a general mechanism in which complement proteins at each step of activation may recruit and activate many additional molecules.

THE ALTERNATIVE PATHWAY: REGULATION

The alternative pathway is also regulated by a variety of proteins and natural processes (Table 1.4). First, the inherently labile C3bBb complex is stabilized by factor P (properdin) as described above[190]. The C3bBb complex is also regulated by:

(1) Factor H, a 150 000 Mr (1213 amino acid) glycoprotein, which is analogous to C4-bp of the classical pathway[79,80,198]. Factor H may disassemble the C3bBb complex or may bind to C3b to produce C3bH, which prevents C3b from binding factor B molecules[199]. The affinity of C3b for factor H is about four times greater than the affinity for factor B[200]. Factor H also serves as a cofactor for factor I.
(2) Factor I inactivates C3b proteolytically to produce iC3b, C3c, C3d, C3f, and C3dg[81–84,201–203], described below in the C3 section.
(3) MCP also serves as a factor I cofactor in the permanent inactivation of C3b but does not dissociate the C3bBb complex[92,93,173–175].
(4) DAF may dissociate C3bBb but does not serve as a factor I cofactor[94,95,176–178].

(5) CR1 dissociates C3bB and serves as a factor I cofactor in the inactivation of C3b[204–206].

Finally, it is important again to recognize that the non-properdin stabilized alternative pathway convertase (C3bBb), similar to the classical pathway convertase (C4b2a), is inherently unstable with a half-life of 3–4 minutes[190]. Thus, multiple factors serve to regulate the formation and decay of the alternative pathway C3 convertase.

Unlike the classical pathway, the alternative pathway is controlled by the surface on which activation occurs. Surfaces onto which the C3bBb complex may attach are either activating surfaces (such as yeast walls and rabbit erythrocytes) or non-activating surfaces (such as sheep erythrocytes)[180, 207]. When C3b is bound to activating surfaces, it forms C3bBb complexes preferentially whereas, on non-activating surfaces, the predisposition is to form C3bH complexes[180,207]. It was once thought that the concentration of sialic acid on the surface plays the predominant role in determining whether a surface is activating or non-activating[180,207–210]. Rabbit erythrocytes, which activate the alternative pathway, have less sialic acid than do sheep erythrocytes, which do not activate this pathway[207]. Treatment of sheep erythrocytes to remove sialic acid renders them able to activate the alternative pathway. The concentration of sialic acid on mouse erythrocytes is inversely related to the ability of these cells to activate complement by the alternative pathway[210]. Studies have shown that the sialic acid content on a membrane determines the affinity of C3b on that surface to interact with factor H but has no effect on the ability of C3b to bind to factor B[200,210]. However, although sialic acid may play an important role in determining whether a surface will activate this pathway of complement, additional mechanisms may also be important in determining whether a surface is activating or non-activating[211].

The mechanisms described above explain how various substances activate the alternative pathway *in vivo*:

(1) Cobra venom factor (CoVF) is like cobra C3b[181]. The CoVFBb complex is very stable with a half-life measured in hours, rather than 3–4 minutes as is seen with the C3bBb complex. In addition, the CoVFBb complex is not susceptible to the decay activity of factor H, allowing the CoVFBb complex to cause brisk and total cleavage of C3[181,212].

(2) C3 nephritic factor (C3NeF), which is found in the serum of about 10% of patients with membranoproliferative glomerulonephritis, is an immunoglobulin directed to the C3bBb complex. Like properdin, C3NeF stabilizes C3bBb, but, unlike the C3bBbP complex, the C3bBbC3NeF complex is relatively resistant to the decay activity of factor H[182–185].

(3) Yeast walls (zymosan) and certain membranes (e.g. rabbit erythrocytes) are activating surfaces where a C3bBb complex is protected from the decay activity of factor H so that the complex remains active[180,207].

(4) IgG may bind to surfaces that activate the alternative pathway and enhance the binding of factor B to C3b[213]. Thus, even though immunoglobulin is not necessary for zymosan activation of the alternative pathway, its presence will increase the activation of this pathway.

C3 (Figure 1.6)

Both the classical and alternative pathways form effective convertases (C4b2a and C3bBb, respectively) that presumably cleave C3 in an identical fashion. C3 cleavage is felt to be the most critical event in the complement cascade because of the important biological events that result from C3 cleavage, including generation of anaphylatoxins and chemotactic factor activity and the induction of opsonization, immune complex clearance, cell adherence, degranulation and lysis. Thus, it is important to understand the nature of the third component of complement and how it interacts with membranes and cell receptors.

C3 is present in plasma in the highest concentration of any complement protein and constitutes 1–2% of the total serum proteins. C3, a glycoprotein (Mr 190 000), contains disulphide-linked alpha (992 amino acids, Mr 118 000) and beta (645 amino acids, Mr 75 000) chains[74,214]. The alpha chain contains all of the known cleavage sites and the binding sites for the interaction of C3 with membranes and receptors[215,216].

Cleavage of C3 by either convertase results in the production of a 77-amino-acid peptide (Mr 9000) from the amino terminal end of C3 called C3a[217]. The remainder of the molecule is then known as C3b. Cleavage of C3 also results in externalization of a labile thiolester bond (the metastable binding site) between the thiol group of cysteine and the gamma carbonyl group of glutamic acid, in the sequence -GLY-CYS*-GLY-GLU-GLX*-, which is found in the C3d region

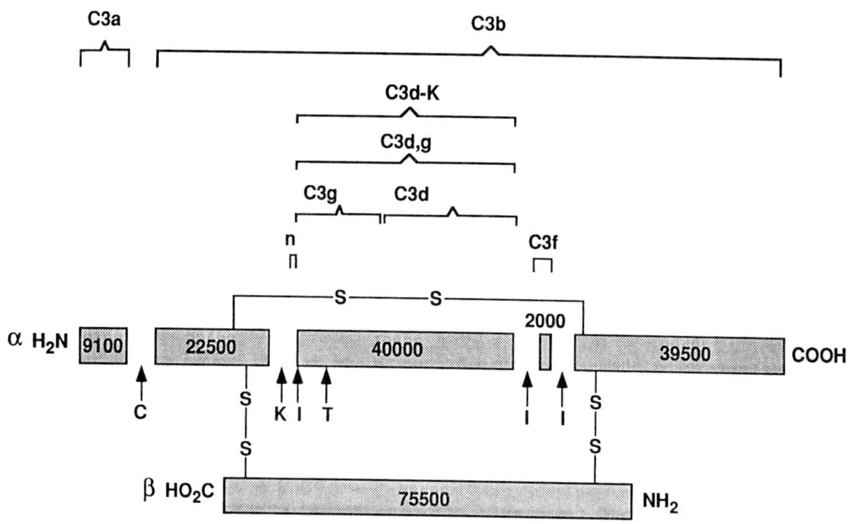

Figure 1.6 The breakdown of C3 leads to a variety of biologically active fragments. Key to this figure: C – convertase; K – kallekrein; I – factor I; T – trypsin. Fragments C3a, C3b, C3d, C3f, C3g, C3d-K and C3dg are clearly defined. C3c is C3b from which C3dg has been removed. C3e has never been mapped. n represents a nonapeptide. The alpha chain contains all the known sites by which C3 interacts with other proteins and substances. The thiolester site is contained on C3d. Interaction with properdin is on the 39 500 fragment

on the alpha chain of C3[218–221]. If a suitable surface is present when this occurs, there is transfer of the acyl group from the thiol to a hydroxyl group on the acceptor molecule resulting in the formation of a covalent bond between C3 and the receptor surface[218–221]. If a suitable surface is not present at the time that C3 cleavage occurs, then the C3b quickly becomes incapable of binding to membranes and remains in the fluid phase in a non-binding form[218]. C3 can also become C3b-like ($C3_{H_2O}$) after treatment with methylamine or after spontaneous hydrolysis. C3b, whether bound to a surface or in the fluid phase, and $C3_{H_2O}$ has the capacity to interact with factor B to form C3 convertase (C3bB or $C3_{H_2O}B$). Then, factor D cleaves B to produce C3bBb and $C3_{H_2O}Bb$.

C3b that is bound to membranes may or may not be degraded by enzymes such as factor I[222,223]. C3b may participate in a variety of reactions, depending upon whether it has been degraded, including: (1) formation of the alternative pathway C3 convertase (C3bBb); (2) formation of the alternative pathway C5 convertase (C3bBb3b)[224] described below; (3) interaction with CR1[138]; (4) induction of various biological activities, such as opsonization and regulation of B cell responses[225,226]; and (5) degradation by enzymes[227–233].

Degradation of C3b has been studied extensively[227–233]. As described above for the regulation of the alternative pathway, C3b first interacts with either factor H, MCP or CR1, which serve as cofactors for the proteolysis of C3b by factor I[212]. Factor I alone can also cause proteolysis of C3b in the absence of a cofactor but this occurs at a very slow rate and is probably inconsequential *in vivo*[212]. In the presence of a cofactor, such as factor H, MCP or CR1, factor I cleaves the alpha chain of C3b at two sites, producing a 17-amino-acid fragment (Mr 3000). The remaining molecule is called iC3b, which is no longer able to interact with factors B, D and P[222,223]. iC3b can then interact with CR3 (CD11b/CD18)[138].

iC3b may undergo further cleavage, perhaps by trypsin-like enzymes or factor I, in the absence of CR1 to produce C3c and C3dg (also called α2D)[227–233]. C3dg, in turn, may also be cleaved by trypsin-like enzymes into C3d and C3g[230–232]. An additional fragment, called 'C3e', has been reported to induce leukocytosis by causing release of cells directly from bone marrow[234–236]. However, the existence of C3e has never been proved or mapped to C3 and may be an artifact of the treatment of C3 preparations with trypsin. Kallikrein treatment of iC3b may also produce C3d-K and a nonapeptide; the nonapeptide has activity similar to C3e in causing release of leukocytes from bone marrow and C3d-K has the capacity to regulate B cells[237,238]. C3dg and C3d interact with CR2, which is also known as the Epstein–Barr virus (EBV) receptor, to regulate B cells[239–243]. C3dg contains the labile thiolester site by which C3b binds covalently to membranes and other surfaces[230]. Consequently, C3dg remains on the surface with the release of C3c into the fluid phase.

SIMILARITIES BETWEEN CLASSICAL AND ALTERNATIVE PATHWAYS

The two activating pathways are very similar although differences are also striking (Table 1.5). Factor D and C1s, which are serine proteases, act on substrates (factor B and C2, respectively) in the zymogen form of each

Table 1.5 Comparison of classical and alternative pathways

	Classical pathway		*Alternative pathway*
C1s	Serine protease that cleaves C4 and C2 Must be activated to C1$\overline{s}$	Factor D	Serine protease that cleaves factor B Circulates in activated form
C4b	Interacts with C2 to form C4b2	C3b	Interacts with factor B to form C3bB
C2	Single chain (Mr 100 000) Structural gene on chromosome 6 Interacts with C4 to form C4b2 Cleaved by C1$\overline{s}$ into C2b and C2a Contains enzymatic site in classical pathway C3 convertase Decays from the C4b2a complex	Factor B	Single chain (Mr 100 000) Structural gene on chromosome 6 Interacts with C3b to form C3bB Cleaved by factor D into Ba and Bb Contains enzymatic site in alternative pathway C3 convertase Decays from the C3bBb complex
C4b2a	Requires Mg^{2+} for binding Half-life is about 3–4 min at 30°C Temperature-dependent decay	C3bBb	Requires Mg^{2+} for binding Half-life is about 3–4 min at 30°C Temperature-dependent decay
Factor I	Inactivates C4b if factor I cofactor is also present	Factor I	Inactivates C3b if factor I cofactor is also present

convertase (C3bB and C4b2, respectively) to produce C3bBb and C4b2a, respectively[75]. The convertases require Mg^{2+} and decay over time dependent upon temperature[5,72,190]. Indeed, the half-life of the non-stabilized alternative pathway C3bBb complex is about the same as that of the classical pathway C4b2a complex[5,190]. C2 probably resulted from gene reduplication of factor B[144]. Each is a single polypeptide chain encoded by a single structural gene on chromosome 6. Each contains an active enzyme site on the larger cleavage fragment (C2a and Bb) and the specificity for C3 cleavage by both these enzymes is thought to be identical[144].

Regulation of these two convertases is also very similar (Table 1.4): factor H causes dissociation of C3bBb and serves in the alternative pathway as a factor I cofactor; C4-bp causes dissociation of C4b2a and serves in the classical pathway as a factor I cofactor. On membranes, DAF causes dissociation of C3bBb and C4b2a and MCP serves as a cofactor for factor I in the regulation of both pathways. In contrast, CR1 serves in both pathways to dissociate the convertase and as a cofactor for factor I.

The differences between the pathways are: (1) there is no C1-INH-like molecule in the alternative pathway; (2) C1s requires activation whereas factor D exists in an activated form in plasma; and (3) there is no properdin-like molecule in the classical pathway to stabilize the C4b2a complex.

MEMBRANE ATTACK COMPLEX (C5–9): ACTIVATION (Figure 1.7)

Classical and alternative pathway C3 convertases (C4b2a and C3bBb, respectively) become C5 convertases by addition of another C3b into the complex (to form C4b2a3b and C3bBb3b, respectively)[224,244,245]. Thus, the addition of a C3b into the complex shifts the specificity from cleavage of C3 to cleavage of C5[224,244,245] although the enzymatic site remains on C2a and Bb, respectively. C5 is thought to be cleaved by both classical and alternative pathway

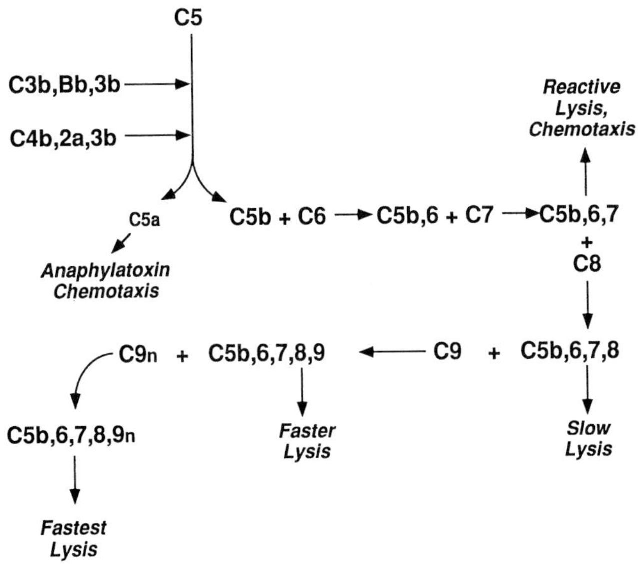

Figure 1.7 Formation of the membrane attack complex (MAC) follows activation by either the classical or alternative pathway and proceeds with the assembly of the terminal complement components

convertases in an identical fashion into C5a and C5b, beginning the formation of the membrane attack complex.

C5, which is similar in structure to C3, is a glycoprotein (1654 amino acids, Mr 196 000) with disulphide-linked alpha (Mr 130 000) and beta (Mr 80 000) chains[246–249]. Cleavage of C5 produces an anaphylatoxin (C5a, Mr 11 000, 74 amino acids) that contains a carboxy terminal arginine[247]. C5a, unlike C3a, contains about 25% carbohydrate. C3a and C5a are susceptible to anaphylatoxin inactivator, which cleaves the carboxy-terminal arginine to produce $C3a_{desarg}$ and $C5a_{desarg}$, respectively[247].

C6 may bind to C5b to produce C5b6. Then, C7 may bind to form C5b67, which can attach itself to membranes and lipid bilayers. When this occurs on a cell that does not otherwise have any complement products upon it, C8 and C9 may then also bind to the cell causing lysis. This is called the innocent bystander phenomenon or reactive lysis[250]. C6 (913 amino acids, Mr 125 000) and C7 (821 amino acids, Mr 120 000) are single-chain molecules that are similar in structure and have probably resulted from gene reduplication[251–254].

Next, C8 may bind to the C5b67 complex to form C5b678, which is capable of causing slow inefficient lysis of non-nucleated cells[255,256]. C8 (Mr 150 000) contains an alpha (Mr 64 000), beta (Mr 64 000) and gamma (Mr 22 000) chain[257–264]. The alpha and gamma chains are disulphide linked and non-covalently linked to the beta chain[257]. The beta chain interacts with the C5b-7 complex and the alpha chain, which is quite hydrophobic, interacts with the membrane on which the C5b-8 complex sits[258].

The beta chain of C8 also interacts with C9 to form C5b6789, which initiates substantial lysis of the cell. As additional C9 molecules are added to the C5b-9 complex, lysis increases[265]. About six C9 molecules are required for maximal lysis of a red blood cell although C5b-9_n complexes may contain between 12 and 28 C9 molecules[266,267]. C9 is a single-chain molecule (537 amino acids, Mr 66 000) that contains the perforin sequence that is also found to play a role in lysis by cytotoxic T lymphocytes[268–271]. The lesion that forms has been likened to the formation of a barrel with the staves represented by the C9 monomers. The lesion in the hydrophobic membrane outer layer has been estimated from electron microscopic studies to be 9–12 nm in diameter[266,267]. Red cells require only one such lesion (consistent with the one hit theory of Mayer[5], whereas nucleated cells may not be destroyed by multiple attacks, probably because the membrane may be repaired before the cellular contents leak out[272–273]. C9 also has a tendency to polymerize spontaneously, a slow process that can be enhanced by the presence of zinc[269].

MEMBRANE ATTACK COMPLEX: REGULATION[274]

The membrane attack complex is regulated by S protein, also called vitronectin, which controls the activity of C5b-7[275–277]. Membrane lysis is also controlled by homologous restriction factor (HRF)[96,97] and CD59 (also called protectin)[98,99]. HRF is a single-chain protein whose sequence has not been reported. CD59 (Mr 18 000) is expressed on the surfaces of many types of cells, including erythrocytes and T cells, and is probably more important than HRF in preventing host cells from being lysed by autologous complement proteins[96–99]. Both HRF and CD59 (as well as DAF) are linked to the membrane by glycophospholipid (GPI) anchors.

BIOLOGICAL ACTIVITIES

Lysis[5]

Lysis of cells and membranes is often thought to be the most important biological activity associated with complement activation. However, lysis is only one of many biological activities and is probably not the most important phenomenon associated with complement activation. Lysis is seen clinically in paroxysmal nocturnal haemoglobinuria, a rare disorder in which membrane proteins – DAF, HRF and CD59 – are deficient[278–280]. Lysis may also be seen in individuals bitten by cobras due to intense fluid-phase complement activation and the occurrence of reactive lysis.

Opsonization[281]

Fragments of C3 are deposited on unwanted substances (such as effete red cells, bacteria and immunoglobulin aggregates). Then phagocytic cells ingest and dispose of these substances that have been opsonized (or marked) for removal.

Anaphylatoxin activity[282,283]

C4a, C3a and C5a are anaphylatoxins; C4a is the weakest and C5a is the most potent. Anaphylatoxins cause: (1) mast cell degranulation with the release of histamine and other mast cell granule mediators; (2) increased vascular permeability; and (3) smooth muscle contraction. Anaphylatoxins are regulated by an inactivator, anaphylatoxin inactivator (carboxypeptidase N), which removes the carboxy-terminal arginine within seconds in serum. Thus, C3a becomes $C3a_{desarg}$, which has no activity as an anaphylatoxin.

Chemotactic activity[284]

C5a and $C5a_{desarg}$ may attract certain cells into the area of inflammation. C5a has both anaphylatoxin and chemotactic activity; C3a and C4a have no chemotactic activity. $C5a_{desarg}$ requires a cofactor, vitamin D binding protein, for this activity.

Neutrophil and monocyte activity[285–287]

C5a and $C5a_{desarg}$ regulate monocyte and neutrophil activity. C5a may cause augmented cell adherence, production of toxic oxygen species, degranulation and release of intracellular enzymes from granulocytes, and initiation of other cellular metabolic events.

Clearance of immune complexes[288]

Complement plays an important role in the clearance of immune complexes. The alternative pathway may increase the solubility of immune complexes and the classical pathway may prevent large insoluble immune complexes from being formed. Immune complexes opsonized by C3b may then be cleared from the blood by binding to erythrocytes by CR1 and being transported to the liver for removal.

Leukocytosis[234–237]

A fragment of C3, called C3e, was once thought to induce leukocytosis. However, this peptide has never been characterized or mapped onto the C3 molecule. Another fragment called C3d-K, which is produced by treating iC3b with kallikrein, also causes leukocytosis and inhibits T-cell responses[238]. C3d-K, which is similar to C3dg, contains an additional 9 amino acids on its amino terminal end. This nonapeptide is thought to be responsible for bone marrow release of leukocytes[237].

Immune response[289,290]

Interaction with CR2 regulates antibody production by a direct effect on B lymphocytes. CR2 is the Epstein–Barr virus receptor. Additional complement components and fragments (such as C4, C3a and C5a) may also play a role in the regulation of antibody production.

Miscellaneous biological activities

Hereditary angio-oedema, which is caused by C1-INH deficiency, may be mediated by a kinin-like substance released from C2[291]. A fragment of factor B may cause increased spreading and adherence of macrophages[292,293]. Complement activation may also neutralize viruses[294].

Assays for complement[5,295,296]

Assays for complement proteins are: (1) antigenic; (2) haemolytic (functional); and (3) genetic. Complement proteins can be measured using antigenic techniques, such as nephelometry, rocket electrophoresis, radial immunodiffusion, enzyme-linked immunosorbent assay (ELISA) or radioimmunoassay (RIA). These assays quantitate the presence of an immunologically reactive protein but provide no information about the functional capacity of that protein.

Haemolytic assays measure the functional capacity of the complement proteins. Global haemolytic assays are: (1) the CH50 or total haemolytic complement assay, which measures the ability of the classical pathway and the membrane attack complex to lyse a sheep red blood cell to which antibody has been attached (E^SA); and (2) the alternative pathway CH50 (rabbit CH50 or APCH50), which measures the ability of the alternative pathway and the membrane attack complex to lyse a rabbit red blood cell (E^R). Specific haemolytic assays are also used to measure the functional activity of specific components of either complement pathway[5].

Recently, molecular biological techniques have allowed the detection of defects in individual complement genes. Restriction fragment length polymorphism and, more recently, the use of polymerase chain reaction have allowed the defects to be mapped and mutations to be identified.

CONCLUSIONS

Complement research has progressed extremely rapidly over the last decade. Virtually all complement proteins and most membrane proteins with complement regulatory activity have been cloned and expressed. Both cDNA sequences and genomic sequences have been obtained for many of these proteins. This work has allowed sophisticated examination of the regulatory aspects of the complement proteins, the nature of complement deficiency states and the role of individual epitopes in interaction with other components within and out of the complement system. Using such techniques as synthetic peptide synthesis and site-directed mutagenesis, it has been possible to begin to examine how the complement proteins interact.

In the next decade, it is likely that studies will examine the tertiary structure of many of these proteins in great detail. Crystallographic studies will be combined with nuclear magnetic resonance studies and with sophisticated molecular modelling to examine in even more detail how the complement proteins interact. In addition, investigators will examine the complex interactions among the various complement proteins with elements of other immune systems, such as T cells and B cells, and non-immune systems, such as the coagulation pathways. It will be important to understand the role of various complement receptors and it is likely that additional receptors will be discovered. These studies will build upon molecular biology studies performed in the 1980s and early 1990s that have provided the map for understanding the role that the complement system plays in health and disease.

References

1. Metchnikoff, E. (1905). *Immunity in Infective Diseases.* (Cambridge: Cambridge University Press)
2. Kolmer, J. A. (1917). *A Practical Text-book of Infection, Immunity and Specific Therapy*, 2nd edn. (Philadelphia: W. B. Saunders)
3. Osborn, T. W. B. (1937). *Complement or Alexin.* (London: Oxford University Press)
4. Maaloe, O. (1946). *On the Relation Between Alexin and Opsonin.* (Copenhagen: Einar Munksgaard)
5. Kabat, E. A. and Mayer, M. M. (1961). *Experimental Immunochemistry*, 2nd edn. (Springfield, IL: Charles C. Thomas)
6. Wolstenholme, G. E. W. and Knight, J. (1965). *Ciba Foundation Symposium: Complement.* (Boston: Little, Brown and Company)
7. Rapp, H. J. and Borsos, T. (1966). Complement research. *J. Am. Med. Assoc.* **198**, 97–104
8. Rapp, H. J. and Borsos, T. (1970). *Molecular Basis of Complement Action.* (New York: Appleton–Century–Crofts)
9. Mayer, M. M. (1970). Highlights of complement research during the past twenty-five years. *Immunochemistry*, **7**, 485–96
10. Schultz, D. R. (1971). The complement system. In Kallös, P., Hasek, M., Inderbitzin, T. M., Miescher, P. A. and Waksman, B. H. (eds.) *Monographs in Allergy*, Vol. 6 (New York: S. Karger)
11. Osler, A. G. (1976). *Complement: Mechanisms and Functions.* (Englewood Cliffs, NJ: Prentice-Hall)
12. Opferkuch, W., Rother, K. and Schultz, D. R. (1978). *Clinical Aspects of the Complement System; International Symposium*, Bochum, October 1976. (Stuttgart: Georg Thieme Publishers; Massachusetts: PSG Publishing Company)
13. Fine, D. P. (1981). *Complement and Infectious Diseases.* (Boca Raton, FL: CRC Press)
14. Mayer, M. M. (1984). Complement: historical perspectives and some current issues. *Complement*, **1**, 2–26
15. Ross, G. D. (1986). *Immunobiology of the Complement System: An Introduction for Research and Clinical Medicine.* (Orlando, FL: Academic Press)
16. Whaley, K. (1987). *Complement in Health and Disease*, 1st edn. (Lancaster: MTP Press)
17. Law, S. K. A. and Reid, K. B. M. (1988). *Complement.* (Oxford: IRL Press Limited)
18. Rother, K. and Till, G. O. (1988). *The Complement System.* (Berlin: Springer–Verlag)
19. Morgan, B. P. (1990). *Complement: Clinical Aspects and Relevance to Disease.* (London: Academic Press)

20. Grohmann, W. (1884). Ueber die Einwirkung des zellenfreien Blutplasma auf einige pfanzliche Microorganismen (Schimmel-Spross, pathogene und nicht pathogene Spaltpilze). Dorpat. C. Mattiesen, p. 34 (quoted in reference 8)
21. Nuttall, G. (1888). Experimente über die bacterienfeindlichen Einflüsse des thierischen Körpers. *Z. Hyg. Infektionskr.*, **4**, 353–95
22. Buchner, H. (1889). Ueber die bakterientödtende Wirkung des zellenfreien Blutserums. *Central. Bakter. Parasit.*, **5**, 817–23
23. Buchner, H. (1889). Ueber die nähere Natur der bakterientödtenden Substanz im Blutserum. *Central. Bakter. Parasit.*, **6**, 561–5
24. Pfeiffer, R. and Issaeff, R. (1894). Ueber die specifische Bedeutung der Choleraimmunität *Z. Hyg. Infektionskr.*, **17**, 355–400
25. Bordet, J. (1896). Sur le mode d'action des sérums préventifs. *Ann. Inst. Pasteur*, **10**, 193–219
26. Bordet, J. (1898). Sur l'agglutination et la dissolution des globules rouges par le serum d'animaux injectés de sang defibriné. *Ann. Inst. Pasteur,* **12**, 688–95
27. Bordet, J. and Gengou, O. (1901). Sur l'Existence de Substances sensibilisatrices; dans la plupart des sérums antimicrobiens. *Ann. Inst. Pasteur*, **15**, 289–302
28. Ehrlich, P. and Morgenroth, J. (1899). Zur Theorie der Lysenwirkung. *Berlin. Klin. Wschr.*, **36**, 6–9
29. Ehrlich, P. (1906). In: *Collected Studies on Immunity*, collected and translated by C. Bolduan, 1st edn., Chapter 1. (New York: Wiley & Sons)
30. Ferrata, A. (1907). Die Unwirksamkeit der komplexen Hämolysine in salzfreien Lösungen und ihre Ursache. *Berlin. Klin. Wschr.*, **44**, 366–8
31. Brand, E. (1907). Ueber das Verhalten der Komplemente bei der Dialyse. *Berlin. Klin. Wschr.*, **44**, 1075–9
32. Ritz, H. (1912). Ueber die Wirkung des Cobragiftes auf die Komplemente. *Z. Immunitaetsforsch.*, **13**, 62–83
33. Coca, A. F. (1914). A study of the anticomplementary action of yeast, of certain bacteria and of cobra-venom. *Z. Immunitaetsforsch.*, **21**, 604–22
34. Gordon, J., Whitehead, H. R. and Wormall, A. (1926). The action of ammonia on complement. The fourth component. *Biochem J.*, **20**, 1028–35
35. Pillemer, L., Ecker, E. E., Oncley, J. L. and Cohn, E. J. (1941). The preparation and physicochemical characterization of the serum protein components of complement. *J. Exp. Med.*, **74**, 297–308
36. Agostoni, A. (1984). Clinical aspects of complement-mediated diseases. *Complement*, **1**, 123–4
37. Complement Receptor Workshop (1984). *Complement*, **1**, 160–76
38. European Meeting on Complement in Human Disease (1986). *Complement*, **3**, 189–222
39. 2nd European Meeting on Complement in Human Disease (1988). *Complement*, **5**, 180–219
40. Rittner, C. and Schneider, P. M. (eds.) (1989). VIth Complement Genetics Workshop and Conference. *Complement Inflamm.*, **6**, 283–304
41. Rittner, C., Hauptmann, G., Mauff, G. and Schneider, P. M. (eds.) (1990). Proceedings of the VIth Complement Genetics Workshop and Conference. *Complement Inflam.*, **7**, 173–318
42. Starsia, Z. and Nydegger, U. (eds.) (1990). 3rd European Meeting on Complement in Human Disease. *Complement Inflamm.*, **7**, 112–62
43. Thompson, R. A. (ed.) (1991). Complement in disease. *Clin. Exp. Immunol.*, **86** (Suppl. 1), 1–64
44. Rapp, H. J. and Borsos, T. (1963). Complement and hemolysis. *Science*, **141**, 738–40
45. Abstracts: Complement Workshop (1966). *Immunochemistry*, **3**, 495–505
46. Abstracts of papers presented at the Third International Complement Workshop, Harvard Medical School, Boston, Massachusetts (1968). *J. Immunol.*, **101**, 810–21
47. Abstracts of papers presented at the Fourth International Complement Workshop, Johns Hopkins University School of Medicine, Baltimore, Maryland (1971). *J. Immunol.*, **107**, 309–24
48. Abstracts of the Fifth International Complement Workshop, Hotel Del Coronado, Coronado, California (1973). *J. Immunol.*, **111**, 286–315
49. Abstracts of papers presented at the Sixth International Complement Workshop, Sarasota, Florida (1976). *J. Immunol.*, **116**, 1727–55
50. Abstracts of papers presented at the Seventh International Complement Workshop, St. Petersburg Beach, Florida (1978). *J. Immunol.*, **120**, 1761–1803
51. Abstracts of papers presented at the Eighth International Complement Workshop, Key Biscayne, Florida (1980). *J. Immunol.*, **124**, 1512–47

52. Abstracts: IXth International Complement Workshop (1982). *Mol. Immunol.*, **19**, 1357–413
53. Abstracts: Xth International Complement Workshop (1983). *Immunobiology*, **164**, 203–324
54. Abstracts: XIth International Complement Workshop (1985). *Complement*, **2**, 3–92
55. Abstracts: XIIth International Complement Workshop (1987). *Complement*, **4**, 123–244
56. Abstracts: XIIIth International Complement Workshop (1989). *Complement Inflamm.*, **6**, 307–425
57. Abstracts: XIVth International Complement Workshop (1991). *Complement Inflamm.*, **8**, 123–247
58. Müller-Eberhard, H. J., Dalmasso, A. P. and Calcott, M. A. (1966). The reaction mechanism of β_{1C}-globulin (C′3) in immune hemolysis. *J. Exp. Med.*, **123**, 33–54
59. Nelson, R. A. Jr., Jensen, J., Gigli, I. and Tamura N. (1966). Methods for the separation, purification and measurement of nine components of hemolytic complement in guinea pig serum. *Immunochemistry*, **3**, 111–35
60. Nomenclature of complement (1968). *Bull. WHO*, **39**, 935–8
61. Nomenclature of complement (1970). *Immunochemistry*, **7**, 137–42
62. Flexner, S. and Noguchi, H. (1902). Snake venom in relation to haemolysis, bacteriolysis and toxicity. *J. Exp. Med.*, **6**, 277–301
63. Pillemer, L., Blum, L., Lepow, I. H., Ross, O. A., Todd, E. W. and Wardlaw, A. C. (1954). The properdin system and immunity: I. Demonstration and isolation of a new serum protein, properdin, and its role in immune phenomena. *Science*, **120**, 279–85
64. Nelson, R. A. Jr. (1958). An alternative mechanism for the properdin system. *J. Exp. Med.*, **108**, 515–35
65. Lepow, I. H. (1980). Presidential address to American Association of Immunologists in Anaheim, California, April 16, 1980. *J. Immunol.*, **125**, 471–8
66. Ratnoff, W. D. (1980). A war with the molecules: Louis Pillemer and the history of properdin. *Persp. Biol. Med.*, **23**, 638–57
67. Götze, O. and Muller-Eberhard, H. J. (1971). The C3-activator system: an alternative pathway of complement activation. *J. Exp. Med.*, **134**, 90s–108s
68. Marcus, R. L., Shin, H. S. and Mayer, M. M. (1971). An alternate complement pathway: C-3 cleaving activity, not due to $\overline{C4,2a}$, on endotoxic lipopolysaccharide after treatment with guinea pig serum; relation to properdin. *Proc. Natl. Acad. Sci. (USA)*, **68**, 1351–4
69. Todd, E. W., Pillemer, L. and Lepow, I. H. (1959). The properdin system and immunity. IX. Studies on the purification of human properdin. *J. Immunol.*, **83**, 418–27
70. Lepow, I. H., Pillemer, L., Schoenberg, M. D., Todd, E. W. and Wedgwood, R. J. (1959). The properdin system and immunity. X. Characterization of partially purified human properdin. *J. Immunol.*, **83**, 428–36
71. Hunsicker, L. G., Ruddy, S. and Austen, K. F. (1973). Alternate complement pathway: factors involved in cobra venom factor (CoVF) activation of the third component of complement (C3). *J. Immunol.*, **110**, 128–38
72. Fearon, D. T., Austen, K. F. and Ruddy, S. (1973). Formation of a hemolytically active cellular intermediate by the interaction between properdin factors B and D and the activated third component of complement. *J. Exp. Med.*, **138**, 1305–13
73. Götze, O. and Müller-Eberhard, H. J. (1974). The role of properdin in the alternate pathway of complement activation. *J. Exp. Med.*, **139**, 44–57
74. Tack, B. F. and Prahl, J. W. (1976). Third component of human complement: purification from plasma and physicochemical characterization. *Biochemistry* **15**, 4513–21
75. Medicus, R. G., Götze, O. and Müller-Eberhard, H. J. (1976). The serine protease nature of the C3 and C5 convertases of the classical and alternative complement pathways. *Scand. J. Immunol.*, **5**, 1049–55
76. LeSavre, P. H. and Müller-Eberhard, H. J. (1978). Mechanism of action of factor D of the alternative complement pathway. *J. Exp. Med.*, **148**, 1498–1509
77. Landerman, N. S., Webster, M. E., Becker, E. L. and Ratcliffe, H. E. (1962). Hereditary angioneurotic edema. II. Deficiency of inhibitor for serum globulin permeability factor and/or plasma kallikrein. *J. Allergy*, **33**, 330–41
78. Donaldson, V. H. and Evans, R. R. (1963). A biochemical abnormality in hereditary angioneurotic edema: absence of serum inhibitor of C′1-esterase. *Am. J. Med.*, **35**, 37–44
79. Whaley, K. and Ruddy, S. (1976). Modulation of the alternative complement pathway by β1H globulin. *J. Exp. Med.*, **144**, 1147 –63

80. Weiler, J. M., Daha, M. R., Austen, K. F. and Fearon, D. T. (1976). Control of the amplification convertase of complement by the plasma protein β1H. *Proc. Natl. Acad. Sci. (USA)*, **73**, 3268–72
81. Lachmann, P. J. and Müller-Eberhard, H. J. (1968). The demonstration in human serum of 'conglutinogen-activating factor' and its effect on the third component of complement. *J. Immunol.*, **100**, 691–8
82. Ruddy, S. and Austen, K. F. (1969). C3 inactivator of man. I. Hemolytic measurement by the inactivation of cell-bound C3. *J. Immunol.*, **102**, 533–43
83. Ruddy, S. and Austen, K. F. (1971). C3b inactivator of man. II. Fragments produced by C3b inactivator cleavage of cell-bound or fluid phase C3b. *J. Immunol.*, **107**, 742–50
84. Ruddy, S., Hunsicker, L. G. and Austen, K. F. (1972). C3b inactivator of man. III. Further purification and production of antibody to C3b INA. *J. Immunol.*, **108**, 657–64
85. Scharfstein, J., Ferreira, A., Gigli, I. and Nussenzweig, V. (1978). Human C4 binding protein. I. Isolation and characterization. *J. Exp. Med.*, **148**, 207–22
86. Fujita, T. and Nussenzweig, V. (1979). The role of C4-binding protein and β1H in proteolysis of C4b and C3b. *J. Exp. Med.*, **150**, 267–76
87. Nelson, D. S. (1963). Immune adherence. *Adv. Immunol.*, **3**, 131–80
88. Fearon, D. T. (1979). Regulation of the amplification C3 convertase of human complement by an inhibitory protein isolated from human erythrocyte membrane. *Proc. Natl. Acad. Sci. (USA)*, **76**, 5867–71
89. Barel, M., Charriaut, C. and Frade, R. (1981). Isolation and characterization of a C3b receptor-like molecule from membranes of a human B lymphoblastoid cell line (Raji). *FEBS Lett.*, **136**, 111–14
90. Lay, W. H. and Nussenzweig, V. (1968). Receptors for complement on leukocytes. *J. Exp. Med.*, **128**, 991–1009
91. Vik, D. P. and Fearon, D. T. (1985). Neutrophils express a receptor for iC3b, C3dg, and C3d that is distinct from CR1, CR2 and CR3. *J. Immunol.*, **134**, 2571–9
92. Seya, T., Turner, J. R. and Atkinson, J. P. (1986). Purification and characterization of a membrane protein (gp45-70) that is a cofactor for cleavage of C3b and C4b. *J. Exp. Med.*, **163**, 837–55
93. Cole, J. L., Housley, G. A., Dykman, T. R., MacDermott, R. P. and Atkinson, J. P. (1985). Identification of an additional class of C3-binding membrane proteins of human peripheral blood leukocytes and cell lines. *Proc. Natl. Acad. Sci. (USA)*, **82**, 859–63
94. Nicholson-Weller, A., Burge, J. and Austen, K. F. (1981). Purification from guinea pig erythrocyte stroma of a decay-accelerating factor for the classical C3 convertase, C4b,2a. *J. Immunol.*, **127**, 2035–9
95. Nicholson-Weller, A., Burge, J., Fearon, D. T., Weller, P. F. and Austen, K. F. (1982). Isolation of a human erythrocyte membrane glycoprotein with decay-accelerating activity for C3 convertases of the complement system. *J. Immunol.*, **129**, 184–9
96. Zalman, L. S., Wood, L. M. and Müller-Eberhard, H. J. (1986). Isolation of a human erythrocyte membrane protein capable of inhibiting expression of homologous complement transmembrane channels. *Proc. Natl. Acad. Sci. (USA)*, **83**, 6975–9
97. Zalman, L. S., Wood, L. M. and Müller-Eberhard, H. J. (1987). Inhibition of antibody-dependent lymphocyte cytotoxicity by homologous restriction factor incorporated into target cell membranes. *J. Exp. Med.*, **166**, 947–55
98. Davies, A., Simmons, D. L., Hale, G., Harrison R. A., Tighe, H., Lachmann, P. J. and Waldmann, H. (1989). CD59, an LY-6-like protein expressed in human lymphoid cells, regulates the action of the complement membrane attack complex on homologous cells. *J. Exp. Med.*, **170**, 637–54
99. Okada, H., Nagami, Y., Takahashi, K., Okada, N., Hideshima, T., Takizawa, H. and Kondo, J. (1989). 20 kDa homologous restriction factor of complement resembles T cell activating protein. *Biochem. Biophys. Res. Commun.*, **162**, 1553–9
100. Müller-Eberhard, H. J. (1984). The membrane attack complex. *Springer Semin. Immunopathol.*, **7**, 93–141
101. Müller-Eberhard, H. J. (1986). The membrane attack complex of complement. *Ann. Rev. Immunol.*, **4**, 503–28
102. Lichtenheld, M. G., Olsen, K. J., Lu, P., Lowrey, D. M., Hameed, A., Hengartner, H. and Podack, E. R. (1988). Structure and function of human perforin. *Nature*, **335**, 448–51

103. Morgan, B. P. (1989). Mechanisms of tissue damage by the membrane attack complex of complement. *Complement Inflamm.*, **6**, 104–11
104. Esser, A. F. (1990). The membrane attack pathway of complement. In Cruse, J. M. and Lewis, R. E. Jr. (eds.) *The Year in Immunology 1989–90*, pp. 229–44 (Basel: Karger)
105. Esser, A. F. (1991). Big MAC attack: complement proteins cause leaky patches. *Immunol. Today*, **12**, 316–18
106. Bhakdi, S. and Tranum-Jensen, J. (1991). Complement lysis: a hole is a hole. *Immunol. Today*, **12**, 318–20
107. (1991). The biology of complement. *Immunol. Today*, **12**, 291–342
108. Subcommittee of the IUIS/WHO Nomenclature Committee (1981) Nomenclature of the alternative activating pathway of complement. *Bull. WHO*, **59**, 489–91
109. Ziccardi, R. J. and Cooper, N. R. (1977). The subunit composition and sedimentation properties of human C1. *J. Immunol.*, **118**, 2047–52
110. Ziccardi, R. J. (1983). Nature of the metal ion requirement for assembly and function of the first component of human complement. *J. Biol. Chem.*, **258**, 6187–92
111. Villiers, C. L., Arlaud, G. J. and Colomb, M. G. (1985). Domain structure and associated functions of subcomponents C1r and C1s of the first component of human complement. *Proc. Natl. Acad. Sci. (USA)* **82**, 4477–81
112. Journet, A. and Tosi, M. (1986). Cloning and sequencing of full-length cDNA encoding the precursor of human complement component C1r. *Biochem. J.*, **240**, 783–7
113. Mackinnon, C. M., Carter, P. E., Smyth, S. J., Dunbar, B. and Fothergill, J. E. (1987). Molecular cloning of cDNA for human complement component C1s. The complete amino acid sequence. *Eur. J. Biochem.*, **169**, 547–53
114. Porter, R. R. and Reid, K. B. M. (1978). The biochemistry of complement. *Nature*, **275**, 699–704
115. Knobel, H. R., Villiger, W. and Isliker, H. (1975). Chemical analysis and electron microscopy studies of human C1q prepared by different methods. *Eur. J. Immunol.*, **5**, 78–82
116. Schumaker, V. N., Poon, P. H., Seegan, G. W. and Smith C. A. (1981). Semi-flexible joint in the C1q subunit of the first component of human complement. *J. Mol. Biol.*, **148**, 191–7
117. Strang, C. J., Siegel, R. C., Phillips, M. L., Poon, P. H. and Schumaker, V. N. (1982). Ultrastructure of the first component of human complement: electron microscopy of the crosslinked complex. *Immunology*, **79**, 586–90
118. Reid, K. B. M. and Thompson, R. A. (1983). Characterization of a non-functional form of Clq found in patients with a genetically linked deficiency of C1q activity. *Mol. Immunol.*, **20**, 1117–25
119. Reid, K. B. M. (1985). Molecular cloning and characterization of the complementary DNA and gene coding for the B-chain of subcomponent C1q of the human complement system. *Biochem. J.*, **231**, 729–35
120. Colomb, M. G., Arlaud, G. J. and Villiers, C. L. (1984). Activation of C1. *Phil. Trans. R. Soc. Lond.*, **306**, 283–92
121. Burton, D. R. (1985). Immunoglobulin G: functional sites. *Mol. Immunol.*, **22**, 161–206
122. Hurst, M. M., Volanakis, J. E., Hester, R. B., Stroud, R. M. and Bennett, J. C. (1974). The structural basis for binding of complement by immunoglobulin M. *J. Exp. Med.*, **140**, 1117–21
123. Hurst, M. M., Volanakis, J. E., Stroud, R. M. and Bennett, J. C. (1975). C1 fixation and classical complement pathway activation by a fragment of the Cμ4 domain of IgM. *J. Exp. Med.*, **142**, 1322–6
124. Hurst, M. M., Volanakis, J. E., Stroud, R. M. and Bennett, J. C. (1976). A comparative analysis of the $C\bar{1}$-binding ability of fragments derived from complement-fixing and noncomplement-fixing IgM proteins. *J. Clin. Invest.*, **58**, 16–21
125. Wright, J. F., Shulman, M. J., Isenman, D. E. and Painter, R. H. (1988). C1 binding by murine IgM. *J. Biol. Chem.*, **263**, 11221–6
126. Dodds, A. W., Sim, R. B., Porter, R. R. and Kerr, M. A. (1978). Activation of the first component of human complement (C1) by antibody–antigen aggregates. *Biochem. J.*, **175**, 383–90
127. Valet, G. and Cooper, N. R. (1974). Isolation and characterization of the proenzyme form of the C1r subunit of the first complement component. *J. Immunol.*, **112**, 1667–73
128. Ziccardi, R. J. and Cooper, N. R. (1976). Physicochemical and functional characterization of the C1r subunit of the first complement component. *J. Immunol.*, **116**, 496–503

129. Porter, R. R. (1980). The complex proteases of the complement system. *Proc. R. Soc. Lond.*, **210**, 477–98
130. Schreiber, R. D. and Müller-Eberhard, H. J. (1974). Fourth component of human complement: description of a three polypeptide chain structure. *J. Exp. Med.*, **140**, 1324–35
131. Seya, T., Nagasawa, S. and Atkinson, J. P. (1986). Location of the interchain disulfide bonds of the fourth component of human complement (C4): evidence based on the liberation of fragments secondary to thiol–disulfide interchange reactions. *J. Immunol.*, **136**, 4152–6
132. Nonaka, M., Nakayama, K., Yeul, Y. D. and Takahashi, M. (1985). Complete nucleotide and derived amino acid sequences of the fourth component of mouse complement (C4). *J. Biol. Chem.*, **260**, 10936–43
133. Gorski, J. P., Hugli, T. E. and Müller-Eberhard, H. J. (1981). Characterization of human C4a anaphylatoxin. *J. Biol. Chem.*, **256**, 2707–11
134. Moon, K. E., Gorski, J. P. and Hugli, T. E. (1981). Complete primary structure of human C4a anaphylatoxin. *J. Biol. Chem.*, **256**, 8685–92
135. Gorski, J. P., Hugli, T. E. and Müller-Eberhard, H. J. (1979). C4a: the third anaphylatoxin of the human complement system. *Proc. Natl. Acad. Sci. (USA)*, **76**, 5299–302
136. Campbell, R. D., Gagnon, J. and Porter, R. R. (1981). Amino acid sequence around the thiol and reactive acyl groups of human complement component C4. *Biochem. J.*, **199**, 359–70
137. Kerr, M. A. (1980). The human complement system: assembly of the classical pathway C3 convertase. *Biochem. J.*, **189**, 173–81
138. Ross, G. D. (1980). Analysis of the different types of leukocyte membrane complement receptors and their interaction with the complement system. *J. Immunol. Methods*, **37**, 197–211
139. Schifferli, J. A. and Paccaud, J-P. (1989). Two isotypes of human C4, C4A and C4B have different structure and function. *Complement Inflamm.*, **6**, 19–26
140. Isenman, D. E. and Young, J. R. (1984). The molecular basis for the difference in immune hemolysis activity of the Chido and Rodgers isotypes of human complement component C4. *J. Immunol.*, **132**, 3019–27
141. Carroll, M. C., Fathallah, D. M., Bergamaschini, L., Alicot, E. M. and Isenman, D. E. (1990). Substitution of a single amino acid (aspartic acid for histidine) converts the functional activity of human complement C4B to C4A. *Proc. Natl. Acad. Sci. (USA)*, **87**, 6868–72
142. Reilly, B. D., Levine, R. P. and Skanes, V. M. (1991). Amino acid residues 1101–1105 of the isotypic region of human C4B is important to the covalent binding activity of complement component C4. *J. Immunol.*, **147**, 3018–23
143. Polley, M. J. and Muller-Eberhard, H. J. (1968). The second component of human complement: its isolation, fragmentation by C′1 esterase, and incorporation into C′3 convertase. *J. Exp. Med.*, **128**, 533–51
144. Campbell, R. D. and Bentley, D. R. (1985). The structure and genetics of the C2 and factor B genes. *Immunol. Rev.*, **87**, 19–37
145. Bentley, D. R. (1986). Primary structure of human complement component C2. *Biochem. J.* **239**, 339–45
146. Horiuchi, T., Macon, K. J., Kidd, V. J. and Volanakis, J. E. (1989). cDNA cloning and expression of human complement component C2. *J. Immunol.*, **142**, 2105–11
147. Gigli, I. and Austen, K. F. (1969). Fluid phase destruction of $C2^{hu}$ by $C1^{hu}$. II. Unmasking by $C4i^{hu}$ of $C\overline{1}^{hu}$ specificity for $C2^{hu}$. *J. Exp. Med.*, **130**, 833–46
148. Villiers, M.-B., Thielens, N. M. and Colomb, M. G. (1985). Soluble C3 proconvertase and convertase of the classical pathway of human complement. *Biochem. J.* **226**, 429–36
149. Nagasawa, S. and Stroud, R. M. (1977). Cleavage of C2 by $C\overline{1}s$ into the antigenically distinct fragments C2a and C2b: demonstration of binding of C2b to C4b. *Proc. Natl. Acad. Sci. (USA)*, **74**, 2998–3001
150. Kerr, M. A. and Porter, R. R. (1978). The purification and properties of the second component of human complement. *Biochem. J.*, **171**, 99–107
151. Rent, R., Ertel, N., Eisenstein, R. and Gewurz, H. (1975). Complement activation by interaction of polyanions and polycations. I. Heparin-protamine induced consumption of complement. *J. Immunol.*, **114**, 120–4
152. Rosenberg, A. M., Prokopchuk, P. A. and Lee, J. S. (1988). The binding of native DNA to the collagen-like segment of C1q. *J. Rheumatol.*, **15**, 1091–6
153. van Schravendijk, M. R. and Dwek, R. A. (1982). Interaction of C1q with DNA. *Mol. Immunol.*, **19**, 1179–87

154. Kaplan, M. H. and Volanakis, J. E. (1974). Interaction of C-reactive protein complexes with the complement system. I. Consumption of human complement associated with the reaction of C-reactive protein with pneumococcal C-polysaccharide and with the choline phosphatides, lecithin and sphingomyelin. *J. Immunol.*, **112**, 2135–47
155. May, J. E. and Frank, M. M. (1973). A new complement-mediated cytolytic mechanism – the C1-bypass activation pathway. *Proc. Natl. Acad. Sci. (USA)*, **70**, 649–52
156. May, J. E. and Frank, M. M. (1973). Hemolysis of sheep erythrocytes in guinea pig serum deficient in the fourth component of complement I. Antibody and serum requirements. *J. Immunol.*, **111**, 1661 -7
157. May, J. E. and Frank, M. M. (1973). Hemolysis of sheep erythrocytes in guinea pig serum deficient in the fourth component of complement II. Evidence for involvement of C1 and components of the alternative complement pathway. *J. Immunol.*, **111**, 1668–76
158. Steuer, K. L. K., Sloan, L. B., Oglesby, T. J., Farries, T. C., Nickells, M. W., Densen P., Harley, J. B. and Atkinson, J. P. (1989). Lysis of sensitized sheep erythrocytes in human sera deficient in the second component of complement. *J. Immunol.*, **143**, 2256–61
159. Farries, T. C., Steuer, K. L. K. and Atkinson, J. P. (1990). Evolutionary implications of a new bypass activation pathway of the complement system. *Immunol. Today*, **11**, 78–80
160. Masaki, T., Matsumoto, M., Yasuda, R., Levine, R. P., Kitamura, H. and Seya, T. (1991). A covalent dimer of complement C4b serves as a subunit of a novel C5 convertase that involves no C3 derivatives. *J. Immunol.*, **147**, 927–32
161. Niven, I. P. and Whaley, K. (1986). Inhibition of C1q binding to antigen–antibody complexes by a factor in rheumatoid arthritis serum. *Rheumatol. Int.*, **6**, 205–8
162. Lopez-Trascasa, M., Bing, D. H., Rivard, M. and Nicholson-Weller, A. (1989). Factor J: isolation and characterization of a new polypeptide inhibitor of complement C1. *J. Biol. Chem.*, **264**, 16214–21
163. Sim, R. B., Arlaud, G. J. and Colomb, M. G. (1979). $C\overline{1}$ inhibitor-dependent dissociation of human complement component $C\overline{1}$ bound to immune complexes. *Biochem. J.* **179**, 449–57
164. Ziccardi, R. J. and Cooper, N. R. (1979). Active disassembly of the first complement component, $C\overline{1}$, by $C\overline{1}$ inactivator. *J. Immunol.*, **123**, 788–92
165. Tosi, M., Duponchel, C., Bourgarel, P., Colomb, M. and Meo, T. (1986). Molecular cloning of human C1 inhibitor: sequence homologies with α_1-antitrypsin and other members of the serpins superfamily. *Gene*, **42**, 265–72
166. Que, B. G. and Petra, P. H. (1986). Isolation and analysis of a cDNA coding for human C1 inhibitor. *Biochem. Biophys. Res. Commun.*, **137**, 620–5
167. Davis, A. E. III, Whitehead, A. S., Harrison, R. A., Dauphinais, A., Bruns, G. A. P., Cicardi, M. and Rosen, F. S. (1986). Human inhibitor of the first component of complement, C1: characterization of cDNA clones and localization of the gene to chromosome 11. *Proc. Natl. Acad. Sci. (USA)*, **83**, 3161–5
168. Davis, A. E. III. (1988). C1 inhibitor and hereditary angioneurotic edema. *Ann. Rev. Immunol.*, **6**, 595–628
169. Fujita, T., Gigli, I. and Nussenzweig, V. (1978). Human C4-binding protein. II. Role in proteolysis of C4b by C3b-inactivator. *J. Exp. Med.*, **148**, 1044–51
170. Villiers, M. B., Thielens, N. M., Villiers, C. L. and Colomb, M. G. (1985). Ultrastructure of human C4-binding protein: proposition for a new model. *Eur. J. Immunol.*, **15**, 941–5
171. Pardo-Manuel, F., Rey-Campos, J., Hillarp, A., Dahlbäck, B. and De Cordoba, S. R. (1990). Human genes for the α and β chains of complement C4b-binding protein are closely linked in a head-to-tail arrangement. *Proc. Natl. Acad. Sci. (USA)*, **87**, 4529–32
172. Hillarp, A. and Dahlbäck, B. (1990). Cloning of cDNA coding for the β chain of human complement component C4b-binding protein: sequence homology with the α chain. *Proc. Natl. Acad. Sci. (USA)*, **87**, 1183–7
173. Seya, T. and Atkinson, J. P. (1989). Functional properties of membrane cofactor protein of complement. *Biochem. J.*, **264**, 581–8
174. Lublin, D. M., Liszewski, M. K., Post, T. W., Arce, M. A., Le Beau, M. M., Rebentisch, M. B., Lemons, R. S., Seya, T. and Atkinson, J. P. (1988). Molecular cloning and chromosomal localization of human membrane cofactor protein (MCP). *J. Exp. Med.*, **168**, 181–94
175. Bora, N. S., Lublin, D. M., Kumar, B. V., Hockett, R. D., Holers, V. M. and Atkinson, J. P. (1989). Structural gene for human membrane cofactor protein (MCP) of complement maps to within 100 kb of the 3′ end of the C3b/C4b receptor gene. *J. Exp. Med.*, **169**, 597–602

176. Fujita, T., Inoue, T., Ogawa, K., Iida, K. and Tamura, N. (1987). The mechanism of action of decay-accelerating factor (DAF). *J. Exp. Med.*, **166**, 1221–8
177. Medof, M. E., Lublin, D. M., Holers, V. M., Ayers, D. J., Getty, R. R., Leykam, J. F., Atkinson, J. P. and Tykocinski, M. L. (1987). Cloning and characterization of cDNAs encoding the complete sequence of decay-accelerating factor of human complement. *Proc. Natl. Acad. Sci. (USA)*, **84**, 2007–11
178. Post, T. W., Arce, M. A., Liszewski, M. K., Thompson, E. S., Atkinson, J. P. and Lublin, D. M. (1990). Structure of the gene for human complement protein decay accelerating factor. *J. Immunol.*, **144**, 740–4
179. Kinoshita, T., Medof, M. E., Hong, K. and Nussenzweig, V. (1986). Membrane-bound C4b interacts endogenously with complement receptor CR1 of human red cells. *J. Exp. Med.*, **164**, 1377–88
180. Fearon, D. T. and Austen, K. F. (1977). Activation of the alternative complement pathway due to resistance of zymosan-bound amplification convertase to endogenous regulatory mechanisms. *Proc. Natl. Acad. Sci. (USA)*, **74**, 1683–7
181. Alper, C. A. and Balavitch, D. (1976). Cobra venom factor: evidence for its being altered cobra C3 (the third component of complement). *Science*, **191**, 1275–6
182. Thompson, R. A. (1972). C3 inactivating factor in the serum of a patient with chronic hypocomplementaemic proliferative glomerulo-nephritis. *Immunology*, **22**, 147–58
183. Daha, M. R., Austen, K. F. and Fearon, D. T. (1978). Heterogeneity, polypeptide chain composition and antigenic reactivity of C3 nephritic factor. *J. Immunol.*, **120**, 1389–94
184. Davis, A. E. III, Ziegler, J. B., Gelfand, E. W., Rosen, F. S. and Alper, C. A. (1977). Heterogeneity of nephritic factor and its identification as an immunoglobulin. *Proc. Natl. Acad. Sci (USA)*, **74**, 3980–3
185. Scott, D. M., Amos, N., Sissons, J. G. P., Lachmann, P. J. and Peters, D. K. (1978). The immunoglobin nature of nephritic factor (NeF). *Clin. Exp. Immunol.*, **32**, 12–24
186. Platts-Mills, T. A. E. and Ishizaka, K. (1974). Activation of the alternate pathway of human complement by rabbit cells. *J. Immunol.*, **113**, 348–58
187. Campbell, R. D. and Porter, R. R. (1983). Molecular cloning and characterization of the gene coding for human complement protein factor B. *Proc. Natl. Acad. Sci. (USA)*, **80**, 4464–68
188. Mole, J. E., Anderson, J. K., Davison, E. A. and Woods, D. E. (1984). Complete primary structure for the zymogen of human complement factor B. *J. Biol. Chem.*, **259**, 3407–12
189. Rosen, B. S., Cook, K. S., Yaglom, J., Groves, D. L., Volanakis, J. E., Damm, D., White, T. and Spiegelman, B. M. (1989). Adipsin and complement factor D activity: an immune-related defect in obesity. *Science*, **244**, 1483–7
190. Fearon, D. T. and Austen, K. F. (1975). Properdin: binding to C3b and stabilization of the C3b-dependent C3 convertase. *J. Exp. Med.*, **142**, 856–63
191. Chapitis, J. and Lepow, I. H. (1976). Multiple sedimenting species of properdin in human serum and interaction of purified properdin with the third component of complement. *J. Exp. Med.*, **143**, 241–57
192. DiScipio, R. G. (1981). The binding of human complement proteins C5, factor B, β_1H and properdin to complement fragment C3b on zymosan. *Biochem. J.*, **199**, 485–96
193. Farries, T. C., Finch, J. T., Lachmann, P. J. and Harrison, R. A. (1987). Resolution and analysis of 'native' and 'activated' properdin. *Biochem. J.*, **243**, 507–17
194. Pangburn, M. K. (1989). Analysis of the natural polymeric forms of human properdin and their functions in complement activation. *J. Immunol.*, **142**, 202–7
195. Nolan, K. F., Schwaeble, W., Kaluz, S., Dierich, M. P. and Reid, K. B. M. (1991). Molecular cloning of the cDNA coding for properdin, a positive regulator of the alternative pathway of human complement. *Eur. J. Immunol.*, **21**, 771–6
196. Schreiber, R. D. and Müller-Eberhard, H. J. (1978). Assembly of the cytolytic alternative pathway of complement from 11 isolated plasma proteins. *J. Exp. Med.*, **148**, 1722–7
197. Schreiber, R. D., Pangburn, M. K., Lesavre, P. H. and Müller-Eberhard, H. J. (1978). Initiation of the alternative pathway of complement: recognition of activators by bound C3b and assembly of the entire pathway from six isolated proteins. *Proc. Natl. Acad. Sci. (USA)*, **75**, 3948–52
198. Ripoche, J., Day, A. J., Harris, T. J. R. and Sim, R. B. (1988). The complete amino acid sequence of human complement factor H. *Biochem. J.*, **249**, 593–602

199. Conrad, D. H., Carlo, J. R. and Ruddy, S. (1978). Interaction of β1H globulin with cell-bound C3b: quantitative analysis of binding and influence of alternative pathway components on binding. *J. Exp. Med.*, **147**, 1792–1805
200. Kazatchkine, M. D., Fearon, D. T. and Austen, K. F. (1979). Human alternative complement pathway: membrane-associated sialic acid regulates the competition between B and β1H for cell-bound C3b. *J. Immunol.*, **122**, 75–81
201. Nicol, P. A. E. and Lachmann, P. J. (1973). The alternate pathway of complement activation. *Immunology,* **24**, 259–75
202. Pangburn, M. K., Schreiber, R. D. and Müller-Eberhard, H. J. (1977). Human complement C3b inactivator: isolation, characterization, and demonstration of an absolute requirement for the serum protein β1H for cleavage of C3b and C4b in solution. *J. Exp. Med.*, **146**, 257–70
203. Catterall, C. F., Lyons, A., Sim, R. B., Day, A. J. and Harris, T. J. R. (1987). Characterization of the primary amino acid sequence of human complement control protein factor I from an analysis of cDNA clones. *Biochem. J.*, **242**, 849–56
204. Wong, W. W. (1990). Structural and functional correlation of the human complement receptor type 1. *J. Invest. Dermatol.*, **94**, 64S–67S
205. Holers, V. M., Chaplin, D. D., Leykam, J. F., Gruner, B. A., Kumar, V. and Atkinson, J. P. (1987). Human complement C3b/C4b receptor (CR1) mRNA polymorphism that correlates with the CR1 allelic molecular weight polymorphism. *Proc. Natl. Acad. Sci. (USA)*, **84**, 2459–63
206. Wong, W. W., Cahill, J. M., Rosen, M. D., Kennedy, C. A., Bonaccio, E. T., Morris, M. J., Wilson, J. G., Klickstein, L. B. and Fearon, D. T. (1989). Structure of the human CR1 gene. *J. Exp. Med.*, **169**, 847–63
207. Fearon, D. T. and Austen, K. F. (1977). Activation of the alternative complement pathway with rabbit erythrocytes by circumvention of the regulatory action of endogenous control proteins. *J. Exp. Med.*, **146**, 22–33
208. Fearon, D. T. (1978). Regulation by membrane sialic acid of β1H-dependent decay – dissociation of amplification C3 convertase of the alternative complement pathway. *Proc. Natl. Acad. Sci. (USA)*, **75**, 1971–5.
209. Pangburn, M. K. and Müller-Eberhard, H. J. (1978). Complement C3 convertase: cell surface restriction of β1H control and generation of restriction on neuraminidase-treated cells. *Proc. Natl. Acad. Sci. (USA)*, **75**, 2416–20
210. Nydegger, U. E., Fearon, D. T. and Austen, K. F. (1978). Autosomal locus regulates inverse relationship between sialic acid content and capacity of mouse erythrocytes to activate human alternative complement pathway. *Proc. Natl. Acad. Sci. (USA)*, **75**, 6078–82
211. Chonn, A., Cullis, P. R. and Devine, D. V. (1991). The role of surface charge in the activation of the classical and alternative pathways of complement by liposomes. *J. Immunol.*, **146**, 4234–41
212. Nagaki, K., Iida, K., Okubo, M. and Inai, S. (1978). Reaction mechanisms of β1H globulin. *Int. Arch. Allergy Appl. Immun.*, **57**, 221–32
213. Nelson, B. and Ruddy, S. (1979). Enhancing role of IgG in lysis of rabbit erythrocytes by the alternative pathway of human complement. *J. Immunol.*, **122**, 1994–9
214. De Bruijn, M. H. L. and Fey, G. H. (1985). Human complement component C3: cDNA coding sequence and derived primary structure. *Proc. Natl. Acad. Sci. (USA)*, **82**, 708–12
215. Lambris, J. D. and Müller-Eberhard, H. J. (1986). The multifunctional role of C3: structural analysis of its interactions with physiological ligands. *Mol. Immunol.*, **23**, 1237–42
216. Volanakis, J. E. (1989). Participation of C3 and its ligands in complement activation. *Curr. Top. Microbiol. Immunol.*, **153**, 1–21
217. Hugli, T. E. (1975). Human anaphylatoxin (C3a) from the third component of complement. *J. Biol. Chem.*, **250**, 8293–301
218. Tack, B. F., Harrison, R. A., Janatova, J., Thomas, M. L. and Prahl, J. W. (1980). Evidence for presence of an internal thiolester bond in third component of human complement. *Proc. Natl. Acad. Sci. (USA)*, **77**, 5764–8
219. Law, S. K., Lichtenberg, N. A. and Levine, R. P. (1980). Covalent binding and hemolytic activity of complement proteins. *Proc. Natl. Acad. Sci. (USA)*, **77**, 7194–8
220. Pangburn, M. K. and Müller-Eberhard, H. J. (1980). Relation of a putative thioester bond in C3 to activation of the alternative pathway and the binding of C3b to biological targets of complement. *J. Exp. Med.*, **152**, 1102–14

221. Law, S. K. and Levine, R. P. (1977). Interaction between the third complement protein and cell surface macromolecules. *Proc. Natl. Acad. Sci. (USA)*, **74**, 2701–5
222. Ross, G. D., Newman, S. L., Lambris, J. D., Devery-Pocius, J. E., Cain, J. A. and Lachmann, P. J. (1983). Generation of three different fragments of bound C3 with purified factor I or serum. II. Location of binding sites in the C3 fragments for factors B and H. Complement receptors, and bovine conglutinin. *J. Exp. Med.*, **158**, 334–52
223. Davis, A. E. III and Harrison, R. A. (1982). Structural characterization of factor I mediated cleavage of the third component of complement. *Biochemistry*, **21**, 5745–9
224. Daha, M. R., Fearon, D. T. and Austen, K. F. (1976). C3 requirements for formation of alternative pathway C5 convertase. *J. Immunol.*, **117**, 630–4
225. Morgan, E. L., Thoman, M. L., Hoeprich, P. D. and Hugli, T. E. (1985). Bioactive complement fragments in immunoregulation. *Immunol. Lett.*, **9**, 207–13
226. Hostetter, M. K., Krueger, R. A. and Schmeling, D. J. (1984). The biochemistry of opsonization: central role of the reactive thiolester of the third component of complement. *J. Infect. Dis.*, **150**, 653–61
227. Conroy, M. C., Ozols, J. and Lepow, I. H. (1976). Structural features and biologic properties of fragments obtained by limited proteolysis of C3. *J. Immunol.*, **116**, 1682–7
228. Harrison, R. A. and Lachmann, P. J. (1980). The physiological breakdown of the third component of human complement. *Mol. Immunol.*, **17**, 9–20
229. Parkes, C., DiScipio, R. G., Kerr, M. A. and Prohaska, R. (1981). The separation of functionally distinct forms of the third component of human complement (C3). *Biochem. J.*, **193**, 963–70
230. Chaplin, H., Monroe, M. C. and Lachmann, P. J. (1982). Further studies of the C3g component of the α2D fragment of human C3. *Clin. Exp. Immunol.*, **51**, 639–46
231. Lachmann, P. J., Pangburn, M. K. and Oldroyd, R. G. (1982). Breakdown of C3 after complement activation. *J. Exp. Med.*, **156**, 205–16
232. Davis, A. E. III, Harrison, R. A. and Lachmann, P. J. (1984). Physiologic inactivation of fluid phase C3b: isolation and structural analysis of C3c, C3dg (α2D), and C3g. *J. Immunol.*, **132**, 1960–6
233. Folkersen, J., Teisner, B., Eggertsen, G. and Sim, R. B. (1986). Immunoblotting analysis of the peptide chain structure of the physiological breakdown products of the third component of human complement. *Electrophoresis*, **7**, 379–86
234. Rother, K. (1972). Leucocyte mobilizing factor: a new biological activity derived from the third component of complement. *Eur. J. Immunol.*, **2**, 550–8
235. Ghebrehiwet, B. and Müller-Eberhard, H. J. (1979). C3e: an acidic fragment of human C3 with leukocytosis-inducing activity. *J. Immunol.*, **123**, 616–21
236. Ghebrehiwet, B. (1984). The release of lysosomal enzymes from human polymorphonuclear leukocytes by human C3e. *Clin. Immunol. Immunopathol.*, **30**, 321–9
237. Hoeprich, P. D. Jr., Dahinden, C. A., Lachmann, P. J., Davis, A. E. III and Hugli, T. E. (1985). A synthetic nonapeptide corresponding to the NH_2-terminal sequence of C3d-K causes leukocytosis in rabbits. *J. Biol. Chem.*, **260**, 2597–600
238. Thoman, M. L., Meuth, J. L., Morgan, E. L., Weigle, W. O. and Hugli, T. E. (1984). C3d-K, a kallikrein cleavage fragment of iC3b is a potent inhibitor of cellular proliferation. *J. Immunol.*, **133**, 2629–33
239. Nemerow, G. R., McNaughton, M. E. and Cooper, N. R. (1985). Binding of monoclonal antibody to the Epstein Barr virus (EBV)/CR2 receptor induces activation and differentiation of human B lymphocytes. *J. Immunol.*, **135**, 3068–73
240. Frade, R., Barel, M., Ehlin-Henriksson, B. and Klein, G. (1985). gp140, the C3d receptor of human B lymphocytes, is also the Epstein–Barr virus receptor. *Proc. Natl. Acad. Sci. (USA)*, **82**, 1490–3
241. Nemerow, G. R., Wolfert, R., McNaughton, M. E. and Cooper, N. R. (1985). Identification and characterization of the Epstein–Barr virus receptor on human B lymphocytes and its relationship to the C3d complement receptor (CR2). *J. Virol.*, **55**, 347–51
242. Weis, J. J., Fearon, D. T., Klickstein, L. B., Wong, W. W., Richards, S. A., De Bruyn Kops, A., Smith, J. A. and Weis, J. H. (1986). Identification of a partial cDNA clone for the C3d/Epstein–Barr virus receptor of human B lymphocytes: homology with the receptor for fragments C3b and C4b of the third and fourth components of complement. *Proc. Natl. Acad. Sci. (USA)*, **83**, 5639–43

243. Weis, J. J. , Toothaker, L. E., Smith, J. A., Weis, J. H. and Fearon, D. T. (1988). Structure of the human B lymphocyte receptor for C3d and the Epstein–Barr virus and relatedness to other members of the family of C3/C4 binding proteins. *J. Exp. Med.*, **167**, 1047–66
244. Vogt, W., Schmidt, G., Von Buttlar, B. and Dieminger, L. (1978). A new function of the activated third component of complement: binding to C5, an essential step for C5 activation. *Immunology*, **34**, 29–40
245. Hong, K., Kinoshita, T., Pramoonjago, P., Kim, Y. U., Seya, T. and Inoue, K. (1991). Reconstitution of C5 convertase of the alternative complement pathway with isolated C3b dimer and factors B and D. *J. Immunol.*, **146**, 1868–73
246. Fernandez, H. N. and Hugli, T. E. (1977). Chemical evidence for common genetic ancestry of complement components C3 and C5. *J. Biol. Chem.*, **252**, 1826–8
247. Fernandez, H. N. and Hugli, T. E. (1978). Primary structural analysis of the polypeptide portion of human C5a anaphylatoxin. *J. Biol. Chem.*, **253**, 6955–64
248. Wetsel, R. A., Lemons, R. S., Le Beau, M. M., Barnum, S. R., Noack, D. and Tack, B. F. (1988). Molecular analysis of human complement component C5: localization of the structural gene to chromosome 9. *Biochemistry*, **27**, 1474–82
249. Haviland, D. L., Haviland, J. C., Fleischer, D. T., Hunt, A. and Wetsel, R. A. (1991). Complete cDNA sequence of human complement pro-C5. Evidence of truncated transcripts derived from a single copy gene. *J. Immunol.*, **146**, 362–8
250. Lachmann, P. J. and Thompson, R. A. (1970). Reactive lysis: the complement-mediated lysis of unsensitized cells. II. The characterization of activated reactor as $C\overline{56}$ and the participation of C8 and C9. *J. Exp. Med.*, **131**, 643–57
251. Podack, E. R., Kolb, W. P. and Müller-Eberhard, H. J. (1976). Purification of the sixth and seventh component of human complement without loss of hemolytic activity. *J. Immunol.*, **116**, 263–9
252. DiScipio, R. G. and Hugli, T. E. (1989). The molecular architecture of human complement component C6. *J. Biol. Chem.*, **264**, 16197–206
253. Haefliger, J.-A., Tschopp, J., Vial, N. and Jenne, D. E. (1989). Complete primary structure and functional characterization of the sixth component of the human complement system. *J. Biol. Chem.*, **264**, 18041–51
254. DiScipio, R. G., Chakravarti, D. N., Müller-Eberhard, H. J. and Fey, G. H. (1988). The structure of human complement component C7 and the C5b-7 complex. *J. Biol. Chem.*, **263**, 549–60
255. Stolfi, R. L. (1968). Immune lytic transformation: a state of irreversible damage generated as a result of the reaction of the eighth component in the guinea pig complement system. *J. Immunol.*, **100**, 46–54
256. Mayer, M. M., Hammer, C. H., Michaels, D. W. and Shin, M. L. (1979) Immunologically mediated membrane damage: the mechanism of complement action and the similarity of lymphocyte-mediated cytotoxicity. *Immunochemistry*, **15**, 813–31
257. Kolb, W. P. and Müller-Eberhard, H. J. (1976). The membrane attack mechanism of complement: the three polypeptide chain structure of the eighth component (C8). *J. Exp. Med.*, **143**, 1131–9
258. Monahan, J. B. and Sodetz, J. M. (1981). Role of the β subunit in interaction of the eighth component of human complement with the membrane-bound cytolytic complex. *J. Biol. Chem.*, **256**, 3258–62
259. Brickner, A. and Sodetz, J. M. (1984). Functions of subunits within the eighth component of human complement; selective removal of the γ chain reveals it has no direct role in cytolysis. *Biochemistry*, **23**, 832–7
260. Kaufman, K. M., Snider, J. V., Spurr, N. K., Schwartz, C. E. and Sodetz, J. M. (1989). Chromosomal assignment of genes encoding the α, β, and γ subunits of human complement protein C8: identification of a close physical linkage between the α and the β loci. *Genomics*, **5**, 475–80
261. Rao, A. G., Howard, O. M. Z., Ng, S. C., Whitehead, A. S., Colten, H. R. and Sodetz, J. M. (1987). Complementary DNA and derived amino acid sequence of the α subunit of human complement protein C8: evidence for the existence of a separate α subunit messenger RNA. *Biochemistry*, **26**, 3556–64
262. Howard, O. M. Z., Rao, A. G. and Sodetz, J. M.(1987). Complementary DNA and derived amino acid sequence of the β subunit of human complement protein C8: identification of a close structural and ancestral relationship to the α subunit and C9. *Biochemistry*, **26**, 3565–70

263. Haefliger, J.-A., Tschopp, J., Nardelli, D., Wahli, W., Kocer, H.-P., Tosi, M. and Stanley, K. K. (1987). Complementary DNA cloning of complement C8β and its sequence homology to C9. *Biochemistry*, **26**, 3551–6
264. Haefliger, J.-A., Jenne, D., Stanley, K. K. and Tschopp, J. (1987). Structural homology of human complement component C8γ and plasma protein HC: identity of the cysteine bond pattern. *Biochem. Biophys. Res. Commun.*, **149**, 750–4
265. Podack, E. R. and Tschopp, J. (1982). Polymerization of the ninth component of complement (C9): formation of poly(C9) with a tubular ultrastructure resembling the membrane attack complex of complement. *Proc. Natl. Acad. Sci. (USA)*, **79**, 574–8
266. Tschopp, J. (1984). Ultrastructure of the membrane attack complex of complement. *J. Biol. Chem.*, **259**, 7857–63
267. Tschopp, J., Engel, A. and Podack, E. R. (1984). Molecular weight of poly(C9). *J. Biol. Chem.*, **259**, 1922–8
268. Hadding, U. and Müller-Eberhard, H. J. (1969). The ninth component of human complement: isolation, description and mode of action. *Immunology*, **16**, 719–35
269. Tschopp, J. (1984). Circular polymerization of the membranolytic ninth component of complement. *J. Biol. Chem.*, **259**, 10569–73
270. DiScipio, R. G., Gehring, M. R., Podack, E. R., Kan, C. C., Hugli, T. E. and Fey, G. H. (1984). Nucleotide sequence of cDNA and derived amino acid sequence of human complement component C9. *Proc. Natl. Acad. Sci. (USA)* **81**, 7298–302
271. Stanley, K. K., Kocher, H.-P., Luzio, J. P., Jackson, P. and Tschopp, J. (1985). The sequence and topology of human complement component C9. *EMBO J.*, **4**, 375–82
272. Hansch, G. M. (1989). The complement attack phase. In Rother, K. and Till, G. O. (eds.) *The Complement System*, pp. 202–30. (Berlin: Springer Verlag)
273. Morgan, B. P., Imagawa, D. K., Dankert, J. R. and Ramm, L. E. (1986). Complement lysis of U937, a nucleated mammalian cell line in the absence of C9: effect of C9 on C5b-8 mediated cell lysis. *J. Immunol.*, **136**, 3402–6
274. Lachmann, P. J. (1991). The control of homologous lysis. *Immunol. Today*, **12**, 312–15
275. Podack, E. R., Kolb, W. P. and Müller-Eberhard, H. J. (1978). The C5b-6 complex: formation, isolation, and inhibition of its activity by lipoprotein and the S-protein of human serum. *J. Immunol.*, **120**, 1841–8
276. Lint, T. F., Behrends, C. L. and Gewurz, H. (1977). Serum lipoproteins and $C\overline{567}$-INH activity. *J. Immunol.*, **119**, 883–8
277. Dahlbäck, B. and Podack, E. R. (1985). Characterization of human S protein, an inhibitor of the membrane attack complex of complement. Demonstration of a free reactive thiol group. *Biochemistry*, **24**, 2368–74
278. Nicholson-Weller, A., Spicer, D. B. and Austen, K. F. (1985). Deficiency of the complement regulatory protein, "decay-accelerating factor", on membranes of granulocytes, monocytes, and platelets in paroxysmal nocturnal hemoglobinuria. *N. Engl. J. Med.*, **312**, 1091–7
279. Medof, M. E., Walter, E. I., Roberts, W. L., Haas, R. and Rosenberry, T. L. (1986). Decay accelerating factor of complement is anchored to cells by a C-terminal glycolipid. *Biochemistry*, **25**, 6740–7
280. Medof, M. E., Gottlieb, A., Kinoshita, T., Hall, S., Silber, T., Nussenzweig, V. and Rosse, W. F. (1987). Relationship between decay accelerating factor deficiency, diminished acetylcholinesterase activity, and defective terminal complement pathway restriction in paroxysmal nocturnal hemoglobinuria erythrocytes. *J. Clin. Invest.*, **80**, 165–74
281. Ballow, M., Shira, J. E., Harden, L., Yang, S. Y. and Day, N. K. (1975). Complete absence of the third component of complement in man. *J. Clin. Invest.*, **56**, 703–10
282. Johnson, A. R., Hugli, T. E. and Müller-Eberhard, H. J. (1975). Release of histamine from rat mast cells by the complement peptides C3a and C5a. *Immunology*, **28**, 1067–80
283. Bitter-Suermann, D. (1987). The anaphylatoxins. In Rother, K. and Till, G. O. (eds.) *The Complement System*, pp. 367–95. (Heidelberg: Springer Verlag)
284. Goldstein, I. M. and Perez, H. D. (1980). Biologically active peptides derived from the fifth component of complement. *Prog. Hemostasis Thromb.*, **5**, 41–77
285. Webster, R. O., Hong, S. R., Johnston, R. B. Jr. and Henson, P. M. (1980). Biological effects of the human complement fragments C5a and $C5a_{des\ Arg}$ on neutrophil function. *Immunopharmacology*, **2**, 201–19

286. Schreiber, R. D., Pangburn, M. K., Bjornson, A. B., Brothers, M. A. and Müller-Eberhard, H. J. (1982). The role of C3 fragments in endocytosis and extracellular cytotoxic reactions by polymorphonuclear leukocytes. *Clin. Immunol. Immunopathol.*, **23**, 335–57
287. Frank, M. M. and Fries, L. F. (1991). The role of complement in inflammation and phagocytosis. *Immunol. Today*, **12**, 322–6
288. Whaley, K. and Ahmed, A. E. E. (1989). Control of immune complexes by the classical pathway. *Behring Inst. Mitt.*, **84**, 111–20
289. Weiler, J. M., Ballas, Z. K., Needleman, B. W., Hobbs, M. V. and Feldbush, T. L. (1982). Complement fragments suppress lymphocyte immune responses. *Immunol. Today*, **3**, 238–43
290. Erdei, A., Füst, G. and Gergely, J. (1991). The role of C3 in the immune response. *Immunol. Today*, **12**, 332–7
291. Cholin, S., Gerard, N. P., Strang, C. J. and Davis, A. E. III (1989). Biologic activity of a C2-derived peptide. Demonstration of a specific interaction with guinea pig lung tissues. *J. Immunol.*, **142**, 2401–4
292. Götze, O., Bianco, C. and Cohn, Z. A. (1979). The induction of macrophage spreading by factor B of the properdin system. *J. Exp. Med.*, **149**, 372–86
293. Sundsmo, J. S. and Götze, O. (1980). Human monocyte spreading induced by factor B of the alternative pathway of complement activation. *Cell. Immunol.*, **52**, 1–17
294. Oldstone, M. B. A. (1975). Virus neutralization and virus-induced immune complex disease. *Progr. Med. Virol.*, **19**, 84–119
295. Gewurz, H. and Suyehira, L. A. (1980). Section C. Complement and immune complexes. In Rose, N. R. and Friedman, H. (eds.) *Manual of Clinical Immunology*, 2nd edn., pp. 163–74. (Washington, D. C.: American Society for Microbiology)
296. Harrison, R. A. and Lachmann, P. J. (1986). Complement technology. In Weir, D. M. (ed.) *Handbook of Experimental Immunology*, pp. 39.1–49. (Oxford: Blackwell Scientific Publications)

2
The phylogeny and evolution of the complement system

A. W. DODDS and A. J. DAY

INTRODUCTION

Since the beginnings of complement research, there has been an interest in the phylogeny of the system. In 1903, Flexner and Noguchi[1] studied the ability of venom from a number of different snakes to activate, probably, the alternative pathway in the sera of various species, and so to bring about lysis of heterologous and homologous erythrocytes. Marshall, in 1904[2], investigated the potency of different mammalian and avian sera in lysing erythrocytes, probably via the classical pathway. In both cases, no real patterns of activity were observed; different sera had widely varying activities which were largely unassociated with their phylogenetic relatedness. Much of the work performed since these earliest studies has concentrated on the demonstration of the presence of haemolytic activities in different species, and on showing differences in functional activity between species[3,4]. It is clear that, to a large extent, the functional variability observed, at least amongst the mammals, is caused by differences in compatibility with components of the assay systems employed, such as the source of the erythrocytes, antibody and other reagents. It probably does not reflect differences in the potency of the complement systems of the species studied against appropriate targets[5]. The problems associated with assays of whole complement activity as well as assays of individual components in different species have been discussed elsewhere[6].

The difficulties encountered in functional studies of the complement systems of the mammals are more pronounced when the lower vertebrates and invertebrates are studied. Not only is there an even greater problem with incompatibility in the assay systems used, there are also non-complement lytic systems present in some species. For example, the serum of the lamprey, a primitive fish, is extremely efficient in lysing mammalian erythrocytes by a mechanism having certain features which are similar to complement[7]. This lytic activity has now been shown to result from the activity of a single component, probably unrelated to complement[8]. However, the same workers have demonstrated the presence of an opsonic system in the lamprey which is undoubtedly related to complement[8]. The presence or absence of lytic activity is therefore a very poor indicator of the existence of a complement-related system.

Together with a comparison of complement systems in different types of animal, insight into the evolutionary history of the complement system can be gained from a complete knowledge of the molecular nature of the components of a single species. There have been great advances in our understanding of the molecular basis of the complement systems of the mammals, notably in mouse and man. The complete primary structures of all of the soluble human components, together with those of a number of receptors, are now available. The chromosomal locations of many of the genes for complement proteins have also been established and show a number of linkage associations between the components. This information indicates that the proteins of the complement system have arisen from diverse evolutionary origins, but also shows that the complexity of the system has been increased by the duplication of certain components[9,10].

Data at the molecular level on other animals are still relatively sparse when compared with the huge amount of information available on mammals. Some aspects of the phylogeny and evolution of the complement system are now receiving attention.These studies have demonstrated that complement-related defence systems definitely exist in all vertebrate classes and that molecules related to complement components are also present in invertebrates, although conclusive evidence of complement-like activation mechanisms in invertebrates is still lacking. Because of the difficulties outlined above in interpreting the significance of purely functional studies, we have limited this review mainly to work at the molecular level.

What is complement?

In the mammals, at least in those studied in detail, complement consists of around 20 plasma proteins together with cell surface receptors and binding proteins, the number of which seems to increase annually. The functions of complement, again in mammals, include: lysis of foreign cells, opsonization of foreign particles, release of biologically active peptides, regulation of the size of immune complexes and regulation of the immune response. A phylogenetically early complement system would be considerably simpler, both in the number of components employed and in the number of functions performed. Since the emergence of the first primitive complement system, evolutionary pressures will have varied in different lineages. Natural selection may have added components to some lines which are different from those found in mammals, removed parts that had become redundant in some species, or found new functions for certain components and so recruited them to systems outside the immediate realm of host defence.

It was proposed by Lachmann[11] that the original complement system would have resembled a simplified alternative pathway consisting of a C3-like and a factor B-like component, together with a receptor on a phagocytic cell. The major function of such a system would therefore have been opsonic rather than lytic. If this notion is true, and evidence from the most primitive vertebrates, the jawless fish, suggests that it may be, the best approach to unravelling the origins of complement may be to look for invertebrate opsonins which resemble C3. On the other hand, it is possible that the original complement system could have been more like the classical pathway in its activation mechanism. The recent finding that this pathway can be activated by the mammalian lectin, mannan binding protein, which resembles C1q in its architecture[12,13], raises the possibility that the classical pathway could have predated the development of antibodies, and hence be more ancient than has been assumed. The possible primitive origins of the complement system are discussed in the final section of this review.

Animal interrelationships

Figure 2.1 shows the major phyla of the animal kingdom and one possible way in which they may be interrelated. For the purposes of this review, only the more

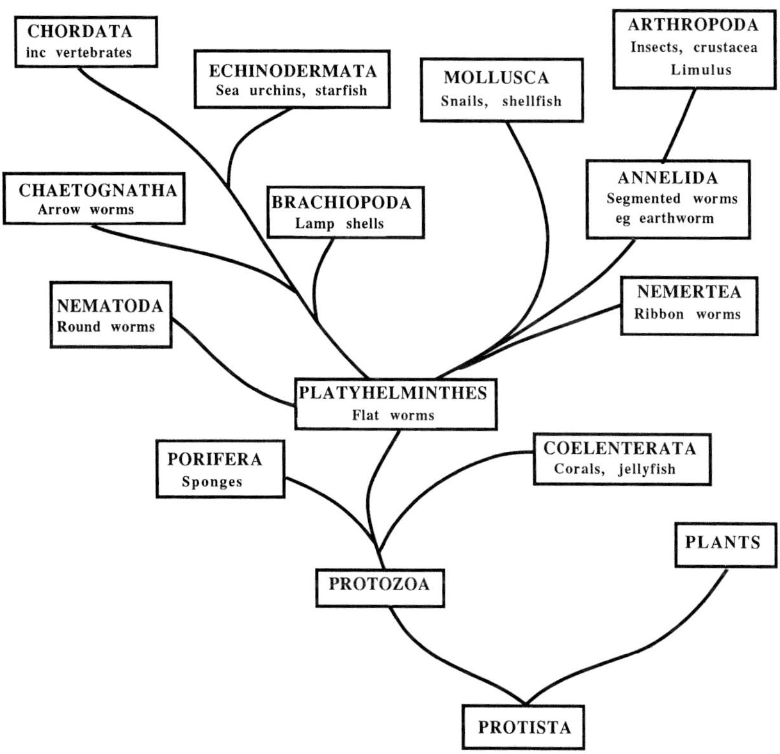

Figure 2.1 Possible relationships amongst the major phyla of the animal kingdom

important phyla have been included. It should, however, be borne in mind that there is virtually no fossil record to give us clues about animal evolutionary history prior to the development of skeletons, shells and exoskeletons, and that this phylogeny is based on shared anatomical features of living examples of the various phyla. The simplest multicellular animals are the sponges, corals and jellyfish. There is no information on the presence in these phyla of complement-related defence mechanisms or proteins. It is generally agreed that an animal with a platyhelminthes-like body plan was likely to have been the ancestor of all of the higher animal phyla. Two major groups are apparent in the scheme shown. The first includes the echinoderms (sea urchins and star fish) and the chordates which incorporates the vertebrates and a number of other species which have a vertebrate-like body plan but lack a skeleton, e.g. *Amphioxus* and sea squirts. The second includes the molluscs (snails and shellfish) and the arthropods (insects, arachnids, crustacea, etc.) which are probably related to the annelids (earthworms and other segmented worms). The relationship of the nematodes to the other phyla is unclear. For discussion of other possible relationships and alternative phylogenies of the animal kingdom, the subject has recently been extensively reviewed by Jefferies[14] and Willmer[15].

Kinships within the vertebrates are clearer since the development of a skeleton has left a fossil record and, in contrast to the case in the invertebrates, it is possible to put a geological time scale upon developments (Figure 2.2). Dates at which the various vertebrate classes diverged are not precise. The earliest vertebrate fossils appear towards the end of the Cambrian period, approximately 500 million years ago (MYA). The simplest extant vertebrates are the Agnatha (jawless fish) which include the lampreys and hagfish. Forms recognizable as cartilaginous fish (sharks and rays) are apparent from Silurian deposits of about 400 MYA and the first bony fish are apparent at the same time or a little later. The earliest amphibians started to colonize the land during the late Devonian, 350 MYA. Reptilian forms are apparent from the middle of the Carboniferous period about 320 MYA and the separate line of reptiles from which the mammals evolved appeared soon afterwards, though species recognizable as mammals did not appear until the Lower Jurassic period. The earliest birds diverged from their reptilian ancestors towards the end of the Jurassic period, about 150 MYA. Their nearest relatives amongst the extant reptiles are probably the crocodiles. The living mammals can be divided into three major groups: monotremes (duck-billed platypus), marsupials (kangaroos, etc.) and placentals are all first evident in the early Cretaceous period. The modern placental orders (rodents, primates, ungulates, etc.) all originated close to the time of the extinction of the dinosaurs in the late Cretaceous and early Tertiary periods, about 65 MYA. For a complete review of vertebrate interrelationships, see Carroll[16].

PHYLOGENY OF COMPLEMENT

Invertebrates

Little new convincing functional evidence on the possibility of complement activity in invertebrates has emerged since the reviews of Gigli and Austen[3] and

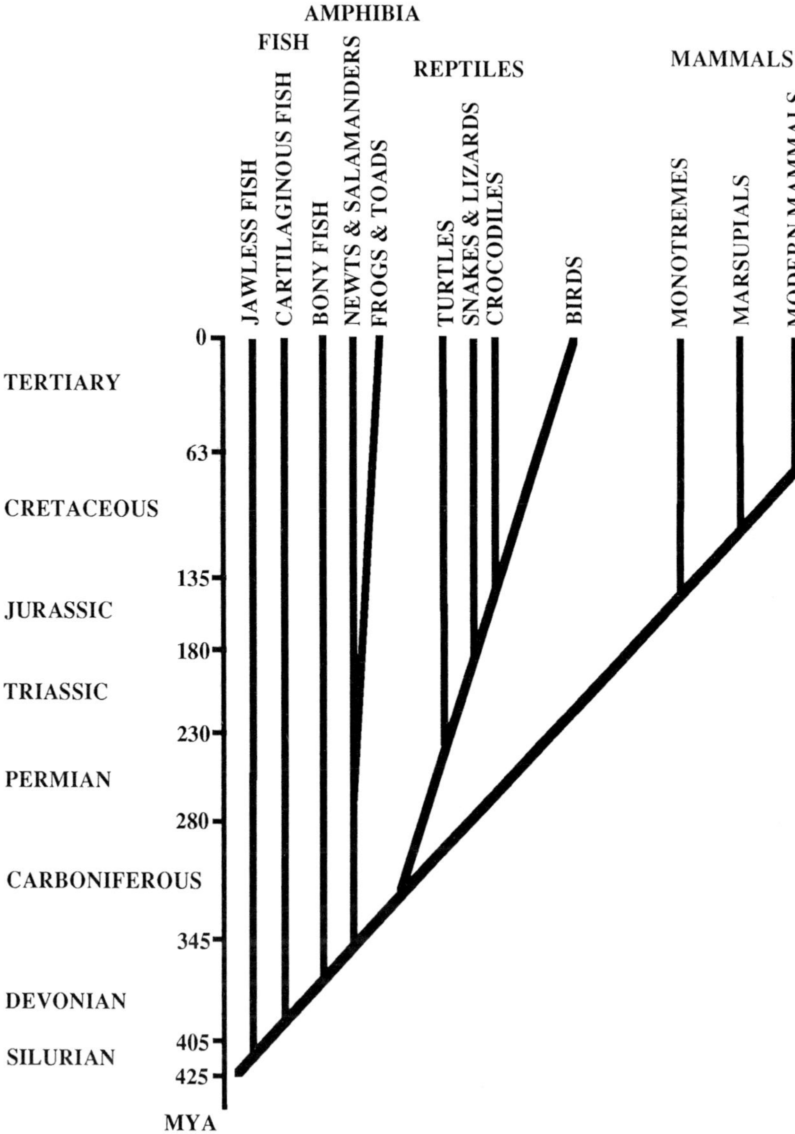

Figure 2.2 The major vertebrate classes

Ballow[4] in the seventies. The haemolymphs of a number of invertebrate species are able to bring about the lysis of vertebrate erythrocytes, either alone or in combination with cobra venom factor and/or vertebrate serum. Some of these lytic mechanisms resemble complement in being heat labile and/or divalent metal ion dependent. Many of the early studies used cobra venom factor which was contaminated with phospholipase; this led to considerable confusion[17].

Much of the more recent literature on complement-like and non-complement-like haemolytic systems in invertebrates is contradictory. As discussed in the introduction, assays of complement lytic activity, even in the mammals, are extremely difficult to interpret. It is unlikely that functional assays of this type, without supporting molecular evidence, will ever be convincing in demonstrating complement in invertebrates. A number of phenomena have, however, been described, indicating the presence of proteins related to vertebrate complement components and molecules from invertebrates that can interact with vertebrate complement.

Thiolester containing proteins

α_2 Macroglobulin (α_2M) is a thiolester containing protein which has a structural and evolutionary relationship to C3, C4 and C5 of the complement system (Figure 2.3), though its function is as a protease inhibitor[18]. α_2M has been described in the horseshoe crab, *Limulus polyphemus*[19,20], the crayfish, *Pacifastcus leniusculus*[21] and in the lobster, *Homorus americanus*[22]. Human α_2M has a molecular mass of 720 kDa and is composed of four identical subunits of 180 kDa. The molecule from the horseshoe crab has a molecular mass of 550 kDa and is suggested by the authors to be a trimer of smaller subunits[20], although a dimer or tetramer would seem more likely. The native α_2M of the lobster is a dimer of molecular mass 342 kDa composed of disulphide-linked subunits of 180 kDa[22]. All three molecules are inhibitors which can act upon a wide range of proteases by limiting access rather than by direct interaction with the active sites of the enzymes with which they react. This can be demonstrated by the fact that the activity of proteases is inhibited only against large substrates; molecules which are small enough to reach the active site of the α_2M–protease complex are cleaved. Inhibition is achieved by the immobilization and steric obstruction of the protease by the α_2M utilizing two mechanisms. A Venus flytrap-like change in conformation of the protein physically captures the protease. Covalent crosslinking of the enzyme to the α_2M can occur through the thiolester bond which becomes reactive upon activation of the inhibitor. Both mechanisms are activated by the proteolytic cleavage of a bait region in the α_2M which has sites susceptible to many proteases. Sequence analysis of the thiolester-containing peptides of lobster, crayfish and horseshoe crab α_2M showed high similarity to the corresponding regions of vertebrate thiolester-containing proteins[21–23]. Nineteen peptides covering 435 residues of the horseshoe crab α_2M have been sequenced; of these, 203 residues could be aligned with corresponding sequences in mammalian α_2M[23].

Lytic proteins

Molecules possibly related to those of the mammalian complement lytic system have been described in the echinoderms. The coelomocytes of *Holothunia polii* contain haemolysins which may be related to mammalian perforin. Two molecules with molecular mass of 80 kDa under non-reducing conditions but which,

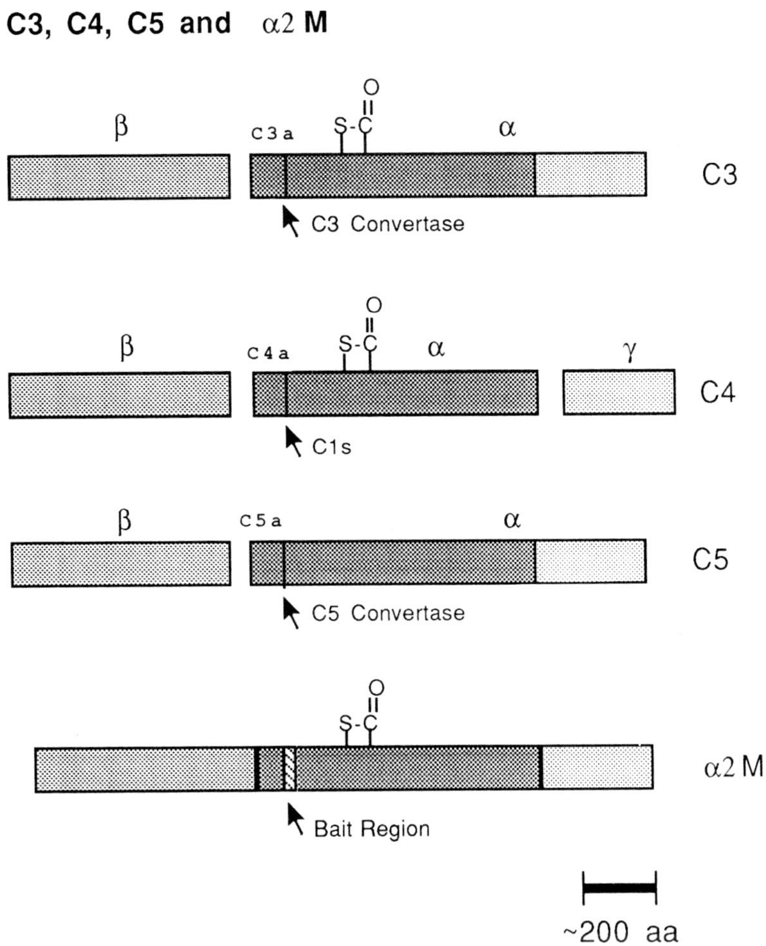

Figure 2.3 The thiolester-containing proteins, C3, C4, C5 and α_2M

on reduction, give apparent molecular masses of 80 and 76 kDa, have been isolated. The apparently smaller form is heat labile and Ca^{2+} dependent, the other is heat stable and Ca^{2+} independent. Antigenically the two forms appear to be identical, antibodies raised against each indivually being mutually fully crossreactive, indicating that the two may be isoforms or that there is variation in post-translational modification[24]. The haemolysins show antigenic cross-reactivity with human perforin and also form lesions in erythrocytes similar to those formed by perforin[25]. Perforin is the lytic molecule found in the granules of mammalian natural killer cells and cytotoxic T-lymphocytes. It shows considerable amino acid sequence similarity to the proposed binding domains of the proteins of the complement membrane attack complex[26] (see Figure 2.6).

A lytic protein from *Trypanosoma cruzi,* the parasitic protozoan responsible for Chagas disease, shows immunological crossreaction with antibodies to denatured C9. By SDS-PAGE analysis, the protein has a molecular mass of 75 kDa under reducing conditions and 80 kDa when non-reduced. This behaviour is extremely reminiscent of that of C9, which is due to the presence of multiple disulphide bonds[27].

Mellitin, a 26-amino-acid haemolytic peptide from bee venom, also shows antigenic crossreactivity with human C9. Residues 8–16 of the mellitin molecule show sequence identity with two segments of C9, residues 292–296 and 527–531. It has been proposed that these two regions of the C9 molecule come together in the three-dimensional structure to form the crossreactive epitope, and also probably a site involved in the lytic activity of the molecules[28]. If this is true, it seems likely to be a case of convergent evolution rather than common ancestry.

Receptors and lectins

Sea urchin, *Strogylocentrotus droebachiensis*, phagocytes can ingest erythrocytes opsonized either with vertebrate sera[29] or with purified human C3[30]. The effect of C3 is greatest when C3b is converted to iC3b, and is lost on conversion to C3d. Fab fragments of anti-C3 antibody considerably inhibit phagocytosis of the C3-coated erythrocytes, indicating that the reaction is probably specific for C3[30]. This evidence points to the possible presence on echinoderm phagocytes of a receptor which can recognize mammalian C3 and presumably a C3-like molecule in sea urchin haemolymph. It should, however, be noted that conglutinin, a soluble mammalian lectin, reacts with iC3b in an extremely similar manner[31]. Conglutinin belongs to the family of collagen-containing lectins which includes mannan-binding protein (MBP) and lung surfactant protein[12,32]. Another species of sea urchin, *Anthocidoris crassispina*, has a soluble lectin, echinoidin, which is found in its coelomic fluid and is believed to be involved in host defence[33]. It is a multimeric protein of 300 kDa composed of approximately 20 kDa subunits which are present as disulphide-linked dimers. Echinoidin shows sequence homology with the type C lectin domains which are also present in MBP[34].

Earthworms, *Lumbricus terrestris*, produce two apparently non-lectin substances which are involved in the opsonization of foreign particles and their ingestion by leukocytes. One appears to be a specific inducible immune molecule, which is comparable with antibody. The second is present in non-immunized worms and may be related to complement. Both molecules have molecular masses below 50 kDa[35]. Recent experiments have shown that sheep erythrocytes sensitized with rabbit IgG, but not those sensitized with IgM, are more easily agglutinated and phagocytosed by earthworm leukocytes than are unsensitized cells. The effect is enhanced by the presence of human C3b on the erythrocyte surface. Conversion of C3b to iC3b or C3d destroys the enhancement. This may indicate the presence of receptors on the leukocytes able to recognize both mammalian IgG and C3b and the presence in earthworms of C3-like molecules[36].

C-reactive protein (CRP) in mammals is an acute-phase protein which can interact directly with micro-organisms in a Ca^{2+}-dependent manner to bring about a number of immune phenomena, including agglutination and complement activation. A CRP-like molecule has been demonstrated in the horseshoe crab[37]. A report of the amino acid sequence of the protein shows it to be related to mammalian CRP[38]. This raises the possibility that CRP-like molecules could be responsible for some of the earlier reports of the presence in invertebrate haemolymph of substances capable of activating mammalian complement and bringing about agglutination in a complement-like manner.

Miscellaneous

It is interesting to note that a partial sequence of factor C[39], a coagulation system serine protease found in the haemolymph of the horseshoe crab, reveals that it contains a protein module (CCP repeat – complement control protein repeat) often associated with C3 and C4 binding in human complement components (see Figure 2.6). The serine protease zymogen, factor C, participates in the initial stages of haemolymph coagulation and its activation leads to the formation of insoluble coagulin gel. Factor C is unusual in that it can apparently be activated by lipopolysaccharides (from bacterial endotoxins) without the presence of any other proteases and thus plays a direct role in host defence.

A protease has been described in the greater wax moth, *Galleria mellonella*, which can interact with cobra venom factor-Sepharose to bring about cleavage of bovine C3. The authors suggest that this demonstrates the presence in insects of factor B- and D-like proteases which can interact with cobra venom factor to form a C3 convertase, implying that insects also have C3[40]. However, a number of mammalian proteases which are not involved in the complement system can also cleave C3, the insect protease could therefore be non-complement related. A haemolytic activity in the greater wax moth appears not to be complement related. Lysis is caused by a single high molecular mass factor (<250 kDa) which appears as two polypeptide chains of 69 and 75 kDa on SDS-PAGE after reduction[41].

Two proteins which can interact with mammalian complement have been purified from the haemolymph of the larval fall army worm, *Spodoptera frugiperda*. The first, a disulphide-linked dimer of 55 kDa subunits, is able either to inhibit or inactivate the alternative pathway reaction of human serum against rabbit erythrocytes. It is not clear at which step in complement activation the molecule is acting[42]. The second is an inhibitor of the mammalian classical pathway, and acts in a manner similar to C4 binding protein (C4-bp). Interestingly, the molecular mass and the proteolytic degradation pattern of the protein also resembles C4-bp[43]. However, no protein sequence has been obtained and therefore it is not known whether this protein contains CCP modules which are found in C4-bp. The protein appears to be involved in storage in the larva.

A protein from the snail, *Helix promatia*, haemolymph, appears to activate human complement in a manner somewhat similar to that seen with cobra venom factor[44].

Jawless fish (Agnatha)

Cobra venom factor can induce lysis of erythrocytes by hagfish serum, while lamprey serum alone can lyse rabbit erythrocytes. However, these activities appear to be heat stable, are only partially inhibited by EDTA, and are not potentiated by antibody[3,7,45]. In the case of the lamprey, the activity is eluted from Sephadex as a single apparently low-molecular-mass component. When chromatographed on Sephacryl, it appears to be a 160 kDa complex composed of subunits of 25 kDa. The inconsistency in these data suggests that the protein probably interacts with the Sephadex matrix[8].

A protein which is a homologue of mammalian C3/C4 has been isolated from lamprey, *Lampreta japonica*, serum[8]. This protein is not involved in the lytic activity present in lamprey serum. The lamprey C3/C4 was shown to bind to zymosan or erythrocytes only when incubated in the presence of lamprey serum. The binding was inhibited by heating or in the presence of EDTA, but it is unclear whether the activation involves a classical- or an alternative-pathway-like mechanism. When bound, the lamprey C3/C4 potentiated phagocytosis by lamprey macrophage-like phagocytes. A thiolester bond was demonstrated by direct incorporation of methylamine and release of a free SH group on activation. The protein has a molecular mass of 190 kDa, similar to that of mammalian C3 and C4, but has a three-chain structure, molecular mass 84 kDa (α), 74 kDa (β) and 32 kDa (γ), similar to that seen in mammalian C4, rather than the two-chain structure seen in mammalian C3 (see Figure 2.3). Following activation, the thiolester containing α-chain was degraded by enzymes in the lamprey serum to give a final hydrolysed thiolester-containing product of 35 kDa, similar in molecular mass to mammalian C3d and C4d, while the β- and γ-chains remained intact.

The above evidence points to the presence of a fully functioning alternative or classical pathway activation mechanism, i.e. a C3/C4-like molecule, and activating enzymes, plus the presence of a control system which can degrade activated C3/C4, as occurs in mammals, utilizing factors I and H or C4 binding protein[9]. The presence of a receptor for the molecule on the phagocytic cells is also implied.

Cartilaginous fish (elasmobranches)

Functional experiments indicated the probable presence of classical, alternative and terminal pathways in elasmobranches[3,4]. Jensen and co-workers[46] have presented evidence for a classical pathway in the nurse shark, *Ginglymostoma cirratum*, comprised of six components named C1n, C2n, C3n, C4n, C8n and C9n. C1n is thought to be equivalent to mammalian C1. It can be separated from nurse shark serum by euglobulin precipitation at low ionic strength. Sheep erythrocytes treated with nurse shark antibody (An) and C1n can be lysed by C1-depleted guinea pig serum, indicating that C1n can cleave guinea pig C4 and C2. Immunoelectrophoresis in the presence of divalent metal ions gave a single precipitin arc against anti-C1n, while, in the presence of EDTA, up to three precipitating proteins were observed. Thus, like mammalian C1, C1n appears to be a divalent metal ion-dependent complex composed of a number of subcomponents[47,48].

C2n may be similar in its function to mammalian C4. EAnC1n2n can be prepared in the presence of divalent cations to form a stable intermediate comparable with mammalian EAC14[46]. The molecular mass of C2n is around 170–180 kDa and it is one of the most cationic proteins in shark plasma, similar to mammalian C4[49]. C3n, when added to EAnC1nC2n, forms an unstable intermediate which may be analogous to mammalian EAC142. The molecular mass of C3n is greater than 200 kDa, larger than mammalian C2 at 110 kDa[46]. Guinea pig C4 and C2, which together are compatible with C1n, are incapable of forming heterologous complexes in any combination with C2n and C3n[49]. The correspondence of C4n to any of the mammalian complement components is unclear. Jensen *et al.*[46] suggested that C4n may play a role in replacing C3, C5, C6 and C7 of the mammalian complement system. However, now that the primary structures of these proteins are known, it is clear that, whilst C3/C5 and C6/C7 are structurally related, there is no structural or functional similarity between the two pairs.

C8n and C9n appear to be analogues of mammalian C8 and C9. The two shark components can lyse EAnC1n-C4n or mammalian EAC1-7. Mammalian C8 and C9 can also lyse EAnC1n-C4n[46,50]. The molecular masses of C8n and C9n are approximately 185 kDa and 200 kDa, higher than the 150 kDa and 70 kDa found for human C8 and C9. The lesions formed by nurse shark complement have a doughnut-like form, similar in size and shape to those formed by mammalian complement[46]. Contrary to the earlier evidence[3], Jensen and coworkers[46] could find no indication for an alternative pathway in the nurse shark.

Bony fish

Evidence from the early literature indicates that the bony fish probably have classical, alternative and lytic pathways directly comparable with those of the mammalian complement systems[3,51]. Most recent studies confirm this. However, Kaastrupp and Koch[52] could find evidence of an alternative pathway only in the carp.

The most detailed studies of fish complement have been performed by Nonaka and colleagues on the rainbow trout, *Salmo gairdneri*[53]. They have demonstrated convincingly classical, alternative, and lytic pathways as follows. One activation mechanism required trout antibody, Ca^{2+} and Mg^{2+} and was blocked by addition of EDTA or EGTA. Pretreatment of serum with LPS, zymosan or inulin destroyed the activity. An antibody-independent activation mechanism which required Mg^{2+} but not Ca^{2+} was also demonstrated. Following activation, membrane attack complexes were isolated and protein components compared with those of the mammalian membrane attack complex using SDS-PAGE. This showed that the components of the mammalian and trout MAC were comparable in number and molecular mass[53]. A partial nucleotide sequence of trout C9 has been determined and shows considerable homology to mammalian C9[54].

As well as demonstrating that trout complement is functionally extremely similar to mammalian complement, trout C5[55] and C3[56] have been purified. The trout C5 is structurally similar to mammalian C5 and becomes incorporated into the MAC. Antibody to the trout C5 fully inhibited haemolysis by either the classical or alternative pathway [53,55]. Trout C5, like its human counterpart (see Figure 2.3) does not contain a thiolester bond (Nonaka, personal communication), while trout C3 was shown to be similar in structure to mammalian C3, and to contain a thiolester bond. Limited sequence analysis of the α- and β-chains showed similarities in primary structure between trout and human C3[56]. Another molecule from trout serum which bears a close structural resemblance to trout C3 has been purified and characterized. The β-chain of this molecule is 2 kDa smaller than that of trout C3. The molecule, which has been termed C3-2, is haemolytically inactive but contains an intact thiolester. Peptide mapping with trypsin indicates that the two molecules are extremely similar. Amino acid sequences of 26 N-terminal residues of the α-chains showed two differences between C3 and C3-2: no differences were found in the 21 N-terminal residues of the two β-chains. All adult and first-generation offspring had both molecules, indicating that two genes are probably present. The sequence data indicate that the two isotypes probably arose by a recent gene duplication, comparable to that seen in human C4, or perhaps, since one form is haemolytically inactive, more like the mouse C4/S1p duplication[57]. C4 has been partially purified from the carp, *Cyprinus carpio*. The molecule has a molecular mass of 170 kDa and is inactivated by hydrazine and ammonia, indicating the probable presence of a thiolester bond. Details of the chain structure of the molecule were not given[58]. C1 has been purified from carp serum; the molecular mass of the complex is over 1000 kDa, somewhat larger than that observed for human C1[59].

In a study of a large number of wide-ranging vertebrate plasmas, Kaidoh and Gigli[60] were able to demonstrate the presence of enzymes which could cleave human C3 and C4, in a manner similar to human factor I and H or I and C4-bp, in most species from mammals to the perciform bony fish. They went on to demonstrate that the activity in the barred sand bass, *Parablax neblifer*, required two protein factors. The first, with a molecular mass of 155 kDa, appears to be related to factor I. The second is a cofactor of 380 kDa which seems similar in function to H or C4-bp[61]. The size of human factor I is 88 kDA, smaller than that of the sand bass molecule. Human H and C4-bp are 150 kDa and 550 kDa respectively, but both are made up of repeating modules (CCPs) of which probably only a small number are functionally active. Therefore, it would not be surprising to find a differing number of CCP repeats in a particular protein from different species. Such a difference is seen in a comparison of the monomer chains of human and mouse C4-bp which have 8 and 6 CCPs respectively[62]. Salmon macrophages have been shown to have receptors able to recognize human C3b and iC3b, but not C3d[63].

Amphibians

Most of the early functional evidence points to the presence of classical, alternative and lytic pathways in the anuran (frogs and toads) amphibians, though the Urodella (newts and salamanders) may lack a classical pathway[3,4].

A number of complement proteins have been purified from frog sera. Alexander and Steiner[64], prepared C1 from the bullfrog, *Rana catesbeina*, and demonstrated it to be functionally similar to mammalian C1. They isolated C1q and showed that the molelcular mass, chain structure and amino acid composition were similar to mammalian C1q, i.e. that it contained collagen-like portions. Electron microscopy of these molecules showed them to have the appearance of a six-headed bunch of tulips, similar to that of human C1q[65].

Clawed frog, *Xenopus laevis*, C3 has been purified and is similar in molecular mass and chain structure to mammalian C3. A denaturation split reaction, which can be inhibited by prior treatment with methylamine, indicates that the *Xenopus* C3 contains a thiolester bond[66]. A partial cDNA clone of *Xenopus* C3 has been obtained. The clone covers the C-terminal third of the α-chain of the molecule. The derived amino acid sequence shows 48–50% identity to human, rabbit and mouse C3[67]. C3 has also been purified from the axolotl, *Ambystoma mexicanum*, an urodellan amphibian. It consists of disulphide-linked chains of 110 and 72 kDa. A thiolester bond has been demonstrated in the α-chain, and limited N-terminal amino acid sequence data on the intact chains and tryptic peptides indicate that the molecule is highly homologous to C3 from other vertebrates[68]. C4 has been purified from *Xenopus*[69]. It is a three-chain protein containing a thiolester bond in the α-chain, and participates in the classical but not the alternative pathway of complement activation. *Xenopus* C4 was further shown to be polymorphic, two major allotypes being recognized. By a combination of allograft rejection, mixed lymphocyte reactions and graft-versus-host reactions, the C4 polymorphism was shown to be closely linked to the *Xenopus* MHC[70]. *Xenopus* macrophages have separate receptors for IgM, IgY (IgG-like antibodies) and C3[71].

Reptiles

The properties of snake venoms in bringing about the destruction of complement activity in mammalian blood have been recognized since the beginning of complement research[1,72]. It is therefore a little surprising that the complement system of the reptiles is probably less studied than any other group of vertebrates.

The component of snake venom responsible for bringing about activation of mammalian complement (cobra venom factor) has been purified and characterized from a number of sources. In both the Indian cobra, *Naja naja*[73], and the Egyptian cobra, *Naja haje*[74], cobra venom factor is a protein consisting of three polypeptide chains of approximately 70, 50 and 30 kDa. A related protein from the Western diamond back rattle snake, *Crotalus atrox*[75], seems to have a similar structure. Cobra venom factor shows antigenic cross-reactivity with human C3[76–78] and with a component of snake serum having a chain structure similar to mammalian C3[77]. However, in contrast to cobra venom factor, cobra C3 is unglycosylated[79]. Evidence of chain structure, limited primary structure and physical parameters, suggests that cobra venom factor is a C3c-like product of a recently duplicated C3 gene, consisting of a β-chain plus two α-chain fragments[73,80]. Two pieces of evidence point to cobra venom factor being a product of a separate gene from the cobra C3 gene. The difference between the glycosylation of the β-chains of the two molecules, makes it unlikely that cobra venom factor is derived directly from plasma C3. Limited N-terminal sequence analysis of the two proteins indicates that there are a number of differences in the primary structures of the molecules[81].

Cobra venom factor is present in the venom; it can very rapidly activate the complement systems of various vertebrates by mimicking C3b to form an alternative pathway C3 convertase which is resistant to control by factors I and H. The function of cobra venom factor in the venom is not clear. It could be acting as a toxin by inducing anaphylactic shock in the prey. An alternative explanation could be that it acts as a digestive aid for the cobra. It has been postulated that the venom of snakes evolved from the salivary system, which was originally required to lubricate the dry food which animals had to swallow following their emergence from the aquatic environment. Enzymes were included in the saliva to facilitate cleaning of the mouth and teeth and also to commence the digestion of food immediately upon ingestion. The arrangement of the jaws in snakes does not allow food to be chewed. The size of the prey which the snake can utilize is therefore limited to the size which it can swallow. Snake venoms probably evolved as toxins in the saliva which could slow the movements of the prey, so increasing the size which could be swallowed. An animal which is wriggling while it is swallowed has a considerably higher effective diameter than one which is still! The injection of extremely powerful venom via fangs has thus evolved to allow larger prey to be swallowed without chewing[82]. This has created a problem for the venomous snakes: the larger the prey, the lower the surface to volume ratio, and hence the greater the difficulty in digesting food via digestive tract enzymes acting from the outside. Snakes therefore inject digestive enzymes into their prey along with the toxins. It is possible that cobra venom factor, by decomplementing the prey, speeds the digestion of the food by allowing internal putrefaction by the prey's own gut organisms, which would otherwise have been inhibited by the complement present in the prey. Interest in the reaction of snake venoms with complement was originally stimulated by the fact that the bodies of snake-bite victims rotted considerably more rapidly than did those whose death had other causes[72]. Whether its function is as a toxin, as a digestive aid or whether it has some other purpose, cobra venom factor is an example of a complement protein for which evolution has found a use outside the immediate area of host defence.

Early studies indicated that classical and alternative pathways of activation were present in snakes and turtles[3,4]. Recent studies by Vogel and Muller-Eberhard have demonstrated that alternative pathway activation in cobra serum is essentially identical to that of mammals except that it is not activated by cobra venom factor[83]. A multicomponent membrane attack complex, consisting of proteins similar in number and molecular mass to those of the mammalian membrane attack complex, is present in the cobra[84]. The probable presence of an antibody-dependent classical pathway in snakes has also been demonstrated[85,86].

Birds

The complement activity of avian sera has proved difficult to study because of incompatibilities between bird complement and mammalian antibody. With the use of avian antibodies, it has been demonstrated that, in the case of chickens, a classical[87] and an alternative pathway[88,89] are present[6,90]. A number of avian complement proteins have been purified and partially characterized. Chicken, *Gallus gallus*, C1q is similar in size and chain structure to mammalian C1q and contains collagenous regions as demonstrated by amino acid analysis and collagenase digestion. The purified protein can be assayed using a system consisting of rabbit antibody, sheep erythrocytes, human C1r and C1s and guinea pig C4, C2 and C-EDTA, showing that it is fully compatible with mammalian antibody and complement[91,92].

C3 has been purified from the Japanese quail, *Coturnix coturnix japonica*, by affinity chromatography using antibodies against zymosan treated with quail serum. The quail C3 has a molecular mass of 184 kDa and consists of two disulphide-linked chains of approximately 110 kDa and 73 kDa. The protein probably forms a covalent complex via ester bonds with zymosan. Quail serum loses haemolytic activity on treatment with methylamine; this can be restored by the addition of purified quail C3, indicating the probable presence of a thiolester bond[93]. Chicken C3 has also been purified and has been shown to be similar in molecular mass and chain structure, and to contain a thiolester bond[94].

Chicken factor B has a molecular mass of 90 kDa and, on activation, is cleaved into two fragments of 33 kDa (Ba) and 67 kDa (Bb)[95]. With the use of monoclonal antibody columns, it has been possible to deplete chicken serum of factor B and this has been shown to deplete alternative pathway activity. However, no classical pathway activity could be detected in the factor B-depleted serum[89]. This has led to the proposal that, in chickens, factor B may have a dual role such that it is also active in the classical pathway, substituting for C2[90]. However, it is also possible that the classical pathway assay system used was defective, since the same authors had difficulty in demonstrating classical pathway activity in the non-depleted serum. Chicken factor B is polymorphic with two common allotypes. This polymorphism is not linked to the chicken MHC, though it is possible that the difference lies in a post-translational modification[96]. There is, however, some linkage between levels of haemolytic activity in chickens and the MHC[97]. Genomic maps of the chicken MHC are now becoming available. These indicate that, unlike the mammalian situation where the MHC class I and class II genes are coded in separate chromosal areas, chicken MHC class I (B-F) and II (B-L) genes are intermingled in the same segment of DNA. Chickens have an extra type of histocompatibility molecule named B-G (class IV) which is also coded in this region. To date, no evidence has been found for any of the recognized mammalian MHC class III genes, though a number of genes other than class I, II and IV are interspersed within the region[98,99]. As mentioned, the nomenclature is a little confused, it should be noted that B-F refers to the chicken MHC class I molecules and should not be mistaken for factor B, or Bf as the geneticists prefer to call it.

Using immunoelectrophoresis and haemolytic overlay assays, genetic polymorphism has been detected in the C6 of a seabird, the Manx shearwater, *Puffinus puffinus*. Two common alleles were found, together with four rarer variants and a null allele[100].

Mammals

The most extensively studied species to date is undoubtedly man, both from the functional and structural viewpoint. With the emergence of the techniques of molecular biology, a large amount of structural data on mouse complement components has become available, although functional studies have been rather limited. Various complement components have been purified and characterized from a number of other mammalian species. While minor variations exist, no major differences from the human components have been observed. The literature on functional aspects is quite extensive[6]. Genetic polymorphisms in various complement components have been described in a number of mammalian species[100], as have descriptions of strains deficient in various components[101]. In the next section, the molecular architecture of the human complement system will be described.

THE PROTEINS OF THE COMPLEMENT SYSTEM

Studies at the molecular level have shown that three of the major arms of the immune system share a common evolutionary origin. The immunoglobulins, T cell receptors and the major histocompatibility systems all consist of proteins which are members of the immunoglobulin superfamily[102]. The evolutionary history of the complement system is very different from that seen in these others. Primary sequence analysis has shown that at least 14 protein structural families, all of which are found in non-complement proteins, are represented together with other motifs and stretches of amino acid sequence which are so far unique to complement.

Many of the complement proteins are mosaic in nature and are thought to have arisen by gene duplication and/or exon shuffling. These are of two major types: those which are composed of a single module type and others which contain a number of different types of module. In general, the smaller modules are each coded by a separate exon, while larger structures, such as the serine protease domain, have their own internal introns. Other complement components do not contain repeating structures nor are they of a mosaic nature. However, all of these non-modular proteins are homologous to non-complement proteins and so can be regarded as members of protein families. These miscellaneous non-modular proteins of human complement will be discussed first, followed by the single-module and the multimodular (mosaic) proteins together. The complement integrins will be discussed separately. Protein modules and mosaic proteins have been reviewed recently[103,104].

The non-modular complement proteins

The complement components C3, C4 and C5 along with α_2M and related protease inhibitors constitute a protein family. On the basis of degrees of amino acid similarity, which extends along the entire length of these sequences, α_2M is believed to be the parental stock from which the others were derived[105]. These proteins are synthesized as single-chain precursors and Figure 2.3 shows a schematic representation of the chain organizations in the mature proteins. C3, C4 and α_2M all contain a thiolester which becomes exposed on proteolytic cleavage. The thiolester then reacts with any nucleophilic species in its vicinity, and C3, C4 or α_2M can thus become covalently attached to protein or carbohydrate on a surface or in the fluid phase[106]. In the case of C3 and C4 (and this is also true for C5), the activating proteases are specific for these proteins (Figure 2.3), whereas α_2M has a 'bait' region which contains cleavage sites for a wide range of proteases. To date, no modular sequences have been identified in these proteins. Until recently, the only tertiary structural data obtained directly for complement system proteins have been the 77-residue C3a fragment[107], which is generated by proteolytic activation of C3 by the C3 convertases (Figure 2.3). C3a and the equivalent regions in C4 and C5 (C4a and C5a), which are likely to share a common tertiary structure, effect inflammatory responses and have been implicated in immune regulation[108]. C3a could therefore be considered as an independently folded domain but is probably not a structural module as this type of amino acid sequence has not been found in any proteins outside the α_2M superfamily. Another member of this family of proteins is pregnancy zone protein which is 60% identical to α_2M[109].

C1q has an unusual shape, being composed of six globular heads, each of which is joined by a collagen-like connecting strand to a central stalk, resembling a 'floral bouquet'[106]. Mannan-binding protein (MBP), lung surfactant protein (SP-A) and conglutinin all have a gross molecular architecture similar to that of C1q[32]. C1q is composed of 18 polypeptide chains, six A, six B and six C chains[110–112]. Each chain is approximately 225 amino acids in length and each contains a region of 81 residues of collagen-like (Gly-X-Y) repeating sequence involved in the binding of the proenzymes, C1r and C1s, starting close to the N-terminal end. One of each of the A, B and C chains combine to form one triple-helix and one globular head. MBP, SP-A and conglutinin also have N-terminal collagen-like regions as shown in Figure 2.4. MBP has been shown to be able to activate the classical pathway of complement without the involvement of C1q and presumably this is mediated via the collagen-like portion of its sequence[12]. It is also believed that C1q, MBP and SP-A all interact with the C1q receptor[113]. This is also thought to be mediated by the collagen-like regions of these proteins[113]. The C-terminal non-collagenous regions of MBP, SP-A and conglutinin are all C-type lectins[32,34]. However, the C-terminal 135 amino acids of C1q is not a lectin domain and has recently been described[114] as having a high degree of sequence identity with the C-terminal globular NC1 domain of type VIII collagen from rabbit corneal endothelial cells[115] and type X collagen from chicken chondrocytes[116]. This is shown schematically in Figure 2.4, and

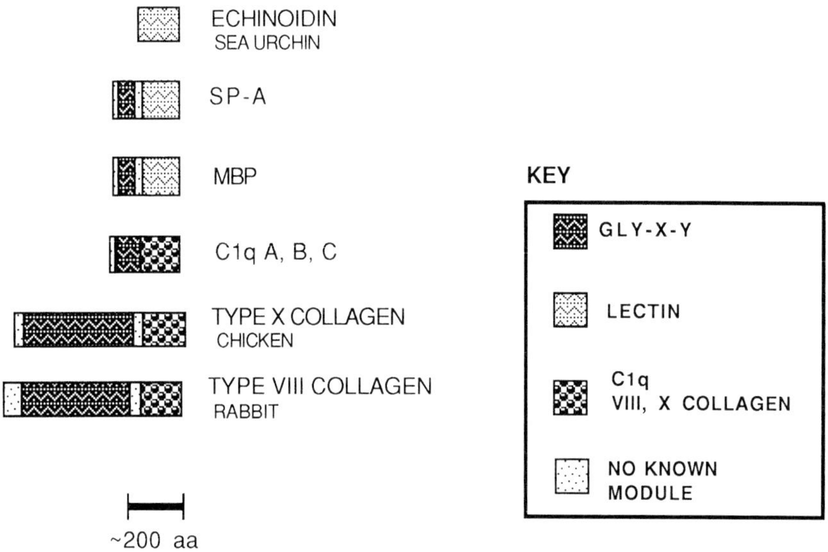

Figure 2.4 The collagen- and C-type-lectin-containing proteins

Figure 2.5 gives an alignment of the amino acid sequences of the type VIII and X collagen NC1 domains with the C1q B chain globular head sequence. It seems very likely that the globular regions of the three C1q chains and the NC1 domains from type VIII and X collagens have evolved from a common ancestral precursor and are likely to have a conserved tertiary structure. The presence of many completely conserved hydrophobic residues (Figure 2.5) is suggestive that these are framework residues and this sequence, therefore, is probably an independently folding domain. Although the biological functions of the type VIII and X collagens are not well defined, they probably play a structural role in the formation of Descemet's membrane, in the cornea, and the development of cartilage, respectively[115,116]. The interactions of these collagens with other molecules of the cellular matrix are not understood. It is possible that, like the C1q globular heads, they may interact with immunoglobulin superfamily domains. Such Ig domains are present in both cartilage-specific proteoglycan core protein[117] and link protein[118].

C1-inhibitor (C1-inh) is 478 amino acid residues in length and about half of its 104 kDa molecular mass is made up of carbohydrate[119,120]. The function of C1-inh is to regulate the classical pathway by binding covalently to activated $C1r_2C1s_2$ and removing them from C1q, thus dissociating the C1 complex. C1-inh is a member of the serine protease inhibitor, or serpin, superfamily[119,120]. Other members of this family include α_1-antitrypsin, α_1-antichymotrypsin, angiotensinogen, heparin cofactor II, α_2-antiplasmin, mouse contrapsin, chicken ovalbumin and barley protein Z[120]. In C1-inh residues 120–479 correspond to the serpin homology and the three-dimensional structure of this domain has been

```
CX      T G M P V S A F T V I L S K A Y P - G A T V P I K F D K I L Y N R Q Q H Y D P R   539-578
CVIII   P A Y E M P A F T A E L T A P F P - P V G A P I K F D R L L Y N G R Q N Y N P Q   611-649
C1Q B   K A T Q K I A F S A T R T I N V P L R R D Q T I R F D H V I T N M N N N Y E P R    90-129

CX      T G I F T C R I P G L Y Y F S Y H V H A K G T N V W V A L Y K N G S P V - - M Y   579-616
CVIII   T G I F T C E V P G V Y Y F A Y H V H C K G G N V W V A L F K N N E P V - - M Y   650-687
C1Q B   S G K F T C K V P G L Y Y F T Y H A S S R G - N L C V N L M R G R E R A Q K V V   130-168

CX      T Y D E Y Q K G Y L D Q A S G S A V I D L M E N D Q V W L Q L P N S E S N G L Y   617-656
CVIII   T Y D E Y K K G F L D Q A S G S A V L L L R P G D R V F L Q M P S E Q A A G L Y   688-727
C1Q B   T F C D Y A Y N T F Q V T T G G M V L K L E Q G E N V F L Q - - A T D K N S L L   169-206

CX      S S E Y V H S S F S G F L F A Q - I       657-673
CVIII   A G Q Y V H S S F S G Y L L Y P - M       728-744
C1Q B   G M E G A N S I F S G F L L F P D M E A   207-226
```

Figure 2.5 Comparison of type X (CX) and type VIII (CVIII) collagen NC1 domains from chicken chrondrocytes and rabbit corneal endothelial cells respectively with the globular head region of human C1q B chain (C1Q B). Gaps are inserted to maximize sequence similarities; identical residues present in all three proteins are boxed and conservative replacements are underlined. Residue number is indicated at the right of the figure

solved for α_1-antitrypsin[121]. The N-terminal ends of C1-inh and other serpins are dissimilar with respect to both length and sequence and it has been suggested that they may represent separate domains evolved from different protein families[120]; however, this region of C1-inh has not been found to be homologous to any other protein to date.

The γ-chain of C8 is 22 kDa, being 182 amino acids in length. Unlike C8α- and β-chains (see below), the γ-chain is not composed of modules. However, C8 is homologous to α_1-microglobulin and protein HC, and the sequence similarity extends along the entire length of their sequences[122]. These proteins belong to the α_1-microglobulin superfamily. It has also been suggested[122] that a region of C8γ (residues 26–41) is homologous to residues 151–171 in C8α but, due to the low level of sequence similarity, it is impossible to judge whether this is significant.

Homologous restriction factor (HRF20/CD59) is a 20 kDa membrane glycoprotein, attached by a glycosylphosphatidylinositol, which inhibits the assembly of homologous complement membrane attack complexes. HRF20 is 103 amino acids in length and has a significant degree of sequence identity (approx 25%) with murine T cell activating protein[123]. Ten out of the 11 cysteines are in identical positions and it seems likely that these proteins will share a common tertiary structure.

The modular complement proteins

In this section, the complement proteins that contain defined modules or domains (Figure 2.6) will be described with each structural type being discussed separately.

The serine protease domain

The serine protease (SP) domain is present in six complement proteins, namely factor D, C1r, C1s C2, factor B and factor I. Factor D (Mr 24 kDa) is the smallest, consisting of a SP domain only, whereas the others are all typical examples of mosaic proteins with various modules N-terminal to their SP domain (Figure 2.6). The SP domain has been well characterized and the tertiary structures of trypsin and chymotrypsin have been determined by X-ray crystallography[124]. At the genomic level, the SP domain is usually split into a number of exons, e.g. eight in factor B[125]. The exon organization in factor B and the C2 gene is very similar to other serine proteases but they contain an extra exon which has no homologous counterpart in other serine proteases, such as trypsin, chymotrypsin and elastase[125] (see Reid and Campbell, Chapter 3). The extra exon in factor B and C2 corresponds to insertions in the protein sequence which may account for the high degree of specificity of these serine proteases for C3 and C5. However, these insertions may also be related to the unusual mode of activation of C2 and factor B. The activation of the SP domains in factor B and C2 does not involve proteolytic cleavage at the N-terminal end of the SP domain and cleavage occurs at the N-terminal end of the von Willebrand factor domain

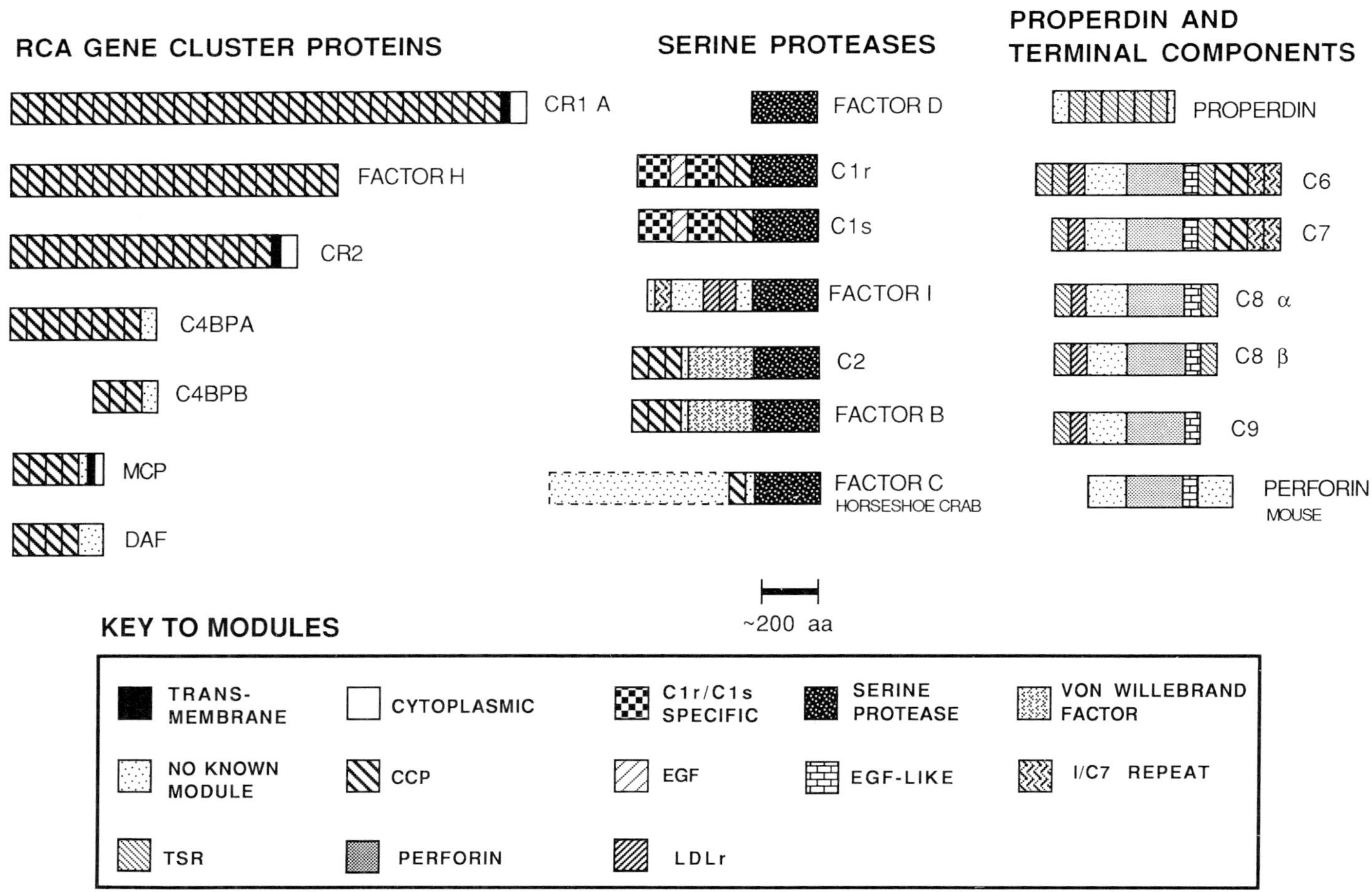

Figure 2.6 The modular structure of the complement components. All the structures shown are from man unless otherwise indicated. Dotted boxes represent areas for which sequence data are not yet available

(Figure 2.6). Thus, the catalytic chains of factor B and C2 are almost twice as long as those of other serine proteases. The SP domains of C1r and C1s are also unusual in that they are encoded by a single exon[126]. The SP-like domain in haptoglobin, which is a haemoglobin-binding serum protein, is also encoded by a discrete exon[127]. Haptoglobin 2 contains two CCP repeats[128] which are almost identical to each other in sequence and, like the second CCP in C1r and C1s (Figure 2.6), to which they are most similar in amino acid sequence, they are encoded by two exons. Thus, it seems likely that C1r, C1s and haptoglobin have evolved from a common ancestral precursor. Factor I is a serine protease of trypsin-like specificity but cleaves only arginyl bonds in its substrates, C3b and C4b. The SP domain of factor I is not particularly similar in sequence to the serine protease regions of the other complement proteases or to plasminogen, factors IX and X or protein C. However, it does appear to be more highly related to the SP domains of tissue plasminogen activator and urokinase which, like factor I, have two additional cysteines, at identical positions, not found in other serine proteases[129].

The complement control protein molecule

The most common structural unit of the complement system is the complement control protein (CCP) module[128,130]. This module was first described as the N-terminal end of factor B and therefore is sometimes referred to as a B-type module[131]. It is often referred to as a short consensus repeat (SCR)[132], although this name could be equally well applied to all the module types found in the complement system. The CCP module is approximately 60 amino acids in length and has a consensus sequence based on four generally invariant cysteines, disulphide bonded in the pattern Cys1-Cys3 and Cys2-Cys4, and other highly conserved residues. The consensus sequence of the CCP module is shown in Figure 2.7. CCP modules are generally encoded by single discrete exons at the gene level[133–136]. However, some CCP modules are encoded by 2 exons[135,137]. The complement control proteins, CR1[132,137], C4b-binding protein (C4-bp)[138,139], membrane cofactor protein (MCP)[140], decay accelerating factor (DAF)[141,142], complement receptor type 2 (CR2)[143] and factor H[144], are composed almost entirely of CCP modules as shown in Figure 2.6. These proteins are encoded in the 'regulation of complement activation' (RCA) gene cluster on human chromosome 1q[145]. The genes for MCP, CR1, CR2, DAF, C4-bpα and C4-bpβ are all located within a megabase of DNA and map to 1q32[146-148] with the factor H locus being 5–10 centimorgans away from this cluster[145,147]. Another CCP-module-containing protein, factor XIIIb subunit (transglutaminase of the blood coagulation system) which consists of 10 CCP repeats[149], has been closely linked to factor H[150] and therefore can be considered as a member of the RCA gene family. Thus, there are at least 112 CCP molecules from 7 proteins encoded in the extended RCA gene cluster. This close association of many CCP modules indicates that these proteins have coevolved by a combination of gene duplication and exon shuffling.

The complement members of the RCA cluster are all involved in the control of C3b and/or C4b. Three CCP modules are also found at the N-termini of the

MODULE	No	Length	CONSENSUS SEQUENCE
CCP	99	~60	xCxxPPxIxNGxIxxxxxxxYxxGExVxYxCxxGYxxxGxxxIxCxxxGxWxxxxPxCxx
TSR	16	~60	DxGWxxWSxWxxCSxTCGxGVxxxRxRxCN-5-10-CxGxxxExxxCxxQxxC
LDLr	5	~40	xxC-2-5-FxCxxxGxCIxxxxxCNGDxDCxDxSxDExxC
EGF	2	~40	C-6-14-CxHxCxxxxxGYxCxCxxxYxLxxxxxxC
EGF-LIKE	6	~30	CxPCxNxGxxxxxxLxGxxCxCxCxxxxxGxAC
I/C7	5	~70	cxxxxCxxWxKcxxxSxCvCxxPxxCxxxxxxxCxxxxxS-4-8-CxxxxxxCxxxxxxxLxxxxC
C1r/C1s	4	~110	cxxxxxxxxGxxxSxxYPxxYPxxxxcxxxIxxxxGxxxxLxxxxxDxExxxxx
C1r/C1s	cont:		CxxDxxxxxxxxxxxGxxCGxxxxxxPxxxxxxxxxxxxxFxTDxxxxxxxxxx

Figure 2.7 Consensus sequences for the modules depicted in Figure 2.6. The length of each module and the number of copies found in the human complement system proteins are indicated. Highly conserved amino acids are shown in one letter code, where x represents a non-conserved amino acid. In the I/C7 and C1r/C1s repeats, c denotes a cysteine residue which is not fully conserved. Dashes indicate regions of variable length

serine proteases, C2 and factor B (Figure 2.6), which are involved in complement activation and their genes are located in the class III region of the MHC on chromosome 6[9]. In C2 and factor B, the CCP module has been shown to be involved in C4b and C3b interaction, respectively. The CCP modules found in C1r and C1s may have a functional role which involves C4-binding. Similarly, the two CCP modules found in the terminal components, C6 and C7, could potentially be involved in the interaction with C5b (homologous to C3b and C4b as discussed above). The CCP module is found in a number of C3b/C4b-binding proteins. However, evidently this structure may be not just associated with C3b/C4b-binding function as these proteins have many CCP modules, but only a few CCP modules in each protein are involved in C3b/C4b-binding. In factor H, the major C3b-binding site is likely to be located between CCP modules 4 and 6[151]. In CR1, two C3b- and one C4b-binding regions have each been localized to within two CCP modules[152]. Similarly, the first two CCP modules of CR2 contain the binding site for C3b[153]. More biochemical data are required to determine which of the individual CCP modules, or pairs of modules, are involved in ligand binding.

There is another cluster of structural genes for proteins containing CCP modules on chromosome 1q in man. This is the 'selectin' family of leukocyte adhesion molecules which consists of granule membrane protein 140 (GMP-140), which has 9 CCP modules[154], endothelial leukocyte adhesion-associated molecule 1 (ELAM-1), with 6 CCP modules[155] and lymphocyte-associated molecule-1 (LAM-1), which has 2 CCP modules[156]. The selectin genes are located within a 300 kb region mapped to 1q21-24[157]. These proteins, which all have a similar organization of modules, mediate the binding of leukocytes to endothelium at inflammatory sites by recognizing carbohydrate determinants[158]. They bind carbohydrate via a single N-terminal type-C lectin domain and this is followed by an epidermal growth factor (EGF) domain, 2–9 CCP modules, a membrane-spanning region and short cytoplasmic sequences. The selectin CCP modules are somewhat unusual in that they contain 2 extra consensus cysteines, which are presumably disulphide bonded.

The CCP module is found in a number of other non-complement human proteins[128,130]. These are β_2-glycoprotein I (β_2I) which has five contiguous CCP modules[159,160], interleukin-2 receptor with two non-contiguous CCP modules, haptoglobin[127] which contains either one or two CCP modules, and a single CCP repeat in thyroid peroxidase[161] and cartilage proteoglycan core protein[162]. Four CCP modules are also found in a 35 kDa protein encoded by vaccinia virus and secreted from cells infected with the virus[163]. These CCP modules have a high degree of sequence similarity with the first four CCP repeats of C4-bp and the vaccinia virus protein has been shown to be capable of down regulating activation of the human complement classical pathway[164]. It is probable that vaccinia virus recruited human genetic material to avoid host defence. CCP modules have also been described in an invertebrate protein, factor C, from the horseshoe crab. Although factor C is a serine protease inhibitor of the coagulation cascade in *Limulus* and has been reported to have five CCP modules as well as type-C lectin and EGF domain[165], the sequence of only one CCP module has been published to date[39]. The CCP module is therefore at least 500 million years old.

Recently the three-dimensional structure of the CCP module has been determined in solution by proton nuclear magnetic resonance spectroscopy[166,167]. The CCP module is based on a β-sandwich arrangement with one face being made up of three β-strands hydrogen-bonded to form a triple-stranded region at its centre and the other face formed from two separate β-strands. Both faces of the sandwich contribute hydrophobic side chains that form a compact core. An analysis of the alignments of all known CCP repeats reveals a high degree of conservation of residues of structural importance (i.e. hydrophobic core residues), whereas insertions and deletions in various repeats are found in loops between elements of the secondary structure. This indicates that many members of the CCP module superfamily can be accurately modelled on the basis of this structure[167]. In this regard, it has been shown that the extra two cysteines, found in each of the CCP modules of the selectin family, can form a disulphide bridge in the tertiary structure model of the CCP module[167]. Similarly, extra disulphide bridges present in the sixth repeat of C4-bp (A chain) and the second CCP module of the interleukin-2 receptor can be accommodated within the consensus structure of the CCP module.

A clear function has not been ascribed to the CCP module in most of the complement and non-complement members of the CCP module superfamily. The CCP module may be important in a wide range of binding specificities, being a structural building block onto which function-related sequence variations can be superimposed, or may, in many cases, have a purely structural role. In this regard, it is known from physical studies that proteins containing many such modules are very elongated and their structures likened to a string of beads[151]. Each bead is an independently folding structure[167] having the dimensions $3.8 \times 2.0 \times 1.0$ nm. Therefore, in cell-surface molecules (e.g. the selectins and complement receptors, CR1 and CR2), CCP modules may act as spacer units, projecting the binding domain away from the cell membrane. At least 136 human CCP modules have been described, and, of these, 112 are encoded on the short arm of chromosome 1. Coordinates are now available for the CCP module structure and this will allow studies to determine the residues involved in CCP module/ligand interactions to be undertaken.

The thrombospondin repeat (TSR)

The second most common motif found in the proteins of the complement system is the thrombospondin repeat (TSR), which was first identified in thrombospondin[168], a 420 kDa adhesion protein secreted from activated platelets. This module is about 60 amino acids long and is largely based on a consensus sequence of 6 cysteines and 3 tryptophan residues. Figure 2.7 shows a consensus sequence for the TSR based on the 3 repeats from thrombospondin itself. At present, the disulphide bond organization in this module is unknown. The TSR module is found in the terminal complement components and properdin as shown in Figure 2.6. The majority of the protein sequence of properdin is composed of six contiguous TSRs[169,170]. The terminal components, C6[171], C7[172], C8α[173], C8β[174,175] and C9[176,177] all contain TSRs as shown in Figure 2.6. These proteins are homologous to each other, with a high degree of amino acid sequence identify along the complete length of the C9 sequence (the shortest amino acid sequence of these proteins). C9 has a single N-terminal TRS, whereas C7, C8α and C8b have an N-terminal TSR and a TSR in the C-terminal half of their polypeptide chains. C6 has an organization of modules similar to that in C7 but has an additional N-terminal TSR. It is interesting to note that the C-terminal TSRs in C6, C7, C8 and C8β are more highly related to the repeats in thrombospondin than to the N-terminal repeats in these proteins[178].

The TSRs in thrombospondin and properdin, like the CCP module and modular structures in general, are usually encoded by discrete exons in their structural genes[179] (K. Nolan, personal communication). This is not the case for the TSR in C9 which is encoded by two exons with the second exon also encoding half the following LDLr domain[180]. It is probable that, in this case, the intron/exon boundary rearrangement has taken place after the duplication of these modules from their respective ancestral genes.

There is no tertiary structural information on the TSR. However, secondary structure prediction and Fourier transform infra-red spectroscopy indicate that TSRs are composed mainly of β-sheet and β-turn structure[181]. Electron microscopy studies on properdin indicate that it has an elongated structure (2.5×36 nm)[182] and that each TSR may have similar dimensions to the CCP module.

The role of the TSRs in thrombospondin, properdin and the terminal components is not known and comparison of the activities of these proteins does not reveal a common function. Properdin, which binds to C3b in the alternative pathway C3 convertase (C3bBb) and thus stabilizes it, presumably interacts with C3b via one or more of its TSRs. There is an interesting sequence similarity between the N-terminal half of TSRs, particularly those of properdin and thrombospondin, and a region from the circumsporozite protein of malaria parasites[169,183]. It has been suggested that this region of the circumsporozite protein, from *Plasmodium falciparum*, may be involved in the attachment of the sporozite (the initial infective stage of malaria) to liver cells and thus may underlie the parasite's ability to enter host cells or evade host defence.

The low-density lipoprotein receptor (LDLr) module

This module was first identified in the low-density lipoprotein receptor (LDLr)[184] and is based on a consensus sequence of 6 invariant cysteines and other highly conserved residues as shown in Figure 2.7. The LDL receptor has 7 contiguous LDLr modules at its N-terminus and also has 3 EGF domains. The α_2M receptor has recently been identified as a previously characterized protein, namely the LDLr-related protein (LRP)[185]. LRP is highly related to the LDLr and has 31 LDLr and 22 EGF modules. The LDLr module is also found in 6 of the complement proteins, i.e. factor I[129], C6[171], C8α[173], C8β[174,175] and C9[176,177], as shown in Figure 2.6. Apart from factor I, which has two, all these proteins contain a single LDLr module. In the structural gene for LDLr, four of the LDLr modules (I, II, VI and VII) are encoded by single discrete exons, whereas the other three modules (III–V) are encoded together in one exon[186]. In C9, the LDLr module is not encoded in a single exon[180], as discussed in the previous section. There is no tertiary structural information available for the LDLr module and the disulphide bond organization is not known. In the first LDLr module of factor I, consensus cysteines 1 and 3 are missing which suggests that these cysteines are disulphide bonded in other LDLr domains.

The epidermal growth factor (EGF) module

This module was first identified in the epidermal growth factor (EGF) precursor which has ten such domains[187,188]. The EGF module, which is probably the best-characterized module type (apart from perhaps the immunoglobulin fold), is found in a large superfamily of diverse proteins[103,189–191]. The EGF module is about 40 amino acids in length and is based on a consensus sequence of six cysteines, disulphide bonded in a pattern of Cys1-3, Cys2-4 and Cys5-6[190], and other highly conserved residues (Figure 2.7). The EGF module structure has been determined for EGF itself and transforming growth factor A (TGFA)[103,189]. The three-dimensional structure of an EGF domain from coagulation factor IX has also been established recently (M. Baron, personal communication). All these structures are similar and consist of anti-parallel β-sheet and β-turns. This observation adds weight to the hypothesis that all members of a module superfamily will have similar global folds.

The complement proteins, C1r[192,193] and C1s[194], which are homologous, having probably arisen by a complete duplication of a common precursor gene, contain a single EGF module sandwiched between two 'C1r/C1s-specific' domains, as shown in Figure 2.6. These EGF modules contain the Ca^{2+} ion consensus, which is found in a large number of EGF modules[103,191], and the evidence available suggests that the formation of the Ca^{2+} ion-dependent tetrameric complex, C1r2C1s2, is mediated via these EGF modules[195,196].

The terminal complement components, C6[171], C7[172], C8α[173], C8β[174,175] and C9[176,177], have all been described as having an EGF module. In Figure 2.6, this domain is designated 'EGF-like' and, in Figure 2.7, the consensus sequence for the EGF-like domain, found in the terminal components, is shown. The degree of sequence similarity between the EGF-like domain and other EGF domains is generally low and the pattern of cysteine residues in these domains is somewhat different. Two out of six cysteines in the EGF-like domains are in different positions from the EGF module consensus sequence (Figure 2.7) and therefore the disulphide bond organization in these domains may be different. The EGF-like domains of the terminal components, although they may have evolved from an ancestral EGF domain, seem to have diverged away from the EGF module structure. It is interesting to note that the EGF-like domain is also found in mouse perforin[197] located at the C-terminal end of a region (approx 220 amino acids) which has extensive sequence similarity to the terminal components as shown in Figure 2.6. Perforin is a cytolytic factor released from cytotoxic T lymphocytes and natural killer cells and is believed to function by binding to target cell membranes and forming a transmembrane channel of perforin polymers. Therefore, perforin is very similar in function to C9 and these proteins have probably evolved from a common ancestral gene which is the progenitor of terminal components C6–C9.

The 'C1r/C1s-specific' repeat

Both C1r and C1s contain two homologous sequences of about 110 amino acids which flank their EGF module as shown in Figure 2.6. The consensus sequence for this domain is shown in Figure 2.7. Until recently, this domain had only been identified in C1r and C1s. It has now been found in single copy in two sea urchin EGF precursor (uEGF) transcripts of a single gene[198]. The two uEGF proteins have an N-terminal EGF module followed by a 'C1r/C1s-specific' domain and 12 or 20 contiguous EGF modules. The C1r/C1s domain and the EGF modules in the uEGF gene are all encoded by single exons separated by phase-1 introns. The C1r/C1s domain is therefore a new type of module, which is old in evolutionary terms (i.e. predating invertebrate/vertebrate divergence), and would be expected to be an independently folded structure. The C1r/C1s module in uEGF is most similar to the second C1r/C1s module in the C1 subcomponents, having four consensus cysteines (rather than just two in the N-terminal C1r/C1s modules of C1r and C1s). It seems likely that an exon encoding the C1r/C1s module and an EGF exon from an ancestral EGF precursor were shuffled together into the gene of an ancestral 'C1rs' component, followed by the subsequent duplication of the C1r/C1s module. There are no data on the possible roles of the C1r/C1s modules in Clr and Cls. One possibility is that these modules are also involved in the dimerization of C1r and C1s along with the Ca^{2+} binding EGF domains.

Factor I/C6/C7-specific repeat

C6[171] and C7[172] both contain two 70 amino acid domains at their C-terminal end and a single domain of this type is found in factor I (Figure 2.6). This domain is based on a consensus sequence of 8 or 10 cysteines and a tryptophan as shown in Figure 2.7. The presence of this domain in C6, C7 and factor I, which also contain LDLr modules, suggests a close relationship between these proteins. However, the significance of these structures being found in these proteins is not known.

The complement integrins (Figure 2.8)

The complement receptors, CR3 (CD18, 11b) and CR4 (CD18, 11c, also known as P150,95), belong to the lymphocyte-function-associated antigen-1 (LFA-1) family of proteins which constitute the β_2 (CD18) subgroup of integrins. These are reviewed by Weitzman and Law (Chapter 10) and therefore will only be described briefly here.

LFA-l, CR3 and CR4 and non-covalently associated heterodimers which share a common β-subunit (CD18) of 95 kDa[199,200] and have related α-subunits of 175, 165 and 150 kDA respectively[201–203]. The α- and β-subunits of CR3 and CR4 do not contain any of the module types described in the previous sections and therefore can be considered to constitute a unique subgroup of complement proteins. However, the α-chains of CR3 and CR4 do contain a von Willebrand factor (vWF) domain (Figure 2.8) which is also found in C2 and factor B

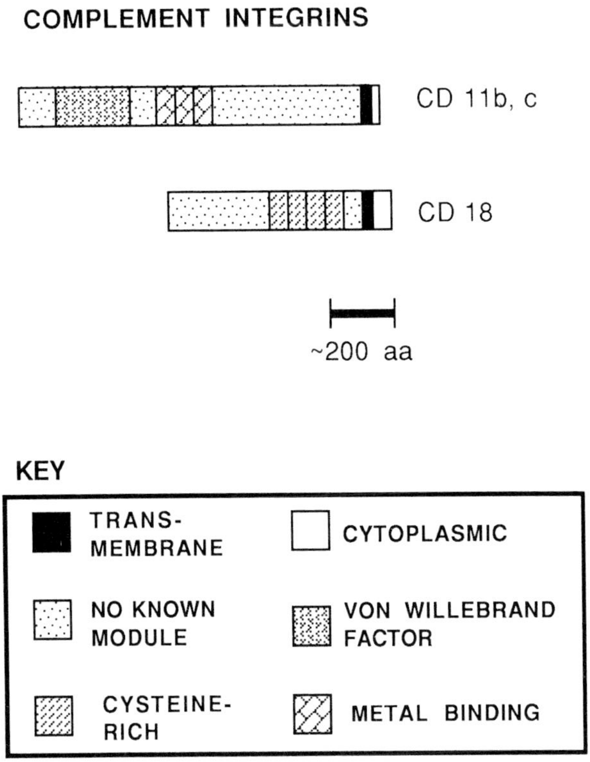

Figure 2.8 The integrin complement receptors, CR3 (above) and CR4 (below)

(Figure 2.6). The domain is about 200 amino acids in length and three examples of this sequence were orginally found in von Willebrand factor[204]. This domain is unique to the β_2-integrin α-chains and is not found in the other integrin subgroups. The possible roles of this vWF domain in CR3 and CR4 could be collagen binding (as it is found in two copies in collagen matrix protein) and/or interaction with iC3b[203].

Evolution of modular proteins

Mosaic proteins are functionally diverse and widespread in multicellular organisms. These proteins are built up from a relatively small pool of modules which are independently folded structures that are mobile evolutionary units, being encoded by discrete 'symmetrical' exons[103,104]. The mechanism of exon-shuffling has been ascribed an important role in the assembly of mosaic proteins from modules[205,206] and Patthy[207] has described some important rules for this process. Only symmetrical exons (i.e. exons that have introns of the same phase class at both their 5′ and 3′ ends) can undergo tandem duplication, deletion or insertion by intronic recombination without disrupting the reading frame. The consequence of this is that only modules of the same intronic phase class can be combined together. Modules encoded by symmetrical exons with phase 1 introns at their 5′ and 3′ ends have been called 'clan 1' modules[207]. All the modules found in the complement system (e.g. CCP, TSR, EGF, LDLr modules) are of the clan 1 type and potentially these (along with other clan 1 modules, e.g. Ig-fold or type-C lectin domain) can be mixed and matched in any combination. However, exon shuffling is not a random sampling of all suitable exons in a genome. Where there is a pre-existing homology between genes, an increased likelihood of further exchange of exons (or cassettes of exons) between those genes (i.e. exon shuffling between members of particular gene families) is strongly preferred. This is clearly illustrated by the RCA gene cluster proteins which have tandem arrays of one module type. Point mutations in the region of modules that confer binding specificity could then lead to a group of proteins with a range of functions.

The serine protease (SP) domains of the blood coagulation and complement system are encoded by a variable number of exons and there is also great variability in the intronic phase between corresponding introns in different SP domains. The 5′ intron, however, is always conserved as a phase 1 intron and therefore can accept any clan 1 module at its N-terminal end. This allows the evolution of serine proteases with different modular recognition domains with exquisite specificity for particular substrates.

The modules described in this review are macromolecular building blocks, with highly conserved structures, onto which function-related sequence elements are superimposed. The genetic and structural features of modules provide an enormous potential for the rapid generation of novel proteins. The evolution of multicellular organisms created new functional niches and provided a driving force for protein evolution. The combination of the functional potential of modular structures with new opportunities may explain the prevalence of mosaic proteins in extracellular environments.

COMPLEMENT EVOLUTION

The unification of the complement system

In the preceding section, we have described the protein domains and structural motifs found in complement components. Each of the various structures described had a separate evolutionary origin, probably outside the immediate area of host defence. They have been integrated into the complement system as it has gradually increased in complexity and sophistication. Following recruitment into the complement system, a number of the original components have undergone gene duplications which have increased the complexity of the system. Examples of components which have arisen by gene duplication are shown in Figures 2.3 and 2.6 Some of these proteins, C1r/C1s, C2/factor B, C3/C4/C5, C6/C7, C8α/C8β and CR3/CR4 α-chains, are sufficiently closely related that their overall structures remain very similar. Other relationships are not so immediately obvious, such as those between the proteins coded in the

RCA locus, where the molecular mass of the individual components can vary by an order of magnitude. However, these proteins are all composed largely of a single small repeating unit (Figure 2.6), but the actual number of repeats in homologous proteins can vary greatly between different species and even within a species. The close proximity of the genes for these proteins in the genome confirms their relatively recent common ancestry.

Although certain components of the system have arisen by common ancestry, it is a mistake to look for a single evolutionary origin for complement. An invertebrate ancestor may have had a number of proteins resembling components of the mammalian complement scheme, but which had not become integrated into an interacting system. This is shown in a totally hypothetical and much simplified form in Figure 2.9. Here we are looking at the integration of just three component parts into a simple complement system; in reality, many more components became incorporated.

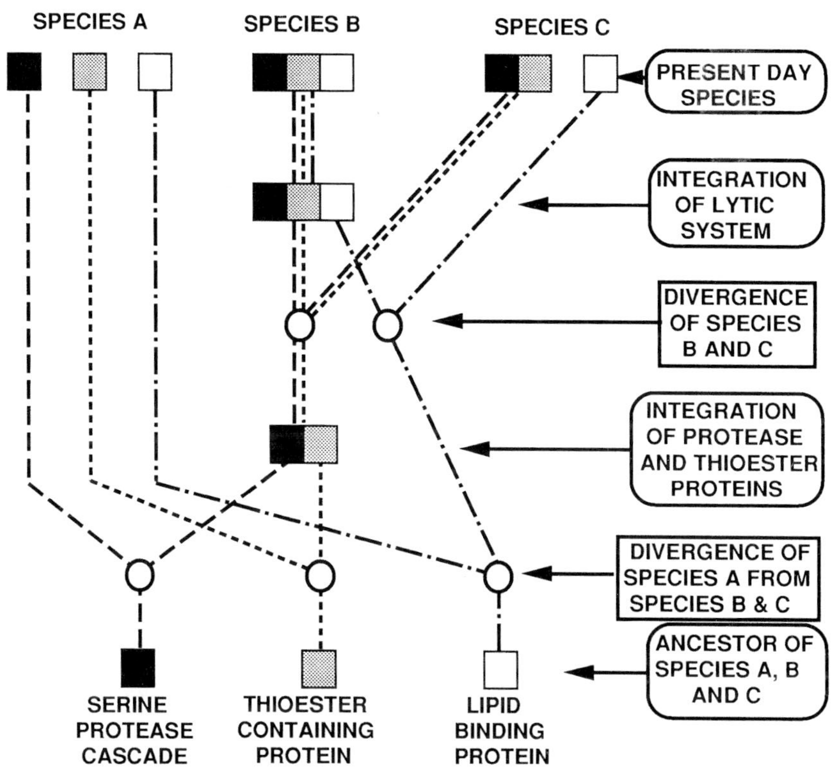

Figure 2.9 A model of the evolution of the complement system. The rectangles represent proteins or groups of proteins and their genes, which, in the ancestral species at the bottom of the figure, are independent and do not interact with one another. Integration of the individual blocks into an opsonic, and eventually a lytic, complement system is represented by the fusion of the rectangles. The circles indicate the points of divergence of the three present-day species at the top of the figure

An ancestral invertebrate can be imagined which had:

1. A serine protease cascade which had evolved, say, to control the release of a biologically active peptide.
2. A thiolester-containing protein which had evolved as a protease inhibitor, together with a receptor to facilitate its clearance.
3. A lipid binding protein which had evolved to control the synthesis of cell membranes.

At some point in evolutionary history between the ancestral invertebrate and the modern mammals, a protease or proteases from the hormone-producing cascade started to interact with the protease inhibitor in a manner which led to the protease inhibitor becoming bound to foreign particles, to form a simple opsonic mechanism. Originally, the two components interacted fortuitously but once they came together to the advantage of the organism, natural selection could begin to refine the specificity and efficiency of the effect and a simple opsonic complement system would have emerged. At some later stage, a protein which had evolved from the lipid-binding protein of the ancient ancestor may, again fortuitously, have begun to interact with the proteins of the opsonic system to bring about direct killing of foreign organisms. Natural selection could refine this into what is now a recognizable lytic complement system. This situation is symbolized in Figure 2.9 by species B. Species A diverged from species B and C prior to the integration of the opsonic system. However, it still has proteins which have evolved from those of the common ancestor. These proteins may now have functions in species A which are unrelated either to the complement system of species B or to the functions of the ancestral proteins. Species C diverged from species B after the integration of the opsonic system but before the incorporation of the lipid-binding protein into the scheme. It therefore has an opsonic mechanism but also a protein related to the lytic protein of the complement system of species B, though this does not interact with the opsonic proteins.

How can the hypothetical outline just described be related to what has been found in the phylogenetic studies discussed earlier? The model described is, of course, much simplified, and takes no account of various complement receptors, control proteins or of the origins of the classical and alternative pathways. Nor does it deal with any of the functions of complement outside the immediate area of opsonization and lysis. However, there are not many phylogenetic data in any of these areas. In the lamprey, the lowest vertebrate studied, there appears to be a complement-like opsonic apparatus. However, the evidence suggests that a lytic mechanism had not yet become incorporated at the time of the divergence of the Agnatha from the remainder of the vertebrates[8]. In the nurse shark, however, there is evidence for complement-like lytic and opsonic mechanisms[46]. It seems possible then that species C in Figure 2.9 could represent the lamprey while species B could be typical of all of the higher vertebrates from the elasmobranches to the mammals. It is possible that a lamprey lytic system does exist, but has yet to be described, or that the lamprey has lost a lytic activity present in its ancestors. None the less, if it is true that the integration of the lytic system did not occur until after the appearance of the vertebrates, then the presence of a lytic system in the invertebrates, which is similar in its overall architecture to complement, is extremely unlikely. This is not to say that lytic proteins in invertebrates could not be related to the lytic proteins of vertebrate complement. Preliminary evidence does suggest that echinoderm coelomocytes bring about killing using a protein that may be related to C9[25].

Echinoderms[30] and anelids[36] appear to have opsonic systems which may be complement related. Species from these phyla could, therefore, be examples of species C in Figure 2.9. If this is the case, then all species higher than the platyhelminthes (Figure 2.1), may also possess similar opsonic mechanisms. It is, however, conceivable that the complement-like opsonic mechanisms in these species have emerged independently of one another and of vertebrate complement. This implies that, after the divergence of species A, the descendants of the serine protease cascade or other proteases and the thiolester protein have become integrated. The observed phenomena could then be the result of parallel evolution based on a number of independent events. Until the molecular basis of these activities is better characterized, it is impossible to draw conclusions.

Possible origins of the complement system

The thiolester-containing proteins

As C3 is central, both to the activation of complement and to its functions, one must conclude that this component was the nucleus around which the complement system evolved. How then could the earliest simple C3-containing complement system have arisen? It is known that the invertebrates, horseshoe crab, crayfish and lobster, each possess protease inhibitors which are related to α_2M and hence to C3. α_2M contains an intrachain thiolester bond, through which it can become covalently attached to enzymes which proteolyse it. The complete amino acid sequences of the invertebrate α_2Ms are not yet available[23]. However, the complete primary structures of the human[208] and rat[209] molecules have been determined. The region in which α_2M is cleaved by the enzymes which it inhibits is in the equivalent position to that in which C3 and C4 are cleaved by their activating enzymes (Figure 2.3). However, while both C3 and C4 has a unique site which is hydrolysed by a very narrow range of enzymes, α_2M has what has been termed a bait region (Figure 2.10). This is a stretch of amino acids of approximately 35 residues in length, including sites which can act as substrates for a wide range of proteases which are subsequently inhibited[210].

Most plasma proteases have evolved in tandem with inhibitors, specific to themselves, as have the complement proteases; that is, C1 has C1-inh, C3 convertases have factors I, H and C4-bp. The role of α_2M in the mammals is probably to remove plasma proteases which are produced in excess of their specific inhibitors, and possibly to inactivate cellular proteases released by tissue damage. α_2M is also able to inhibit novel proteases never before encountered by the organism and hence having no specific inhibitors to deal with them. A major source of such novel proteases could be invading microorganisms. It is tempting to speculate that this could be a major role for α_2M in the invertebrates, as part of their defence systems.

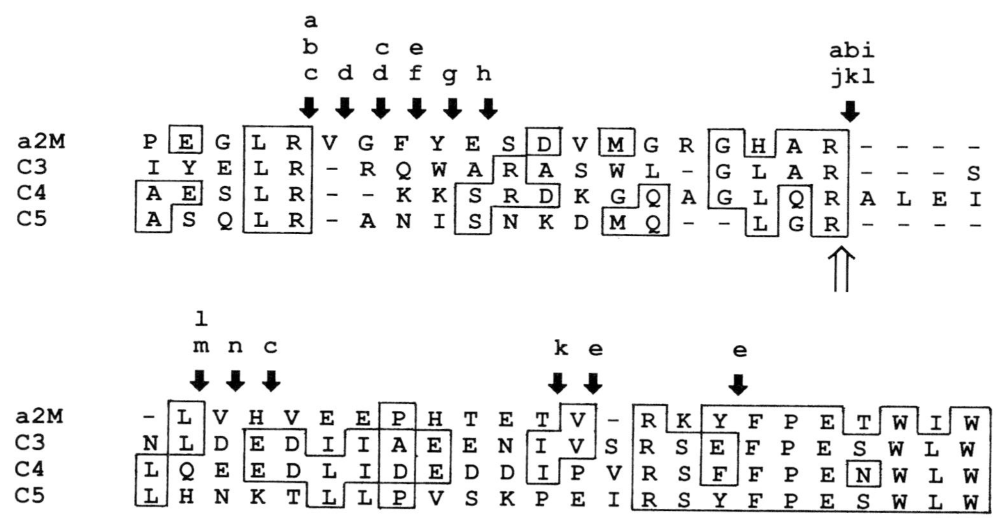

a=bovine trypsin; b=*Streptomyces griseus* trypsin; c=papain; d=porcine pancreatic elastase; e=calf chymosin; f=human cathepsin G; g=bovine chymotrypsin; h=*Staphylococcus aureus* V-8 protease; i=human plasmin; j=bovine thrombin; k=thermolysin; l=subtilisin; m=*Streptomyces griseus* proteinase B; n=human leukocyte elastase; ⇑=site of cleavage of C3, C4 and C5

Figure 2.10 The primary structure of the bait region of α_2 macroglobulin (α2M) and its sites of cleavage by various proteases, compared with the sites cleaved in C3, C4 and C5 during complement activation

Once a protease has reacted with α_2M, either covalently via the thiolester or non-covalently by the Venus fly-trap-like mechanism, it is cleared from the circulation by receptors, specific for the activated form of the molecule, located on macrophages and in other tissues. The α_2M receptor (Mr >500 kDa) has been purified from human placenta and rat liver and shown to comprise three polypeptide chains (420 kDa, 84 kDa and 40 kDa)[211-213] and to require Ca^{2+} for binding to α_2M[214]. It has recently been demonstrated that the receptor is a previously characterized protein called low-density lipoprotein receptor-related protein (LRP)[185]. The 420 kDa and 85 kDa chains are derived from a single 4525 amino acid precursor, in which the lower molecular mass component is C-terminal[215,216]. The 85 kDa polypeptide contains a membrane-spanning segment and a 100-residue cytoplasmic tail; the 420 kDa chain is non-covalently attached to the smaller fragment and contains the α_2M binding site(s). The complete extracellular portion of the molecule is composed of a total of 93 repeating motifs of three types. There are 31 LDL receptor repeats, 22 EGF repeats and 40 copies of the YWTD repeat an approximately 50-residue-long motif characterized by the largely conserved sequence Tyr-Trp-Thr-Asp as well as other residues, though conserved cysteines are lacking. The 40 kDa component of the receptor does not bind to α_2M[213] and may bind other ligands, such as lipoproteins, which have been shown to have affinity for the receptor[185].

The finding that α_2M receptor is apparently unrelated to any of the recognized C3/C4 receptors is perhaps a little surprising from the evolutionary point of view. It may have been expected that, when the thiolester-containing complement components diverged from the protease inhibitors, the receptor would have diverged at the same time. The current evidence suggests that this was not the case, although it should be remembered that C3 has at least four distinct receptors plus the anaphylatoxin receptors, each of which has a different function on different cell types. It is possible that as-yet-uncharacterized α_2M receptors exist which resemble the complement receptors, or that LDL-receptor-like complement receptors exist. Two copies of the LDL receptor domain are present in factor I and one copy is also present in each of the terminal components, C6–C9 (Figure 2.6). EGF domains are present in C1r and C1s and structures which may be related are found in the terminal components (EGF-like in Figure 2.6). Factor I interacts with C3 and C4 to bring about inactivation, while C1s is involved in the activation of C4. The terminal components interact with activated C5 to form the membrane attack complex. Alternatively, these domains could be involved in the interaction of these components with the lipid membrane. Whether these domains are involved in any way in these interactions is as yet unknown.

It is possible that α_2M could have gone one step further than its proposed role as a bacterial protease inhibitor. Some of the molecules could, upon activation, have become covalently attached, not to the protease, but to the nearby protease-producing organism. The first opsonic complement system could have consisted of only two components; an α_2M/C3-like molecule plus a cell surface receptor. The activation mechanism of such a system would rely upon the proteases produced by the microorganisms themselves. The next major step in such an evolutionary scheme may have been the incorporation of a factor-B/C2-like protease which could bind specifically to the α_2M/C3 attached to the bacterial surface. Such an enzyme could form a C3/α_2M convertase, so causing more of the opsonic molecules to be deposited around the original site of activation, greatly increasing the efficiency of receptor–ligand interaction.

An additional point which should perhaps be considered in the context of the relationship between the thiolester-containing protease inhibitors and the complement components is that there is a fundamental difference in the nature of the two types of reaction. When the protease inhibitors are activated by the cleavage of the bait region, the reactive thiolester is in such an orientation in relation to the activating enzyme that a high degree of covalent bond formation occurs between the two molecules. In the case of the activating enzymes for C4 and C3, that is C1s and C2/factor B, no evidence of crosslinking via the thioleser to the activating enzyme has been observed. Furthermore, purified C4 and C3 are extremely susceptible to activation by minute traces of contaminating proteases, indicating that no inhibitory activity is evident. This may indicate that the thiolester bond in the complement components is oriented away from the activating enzyme and towards the desired receptor, that is the cell surface. If this is so, it requires that a major change in the topology of the molecule must have occurred during evolution, with the result that the cleavage and binding sites have moved from being in the same plane in the inhibitors to being on opposite sides of the molecule in the complement proteins.

Enzyme cascades

Macfarlane[217,218] used the term enzyme cascade to describe a number of mechanisms in vertebrate blood. These include clotting, fibrinolysis, angiotensin and kinin formation and complement. These systems are all dependent on the sequential activation of proteolytic zymogens triggered by changes in the homeostasis of blood. Complement is the most complex of these, though blood clotting involves more proteolytic steps. The complexity results from two conflicting requirements of these systems; rapid amplification is necessary for effective defence, but stringent controls are essential to combat the danger to the organism should these mechanisms misfire. Hence the need for a number of steps in the reaction, each of which can bring about amplification but which is also under the control of inhibitors and other factors, such as the rapid decay of enzyme activity. Zymogen cascades have been described in a number of invertebrate systems.

All vertebrates and many invertebrates have clotting mechanisms whereby they can prevent loss of body fluids in case of injury, but also, in the case of some invertebrates, as a defence against invading microbes. Clotting systems in all vertebrates back to the Agnatha have a similar architecture to that found in mammals, and involve, ultimately, the conversion of fibrinogen by thrombin to form a fibrin clot[219]. The clotting mechanisms of most invertebrates have not yet been elucidated but the final clot-forming proteins do not appear to be related to fibrinogen[220]. The most detailed studies of invertebrate clotting have been performed on the horseshoe crab. Clotting in horseshoe crab requires the sequential activation of three serine protease zymogens and a clot-forming protein. The first of these zymogens, factor C, is induced to autoactivate by the binding of lipopolysaccharide. It, in turn, activates factor B, which then cleaves the clotting enzyme precursor and the resultant clotting enzyme proteolyses coagulogen to form coagulin which produces the clot. Evidence from chain structure and limited sequence analysis indicates that factor C may be related to factor B and C2 of the complement system in that it contains CCP domains[35,145].

The prophenol oxidase system of the arthropods is a mechanism by which these organisms protect themselves against wounding and microbial attack. The enzyme, phenol oxidase, brings about melanization by the oxidation of phenols to quinones, which then react spontaneously to form melanin. Melanin is toxic and opsonic to bacteria and fungi and can physically repair damage. The zymogen form, prophenol oxidase, is present in haemolymph, and its activation involves proteolytic cleavage by a serine protease which is itself present as a zymogen. The activation of this molecule requires binding of microbial carbohydrate or lipopolysaccharide, possibly to yet another enzyme. It has been proposed that this cascade could have an evolutionary relationship to the complement system[221].

Even if the two cascades described are not directly related to the complement system, their presence in invertebrates indicates that systems similar in their mechanism of activation to complement have evolved in species far removed from the direct line to the vertebrates.

C1q and the lectins

It has been proposed that the original role of C1q was to opsonize IgM-sensitized particles. IgM appears to be the most ancient immunoglobulin type; alone it can bring about agglutination, but since effector cells lack IgM receptors, C1q and its receptor could have contributed the required bridge between the humoral and cellular immune systems[222].

Lectins are non-immune carbohydrate-recognizing molecules which are present in plants as well as animals. They can agglutinate cells and precipitate molecules bearing specific carbohydrate structures. A number of mammalian proteins have lectin domains, including mannan binding protein (MBP) and conglutinin, both of which resemble C1q in having triple-helical collagen-like domains and in being multimeric. Although C1q has some lectin-like activity, it does not have a standard lectin domain[32]. Both MBP and conglutinin can interact directly with the mammalian complement system. MBP, when bound to mannan-bearing surfaces, such as yeast or certain bacteria, can replace C1q as a binder and activator of C1r and C1s, and hence as an activator of the classical pathway, in the absence of antibody[12,13]. Conglutinin is present at variable levels in bovine sera but also at lower levels in humans[223]. It recognizes and binds to determinants on cell-bound iC3b (C3b which has been inactivated by factor I) and so brings about agglutination of the cells[31]. The lectin domains found in MBP and conglutinin are members of the type-C lectin family, examples of which have also been described in the acorn barnacle, *Megabalanus rosa*[224], the flesh fly, *Sarcophaga peregrina*[225] and in a sea urchin, *Anthocidaris crassispina*[33]. To date, no molecules have been described in invertebrates which have lectin and collagen-like domains. The receptor for C1q, which is present on a number of cell types[226], has not yet been fully characterized, although molecules with monomer molecular masses of 56–80 kDa have been purified. The native receptor is thought to be a non-covalently associated dimer[113,226].

Another group of lectins which interact with the complement system are the pentraxins (C-reactive protein family). These proteins have been characterized in species as far back as horseshoe crab[37,38]. These ancient molecules have a role in defence and predate antibody in being able to discriminate foreign particles[227,228]. C-reactive protein (CRP) is an acute phase protein which can interact, in a Ca^{2+}-dependent manner, with the C-polysaccharide which is present in pneumococcus and in a range of other pathogens. The protein has been described in mammals, birds, bony and cartilaginous fish, and in the invertebrates, horseshoe crab[227] and the tunicate, *Didemnum candidum*[229]. In vertebrates, the plasma form of the protein is disk shaped and is composed of five identical non-covalently associated subunits of approximately 21 kDa. This pentameric structure imparts the multivalency required for precipitin formation. The CRP from horseshoe crab is somewhat different in that three different subunits of around 20 kDa form hexamers, probably consisting of two copies of each subunit type. The three subunits of horseshoe crab CRP are approximately 90% identical in sequence, and show around 25% identity to their human counterpart, suggesting that these molecules have a common evolutionary origin[38].

Human CRP complexed to C-polysaccharide is able to activate the classical pathway of complement in a manner similar to that seen with antibody–antigen aggregates. The alternative pathway does not appear to be directly involved, although, once classical pathway activation has commenced, alternative pathway amplification convertases may be formed. The deposition of C3b onto the surfaces of invading microorganisms leads to opsonization, and complement activation can proceed through to the formation of a membrane attack complex and killing[228,230]. Serum amyloid P (SAP) is closely related to CRP. The plasma form of the protein consists of a stack of two pentameric disks. SAP does not activate complement but may interact with C4 binding protein and with C1q. Whether either of these interactions has any physiological significance is not known[231,232].

Activation of the classical pathway in mammals necessitates the binding of C1q to antibody. It has therefore been suggested that the classical pathway must have evolved after the appearance of antibody, and hence must be a relatively recent addition to an older alternative pathway[11,222]. The ability of a number of different lectins to activate complement, either directly as in the case of MBP or via C1 binding as in the case of CRP, raises the possibility that the alternative pathway activation mechanism, which requires that the complement proteins themselves must discriminate self from non-self, may have been predated by a system in which another molecule acted as the recognition unit, in other words a system more akin to the classical pathway. With the development of antibody, the ancestral C1q molecule may have lost its lectin recognition unit and gained an Fc binding domain. In this context, it is interesting to note that, in their studies of the nurse shark, Jensen and colleagues[46] found evidence for a complement activation mechanism more reminiscent of the classical than of the alternative pathway.

The pore forming proteins

Perforin is a lytic protein present in cytotoxic T cells and natural killer cells. This molecule shows sequence homology with the membrane insertion domains of the proteins of the membrane attack complex, C6, C7, C8 and C9. All these proteins have a mosaic nature (Figure 2.6) and consist of a central, probably membrane-insertable, section to which other domains have been appended to specify their interactions with one another and the membrane. The description of molecules which may be C9/perforin analogues in a protozoan[27] and an echinoderm[25] raises the possibility that the protein structures involved in membrane attack may be very ancient. However, it should be remembered that a lytic peptide from bee venom, which is probably not evolutionarily related, also shows antigenic crossreactivity with these proteins[28]. It is possible that a short sequence which is particularly efficient at membrane insertion has been 'discovered' by natural selection on a number of separate occasions.

SUMMARY

We have described the molecular evidence which indicates that complement exists as a defence mechanism in all vertebrate classes. The system has a similar architecture in all species, from the bony fish to the mammals, though minor differences will almost certainly be found as our knowledge increases. A very similar system appears to be present in the cartilaginous fish, though the evidence points to be a scheme with fewer components than found in the higher vertebrates. The shark complement system seems to resemble the classical pathway more closely than the alternative pathway in its mechanism of activation. In the jawless fish, there is evidence for an opsonic system which involves the binding of a C3-like molecule to pathogens and its recognition by a receptor on phagocytic cells. The mechanism of activation of the C3-like molecule is yet to be established. These animals seem to lack the late-acting complement components which bring about cell lysis. In the invertebrates, evidence for complement-like defence mechanisms is still inconclusive although a number of proteins which are evolutionarily related to complement components are definitely present.

The proteins of the complement system have diverse evolutionary origins. We have described the range of protein motifs found in mammals and have indicated, where possible, comparable structures in lower animals. All of the complement proteins, including those that do not contain modules, have homology to non-complement proteins and belong to established superfamilies. This suggests that the integrated complement system we see today in mammals is relatively young in evolutionary terms, with complete genes and/or individual modules having been borrowed promiscuously from older non-complement proteins. We have presented a much simplified model which partially describes how these diverse proteins could have become integrated to form the complex system found in the higher vertebrates. Whilst the complexity of the system has been somewhat increased by gene duplication, the underlying trend in its evolution appears to have been the assimilation of unrelated proteins which have interacted fortuitously and to the advantage of ancestral organisms.

The simplest 'complement' system which can be imagined would require two components: a recognition molecule and a receptor on an effector cell. We have proposed two possible systems based on known mammalian proteins which fit these requirements. The protease inhibitor α_2M is found in invertebrates and may have a role in defence against bacterial enzymes. An α_2M-like molecule, activated by bacterial proteases, could become bound to the microorganism, so bringing about opsonization, and clearance through receptors. A molecule similar in architecture to C1q but with lectin rather than Fc recognition units could also have acted as an agglutinin and opsonin. In invertebrates, proteins have been described which could be related to the zymogen cascades and to the lytic proteins of the complement system.

Acknowledgements

We would like to thank Ken Reid, Alex Law, Bob Sim, Duncan Campbell, Paul Levine, John Atkinson, Craig Lobb and Sylvia Smith for their helpful discussion and advice, and Alison Marsland for secretarial assistance.

NOTE ADDED IN PROOF

A haemolytic system in the horseshoe crab has been shown to involve the participation of α_2M. The α_2M becomes bound to erythrocytes during this process and it has been proposed that this molecule has a dual role, acting as a protease inhibitor via the Venus flytrap mechanism, and as a C3-like molecule via the thiolester bond[233]. The complete sequence of factor C of the horseshoe crab clotting system has been determined[254]. The cDNA sequences have been reported for the C3-like molecules in two jawless fish, the lamprey[235] and the hagfish[236].

References

1. Flexner, S. and Noguchi, H. (1903). Snake venom in relation to haemolysis, bacteriolysis and toxicity. *J. Exp. Med.*, **6**, 277–301
2. Marshall, H. T. (1904). Studies in haemolysis with special reference to the properties of the blood and body fluids of human beings. *J. Exp. Med.*, **6**, 347–75
3. Gigli, I. and Austen, K. F. (1971). Phylogeny and function of the complement system. *Ann. Rev. Microbiol.*, **25**, 309–32
4. Ballow, M. (1977). Phylogenetics and ontogenetics of the complement system. In Day, N. K. and Good, R. A. (eds.) *Biological Amplification Systems*, pp. 183–204. (New York: Plenum)
5. Hilderman, W. (1978). On the lore of complementology: artefact versus reality. *Dev. Comp. Immunol.*, **2**, 45–50
6. Linscott, W. D. (1986). Biochemistry and biology of the complement system in domestic animals. *Prog. Vet. Microbiol. Immunol.*, **2**, 54–77
7. Fujii, T. and Murakawa, S. (1981). Immunity in lamprey. III Occurrence of complement-like activity. *Dev. Comp. Immunol.*, **5**, 251–9
8. Nonaka, M., Fujii, T., Kaidoh, T., Natsuume-Sakai, S., Yamaguchi, N. and Takahashi, M. (1984). Purification of a lamprey component protein homologous to the third component of mammalian complement system. *J. Immunol.*, **133**, 3242–9

9. Campbell, R. D., Law, S. K. A., Reid, K. B. M. and Sim, R. B. (1988). Structure, organization and regulation of the complement genes. *Annu. Rev. Immunol.*, **6**, 161–95
10. Law, S. K. A. and Reid, K. B. M. (1988). Complement. In Male, D. (ed.) *In Focus* series, pp. 1–72. (Oxford, UK: IRL Press)
11. Lachmann, P. J. (1979). An evolutionary view of the complement system. *Behring. Inst. Mitt.*, **63**, 25–37
12. Lu, J., Thiel, S., Wiedemann, H., Timpl, R. and Reid, K. B. M. (1990). Binding of the pentamer/hexamer forms of mannan-binding protein to zymosan activates the proenzyme $C1r_2$ $C1s_2$ complex, of the classical pathway of complement, without involvement of C1q. *J. Immunol.*, **144**, 2287–94
13. Ohta, M., Okada, M., Yamashina, I. and Kawasaki, T. (1990). The mechanism of carbohydrate mediated complement activation by the serum mannan binding protein. *J. Biol. Chem.*, **265**, 1980–4
14. Jefferies, R. P. S. (1986). *The Ancestry of the Vertebrates* (London: British Museum)
15. Willmer, P. (1990). *Invertebrate Relationships; Patterns in Animal Evolution* (Cambridge University Press)
16. Carroll, R. L. (1988). *Vertebrate Paleontology and Evolution.* (New York: Freeman)
17. Hall, J. L., Rowlands, D. G. and Nilsson, U. R. (1972). Complement-unlike hemolytic activity in lobster hemolymph. *J. Immunol.*, **109**, 816–23
18. Sottrup-Jensen, L., Stepanik, T. M., Kristensen, T., Lonblad, P. B., Jones, C. M., Wierzbick, D. M., Magnusson, S., Domdey, H., Wetsel, R. A., Lundwall, A., Tack, B. F. and Fey, G. H. (1985). Common evolutionary origin of α2-macroglobulin and complement components C3 and C4. *Proc. Natl. Acad. Sci. USA*, **82**, 9–13
19. Quigley, J. P. and Armstrong, P. B. (1983). An endopeptidase inhibitor found in *Limulus plasma*: an ancient form of α2 macroglobulin. *Ann. N. Y. Acad. Sci.*, **421**, 119–23
20. Quigley, J. P. and Armstrong, P. B. (1985). A homologue of α2 macroglobulin purified from the haemolymph of the horseshoe crab *Limulus polyphemus*. *J. Biol. Chem.*, **260**, 12715–19
21. Hall, M., Soderwall, K. and Sottrup-Jensen, L. (1989). Amino acid sequence around the thioester of α2 macroglobulin from plasma of the crayfish *Pacifastacus leniusculus*. *FEBS Lett.*, **254**, 111–14
22. Spycher, S. E., Arya, S., Isenman, D. E. and Painter, R. H. (1987). A functional thiolester containing α2 macroglobulin homologue isolated from the haemolymph of the American lobster *Homarus americanus*. *J. Biol. Chem.*, **262**, 14606–11
23. Sottrup-Jensen, L., Bortl, W., Hall, M., Quigley, J. P. and Armstrong, P. B. (1990). Sequence similarity between α2 macroglobulin from the horseshoe crab *Limulus polyphemus* and proteins of the α2 macroglobulin family from mammals. *Comp. Biochem. Physiol.*, **96B**, 621–5
24. Canicatti, C. and Ciulla, D. (1988). Studies on *Holothuria polli* (Echinodermata) coelomocyte lysate. II Isolation of coelomocyte hemolysins. *Dev. Comp. Immunol.*, **12**, 55–64
25. Canicatti, C. and Tschopp, J. (1989). Relationship between vertebrate channel-forming proteins and invertebrate haemolysins. *Dev. Comp. Immunol.*, **13**, 377
26. Stanley, K. and Luzio, P. (1987). A family of killer proteins. *Nature*, **334**, 475–6
27. Andrews, N. W., Abrams, C. K., Slatin, S. L. and Griffiths G. (1990). A *T. cruzi* secreted protein immunologically related to the complement component C9: evidence for membrane pore forming activity at low pH. *Cell*, **61**, 1277–87
28. Laine, R. O., Morgan, B. P. and Esser, A. P. (1988). Comparison between complement and melittin haemolysis: anti melittin antibodies inhibit complement lysis. *Biochemistry*, **27**, 5308–14
29. Bertheussen, K. and Seljelid, R. (1982). Receptors for complement of echinoid phagocytes. I The opsonic effect of vertebrates sera on echinoid phagocytosis. *Dev. Comp. Immunol.*, **6**, 423–31
30. Bertheussen, K. (1982). Receptors for complement on echinoid phagocytes purified human complement mediates echinoid phagocytosis. *Dev. Comp. Immunol.*, **6**, 635–42
31. Lachmann, P. J. (1973). Complement. In Porter, R. R. (ed.) *Defence and Recognition*, pp. 361–97. (Lancaster, UK: Butterworth)
32. Thiel, S. and Reid, K. B. M. (1989). Structures and functions associated with the group of mammalian lectins containing collagen-like sequences. *FEBS Lett.*, **250**, 78-84
33. Giga, Y., Ikai, A. and Takahashi, K. (1987). The complete amino acid sequence of Echinoidin, a lectin from the coelomic fluid of the sea urchin *Anthocidoris crassispina*. *J. Biol. Chem.*, **262**, 6197–203

34. Drickamer, K. (1988). Two distinct classes of carbohydrate-recognition domain in animal lectins. *J. Biol. Chem.*, **263**, 9557–60
35. Lestage, J., Laulan, A. and Chateaureynaud-Duprat, P. (1983). Nouvelles donnees sur les reactions de defense chez un lumricien *Lumbricus terrestris*. *CR Acad. Sci. Paris*, **296**, 19–24
36. Laulan, A., Lestage, J., Bouc, A. M. and Chateaureynaud-Duprat, P. (1988). The phagocytic activity of *Lumbricus terrestris* leukocytes is enhanced by the vertebrate opsonins IgG and complement C3b fragment. *Dev. Comp. Immunol.*, **12**, 269–78
37. Robey, F. A. and Liu, T. Y. (1981). Limulin: a C-reactive protein from *Limulus polyphemus*. *J. Biol. Chem.*, **256**, 969–75
38. Nguyen, N. Y., Suzuki, A., Boykins, A. and Liu, T. Y. (1986). The amino acid sequence of *Limulus* C-reactive protein. *J. Biol. Chem.*, **261**, 10456–9
39. Tokunaga, F., Miyata, T., Nakamura, T., Morita, T., Kuma, K. and Iwanaga, S. (1987). Lipopolysaccharide-sensitive serine-protease zymogen (factor C) of horseshoe crab hemocytes. *Eur. J. Biochem.*, **167**, 405–16
40. Phipps, D., Menger, M., Chadwick, J. S. and Aston, W. P. (1987). A cobra venom factor (CVF) induced C3 convertase activity in the haemolymph of *Galleria mellonella*. *Dev. Comp. Immunol.*, **11**, 37-46
41. Phipps, D. J., Chadwick, J. S., Leeder, R. G. and Aston, W. P. (1989). The haemolytic activity of *Galleria mellonella* haemolymph. *Dev. Comp. Immunol.*, **13**, 103–11
42. D'Cruz, O. J. M. and Day, N. K. (1984). Purification of a human alternative complement pathway inhibitor from the haemolymph of larval fall army worm (*Spodoptera frugiperda*). *Biochem. Biophys. Res. Commun.*, **122**, 1426–33
43. D'Cruz, O. J. M. and Day, N. K. (1985). Structural and functional similarities between the major haemolymph protein of the fall army worm and cat C4-bp of the complement system. *Dev. Comp. Immunol.*, **9**, 541–50
44. Koch, C. and Nielsen, H. E. (1984). Activation of vertebrate complement by *Helix pomatia* haemolymph. *Dev. Comp. Immunol.*, **8**, 15-22
45. Gewurz, H., Finstad, J., Muschel, L. H. and Good, R. A. (1966). Phylogenic inquiry into the origins of the complement system. In Smith, R. T., Miescher, P. A. and Good, R. A. (eds.) *Phylogeny of Immunity*, pp. 105–17. (Gainesville: University of Florida Press)
46. Jensen, J. A., Festa, E., Smith, D. S. and Cayer, M. (1981). The complement system of the nurse shark: hemolytic and comparative characteristics. *Science*, **214**, 566–9
47. Ross, G. D. and Jensen, J. A. (1973). The first component (C1n) of the complement system of the nurse shark. I. Hemolytic characteristics of partially purified C1n. *J. Immunol.*, **110**, 175–82
48. Ross, G. D. and Jensen, J. A. (1973). The first component (C1n) of the complement system of the nurse shark. II. Purification of the first component by ultracentrifugation and studies of its physicochemical properties. *J. Immunol.*, **110**, 911–18
49. Hyder Smith, S. and Jensen, J. A. (1986). The second component (C2n) of the nurse shark complement system: purification, physico-chemical characterisation and functional comparison with guinea pig C4. *Dev. Comp. Immunol.*, **10**, 191–206
50. Jensen, J. A., Fuller, L. and Iglesia, E. (1973). The terminal components of the nurse shark (*Ginglymostoma cirratum*) C system. *J. Immunol.*, **111**, 306–7
51. Rijkers, G. T. (1982). Non lymphoid defence mechanisms in fish. *Dev. Comp. Immunol.*, **6**, 1–13
52. Kaastrup, P. and Koch, C. (1983). Complement in the carp fish. *Dev. Comp. Immunol.*, **7**, 781–2
53. Nonaka, M., Yamaguchi, N., Natsuume-Sakais, S. and Takahashi, M. (1981). The complement system in the rainbow trout (*Salmo gairdneri*). *J. Immunol.*, **126**, 1489–94
54. Stanley, K. K., Herz, J. and Dickson, J. (1987). Topological mapping of complement component C9 by recombinant DNA techniques suggests a novel mechanism for its insertion into target membranes. *EMBO J.*, **6**, 1951–7
55. Nonaka, M., Natsuume-Sakai, S. and Takahashi, M. (1981). The complement system of the rainbow trout. II. Purification and characterisation of the fifth component. *J. Immunol.*, **126**, 1495–8
56. Nonaka, M., Iwaki, M., Nakai, C., Nozaki, M., Kaidoh, T., Natsuume-Saki, S. and Takahashi, M. (1984). Purification of a major serum protein of rainbow trout (*Salmo gairdneri*) homologous to the third component of mammalian complement. *J. Biol. Chem.*, **259**, 6327–33
57. Nonaka, M., Irie, M., Tanabe, K., Kaidoh, T., Natsuume-Sakai, S. and Takahashi, M. (1985). Identification and characterisation of a variant of the third component of complement (C3) in rainbow trout (*Salmo gairdneri*) serum. *J. Biol. Chem.*, **260**, 809–15

58. Nakao, M., Yano, T. and Matsuyama, H. (1988). Partial purification and characterisation of the fourth component (C4) of carp complement. *Fish. Pathol.*, **23**, 243–50
59. Yano, T., Matsuyama, H. and Nakao, M. (1988). Isolation of the first component of complement (C1) from carp serum. *Nippon Suisan Gadkaishi,* **54**, 851–9
60. Kaidoh, T. and Gigli, I. (1987). Phylogeny of C4b-C3b cleaving activity: similar fragmentation patterns of human C4b and C3b produced by lower animals. *J. Immunol.*, **139**, 194-201
61. Kaidoh, T. and Gigli, I. (1989). Phylogeny of regulatory proteins of the complement system. Isolation and characterisation of a C4b/C3b inactivator and cofactor from sand bass plasma. *J. Immunol.*, **142**, 1605–13
62. Kristensen, T., D'Eustachio, P., Ogata, R. T., Chung, L. P., Reid, K. B. M. and Tack, B. F. (1987). The superfamily of C3b/C4b-binding proteins. *Fed. Proc.*, **46**, 2463–9
63. Johnson, H. and Smith, P. (1984). Attachment and phagocytosis by salmon macrophages of agarose beads coated with human C3b and iC3b. *Dev. Comp. Immunol.*, **8**, 623–30
64. Alexander, R. G. and Steiner, L. A. (1980). The first component of complement from the bullfrog, *Rana catesbeina*: functional properties of C1 and isolation of subcomponent C1q. *J. Immunol.*, **124**, 1418–25
65. Slayter, H. S., Alexander, R. J. and Steiner, L. A. (1983). Electron microscopy of complement protein C1q from the bull frog *Rana catesbiena*. *Eur. J. Immunol.*, **13**, 102–6
66. Sekizawa, A., Fujii, T. and Katagiri, C. (1984). Isolation and characterisation of the third component of complement of the serum of the clawed frog *Xenopus laevis*. *J. Immunol.*, **133**, 1436–43
67. Grossberger, D., Marcuz, A., Du Pasquier, L. and Lambris, J. D. (1989). Conservation of structural and functional domains in complement component C3 of *Xenopus* and mammals. *Proc. Natl. Acad. Sci. USA,* **86**, 132–7
68. Avila, D. and Lambris, J. D. (1990). Isolation and characterisation of the third complement component of axolotl (*Ambystoma mexicanum*). *Comp. Biochem. Physiol.*, **95B**, 839–45
69. Fujii, T., Sekizawa, A. and Katagiri, C. (1985). Characterisation of the fourth component of complement in the serum of the clawed frog *Xenopus laevis*. *Immunology*, **56**, 743–50
70. Nakamura, T., Sekizawa, A.. Fujii, T. and Katagini, C. H. (1986). Cosegregation of the polymorphic C4 with the MHC in the frog *Xenopus laevis*. *Immunogenetics*, **23**, 181–6
71. Sekizawa, A., Fujii, T. and Tochinai, S. (1984). Membrane receptors on *Xenopus* macrophages for two classes of immunoglobulins (IgM and IgY) and the third complement component (C3). *J. Immunol.*, **133**, 1431–5
72. Ewing, C. B. (1884). The action of rattlesnake venom upon the bacteriocidal power of the blood serum. *Lancet*, 1236–8
73. Eggertsen, G., Lind, P. and Sjoquist, J. (1981). Molecular characterisation of the complement activating protein in the venom of the Indian cobra (*Naja naja siamensis*). *Mol. Immunol.*, **18**, 125–33
74. Von Zabern, I., Przyklienk, H. and Vogt, W. (1982). Chain structure of cobra venom factor from *Naja naja* and *Naja haje* venom. *Scand. J. Immunol.*, **15**, 357–62
75. Minta, J. O. and Man, D. (1980). Immunological structural and functional relationships between an anti complementary protein from *Crotalus atrox* venom, cobra venom factor and human C3. *Immunology*, **39**, 503–9
76. Alper, C. A. and Balavitch, D. (1976). Cobra venom factor: evidence for its being altered cobra C3 (the third component of complement). *Science*, **191**, 1275–6
77. Eggertsen, G. E., Lundwall, A., Hellman, O. and Sjoquist, J. (1983). Antigenic relationships between human and cobra complement factor 3 and cobra venom factor (CVF) from Indian cobra (*Naja naja*). *J. Immunol.*, **131**, 1920–3
78. Grier, A. H., Schultz, M. and Vogel, C. W. (1987). Cobra venom factor and human C3 share carbohydrate antigenic determinants. *J. Immunol.*, **139**, 1245–52
79. Petrella, E. C., Bredenhorst, R. and Vogel, C. W. (1989). Purification of cobra C3: initial characterisation and comparison to cobra venom factor. *Complement Inflamm.*, **6**, 386–7
80. Vogel, C. W., Smith, C. A. and Muller-Eberhard, H. J. (1984). Cobra venom factor: structural homology with the third component of human complement. *J. Immunol.*, **133**, 3235–41
81. Becherer, J. D., Alsenz, J. and Lambris, J. D. (1989). Molecular aspects of C3 interactions and structural functional analysis of C3 from different species. *Curr. Top. Microbiol. Immunol.*, **153**, 45–72
82. Gans, C. (1978). Reptilian venoms: some evolutionary considerations. In Gans, C. (ed.) *Biology of the Reptilia*, pp. 1–42. (London: Academic Press)

83. Vogel, C. W. and Muller-Eberhard, H. J. (1985). The cobra complement system. I. The alternative pathway of activation. *Dev. Comp. Immunol.*, **9**, 311–25
84. Vogel, C. W. and Muller-Eberhard, H. J. (1985). The cobra complement system. II. The membrane attack complex. *Dev. Comp. Immunol.*, **9**, 327–33
85 Kawaguchi, S., Muramatsu, S. and Mitsuhashi, S. (1978). Natural haemolytic activity of snake serum. Natural antibody and complement. *Dev. Comp. Immunol.*, **2**, 287–96
86. Kawaguchi, S., Muramatsu, S. and Mitsuhashi, S. (1978). Natural hemolytic activity of snake serum. II. Heterogeneity of putative natural antibody and levels of hemolytic activity. *Dev. Comp. Immunol.*, **2**, 461–8
87. Barta, O. and Barta, V. (1975). Chicken (*Gallus gallus*) hemolytic complement: optimal conditions for its titration. *Immunol. Commun.*, **4**, 337–51
88. Koch, C., Josephsen, J., Nicolaisen, E. M. and Simonsen, M. (1982). Complement mediated lysis in chickens. *Dev. Comp. Immunol.*, **6**, 141–9
89. Koch, C., Kongerslev, L. and Jensen, L. B. (1983). The alternative complement pathway in chickens. *Dev. Comp. Immunol.*, **7**, 785–6
90. Koch, C. (1986). Complement system in avian species. In Toivanen, A. and Toivanen, P. (eds.) *Avian Immunology: Basis and Practice*, pp. 43–55. (CRC Press)
91. Yonemasu, K. and Sasaki, T. (1986). Purification, identification and characterisation of chicken C1q, a subcomponent of the first component of complement. *J. Immunol. Meth.*, **88**, 245–53
92. Yonemasu, K. and Sasaki, T. (1989). C1q a subcomponent of the first complement component: methods for the isolation from various animals. *Rev. Immunoassay Technol.*, **3**, 17–35
93. Kai, C. Y., Yoshikawa, Y., Yamanouchi, K. and Okada, H. (1983). Isolation and identification of the third component of complement of Japanese quails. *J. Immunol.*, **130**, 2814–20
94. Laursen, I. and Koch, C. (1989). Purification of chicken C3 and a structural and functional characterisation. *Scand. J. Immunol.*, **30**, 529–38
95. Koch, C. (1986). The alternative complement pathway in chickens. Purification of factor B and production of a monospecific antibody against it. *Acta Pathol. Microbiol. Scand.*, **94c**, 253–9
96. Koch, C. (1986). A genetic polymorphism of the complement component factor B in chickens not linked to the major histocompatibility complex. *Immunogenetics*, **23**, 364–7
97. Chanh, T. C., Benedict, A. A. and Abplanalp, H. (1976). Association of haemolytic levels with the major histocompatibility complex in chickens. *J. Exp. Med.*, **144**, 555–61
98. Guillemot, F., Billault, A., Pourquie, O., Behar, G., Chausse, A. M., Zoorob, R., Kreibich, G. and Auffray, C. (1988). A molecular map of the chicken major histocompatibility complex: the class II b genes are closely linked to the class I genes and the nucleolar organiser. *EMBO J.*, **7**, 2775–85
99. Kroemer, G., Bernot, A., Behar, G., Chausse, A. M., Gastinel, L. N., Guillemot, F., Park, I., Thoraval, P., Zoorob, R. and Auffray, C. (1990). Molecular genetics of the chicken MHC: current status and evolutionary aspects. *Immunol. Rev.*, **113**, 119–45
100. Whitehouse, D. B. (1988). Genetic polymorphism of animal complement components. *Expl. Clin. Immunogenet.*, **5**, 143–64
101. Rother, K. (1988). Complement deficient animals. In Rother, K. and Till, G. O. (eds.) *The Complement System*, pp. 444–51. (Berlin: Springer Verlag)
102. Williams, A. F. and Barclay, A. N. (1988). The immunoglobulin super family domains for cell surface recognition. *Annu. Rev. Immunol.*, **6**, 381–405
103. Baron, M., Norman, D. G. and Campbell, I. D. (1991). Protein modules. *Trends Biochem. Sci.*, **16**, 13–17
104. Day, A. J. and Baron, M. (1991). Structure/function inter-relationships of mosaic proteins. *J. Biomed. Sci.*, **1**, 153–63
105. Doolittle, R. F. (1985). The genealogy of some recently evolved vertebrate proteins. *Trends Biochem. Sci.*, **10**, 233–7
106. Reid, K. B. M. (1986). Activation and control of the complement system. *Essays Biochem.*, **22**, 27–68
107. Huber, R., Scholze, H., Paques, E. P. and Deisenhofer, J. (1980). Crystal structure analysis and molecular model of human C3a anaphylatoxin. *Hoppe-Seyler's Z. Physiol. Chem.*, **361**, 1389–99
108. Hugli, T. E. (1981). The structural basis for anaphylatoxin and chemotactic functions of C3a, C4a and C5a. *CRC Crit. Rev. Immunol.*, **1**, 321–51
109. Sottrup-Jensen, L., Folkersen, J., Kristensen, T. and Tack, B. F. (1984). Partial primary structure of human pregnancy zone protein: extensive sequence homology with human α2 macroglobulin. *Proc. Natl. Acad. Sci. USA*, **81**, 7353–7

110. Reid, K. B. M., Gagnon, J. and Frampton, J. (1982). Completion of the amino acid sequences of the A and B chains of subcomponent C1q of the first component of human complement. *Biochem. J.*, **203**, 559–69
111. Reid, K. B. M. (1985). Molecular cloning and characterization of the complementary DNA and gene coding for the B-chain of subcomponent C1q of the human complement system. *Biochem. J.*, **231**, 729–35
112. Sellar, G. C., Blake, D. J. and Reid, K. B. M. (1991). Characterization and organisation of the genes encoding the A-, B- and C-chains of human complement subcomponent C1q. *Biochem. J.*, **274**, 481–90
113. Malhotra, R., Thiel, S., Reid, K. B. M. and Sim, R. B. (1990). Human leukocyte C1q receptor binds other soluble proteins with collagen domains. *J. Exp. Med.*, **172**, 955–9
114. Reid, K. B. M. and Day, A. J. (1990). Ig-binding domains of C1q. *Immunol. Today*, **11**, 387–8
115. Yamaguchi, N., Benya, P. D., van der Rest, M. and Nimomiya, Y. (1989). The cloning and sequencing of α1 (VIII) collagen cDNAs demonstrate that the type VIII collagen is a short chain collagen and contains triple helical and carboxyl-terminal non-triple-helical domains similar to those of type X collagen. *J. Biol. Chem.*, **264**, 16022–9
116. Ninomiya, Y., Gordon, M., van der Rest, M., Schmid, T., Linsenmayer, T. and Olsen, B. R. (1986). The developmentally regulated type X collagen gene contains a long open reading frame without introns. *J. Biol. Chem.*, **261**, 5041–50
117. Doege, K., Sasaki, M., Horigan, E., Hassell, J. R. and Yamada, Y. (1987). Complete primary structure of the rat cartilage proteoglycan core protein deduced from cDNA clones. *J. Biol. Chem.*, **262**, 17757–67
118. Bonnet, F., Perin, J. P., Lorenzo, F., Jolles, J. and Jolles, P. C. (1986). An unexpected sequence homology between link proteins of the proteoglycan complex and immunoglobulin like proteins. *Biochim. Biophys. Acta*, **873**, 152–5
119. Carrell, R. and Travis, J. (1985). α1 Antitrypsin and the serpins: variation and counter variation. *Trends Biochem. Sci.*, **10**, 20–4
120. Bock, S. C., Shriver, K., Nielsen, E., Thogersen, H. C., Wiman, B., Donaldson, V. H., Eddy, R. L., Marrinan, J., Radziejewska, E., Huber, R., Shows, T. B. and Magnusson, S. (1986). Human C1 inhibitor. Primary structure, cDNA cloning and chromosomal localization. *Biochemistry*, **25**, 4292–301
121. Loebermann, H., Tokuoka, R., Deisenhofer, J. and Huber, R. (1984). Human α1-proteinase inhibitor: crystal structure analysis of two crystal modifications, molecular model and preliminary analysis of the implications for function. *J. Mol. Biol.*, **177**, 531–56
122. Luzio, J. P. and Stanley, K. K. (1988). Sequence homology of complement C8γ chain with α1 microglobulin and its implications for C8 structure and function. *Mol. Immunol.*, **25**, 513–16
123. Okada, H., Nagami, Y., Takahashi, K., Okada, N., Hideshima, T., Takizawa, H. and Kondo, J. (1989). 20 kDa homologous restriction factor of complement resembles T cell activating protein. *Biochem. Biophys. Res. Commun.*, **162**, 1553–9
124. Young, C. L., Barer, W. C., Tomaselli, C. M. and Dayhoff, M. O. (1978). Serine proteases. In Dayhoff, M. O. (ed.) *Atlas of Protein Sequence and Structure*, pp. 73–93. (Washington DC: National Biomedical Research Foundation)
125. Bentley, D. R. and Campbell, R. D. (1986). C2 and factor B: Structure and genetics. *Biochem. Soc. Symp.*, **51**, 7–18
126. Tosi, M., Journet, A., Duponchel, C., Tosi-Couture, E. and Meo, T. (1989). Human complement C1r and C1s proteins and genes: studies with molecular probes. *Behring. Inst. Mitt.*, **84**, 65–71
127. Maeda, N., Yang, F., Barnett, D. R., Bowman, B. H. and Smithies, O. (1984). Duplication within the haptoglobin Hp2 gene. *Nature* , **309**, 131–5
128. Reid, K. B. M. and Day, A. J. (1989). Structure–function relationships of the complement components. *Immunol. Today*, **10**, 177–80
129. Catterall, C. F., Lyons, A., Sim, R. B., Day, A. J. and Harris, T. J. R. (1987). Characterization of the primary amino acid sequence of human complement control protein factor I from an analysis of cDNA clones. *Biochem. J.*, **242**, 849–56
130. Day, A. J., Campbell, R. D. and Reid, K. B. M. (1989). The mosaic nature of the complement proteins. In Melchers, F. (ed.) *Progress in Immunology VII*, pp. 209–12 (Berlin/Heidelberg: Springer-Verlag)
131. Patthy, L. (1987). Detecting homology of distantly related proteins with consensus sequences. *J. Mol. Biol.*, **198**, 567–77

132. Klickstein, L. B., Wong, W. W., Smith, J. A., Weis, J. H., Wilson, J. G. and Fearon, D. T. (1987). Human C3b/C4b receptor (CR1). Demonstration of long homologous repeating domains that are composed of the short consensus repeats characteristic of C3/C4 binding proteins. *J. Exp. Med.*, **165**, 1095–112
133. Campbell, R. D., Bentley, D. R. and Morley, B. J. (1984). The factor B and C2 genes. *Phil. Trans. R. Soc. Lond. B.*, **306**, 367–78
134. Leonard, W. J., Depper, J. M., Kanehisa, M., Kronke, M., Peffer, N. J., Svetlik, P. B., Sullivan, M. and Greene, W. C. (1985). Structure of the human interleukin-2 receptor gene. *Science*, **230**, 633–9
135. Vik, D. P., Keeney, J. B., Munoz-Canoves, P., Chaplin, D. D. and Tack, B. F. (1988). Structure of the murine complement factor H gene. *J. Biol. Chem.*, **263**, 16720–4
136. Ord, D. C., Ernst, T. J., Zhou, L. J., Rambaldi, A., Spertini, O., Griffin, J. and Tedder, T. F. (1990). Structure of the gene encoding the human leukocyte adhesion molecule-1 (TQ1, Leu-8) of lymphocytes and neutrophils. *J. Biol. Chem.*, **265**, 7760–7
137. Hourcade, D., Meisner, D. R., Atkinson, J. P. and Holers, V. M. (1988). Identification of an alternative polyadenylation site in the human C3b/C4b receptor (complement receptor type 1) transcriptional unit and prediction of a secreted form of complement receptor type 1. *J. Exp. Med.*, **168**, 1255–70
138. Chung, L. P., Bentley, D. R. and Reid, K. B. M. (1985). Molecular cloning and characterisation of the cDNA coding for C4b-binding protein, a regulatory protein of the classical pathway of the human complement system. *Biochem. J.*, **230**, 133–41
139. Hillarp, A. and Dahlback, B. (1990). Cloning of cDNA coding for the b chain of human complement component C4b-binding protein: sequence homology with the a chain. *Proc. Natl. Acad. Sci. USA*, **87**, 1183–7
140. Lublin, D. M., Liszewski, M. K., Post, T. W., Arce, M. A., Le Beau, M. M., Rebentische, M. B., Lemons, R. S., Seya, T. and Atkinson, J. P. (1988). Molecular cloning and chromosomal localization of human membrane cofactor protein (MVP). Evidence for inclusion in the multigene family of complement-regulatory proteins. *J. Exp. Med.*, **168**, 181–94
141. Medof, M. E., Lublin, D. M., Holers, V. M., Ayers, D. J., Getty, R. R., Leykam, J. K., Atkinson, J. P. and Tykocinski, M. L. (1987). Cloning and characterization of cDNAs encoding the complete sequence of decay-accelerating factor of human complement. *Proc. Natl. Acad. Sci. USA*, **84**, 2007–11
142. Caras, I. W., Davitz, M. A., Rhee, L., Weddell, G., Martin, D. W. and Nussenzweig, V. (1987). Cloning of decay-accelerating factor suggests novel use of splicing to generate two proteins. *Nature*, **325**, 545–9
143. Weis, J. J., Toothaker, E., Smith, J. A., Weis, J. H. and Fearon, D. T. (1988). Structure of the human B lymphocyte receptor for C3d and the Epstein–Barr virus and relatedness to other members of the family of C3/C4 binding proteins. [Published erratum appears in *J. Exp. Med.* 1988 Nov 1; **168** (5): 1953–4.] *J. Exp. Med.*, **167**, 1047–66
144. Ripoche, J., Day, A. J., Harris, T. J. R. and Sim, R. B. (1988). The complete amino acid sequence of human complement factor H. *Biochem. J.*, **249**, 593–602
145. Rodriguez de Cordoba, S. and Rubinstein, P. (1987). New alleles of C4-binding protein and factor H and further linkage data in the regulator of complement activation (RCA) gene cluster in man. *Immunogenetics*, **25**, 267–8
146. Carroll, M. C., Alicot, E. M., Katzman, P. J., Klickstein, L. B., Smith, J. A. and Fearon, D. T. (1988). The organization of the gene encoding complement receptors type 1 and 2, decay-accelerating factor, and C4-binding protein in the RCA locus on human chromosome 1. *J. Exp. Med.*, **167**, 1271–80
147. Rey-Campos, J., Rubinstein, P. and Rodriguez de Cordoba, S. (1988). A physical map of the human regulator of complement gene cluster linking the complement genes CR1, CR2, DAF, and C4-bp. *J. Exp. Med.*, **167**, 664–9
148. Pardo-Manuel, F., Rey-Campos, J., Hillarp, A., Dahlback, B. and Rodriquez de Cordoba, S. (1990). Human genes for the a and b chains of the complement C4b-binding protein are closely linked in a head-to-tail arrangement. *Proc. Natl. Acad. Sci. USA*, **87**, 4529–32
149. Ichinose, A., McMullen, B. A., Fujikawa, K. and Davie, E. W. (1986). Amino acid sequence of the b subunit of human factor XIII, a protein composed of ten repetitive segments. *Biochemistry*, **25**, 4633–8
150. Rodriguez de Cordoba, S., Rey-Campos, J., Dykes, D. D., McAlpine, P. J., Wong, P. and Rubinstein, P. (1988). Coagulation factor XIII B subunit is encoded by a gene linked to the

regulator of complement activation (RCA) gene cluster in man. *Immunogenetics*, **28**, 452–4

151. Sim, R. B. and Perkins, S. J. (1990). Molecular modelling of C3 and its ligands. *Curr. Top. Microbiol.*, **153**, 209–22
152. Klickstein, L. B., Bartow, T. J., Miletic, V., Rabson, L. D., Smith, J. A. and Fearon, D. T. (1988). Identification of distinct C3b and C4b recognition sites in the human C3b/C4b receptor (CR1, CD35) by deletion mutagenesis. *J. Exp. Med.*, **168**, 1699–717
153. Carel, J. C., Myones, B. L., Frazier, B. and Holers, V. M. (1990). Structural requirement for C3dg/Epstein–Barr virus receptor (CR2/Cd21) ligand binding, internalization, and viral infection. *J. Biol. Chem.*, **265**, 12293–9
154. Johnson, G. I., Cook, R. G., Le Beau, M. M. and McEver, R. P. (1989). Cloning of GMP-140, a granule membrane protein of platelets and endothelium: sequence similarity to proteins involved in cell adhesion and inflammation. *Cell*, **56**, 1033–44
155. Bevilacqua, M. P., Stengelin, S., Gimbrone, M. A. and Seed, B. (1989). Endothelial leukocyte adhesion molecule 1: an inducible receptor for neutrophils related to complement regulatory proteins and lectins. *Science*, **243**, 1160–5
156. Lasky, L., Singer, M. S., Yednock, T. A., Dowbenko, D., Fennie, C., Rodriguez, H., Nguyen, T., Stachel, S. and Rosen, S. D. (1989). Cloning of a lymphocyte homing receptor reveals a lectin domain. *Cell*, **54,** 1045–55
157. Watson, M. L., Kingsmore, S. F., Johnson, G. I., Siegelman, M. H., Le Beau, M. M., Lemons, R. S., Bora, N. S., Howard, T. A., Weissman, I. L., McEver, R. P. and Seldin, M. F. (1990). Genomic organisation of the selection family of leukocyte adhesion molecules on human and mouse chromosome 1. *J. Exp. Med.*, **172**, 263–72
158. Springer, T. A. (1990). Adhesion receptors of the immune system. *Nature*, **346**, 425–34
159. Lozier, J., Takahshi, N. and Putman, F. W. (1984). Complete amino acid sequence of human plasma β_2-glycoprotein I. *Proc. Natl. Acad. Sci. USA*, **81**, 3640–4
160. Steinkasserer, A., Estaller, C., Weiss, E. H., Sim, R. B. and Day, A. J. (1991). Complete nucleotide and deduced amino acid sequence of human β_2-glycoprotein I. *Biochem. J.*, **277**, 387–91
161. Libert, F., Ruel, J., Ludgate, M., Swillens, S., Alexander, N., Vassart, G. and Dinsart, C. (1987). Thyroperoxidase, an auto-antigen with a mosaic structure made of nuclear and mitochondrial gene modules. *EMBO J.*, **63**, 4193–6
162. Baldwin, C. T., Reginato, A. M. and Prockop, D. J. (1989). A new epidermal growth factor-like domain in the human core protein for the large cartilage-specific proteoglycan. Evidence for alternative splicing of the domain. *J. Biol. Chem.*, **264**, 15747–50
163. Kotwal, G. J. and Moss, B. (1988). Vaccinia virus encodes a secretory polypeptide structurally related to complement control proteins. *Nature*, **335**, 176–8
164. Kotwal, G. J., Isaacs, S. N., McKenzie, R., Frank, M. M. and Moss, B. (1990). Inhibition of the complement cascade by the major secretory protein of vaccinia virus. *Science*, **250**, 827–30
165. Muta, T., Miyata, T., Tokunaga, T., Nakamura, T. and Iwanaga, S. (1990). Molecular mechanism of haemolymph clotting system in Limulus. *Dev. Comp. Immunol.*, **14**, III
166. Barlow, P. N., Baron, M., Norman, D. G., Day, A. J., Willis, A. C., Sim, R. B. and Campbell, I. D. (1991). Secondary structure of the complement control protein module by two-dimensional ^{1}H NMR. *Biochemistry*, **30**, 997–1004
167. Norman, D. G., Barlow, P. N., Baron, M., Day, A. J., Sim, R. B. and Campbell, I. D. (1991). The three-dimensional structure of a complement control protein module in solution. *J. Mol. Biol*, **219**, 717–25
168. Lawler, J. and Hynes, R. O. (1986). The structure of human thrombospondin, an adhesive glycoprotein with multiple calcium-binding sites and homologies with several different proteins. *J. Cell. Biol.*, **103**, 1635–48
169. Goundis, D. and Reid, K. B. M. (1988). Properdin, the terminal complement components, thrombospondin and the circumsporozoite protein of malaria parasites contain similar sequence motifs. *Nature*, **335**, 82–5
170. Nolan, K. F., Schwaeble, W., Kaluz, S., Dierich, M. P. and Reid, K. B. M. (1991). Molecular cloning of a cDNA coding for properdin, a positive regulator of the alternative pathway of human complement. *Eur. J. Immunol.* **21**, 771–6
171. DiScipio, R. G. and Hugli, T. E. (1989). The molecular architecture of human complement component C6. *J. Biol. Chem.*, **264**, 16197–206

172. DiScipio, R. G., Chakravarti, D. N., Müller-Eberhard, H. J and Fey, G. H. (1988). The structure of human complement component C7 and C5b-7 complex. *J. Biol. Chem.*, **263**, 549–60
173. Rao, A. G., Howard, Z., Ng, S. C., Whitehead, A. S., Colten, H. R. and Sodetz, J. M. (1987). Complementary DNA and derived amino acid sequence of the alpha subunit of human complement protein C8: evidence for the existence of a separate alpha subunit messenger RNA. *Biochemistry*, **26**, 3556–64
174. Haefliger, J. A., Tschopp, J., Naedelli, D., Wahli, W., Kocher, H. P., Tosi, M. and Stanley, K. K. (1987). Complementary DNA cloning of complement C8 beta and its sequence homology to C9. *Biochemistry*, **26**, 3551–6
175. Howard, O. M., Rao, A. G. and Sodetz, J. M. (1987). Complementary DNA and derived amino acid sequence of the beta subunit of human complement protein C8: identification of a close structural and ancestral relationship to the alpha subunit and C9. *Biochemistry*, **26**, 3565–70
176. DiScipio, R. G., Gehring, M. R., Podack, E. R., Kan, C. C., Hugli, T. E. and Fey, G. F. (1984). Nucleotide sequence of cDNA and derived amino acid sequence of human complement component C9. *Proc. Natl. Acad. Sci. USA*, **81**, 7298–302
177. Stanley, K. K., Kocher, H. P., Luzio, J. P., Jackson, P. and Tschopp, J. (1985). The sequence and topology of human complement component C9. *EMBO J.*, **4**, 375–82
178. Patthy, L. (1988). Detecting distant homologies of mosaic proteins. *J. Mol. Biol.*, **202**, 689–96
179. Wolf, F. W., Eddy, R. L., Shows, T. B. and Dixit, V. M. (1990). Structure and chromosomal localization of the human thrombospondin gene. *Genomics*, **6**, 685–91
180. Marazziti, D., Eggertsen, G., Fey, G. H. and Stanley, K. K. (1988). Relationships between the gene and protein structure in human complement. *Biochemistry*, **27**, 6529–34
181. Perkins, S. J., Nealis, A. S., Haris, P. I., Chapman, D., Goundis, D. and Reid, K. B. M. (1989). Secondary structure in properdin of the complement cascade and related proteins: A study by Fourier transform infrared spectroscopy. *Biochemistry*, **28**, 7176–82
182. Smith, C. A., Pangburn, M. K., Vogel, C. and Müller-Eberhard, H. J. (1984). The molecular architecture of human properdin, a positive regulator of the alternative pathway of complement. *J. Biol. Chem.*, **259**, 4582–8
183. Robson, K. J. H., Hall, J. R. S., Jennings, M. W., Harris, T. J. R., Marsh, K., Newbold, C. I., Tate, V. E. and Weatherall, D. J. (1988). A highly conserved amino-acid sequence in thrombospondin, properdin and in proteins from sporozoites and blood stages of a human malaria parasite. *Nature*, **335**, 79–82
184. Yamamoto, T., Davis, C. G., Brown, M. S., Schneider, W. J., Casey, M. L., Goldstein, J. L. and Russell, D. W. (1984). The human LDL receptor: a cysteine-rich protein with multiple Alu sequences in its mRNA. *Cell*, **39**, 27–38
185. Strickland, D. K., Ashcom, J. D., Williams, S., Burgess, W. H., Migliorini, M. and Argraves, W. S. (1990). Sequence identity between the α2 macroglobulin receptor and low density lipoprotein receptor related protein suggests that this molecule is a multifunctional receptor. *J. Biol. Chem.*, **265**, 17401–4
186. Sudhof, T. C., Goldstein, J. L., Brown, M. S. and Russell, D. W. (1985). The LDL receptor gene: a mosaic of exons shared with different proteins. *Science*, **228**, 815–22
187. Scott, J., Urdea, M., Quiroga, M., Sanchez-Pescador, R., Fong, N., Selby, M., Rutter, W. J. and Bell, G. I. (1983). Structure of a mouse submaxillary messenger RNA encoding epidermal growth factor and seven related proteins. *Science*, **221**, 236–40
188. Doolittle, R. F., Feng, D. F. and Johnson, M. S. (1984). Computer-based characterization of epidermal growth factor precursor. *Nature*, **307**, 558–60
189. Campbell, I. D., Cooke, R. M., Baron, M., Harvey, T. S. and Tappin, M. J. (1989). The solution structures of epidermal growth factor and transforming growth factor alpha. *Prog. Growth Factor Res.*, **1**, 13–22
190. Appella, E., Weber, I. T. and Blasi, F. (1988). Structure and function of epidermal growth factor-like regions in proteins. *FEBS Lett.*, **231**, 1–4
191. Rees, D. J. G., Jones, I. M., Handford, P. A., Walter, S. J., Esnouf, M. P., Smith, K. J. and Brownlee, G. G. (1988). The role of β-hydroxyaspartate and adjacent carboxylate residues in the first EGF domain of human factor IX. *EMBO J.*, **7**, 2053–61
192. Leytus, S. P., Kurachi, K., Sakariassen, K. S. and Davie, E. E. (1986). Nucleotide sequence of the cDNA coding for human complement C1r. *Biochemistry*, **25**, 4855–63
193. Journet, A. and Tosi, M. (1986). Cloning and sequencing of full-length cDNA encoding the precursor of human complement component C1r. *Biochem. J.*, **240**, 783–7

194. Mackinnon, C. M., Carter, P. E., Shyth, S. J., Dunbar, B. and Fothergill, J. E. (1987). Molecular cloning of cDNA for human complement component C1s. The complete amino acid sequence. *Eur. J. Biochem.*, **169**, 547–53
195. Thielens, N. M., Aude, C. A., Larcroix, M. B., Gagnon, J. and Arlaud, G. J. (1990). Ca^{2+} binding properties and Ca^{2+}-dependent interactions of the isolated NH_2-terminal alpha fragments of human complement proteases C1-r and C1-s. *J. Biol. Chem.*, **265**, 14469–75
196. Thielens, N. M., Van Dorsselaer, A., Gagnon, J. and Arlaud, G. J. (1990). Chemical and function characterization of a fragment of C1-s containing the epidermal growth factor homology region. *Biochemistry*, **29**, 3570–8
197. Shinkai, Y., Takio, K. and Okumura, K. (1988). Homology of perforin to the ninth component of complement (C9). *Nature*, **334**, 525–7
198. Delgadillo-Reynoso, M. G., Rollo, D. R. and Raff, R. A. (1989). Structural analysis of the uEGF gene in the sea urchin *Strongylocentrotus purpuratus* reveals more similarity to vertebrate than to invertebrate genes with EGF-like repeats. *J. Mol. Evol.*, **29**, 314–27
199. Law, S. K. A., Gagnon, J., Hildreth, J. E. K., Wells, C. E., Willis, A. C. and Wong, A. J. (1987). The primary structure of the β-subunit of the cell surface adhesion glycoproteins LFA-1, CR3 and p150,95 and its relationship to the fibronection receptor. *EMBO J.*, **6**, 915–19
200. Kishimoto, T. K., O'Connor, K., Lee, A., Roberts, T. M. and Springer, T. A. (1987). Cloning of the beta subunit of the leukocyte adhesion proteins: homology to an extracellular matrix receptor defines a novel supergene family. *Cell*, **48**, 681–90
201. Larson, R. S., Corbi, A. L., Berman, L. and Springer, T. (1989). Primary structure of the leukocyte function-associated molecule-1 alpha subunit: an integrin with an embedded domain defining a protein superfamily. *J. Cell. Biol.*, **108**, 703–12
202. Corbi, A. L., Miller, L. J., O'Connor, K., Larson, R. S. and Springer, T. A. (1987). cDNA cloning and complete primary structure of the α subunit of a leukocyte adhesion glycoprotein, p150,95. *EMBO J.*, **6**, 4023–8
203. Pytela, R. (1988). Amino acid sequence of the murine MAC-1 alpha chain reveals homology with the integrin family and an additional domain related to von Willebrand factor. *EMBO J.*, **7**, 1371–8
204. Shelton-Inloes, B. B., Titani, K. and Sadler, J. E. (1986). cDNA sequences for human von Willebrand factor reveal five types of repeated domains and five possible protein sequence polymorphisms. *Biochemistry*, **25**, 3164–71
205. Patthy, L. (1985). Evolution of the proteases of blood coagulation and fibrinolysis by assembly from modules. *Cell*, **41**, 657–63
206. Gilbert, W. (1985). Genes-in-pieces revisited. *Science*, **228**, 823–4
207. Patthy, L. (1987). Intron-dependent evolution: preferred types of exons and introns. *FEBS Lett.*, **214**, 1–7
208. Sottrup-Jensen, L., Stepanik, T. M., Wierzbicki, D. M., Jones, C. M., Lonblad, P. B., Kirstensen. T., Mortensen, S. B., Petersen, T. E. and Magnusson, S. (1983). The primary structure of α2 macroglobulin and localization of a factor XIII cross linking site. *Ann. N. Y. Acad. Sci.*, **421**, 41–60
209. Gehring, M. R., Shiels, B. R., Northemann, W., de Brujin, M. H. L., Kan, C. C., Chain, A. C., Noonan, D. J. and Fey, G. H. (1987). Sequence of rat liver α2 macroglobulin and acute phase control of its messenger RNA. *J. Biol. Chem.*, **262**, 446–54
210. Roberts, R. C. and Hall, P. K. (1983). Specificity of proteinases for the bait region of α2 macroglobulin. *Ann. N. Y. Acad. Sci.*, **421**, 61–8
211. Jensen, P. H., Moestrup, S. K. and Gliemann, J. (1989). Purification of the human placental α2 macroglobulin receptor. *FEBS Lett.*, **255**, 275–80
212. Moestrup, S. K. and Gliemann, J. (1989). Purification of rat hepatic α2 macroglobulin receptor as an approximately 400 kDa single chain protein. *J. Biol. Chem.*, **264**, 15574–7
213. Ashcom, J. D., Tiller, S. E., Dickerson, K., Cravens, J. L., Argraves, W. S. and Strickland, D. K. (1990). The human alpha 2 macroglobulin receptor: identification of a 420 kd surface glycoprotein specific for activated conformations of alpha 2 macroglobulin. *J. Cell Biol.*, **110**, 1041–8
214. Moestrup, S. K., Kaltoft, K., Sottrup-Jensen, L. and Gliemann, J. (1990). The human α2M receptor contains high affinity calcium binding sites important for receptor conformation and ligand recognition. *J. Biol. Chem.*, **265**, 12623–8
215. Herz, J. J., Hamann, U., Rogne, S., Mylebost, O., Gausepohl, H. and Stanley, K. K. (1988). Surface location a high affinity for calcium of a 500 kd liver membrane protein closely related

to the LDL receptor suggest a physiological role as a lipoprotein receptor. *EMBO J.*, **7**, 4119–27

216. Herz, J., Kowal, R. C., Goldstein, J. L. and Brown, M. S. (1990). Proteolytic processing of the 600 kd low density lipoprotein receptor-related protein (LRP) occurs in the trans-Golgii. *EMBO J.*, **9**, 1769–6
217. Macfarlane, R. G. (1964). An enzyme cascade in the blood clotting mechanism, and its function as a biochemical amplifier. *Nature*, **202**, 498–9
218. Macfarlane, R. G. (1969). A discussion on triggered enzyme systems in blood plasma: general introduction. *Proc. R. Soc. B.*, **173**, 259
219. Doolittle, R. F. and Feng, D. F. (1987). Reconstructing the evolution of vertebrate blood coagulation from a consideration of the amino acid sequences clotting proteins. *Cold Spring Harbor Symp. Quant. Biol.*, **52**, 869–74
220. Ratnoff, O. D. (1987). The evolution of hemostatic mechanisms. *Perspect. Biol. Med.*, **31**, 4–33
221. Soderhall, K. and Smith, V. J. (1986). Prophenoloxudase-activating cascade as a recognition and defence system in arthropods. In Grupta, A. P. (ed.) *Hemolytic and Humoral Immunity in Arthropods*, pp. 251–85. (New York: John Wiley)
222. Farries, T. C., Steuer, K. L. and Atkinson, J. P. (1990). Evolutionary implications of a new bypass activation pathway of the complement system. *Immunol. Today*, **11**, 78–80
223. Thiel, S., Baatrup, G., Friis-Christiansen, P., Svehag, S. E. and Jensenius, J. C. (1987). Characterisation of a lectin in human plasma analogous to bovine conglutinin. *Scand. J. Immunol.*, **26**, 461–8
224. Muramoto, K. and Kaniya, H. (1986). The amino acid sequence of a lectin of the acorn barnacle *Megabalanus rosa*. *Biochim. Biophys. Acta*, **874**, 285–95
225. Takahashi, H., Komano, H., Kawaguchi, N., Kitamujra, N., Nakanishi, S. and Natori, S.(1985). Cloning and sequencing of cDNA of *Sarcophaga peregrina* humoral lectin induced on injury of the body wall. *J. Biol. Chem.*, **260**, 12228–33
226. Ghebrehiwet, B. (1987). C1q receptor. *Meth. Enzymol.*, **150**, 558–78
227. Baltz, M. L., De Beer, F. C., Feinstein, A., Munn, E. A., Milstein, C. P., Fletcher, T. C., March, J. F., Taylor, J., Bruton, C., Clamp, J. R., Davies, A. J. S. and Pepys, M. B. (1982). Phylogenic aspects of C reactive protein and related proteins. *Ann. N. Y. Acad. Sci.*, **389**, 49–73
228. Mold, C., Du Clos, T. W., Nakayama, S., Edwards, K. M. and Gewurz, H. (1982). C reactive protein reactivity with complement and effects on phagocytosis. *Ann. N. Y. Acad. Sci.*, **389**, 251–9
229. Vasta, G. R., Hunt, J. C., Marchelonis, J. J. and Fish, W. W. (1986). Galactosyl binding lectins from the tunicate *Didemnum candidum*. Purification and physiochemical characterisation. *J. Biol. Chem.*, **261**, 9174–81
230. Volanakis, J. E. (1982). Complement activation by C-reactive protein. *Ann. N. Y. Acad. Sci.*, **389**, 235–49
231. Pepys, M. B., Baltz, M. L., De Beer, F. C., Dyck, R. F., Holford, S., Breathnach, S. M., Black, M. M., Tribe, C. R., Evans, D. J. and Feinstein, A. (1982). Biology of serum amyloid P component. *Ann. N. Y. Acad. Sci.*, **389**, 286–7
232. Bristow, C. L. and Boackle, R. J. (1986). Evidence for the binding of human serum amyloid P component to C1q and Fab. *Mol. Immunol.*, **23**, 1045–52
233. Enghild, J. J., Thogersen, I. B., Salvesen, G., Fey, G. H., Figler, N. L., Gonias, S. L. and Pizzo, S. V. (1990). α-Macroglobulin from *Limulus polyphemus* exhibits proteinase inhibitory activity and participates in a hemolytic system. *Biochemistry*, **29**, 10070–80

234 Muta, T., Miyata, T., Misumi, Y., Tokunaga, F., Nakamura, T., Toh, Y., Ikehara, Y. and Iwanaga, S. (1991). Limulus factor C. An endotoxin sensitive serine protease zymogen with a mosiac structure of complement-like, epidermal growth factor-like and lectin like domains. *J. Biol. Chem.*, **266**, 6554–61

235 Nonaka, M. and Takahashi, M.(1992). Complete complementary DNA sequence of the third component of complement of lamprey. *J. Immunol.*, **148**, 3290–5

236 Ishiguro, H., Kobayashi, K., Suzuki, M., Titani, K., Tomonaga, S. and Kurosawa, Y. (1992). Isolation of a hagfish gene that encodes a complement component. *EMBOJ.*, **11** 829-37

3
Structure and organization of complement genes

K. B. M. REID and R. D. CAMPBELL

INTRODUCTION

Most of the proteins and receptors associated with the activation and control of the complement system have now been cloned at both the cDNA and genomic levels and chromosome assignments are available for the majority of the genes (Table 3.1). There are two distinct clusters of complement genes: the C2, C4 and factor B genes on human chromosome 6 at 6p21.3, which constitute the MHC class III complement genes; the factor H, C4-bp (α and β), CR1, CR2, MCP and DAF genes, present on human chromosome 1 at 1q32, which constitute the regulators of complement activation (RCA) cluster. Apart from the genes encoding the closely related A-, B- and C-chains of human C1q (on 1p34-1p36.3) and pairs of genes, such as components C6 and C7 (on 5q), the C8α and C8β chains (1p34) and the human C1r and C1s proenzymes (on 12p13), the genes for other complement proteins and receptors are distributed on quite a wide variety of different chromosomes. In view of the structural and functional similarity between the terminal components of complement C6, C7, C8α, C8β, C9 and perforin, it might have been expected that they would perhaps all be linked, but this does not appear to be the case.

The class III MHC complement genes show a relatively high degree of polymorphism and this is especially true for C4 which is encoded by two separate loci, C4A and C4B, with at least 33 allotypes being assigned to date. As outlined later in this chapter, certain alleles of C4 are clearly linked with susceptibility to autoimmune diseases, such as systemic lupus erythematosus. The other complement genes do not display a high degree of polymorphism but genetic deficiencies of most of the components (except factor B) have been reported and, in many cases, the primary basis for the defect has been analysed by use of the available cDNA and genomic probes and sequencing of the defective gene.

Table 3.1 Chromosomal localization of proteins and receptors associated with the activation and control of the human serum complement system

Component	*Chromosomal localization*
Plasma components	
Classical pathway	Chromosomal localization
C1q (A, B and C chains)	1p34-1p36.3
C1r } close linkage	12p13
C1s } close linkage	12p13
C4	6p21.3
C2	6p21.3
Alternative pathway	
Factor B	6p21.3
Factor D	Unknown
C3	19
Terminal pathway	
C5	9q32-9q34
C6	5q
C7	5q
C8 (α and β linked)	1p34
C8γ	9q
C9	5p13
Regulatory proteins	
Plasma	
Properdin	Xp11.23-Xp11.3
C1 inhibitor	11p11.2-11q13
Factor I	4q24-4q26
C4b-binding protein (α and β chains)	1q32
Factor H	1q
Sprotein/vitronectin	Unknown
Sp40,40	Unknown
Anaphylatoxin inactivator	Unknown
Membrane bound	
DAF (CD55)	1q32
MCP (CD46)	1q32
HRF (65 kDa homologous restriction factor)	Unknown
CD59 (protectin, HRF20, MACIF)	11p
Complement receptors	
CR1 (CD35)	1q32
CR2 (CD21)	1q32
CR3 (CD11b/CD18)	16p11-16p13.1 (CD11a, b, and c)
CR4 (CD11c/CD 18)	21q22.1 (CD18)
CR5	Unknown
C5a receptor	Unknown
C3a receptor	Unknown
C1q receptor	Unknown

In this chapter, a brief description of the structure and function of each component/control protein/receptor is given and this is related to what is known, in each case, about the gene structure, chromosomal localization and genetic deficiency.

THE C1 COMPLEX

C1, the first component of complement, is composed of subcomponent C1q (460 kDa) and the Ca^{2+}-dependent $C1r_2$:$C1s_2$ proenzyme complex (360 kDa). The C1q molecule plays a recognition role in classical pathway activation by binding, via its globular heads, to immune complexes containing IgM and certain subclasses of IgG. This binding brings about the activation of the $C1r_2$:$C1s_2$ proenzyme complex which is located on collagen-like regions present in the C1q molecule.

The A-, B- and C-chains of C1q

The human C1q molecule is composed of six A-, six B- and six C-chains, the three types of chains having a similar overall structure, i.e. a collagen-like region of approximately 81 residues located near the N-terminus and a C-terminal globular region of approximately 136 residues[1]. When viewed in the electron microscope, C1q is seen to have a hexameric structure in which six triple-helical regions are formed between the collagen-like sequences in the A-, B- and C-chains to yield a fibril-like central region and six collagen-like 'stalks'. A globular 'head', formed by association of the C-terminal regions of the A-, B- and C-chains, is found at the end of the stalks[2,3]. Amino acid sequence and cDNA studies established the primary sequences of the entire A- and B-chains and the collagen-like region of the C-chain[4–7]. The isolation of overlapping cosmid clones allowed the derivation of the entire primary amino acid sequence of the C-chain and the mapping and alignment of the genes encoding the A-, B- and C-chains of human C1q[7,8]. The genes are aligned $5' \rightarrow 3'$, in the same orientation, in the order of A-C-B on a 24 kb stretch of DNA on the 1p34.1-1p36.3 region of chromosome 1[8–10]. The A-, B- and C-chain genes are approximately 2.5, 2.6 and 3.2 kb long, respectively, and each contains one intron which is located within a codon for a glycine residue positioned half way along the collagen-like region present in each chain. These glycine residues are located just prior to the point where the triple-helical portions of the C1q molecule are interrupted and appear to 'bend' when viewed in the electron microscope and thus the positioning of the introns implies conservation of an important structural feature in the molecule. There is a structural similarity at both the DNA[11] and protein levels[12] between the chains of C1q and those of mannan-binding protein (MBP), a lectin found in serum. The collagen-like regions of the chains of MBP are also interrupted about half way along their length, at the protein level by disruption of the Gly-X-Y-repeating sequence and at the DNA level by the presence of an intron. MBP can mimic C1q function by binding to suitable carbohydrate structures and activating the $C1r_2$ $C1s_2$ complex, thus causing efficient antibody-independent activation of the classical pathway[12] which may be of considerable importance in conditions where there is little or no antibody response to a pathogenic organism in the blood[13].

Southern blot analyses on genomic DNA from a number of normal individuals, using probes from each of the three chains, indicate that there is only one gene per chain. Although the first cDNA clone for a chain of C1q (the B-chain; Reid, 1985[7]) was isolated from a liver cDNA library, the use of both human and mouse cDNA probes indicates that macrophages are likely to be the primary source of serum C1q. Northern blot analysis of mRNA isolated from human monocytes, which showed macrophage-like adherent properties after 3–7 days culture, gave strong signals at approx. 1.4 kb with probes for all three chains, while mRNA from liver gave a very weak signal and no signal at all was obtained from mRNA isolated from non-adherent monocytes and the U937 cell line. Studies on the source of synthesis of mouse C1q by Northern blot analysis, using mouse A- and B-chain cDNA probes, gave strong signals from mRNA isolated from peritoneal macrophages (both activated and unactivated), moderate signals from spleen, thymus and heart, and very weak signals from liver, kidney, lung and intestine[14,15]. This apparent tissue specificity in expression of C1q is consistent with the finding of efficient synthesis and release of C1q by three-day cultures of human or mouse macrophages[16–18].

Use of the cDNA and genomic probes, coding for the chains of C1q, in Southern blot analysis of genomic DNA from C1q-deficient patients from three families showed that none of these individuals possessed any large deletions or insertions within the structural genes for the C1q chains[8]. Only in one case of C1q deficiency has the probable defect been located: in this patient, there is a loss of a Taq I restriction site within the B-chain by virtue of a homozygous point mutation in the DNA, at the position coding for residue 150 in the chain, which results in the generation of a termination codon[19]. Since no material corresponding to the A- and C-chains, or a truncated B-chain, was found in the patient's serum, it seems likely that a virtually complete B chain must be synthesized before assembly and secretion of even a modified form of C1q takes place. Preliminary studies on three individuals of another C1q-deficient family have revealed the lack of two Sty I restriction enzyme sites in the C-chain gene, and one of these sites lies within the coding sequence for the C-chain[14]. From the data available at present, it seems probable that genetic deficiency of C1q may be due primarily to a number of different point mutations, or small deletion or insertion events, within any of the A-, B- or C-chain genes. In normal individuals, no evidence for extensive polymorphism of the chains has been detected with only one Pst I restriction enzyme polymorphic site (probably present in the non-coding region of the B-chain gene) being seen on examination of genomic DNA from about 50 normal individuals with 12 common restriction enzymes.

C1r and C1s

The single-chain mature forms of proenzymes C1r and C1s are activated by splitting of one peptide bond, in either case, to yield non-catalytic A-chains of approximately 56 kDa disulphide-bonded to catalytic B-chains of approximately 27 kDa. On the basis of primary amino acid sequence data, the analysis of fragments produced by limited proteolysis, and positioning of intron/exon boundaries in the genes, both C1r and C1s can be clearly divided into six well-defined domains. The N-terminal A-chains contain domains I to V while the C-terminal catalytic B-chains are composed of typical serine proteinase domains. Domains I and III show approximately 30% identity to each other and, so far, this amino acid sequence motif has only been found in C1r and C1s which is suggestive that they may be involved with a highly specific C1r-C1s function, such as the interaction of the $C1r_2$-Ca^{2+}-$C1s_2$ complex with the collagen regions of C1q. Domain II is similar in sequence to the motif found in epidermal growth factor (EGF) and this region in C1r and C1s may be involved in calcium binding within the $C1r_2$-Ca^{2+}-$C1s_2$ complex. The C-terminal halves of the A-chains of activated C1r, or C1s, contain two similar domains (IV and V) which are members of the group of short consensus repeats (SCRs) – sequence motifs which are 60 amino acids long and have four highly conserved cysteine residues and which are found in a number of complement proteins (especially in the control proteins of the RCA cluster, as discussed later) which interact with C3b or C4b. Each of the C1r and C1s proenzymes contains two SCRs; thus, in the $C1r_2$-Ca^{2+}-$C1s_2$ complex, eight SCRs could be aligned to provide a site for the binding of C4 prior to its activation to C4b by activated C1s.

Full-length cDNA clones have been isolated from human liver cDNA libraries for both C1r[20,21] and C1s[22]. In 1988, Kusumoto *et al.*[23] showed that the C1r and C1s genes are orientated 3′ to 3′, with the distance between their 3′ ends being only 9.5 kb. The genes have been shown to be present on chromosome 12 by the use of mouse/human somatic cell hybrids and further localization to the 12p13 region was achieved by *in situ* hybridization studies[24]. Both the C1r and C1s genes are approximately 10–12 kb long and initial studies on the intron/exon boundaries of the C1r gene indicate that each of the domains I to V in the non-catalytic A-chain may be encoded by separate exons while the entire catalytic B-chain, the serine proteinase domain, is encoded by a single exon. The human C1s gene contains 12 exons as gauged by electron microscopy analysis of heteroduplex molecules produced by hybridization of a full-length genomic clone and a full-length cDNA clone[25]. An unusual feature of the gene structure is the finding that the two SCRs in C1s are both encoded by two exons rather than a single exon. As for C1r, the catalytic B-chain of C1s is encoded by one exon, which again is unusual since, in other vertebrate serine proteinase genes which have been examined, the serine, aspartic acid and histidine residues which form the catalytic site are usually found in separate exons.

The liver appears to be the major site of synthesis of C1r and C1s although they have been shown to be synthesized by a wide variety of tissues and cell lines[26,27]. They appear to be expressed and secreted in equimolar amounts which is consistent with their tight linkage on chromosome 12. There does not appear to be coordination of C1q synthesis with the synthesis of C1r and C1s since, under certain studies, C1q synthesis was found to exceed that of C1r and C1s while, in other studies, the converse was seen[28,29]. Recombinant C1r has been produced in cultured insect cells at levels of approximately 1 mg/L of culture medium[30] and this material was shown to be haemolytically active. The expression of mutant forms of C1r lacking one or more of the N-terminal domains found in the B-chain should provide a powerful tool for examining structure–function relationships within the C1 complex[30].

Genetic deficiency of C1r and C1s appears to be quite rare with, in the few cases described[31], there being a loss of function of both genes, which might be expected in view of their close linkage and observed coordinated synthesis.

THE C2, C4 AND FACTOR B GENES

Proenzyme C2 and component C4 of the classical activation pathway, and proenzyme factor B of the alternative activation pathway, are encoded by genes which map to the class III region of the human major histocompatibility complex (MHC) on the short arm of chromosome 6. The genes have been aligned with respect to one another in a series of overlapping cosmid clones isolated using the corresponding cDNA clones[32]. The single C2 and factor B genes are very closely linked, with the transcriptional start site of the factor B gene lying only 421 bp from the polyadenylation site of the C2 gene[33]. Approximately 30 kb from the factor B gene is the first of the two C4 loci, separated from each other by ~10 kb. Hybridization of C4A- and C4B-specific oligonucleotides to the cosmid clones has shown that the C4A gene lies closest to the factor B gene[34].

The complement genes are contained in a 120 kb stretch of DNA[32] in the order cen-C4B-C4A-Bf-C2-tel, with the C4B gene lying ~400 kb from DRA while the C2 gene lies ~600 kb from HLA-B[35]. This cluster also contains the CYP21 gene and the CYP21P pseudogene which lie immediately 3′ of the C4B and C4A genes, respectively[36–39]. Recently, three novel genes have been located in the complement gene cluster, the RD, G11 and OSG genes[40–42] (Figure 3.1).

On the basis of DNA sequence conservation across animal species, Levi-Strauss *et al.*[40] identified the RD gene that encodes a novel 42 kDa intracellular protein with a central repeated core sequence and which maps immediately adjacent to the 3′ end of the factor B gene (Figure 3.1). The RD gene is organized in the opposite transcriptional orientation to the other genes in this gene cluster. The function of the RD protein is unknown though the mRNA has been detected in all cell lines so far examined, thereby indicating that it may encode a housekeeping protein.

The OSG gene, which is expressed in a number of different cell types, has been located immediately adjacent to the CYP21 gene[42,43]. In this case, the gene is encoded on the opposite strand to that encoding CYP21 and overlaps with the 3′ end of the CYP21 gene. A 2.7 kb incomplete cDNA clone appears to specify a protein characterized by the presence of repeating fibronectin type III repeats

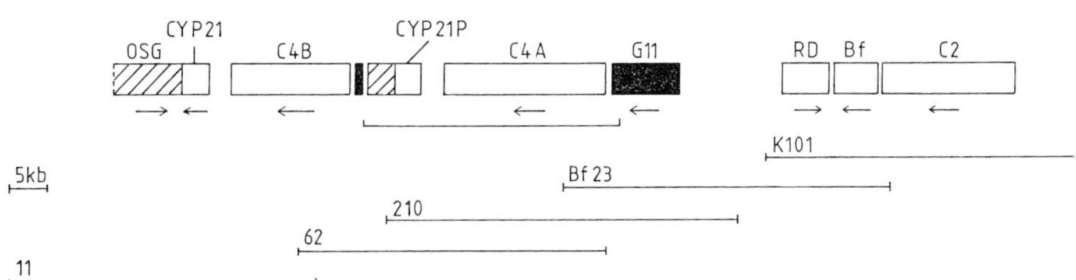

Figure 3.1 Alignment of the complement genes in the class III region of the human MHC in a series of overlapping cosmid clones. Also shown are the recently mapped novel genes, RD, G11 and OSG. Arrows indicate the direction of transcription of the genes. The unit of duplication of the C4 genes is indicated. The cross-hatched box between the CYP21P and C4B genes indicates that a portion of the OSG gene has duplicated as it is part of the unit of duplication. Likewise, the black box between the CYP21P and C4B genes indicates that a portion of the G11 gene has duplicated as it is also part of the unit of duplication.

that show significant homology to tenascin[44], a large glycoprotein found in extracellular matrices. The OSG gene is part of the unit of duplication at the C4 loci and part of the sequence is contained between the CYP21P and C4B genes[43]. This segment of DNA appears to be expressed as a 2.6 kb mRNA in adrenal tissue only. Whether this transcript is translated into protein remains to be established.

The third novel gene, G11, has been located immediately upstream of the C4A gene[41] (Figure 3.1). In this case, the gene was identified by establishing the location of an HTF-island ~10 kb telomeric of the C4A gene. Isolation of cDNA clones revealed that the gene spans ~9.5 kb of DNA and encodes a 1.4 kb mRNA expressed in monocytes, macrophages, T cells, B cells and other cells. The G11 gene encodes a 28 kDa protein, but its function is not known. The 3′ end of the G11 gene is part of the unit of duplication of the C4 genes and ~0.9 kb of the gene is located immediately upstream of the C4B gene[45,46]. In this case, it is not clear whether this segment of sequence is expressed at the mRNA level.

In addition, an extensive search for potential coding sequences in 700 kb of class III region genomic DNA isolated in overlapping cosmids has indicated that the region contains at least 25 previously unidentified genes including genes for the major heat shock protein HSP70 and valyl-tRNA synthetase[41,47–51]. It is, therefore, clear that the complement genes together with CYP21, for so long thought of as the only genes in the class III region, form only a small proportion of a large number of unrelated MHC-linked genes present in this region.

The factor B and C2 genes

The factor B gene, which is 6 kb in length, is organized into 18 exons[52]. The first exon encodes the 5′ untranslated region and 21 of the 25 amino acids which make up the leader peptide. Exons 2, 3, 4 and 5 encode amino acids –4 to 228 which form the bulk of the Ba fragment. Exons 2, 3, and 4 also precisely encode the three SCRs which are a feature of this fragment[53].

The Bb fragment is encoded by 13 exons. Exons 6–10 encode amino acids 229–444 which share significant homology with the A domains of von Willebrand factor (vWF), and homologous domains in the α chain of some integrins (called the ‘I’ domain) and the cartilage matrix protein (CMP). Recently, the genes encoding vWF[54], CMP[55] and the α chain of the integrin p150,95[56] have been reported. In the vWF gene, the A3 domain is encoded by 4 exons, while the A1 and A2 domains are encoded by a single exon. The I domain of the α chain of p150, 95 is also encoded by 4 exons, and, in CMP, the homologous domains are encoded by 2 exons. Comparison of the genomic organization of this region of the factor B gene with the corresponding regions of the vWF gene, the CMP gene and the α chain gene of the p150,95, has shown that there is little consensus on the position of the splice sites within the domain. However, the splice sites at the beginning and end of the domain are conserved as phase 1 introns in each of the genes. This supports the idea that this domain has been inserted as a unit into a diverse range of proteins during evolution, and then has subsequently undergone various modifications, which presumably include duplications and intron insertions/deletions, as well as splice junction sliding.

Exons 11–18 encode amino acids 445–739 which share significant homology with other serine proteinases[57]. The three active site residues, His-501, Asp-551 and Ser-674, the residue-determining specificity in the binding pocket (probably Asp-666), and the Ser-Trp-Gly triplet that forms the secondary binding site, are all encoded in separate exons[58]. This fragmented genomic organization of a serine proteinase domain is not unusual, and, in most cases where the structural organization of the serine proteinase gene has been determined, all of the active site residues and the residue determining specificity in the binding pocket are encoded by separate exons. The exceptions to this are the genes encoding C1r and C1s, and some of the vitamin K-dependent subfamily of serine proteinases, including factor VII, factor IX, factor X and protein C where the active site Asp and Ser residues are encoded in a single exon[59].

The organization of the C2 gene, which is also split into 18 exons, closely resembles that of the factor B gene[33,60,61]. However, in this case, the C2 gene spans 18 kb of DNA due to the presence of larger introns. The overall similarity in structure and function and the close linkage of C2 and factor B suggests that these loci arose by duplication of an ancestral gene. However, the marked divergence in intron lengths between the two genes suggests that the duplication event is not recent.

Phenotypic genetics have established that C2 and factor B are polymorphic[62]. In the case of factor B, the polymorphism which results in the F and S allotypes is due to a G→A transition in the second position of the codon for amino acid 7 of the mature polypeptide[63]. This results in a charge difference between the two allotypes with the F allotype having Glu at this position while the S allotype has Arg.

In Caucasian populations, most chromosomes carry the common allele of C2, C2C. At the genomic level, this allele has been extensively subdivided due to the presence of a multiallelic polymorphism in intron 3 of the gene[64–66]. When the enzyme Sst I and a 300 bp genomic probe are used, Sst I fragments of 2.75, 2.7, 2.65, 2.6 and 2.4 kb are detected. This polymorphism is of particular interest as it allows subdivision of haplotypes carrying the C2C allele. Sequence analysis of the polymorphic fragments of the two most frequently observed alleles (2.7 and 2.4 kb Sst I fragments) has demonstrated that a VNTR is present in intron 3[67]. The data also indicate that the repeated nucleotide sequences constitute part of a non-viral retroposon, apparently derived from a human endogenous retrovirus, HERV-K10, which is homologous to the mouse mammary tumour virus.

RFLPs have also been defined using the factor B cDNA probes. An Msp I polymorphism due to the nucleotide difference in codon 7 is informative for the F and S alleles[63], while two others detected using Rsa I and Taq I are found associated with only some of the F alleles[63,68,69].

Deficiency of C2 in plasma is one of the most common complement protein deficiencies found in man (approximately 1 in 10 000 showing homozygous deficiency). Two types of C2 genetic deficiency have been described: type I, where no C2 protein translation is detected; and type II, in which there is a selective block in C2 secretion. The molecular defect in type I deficiency has been elucidated by study of the C2 gene and cDNA from a homozygous type I C2-

deficient individual[61] who had the common complotype/haplotype – HLA-A25, B18, C2QO, BfS, C4A4, C4B2, DR2, which occurs in over 90% of C2-deficient individuals. The study showed that type I C2 deficiency, in this individual, is caused by a 28 bp genomic deletion that results in skipping of exon 6 during RNA splicing, thus leading to generation of a premature termination codon. The 28 bp deletion is strongly associated with the common complotype/haplotype seen in C2 deficiency which strongly suggests that all type I C2-deficient individuals will show this deletion. The molecular defect in type II C2 deficiency is not yet known.

The C4 genes

The duplicated C4 genes are ~10 kb apart and are organized in the same transcriptional orientation[36]. The C4A (or locus I) gene is ~22 kb in length and is split into 41 exons[70]. It is highly likely that the C4B (or locus II) gene is also split into 41 exons. However, in this case the locus II gene can either be 22 kb in size, similar to the locus I gene, or 16 kb in size. The basis of the size difference is in the length of the intron that separates exons 9 and 10. In long genes, this intron is ~6.5 kb in length, while in short genes the intron is only ~0.35 kb in length (Anderson and Campbell, unpublished).

Both C4 genes are transcribed into mRNA molecules of ~5.5 kb. The two isotypes, C4A and C4B, exhibit extensive structural polymorphism[71]. However, determination of C4A and C4B cDNA sequences has revealed that the two isotypes differ in only a limited number of positions, most of which are located in the C4d fragment[72–74]. Comparison of the available sequences has allowed the location of those residues which are related to the Rg and Ch serological determinants to be deduced[75]. In addition, the comparison has identified four amino acids which are specific to either C4A or C4B[76]. Between residues 1101 and 1106, C4A has the sequence *PC*PV*LD* while C4B has the sequence *LS*PV*IH*. Thus it is these residues which define the isotypes and which are responsible for the functional differences between C4A and C4B[76,77].

An intriguing feature in the genetics of C4 is the unusually high frequency of null alleles forming half-null C4A or C4B haplotypes[78–80]. The frequency of C4A null alleles is 5–15% with about 60% being due to gene deletion, while the frequency of C4B null alleles is 10–20%.

Duplication of one of the loci is also relatively common and is estimated[81] to have a frequency of 8%. Thus, haplotypes have been characterized which have one, three and even four C4 genes, in addition to the common situation with two C4 genes[82,83]. These differences in gene number, and also the difference in gene size due to the size of intron 9, can be observed directly on different haplotypes using pulsed field gel electrophoresis[83].

Characterization of the C4QO phenotype has revealed that it consists of three distinct components. The first is gene deletion which usually occurs together with the flanking CYP21 gene[36,84,85]. The second is non-expression of a defective mutant C4 gene[86]. Presumably, in this case, the defect is due to non-expression from a defective promoter, or point mutations or base deletions/insertions which result in abnormalities in transcription or translation. The third case is homoexpression, the expression of identical allotypes from the two C4 loci[87]. In this case, the expression of an identical allotype from the C4B locus would be masked by the expression of the same allotype from the C4A locus, thus giving the impression of a silent allele at the C4B locus. The initial description of this was on the HLA haplotype B44 C4A3 C4BQO DR6 where the C4BQO allele was found to encode the C4A isotypic residues[87]. Amplification by PCR of other C4BQO alleles has also revealed that most encode the C4A residues[88–90]. Thus, if expressed, these C4BQO alleles would encode a C4 molecule with the properties of the C4A isotype. Isoexpression involves the expression of C4 molecules of the same isotype from the two C4 loci, but different allotype. Haplotypes expressing two different C4A allotypes, such as C4A3 C4A2 or C4A5 C4A2, have been found in several studies[91–94]. Haplotypes expressing two different C4B allotypes have also been reported where the long locus I (C4A) gene, instead of encoding a C4A isotype, encodes a C4B isotype[95,96].

A number of restriction fragment length polymorphisms (RFLPs) have been defined at the human C4 loci[36,85,87,91,97–102]. In particular, the Taql polymorphism at the 5′ end of the genes[85,87,91], and the NIaIV and Eco0109 polymorphic patterns[87] can give information about the nature and characteristics of the two C4 loci. These include whether the ~6.5 kb or the ~0.35 kb intron is present, whether they express the C4A or C4B isotype, and whether they would express the Rg1 or Ch1 antigenic determinants.

C1 INHIBITOR

C1 inhibitor is the major protein involved in the control of the activated C1 complex which it does by virtue of its ability to covalently bind to the activated forms of C1r and C1s and rapidly free them from their interaction with the C1q-classical activator complex. The molecular genetics of C1 inhibitor are discussed in Chapter 9 (Tosi) and C1 inhibitor deficiency is discussed in Chapter 8 (Frank).

FACTOR D

Factor D is synthesized as a single-chain serine esterase proenzyme of 24 kDa but appears to circulate in the blood primarily in its activated form. Since it does not circulate in blood as a proenzyme, regulation of factor D enzymatic activity is provided by its extremely restricted substrate specificity, i.e. it will split a single arginyl–lysine bond in proenzyme factor B after the factor B has associated in a Mg^{2+}-dependent complex with C3b. Thus, factor D plays a very specific and essential role in the generation of the C3bBb complex of the alternative pathway. The sequence of factor D, as established by protein sequencing[103,104] and cDNA cloning studies[105], showed that it belongs to the serine proteinase superfamily[106] with 60 of the 113 normally conserved residues being found in factor D, which included 26 of the 29 ‘invariable’ residues. The His,

Asp and Ser residues forming the serine proteinase charge-relay system were found in the expected positions, as was an aspartic acid residue in the specificity determining position which is consistent with factor D showing a tryptic-like specificity.

Although factor D has been found to be synthesized by U937 cells, human blood macrophages and HepG2 cells[107], it appears from recent cDNA cloning studies[105] that factor D is identical to adipsin and that the major site of synthesis of adipsin is adipocytes. The human adipsin/factor D cDNA was found to code for a precursor protein having a secretory signal peptide, a five-residue-long activation peptide and the mature protein of 228 amino acids[105]. Several apparent differences between the sequences for factor D which were derived by protein sequencing[103,104] and sequence predicted for adipsin/factor D from the cDNA study could be ascribed to incompleteness of the protein data. Further confirmation of identity of adipsin and factor D was shown by the fact that antisera raised against synthetic peptides designed from the human adipsin cDNA sequence reacted with purified factor D. The use of the cDNA confirmed, by Northern blot analyses, that adipsin/factor D was expressed at high levels in human lung and adipose tissue while low levels were found in U937 cells (after stimulation with TPA) and in peripheral mononuclear leukocytes, but no signal was detected in liver mRNA samples. Although the mouse adipsin gene has been characterized[108] no data are yet available regarding the cloning of the human adipsin/factor D gene and its chromosomal location.

Reports of factor D deficiency are rare, with one family with a partial deficiency of factor D activity[109] and another with a case of homozygous deficiency[110] having been reported. In the partial deficiency family, two sisters suffered from recurrent respiratory tract bacterial infections and had factor D functional activity of less than 10% of normal, while their mother, brother and sister had normal values. It was not clear whether the deficiency was due to a dysfunctional protein and the genetic defect was not established. Recurrent Neisserial infections were seen in the homozygous deficient family; no information is yet available concerning the nature of the defect at the molecular level. In an animal model of obesity, decreased serum levels of factor D are found (58–80% of those seen in lean controls), which argues for a second role for factor D, other than activation of factor B, or indicates that malfunction of the alternative pathway of complement in adipocytes may be of importance in this model system[111]. The promotor of the mouse adipsin/factor D gene has been characterized in transgenic animals and it has been observed that the 950 bp of the 5′ flanking region of the gene carries information that specifies both expression in adipose tissue and a response to a gene product or chemical that induces obesity[108].

PROPERDIN

Properdin is found in plasma as a polydisperse mixture of cyclic polymers, mainly dimers, trimers and tetramers in the ratio 20:54:26, formed by the interactions of a single 53 kDa asymmetric monomer[112]. The monomer is not seen in plasma and its polymerization into oligomers of defined size is probably carefully controlled in order to maintain an optimal functional ratio of the different polymeric forms of properdin and prevent anomalous aggregates forming[113,114]. Properdin is a positive regulator of the alternative pathway and it achieves this role by virtue of its ability to bind and stabilize the inherently labile C3 and C5 convertase enzyme complexes (C3bBb and $C3b_nBb$). The binding of properdin results in a decreased rate of dissociation of the Bb catalytic subunit and may also protect the complexes from the negative regulatory proteins, factors I and H[115].

cDNA clones have been isolated for mouse[116] and human[117] properdin and the complete structure of the approximately 6 kb-long human gene has been established[118]. The derived amino acid sequences show that, in both the mouse and in humans, the 441-amino-acid-long chain of properdin is composed mainly of six repeating motifs, each of about 60 amino acids, of a type first found in thrombospondin[119]. In properdin, these six repeating motifs, designated TSRs, are flanked by distinct N-terminal and C-terminal domains of about 50 amino acids. The major site of synthesis of properdin in humans has not been established but macrophage-type cells have been shown to synthesize properdin in *in vitro* studies and the mouse and human cDNA clones were isolated from macrophage- and PMA-stimulated U937 cells, respectively. Northern blotting studies, using mRNA from mouse tissues, indicated that spleen was a good source of properdin mRNA while no signal could be seen in liver mRNA[116].

The human properdin gene spans ~6.0 kb of DNA and is organized into ten exons (Figure 3.2)[118] as judged by the complete sequence determination of 8.2 kb of cloned genomic DNA containing the gene. Transcription can start at either of two positions, resulting in a 5′ untranslated region of 238 or 242 bases in the mRNA[118]. No TATA- or CAAT-boxes were found in the vicinity of the transcription start sites but it has been noted that there are four regions of similarity to the Alu family of repetitive sequences, three being upstream of the gene and one located within the final intron of the gene[118]. The first exon of the properdin gene contains sequence which is transcribed but not translated, whilst the second exon contains 65 bases of untranslated sequence, the translation start site and sequence encoding 24 amino acids of the 27-amino-acid-long leader peptide. The third exon encodes the last three amino acids of the leader peptide and the 49 amino acid N-terminal region of the mature protein. The next five exons, exons three to eight, precisely encode the TSR modules 1 to 5 found in properdin and this relationship between gene structure and protein structure is discussed in the following paragraph. The first 38 amino acids of TSR 6 are encoded by exon nine while the remainder of TSR 6 and the 29-amino-acid-long C-terminal region are encoded in the final exon. Both phase 1 and phase 2 intron/exon boundaries are present in the gene and it is notable that the TSRs 2 to 5 are encoded by symmetrical, phase 1-1, exons while the remaining exons are asymmetrical.

The TSR 60-amino-acid-long consensus sequence is based primarily upon the presence of six cysteine and three tryptophan residues and it seems likely that these cysteines will form intramodular disulphide bridges, thus ensuring that each TSR sequence yields an independently folding unit. These TSR modules have been identified in the complement proteins, C6, C7, C8 (α and β), and C9, as well as thrombospondin (Figure 3.2) and the circumsporozoite protein of a number of species of malaria parasites. These proteins are all involved in interactions at the cell surface and it is possible that cell binding takes place via the presence of a Val-Thr-Cys-Gly sequence motif found in certain TSRs, with the membrane protein CD36 being implicated as the potential receptor (reviewed by Frazier[120]). This sequence motif is present in TSR4 of both human and mouse properdin but it is not yet known whether it is of functional importance. The finding that TSR modules 2 to 5 of human properdin are encoded by discrete exons which are symmetrical with respect to the phase of their boundaries (phase 1-1) is consistent with the hypothesis that exon shuffling was involved in the evolutionary positioning of these modules[121]. The introduction of independently folding units minimized possible folding problems in a new protein environment. Also, symmetrical exons could be shuffled into, or from, introns of the same phase class without disruption of the reading frame. There is a clear bias for the use of phase 1-1 exons, as found in TSRs 2–5, in modular proteins such as properdin. However, it seems likely that evolution of the properdin gene since the exon shuffling events has resulted in the generation of the asymmetrical exons encoding TSR1, and the N-terminal half of TSR6, of properdin[118].

Three forms of properdin deficiency have been reported (as reviewed by Sjoholm[122] and Figueroa and Densen[123]): type 1, total deficiency with zero or low (<2% of normal) levels of properdin; type II, partial deficiency, with a level of properdin approximately 10% of normal with the properdin being functionally active; and type III with a dysfunctional form of properdin present at close to normal antigenically-determined levels. All these forms of properdin deficiency are X-linked recessive and carry a high risk of fatal fulminant meningococcal infections. The mapping of the properdin structural gene, on the short arm of the X chromosome, to Xp11.3-Xp11.23 <100 kb distal to TIMP[124] is consistent with the X-linked nature seen in the families with properdin deficiency[125]. The characterization of two dinucleotide repetitive sequences ($(dC\text{-}dA)_n(dG\text{-}dT)_n$) less than 15 kb downstream of the properdin structural gene[118,124] has allowed the identification of carrier status with respect to properdin deficiency[126]. Three families, with seven properdin-deficient individuals, were investigated using ELISA, haemolytic assays and a PCR-based technique for the detection of microsatellite repetitive sequences. There was complete agreement between the function and immunological assessment of deficient individuals. However, probable and definite carriers of the deficiency showed functional and immunochemical levels in the normal range. No recombinants between the microsatellite loci and properdin deficiency were detected. Therefore, the defective allele could be traced through the generations in all three families, thus providing a rapid method of detection of carrier status and prenatal diagnosis[126].

The precise molecular defect, for any of the types of properdin deficiencies, remains to be established but it is clear from Southern blot analysis of genomic DNA from three properdin-deficient families, and sequencing of extended regions of the 5′ end of the properdin gene of one patient, that it is unlikely that there are any large deletions or insertions within the structural gene of properdin-deficient individuals.

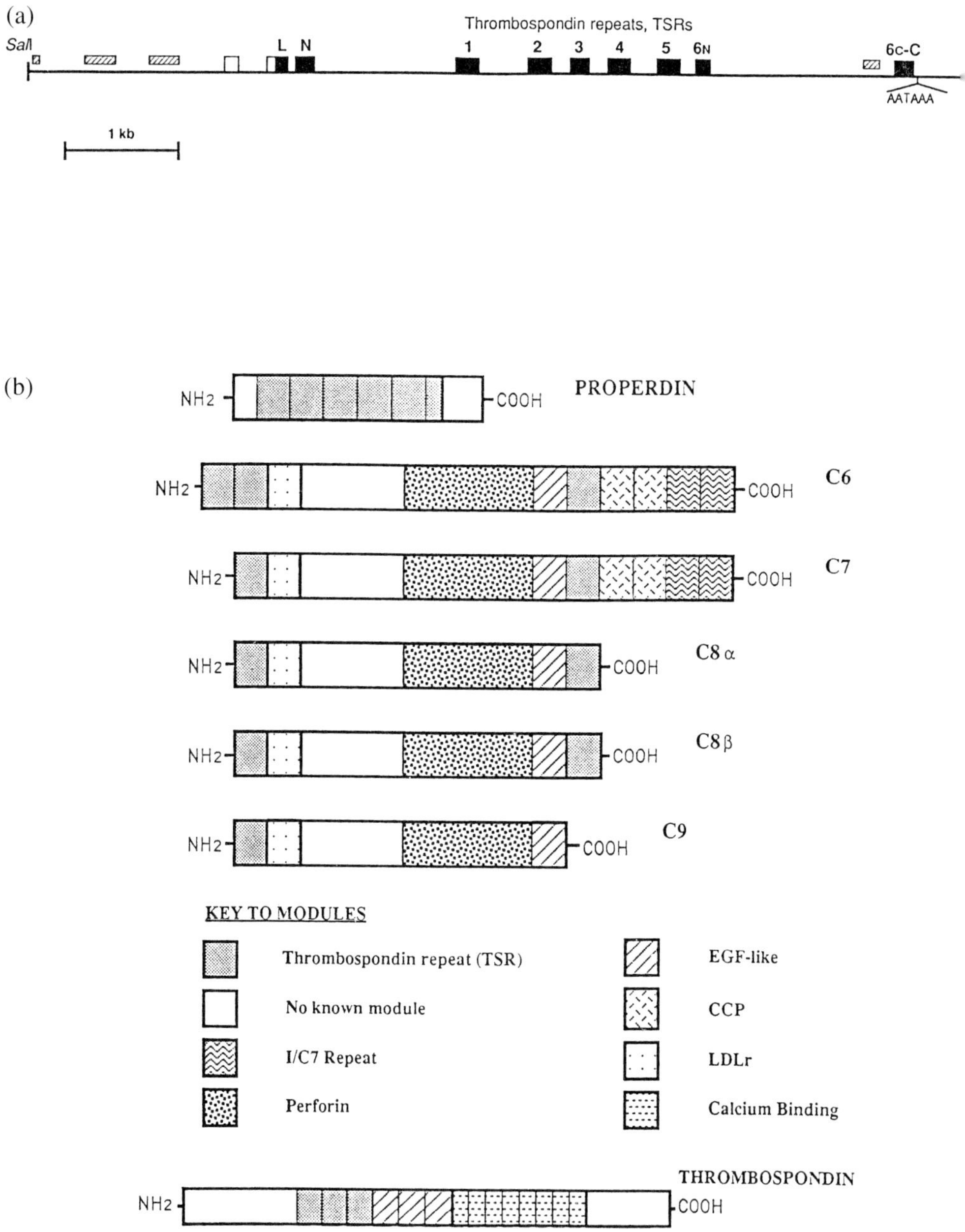

Figure 3.2 (a) Schematic representation of the human properdin gene structure. Approximately 8.2 kb of DNA, of a ~40 kb cosmid, was sequenced to establish the entire coding structure of the human properdin gene. Exons which are translated are represented by filled boxes, with the region of protein encoded by the exon indicated above the box (L, leader; N, N-terminus; 6N, N-terminal region of TSR6; 6C, C-terminal region of TSR6; C, C-terminus). Exons which are not translated are

Figure 3.2 (*contd*) represented as open boxes. No TATA- or CAAT-boxes were identified in the vicinity of the transcription start site, but two complete and two partial repetitive Alu sequences were identified, located in the 5′ upstream sequence and in the final intron and are indicated as hatched rectangles. The stop codon is followed 43 bp downstream by a typical polyadenylation signal, AATAAA. (**b**) Schematic representation of the primary structures of the complement proteins and cell adhesion protein thrombospondin. TSR modules were first described as type 1 modules in the cell adhesion protein, thrombospondin (420 kDa). These modules have subsequently been identified in a diverse range of proteins including the complement proteins, properdin (53 kDa), C6 (120 kDa), C7 (110 kDa), C8α (64 kDa), C8β (64 kDa) and C9 (71 kDa) (see text for references)

FACTOR I

As judged by analysis of cDNA clones, factor I is synthesized as a single-chain proenzyme of 583 amino acids which includes an 18-long leader sequence[127,128]. The major sites of synthesis are the liver and monocytes, the mRNA size in liver being 2.4 kb[127]. The single-chain proenzyme is processed, mainly intracellularly, to the active form consisting of a heavy chain of 43 kDa and a light catalytic chain of 39 kDa. However, in the HepG2 cell-line, a processing defect has been reported[128] which results in the secretion of a single-chain form. The gene has been mapped to chromosome 4 by the use of somatic cell hybrids[128] and the position refined to 4q24-26 by *in situ* hybridization studies[129,130]. Pulsed field gel electophoresis studies, covering approximately 3 Mbp of chromosome 4q, have linked the factor I gene and epidermal growth factor genes to within 250 kb of 4q25[130]. Factor I deficiency is rare and inheritance has been reported to be autosomal codominant[131]. In a study of 8 factor I-deficient individuals and their families, it was found that factor I QO chromosomes showed RFLP profiles in pedigree-specific five point haplotypes, thus allowing carrier detection of the factor I QO allele in all the families studied[130]. These results indicate that factor I deficiency may be caused by heterogeneous mutations in the structural gene.

C3 AND C5

C3 and C5 show significant homology to one another as well as to C4 suggesting that they are descended from a common ancestral protein. However, the genes encoding C3 and C5 do not lie within the MHC. The single copy C3 gene is located on chromosome 19[132], while the single copy C5 gene is located on chromosome 9 in the region q32-34[133].

C3 is the most abundant (~1 g/L) of the complement proteins in plasma and it plays a crucial central role in the activation of the system since it participates in both pathways. Many of the inflammatory and clearance activities associated with complement are mediated by fragments of C3 generated during its activation and regulation by specific complement enzymes and other tryptic-like proteases. C3 is synthesized as a single-chain pro-C3 of 185 kDa (~1.7% carbohydrate). The pro-C3 is processed to yield the α-chain (115 kDa)–β-chain (70 kDa) disulphide linked dimer present in plasma. Activation of C3, by the C3 convertases of either pathway, yields the anaphylatoxin C3a (9 kDa) and the large C3b fragment (176 kDa) which contains the thiolester bond utilized in the covalent attachment of C3b to suitable surfaces. The bound C3b acts as a focus for the formation of the C5 convertase or it is degraded to iC3b and thus becomes a ligand for the CR1 and CR3 complement receptors.

The C3 gene is approximately 42 kb in length and is split into 41 exons which range in size from 52 bp to 213 bp[134–136]. The major transcription initiation site is located –61 bases from the signal peptide and the putative TATA box is probably located at –85 bases, although a second TATA box motif is present 330 bases upstream from the first. A number of regions which show homology to known regulatory sequences were found within 1 kb upstream of the transcription start site. These regions indicated the presence of potential responsive elements for interferon γ, interleukin-6, nuclear factor kB, oestrogen, glucocorticoids and thyroid hormone, which is consistent with C3 synthesis and mRNA levels being affected by many of these agents. The C3 β-chain is encoded by 13 kb of DNA involving exons 1–16. Exon 16 codes for portions of both the β- and α-chains. The C3 α-chain is encoded by 28 kb of DNA involving exons 16–41. On comparison of analogous exons present in C3 and C4 gene structures, 39 out of the 41 exons were found to be of similar size which strongly supports the view that C3 and C4 arose from a common ancestor. An analysis of the intron–exon phase boundaries in the C3 gene has shown that within the β-chain region of the gene, the distribution of intron types is in agreement with the overall average composition of 54%, 27% and 18% for types 0, 1 and 2 respectively, but that, in the α-chain, type 1 predominates (48%). In this context, it is of interest to note that exons 23 and 24 are both symmetrical class 1-1 exons which appear to be preferred when there is an involvement of exon shuffling between different genes. This point may be relevant to the conservation of the thiolester domain in C3, C4 and α_2-macroglobulin.

Patients with inherited homozygous C3 deficiency suffer from recurrent pyogenic infections and are susceptible to rashes and nephritis. The molecular basis for the deficiency has been established in two of the fifteen reported cases of homozygous C3 deficiency[137,138]. In one case, a splice site mutation was the cause of the deficiency in a 10-year-old English boy[137]. In the other case, an Afrikaans patient, there was a deletion of 800 bp from the region of the C3 gene encoding the α-chain[138]. The deletion included two coding regions (exons 22 and 23) which resulted in the generation of a stop codon 19 bp downstream from the deletion. The deletion is considered to have arisen from homologous recombination between two flanking Alu repeats, and the mutant allele was found to have reached a relatively high frequency (0.0057) in the Afrikaaner population in South Africa[138].

C5, like C3 and C4, is synthesized as a single-chain precursor which is subsequently processed to form the plasma form of the molecule – an α-chain (115 kDa) disulphide linked to a β-chain (75 kDa). Unlike C3 and C4, C5 does not contain a thiolester and therefore does not show covalent binding activity upon activation, but freshly activated C5 does have an affinity for C6 and thus serves as the nucleus for the self-assembly of the membrane-attack complex. The complete cDNA sequence of human pro-C5 has been determined[139] and the derived protein sequence shows a strong degree of homology to those of C3, C4 and α_2-macroglobulin, thus illustrating their common evolutionary origin. The C5 gene is at least 50 kb in length and is located on chromosome 9q 32–34[133].

PROTEINS OF THE MEMBRANE ATTACK COMPLEX – THE TERMINAL COMPONENTS OF COMPLEMENT C5b TO C9

The molecular biology of the C5 gene and the similarity of the C5 protein, in terms of activation and overall structure, to the role of the C3 and C4 components is covered in the previous section on C3, C4 and C5.

Upon activation by the convertases of either pathway, the C5a anaphylatoxin (11 kDa) is liberated from the N-terminal end of the α-chain of C5 by cleavage of a single arginyl bond (Arg_{74}-Leu_{75}), leaving the large C5b fragment (185 kDa) which is involved in the formation of the membrane attack complex (MAC). The freshly activated C5b fragment has a metastable binding site for C6 which is probably due to the transient expression of hydrophobic residues. Apart from C5, the components of the MAC clearly belong to a family of proteins which are structurally, antigenically and functionally related. The serum glycoproteins, C6, C7, C8α, C8β and C9 (along with perforin, which is found in the granules of cytolytic T cells) form a well-defined group of membrane disrupting proteins which are all soluble hydrophilic molecules which can undergo a remarkable hydrophilic–amphiphilic transition to form the MAC (or similar type of lesion in the case of perforin) which behaves as an integral membrane component.

Full-length cDNA sequences have been reported for C6[140,141], C7[142], C8α[145], C8β[146,147] and C9[143,144], and show approximately 21–26% identity between any pair of sequences. A striking feature which emerges is the mosaic nature of the structures of these proteins in that all five chains contain a large internal domain, almost free of Cys residues, which is similar to that found in perforin[148–150] along with a variety of other domains, such as those found in thrombospondin (thrombospondin repeat, TSR), the low-density lipoprotein receptor (the LDLr motif), epidermal growth factor (EGF motif) and the complement regulatory proteins, such as factor H (containing the short consensus repeats SCRs). C6 is a good example of this mosaic structure (Figure 3.2), being composed of two TSRs at the N-terminal end followed by an LDLr motif, the perforin/C9 domain, an EGF motif, a third TSR, two SCRs and finally, at the C-terminus, two motifs as yet found only in C6, C7 and factor I. The C7, C8α, C8β, C9 and perforin chains show an overall similarity to C6 and it might be expected that most of the motifs which appear as independently folding domains will be precisely encoded by separate exons. The C8γ chain differs from the other chains of the terminal components in that cDNA studies, yielding the derived amino acid sequence, show that it belongs to the lipocalin protein family which can bind small hydrophobic ligands, i.e. retinol and retinoic acid in the case of C8γ.

The liver is the primary site of synthesis of C6 found in plasma and, since most of the cDNA clones encoding the components C5 to C9 have been isolated from liver cDNA libraries, this tissue is considered to be the primary site of synthesis of all terminal components. The C6 and C7 loci appear to be only a few hundred kb apart, as judged by preliminary mapping studies, using the C6 and C7 cDNA probes[151], which is consistent with earlier studies suggesting that they were closely linked, i.e. the finding of two families with an inherited combined C6 and C7 deficiency[152,153] and from family studies of genetic polymorphisms found in C6 and C7. Deficiency of C6 appears associated with susceptibility to Neisserial infections[154,155]. In most cases of C6 deficiency alone, or C7 deficiency alone, there appears to be C6, or C7, present in the serum but at very low concentrations[156]. The use of the cDNA probes indicates that both C6 and C7 are normally single copy genes although there may possibly be duplication at the C6 locus. Southern blotting of DNA from individuals with C6 or C7 deficiency, including one with a combined deficiency, indicates that there are no large deletions within the coding regions of the genes but there is preliminary evidence for a small deletion within the 5′ region of the C6 gene[151]. The C6 and C7 genes have been mapped to chromosome 5q[157].

Initial characterization of genomic clones covering the entire C8α gene indicates that it is approximately 30 kb long and Southern blot analysis has shown that the C8α gene is within 2.5 kb of the C8β gene in a 5′α–3′β orientation[158]. Chromosomal assignments, made by analysis of somatic cell hybrids, show that the α- and β-chain genes lie on chromosome 1 at 1p34[158] while the γ locus has been assigned to chromosome 9q. Three types of C8 deficiency have been reported, one in which there is an absence of the β-chain, another in which there is a deficiency of the α–γ subunit and only the free β-chain is found in the serum, and a third where there is a dysfunctional β-chain present[159–161]. Use of the deficient sera showed the presence of polymorphism in the α–γ and β subunits and provided the initial demonstration that genes encoding the α- and β-chains are linked to each other and chromosome 1 markers. In a general study of C8β protein and mRNA in ten related C8β-deficient families, it was found that monocytes and fibroblasts from homozygous C8 gene-deficient individuals contain reduced amounts of C8β mRNA[162]. This suggests that a transcriptional defect may be the reason for the deficiency since the C8β gene appears intact in C8β-deficient individuals as judged by Southern blot analysis[163]. A deficiency of the β subunit of mouse C8 has been reported[164] which has allowed the assignment of the gene encoding this subunit to mouse chromosome 4, by the typing of recombinant mice. A C8, α–γ subunit deficiency has been reported in the rabbit[165] which is similar to the human deficiency in that only the free β-chain is found in the serum.

Initial studies on the structure of the human C9 gene indicate that the coding region for this 70 kDa glycoprotein is covered by 12 exons over at least 80 kb of DNA[166]. One unexpected finding was that the Cys-rich regions present in C9 are not encoded by discrete exons despite this being the case in other proteins, such as the LDL receptor, which are homologous to C9 over these regions. The human C9 gene has been mapped to chromosome 5 at position 5p13 by use of the polymerase chain reaction[167]. Deficiency of C9 appears to be quite common in Japan but rare in Western countries[168].

THE REGULATORS OF COMPLEMENT ACTIVATION (RCA) CLUSTER

Control of the complement system is mediated in a number of different ways to prevent damage to one's own tissue. The classical and alternative pathway C3 and C5 convertases are regulated by a number of proteins found in plasma or on cell membranes. These proteins include factor H, C4b binding protein, CR1, DAF and MCP, and interact with the activation fragments of C3 or C4 (C3b or C4b), either to cause dissociation of the convertase and/or to mediate breakdown of C3b and C4b by the serine protease factor I.

The linkage of the genes encoding factor H, C4-bp and CR1 was established by the definition of genetic polymorphism in these proteins, which has been demonstrated by electrophoretic techniques. Three C4-bp variants have been identified which are due to the presence of three alleles at a single autosomal locus. Five factor H alleles at a single locus have been identified, as have 4 alleles at the CR1 locus. Family segregation data of the genetic variants indicated that the factor H gene was linked to C4-bp and CR1 genes[169]. Subsequently, analysis of human–mouse somatic cell hybrids using probes for C4-bp and factor H indicate that the genes are located on chromosome 1. *In situ* hybridization studies have placed the CR1 and CR2 genes on the long arm of chromosome 1 in the q32 region[170]. This linkage group has been termed the 'regulator of complement activation cluster' and is now known to include the genes for factor H, C4-bp, CR1, DAF, MCP and the complement receptor CR2.

Short consensus repeat (SCR), also known as B-type module or complement control protein (CCP) module

A feature of the proteins of the RCA cluster is that they are almost entirely composed of independently folding domains, or modules, which each contain approximately 60 amino acids with 4, generally invariant, cysteines and several other highly conserved residues which yield a compact 'framework' structure ($3.8 \times 2.0 \times 10$ nm) containing three β-strands hydrogen-bonded to form a triple-stranded region at its centre with the other face formed from two separate β-strands[171]. This structure is also present in other non-RCA complement proteins, such as C1r, C1s, C2, factor B and the terminal components as well as a wide variety of non-complement proteins[172]. The module was first described in factor B and therefore is sometimes called a B-type module, and, in view of its common occurrence in the complement control proteins, it is often referred to as a complement control protein (CCP) module.

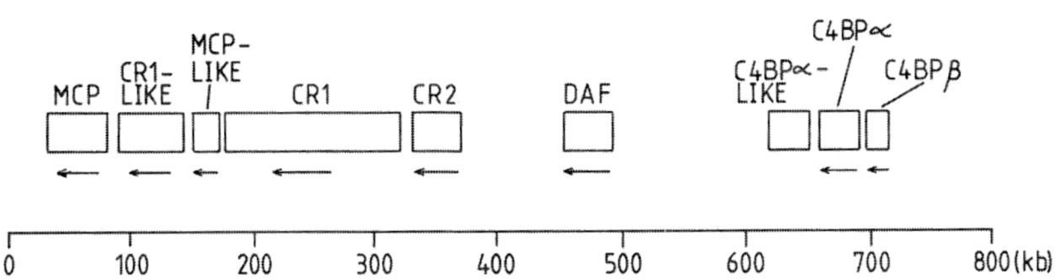

Figure 3.3 Alignment of the genes in the RCA cluster on human chromosome 1.

Molecular mapping of RCA cluster

Physical mapping using PFGE and genomic cloning in yeast artificial chromosomes (YACs) has established the organization of the RCA gene cluster in man[173–176] (Figure 3.3). The initial mapping using PFGE established that four of the genes, CR1, CR2, C4-bp and DAF, were clustered in an ~700 kb segment of DNA in the order CR1-CR2-DAF-C4-bp[174,175]. Subsequently, the gene encoding MCP was located -70 kb from the CR1 gene, while the gene encoding the C4-bpβ chain was located within 5 kb of the C4-bpα chain[176]. In addition, a C4-bp-like gene has been mapped adjacent to the 3′ end of the C4-bpβ gene, a CR1-like gene has been mapped adjacent to the 3′ end of the CR1 gene, while an MCP-like sequence has been mapped between the CR1-like and CR1 genes. All of the genes are orientated in the same 5′ to 3′ direction, which is likely to be a result of evolution of the RCA gene cluster by extensive gene duplication. Several regions of the RCA cluster have been cloned in overlapping YAC clones. The longest mapped region spans ~ 900 kb of DNA and extends from the MCP gene to the C4-bpα gene. YAC clones have also been isolated that include the factor H gene, at least two factor H-related homologies and the factor XIIIb gene. However, no information is yet available on the precise location of the factor H gene relative to the MCP, CR1, CR2, DAF or C4-bp genes, since it appears to be at least 500 kb away from the other members of the RCA cluster[174,175].

C4-bp

C4-bp acts as a regulator of the classical pathway by accelerating the decay of the C3 convertase, C4b2a, and also by acting as cofactor for the degradation of C4b by factor I. The major form of C4-bp has a molecular weight of 570 kDa and is composed of seven identical α-chains (each 70 kDa) and one β-chain (45 kDa)[177] but minor forms, with compositions of $\alpha_7\beta_0$ and $\alpha_6\beta_1$, are also found. Both chains are composed primarily of SCRs, there being 8 in the α-chain and three in the β-chain[178]. The β-chain in C4-bp is involved in the binding of protein S and thus C4-bp appears to also play a regulatory role in the coagulation system since free protein S (but not C4-bp-bound protein) is a cofactor for activated protein C in the degradation of activated factors V and VIII[177].

The C4-bpα gene spans ~30 kb of DNA and is split into 12 exons[179]. Each of the SCRs defined at the protein level is encoded by a separate exon. The gene encodes a single mRNA of ~2.5 kb which is found in liver. Four possible polymorphic sites in C4-bpα were identified by sequence analysis though their relationship to the charge variants has not been established. Characterization of the C4-bpβ-chain gene has revealed that it spans 13 kb of DNA and is split into 7 exons. Exon 1 encodes the 5′-untranslated region and exon 2 the leader peptide. Exons 3 and 4 each encode a complete SCR (SCRI and II, respectively) while SCRIII is split over exons 5 and 6. The exon/intron boundary within SCR III is at the same position as has been reported for other SCRs encoded by two exons. Exon 7 encodes the C-terminal region of the protein and the 3′-untranslated region.

Factor H

Factor H is a 150 kDa single-chain glycoprotein which serves, in plasma, as a cofactor for the regulation of C3b by the enzyme factor I. Analysis of protein sequence and cDNA data[180] has shown that the 150 kDa protein, which is encoded by a 4.3 kb mRNA transcript, is entirely composed of 20 SCRs. Northern blot analysis has shown that, in addition to the 4.3 kb mRNA transcript, transcripts of 1.8 kb and 1.4 kb can be detected in human liver mRNA by use of factor H cDNA probes. The 1.8 kb transcript encodes a 43 kDa factor H-like polypeptide, coding for the N-terminal 431 residues of factor H, and considered to be derived from the factor H gene by alternative splicing[181,182]. The cDNA, corresponding to the 1.4 kb mRNA, appears to be transcribed from a gene distinct from, but related to, factor H[183]. The derived protein sequence data indicate that the polypeptide encoded by this message is composed of five SCRs with SCRs 1 and 2 not showing any significant similarity to factor H whereas SCRs 3 to 5 are very similar to SCRs 18 to 20 of factor H. Due to different usage of glycosylation sites, two glycoproteins, of 42 kDa and 37 kDa, are seen in plasma and are products of the 1.4 kb mRNA[183]. Two further plasma proteins, of 29 kDa and 24 kDa, which are made in liver have been characterized at the cDNA level. These proteins are composed of 4 SCRs with their SCRs 1 and 2 being similar to SCRs 1 and 2 of the 42 kDa and 27 kDa and their SCRs 3 and 4 showing a strong similarity to SCRs 19 and 20 of the 150 kDa factor H[183]. Thus, there appears to be a gene family composed of the factor H gene plus, at least, two factor H-related genes. Deficiency of factor H appears to be rare since only two cases of homozygous deficiency have been reported. These patients suffered from recurrent pyogenic infections and membranoproliferative glomerulonephritis but the molecular defect(s) responsible for the deficiencies is not known.

Complement receptor type 1 (CR1, CD35)

CR1 is a single-chain integral membrane glycoprotein which is found on erythrocytes, monocytes/macrophages, neutrophils, B lymphocytes, some T lymphocytes and podocytes. It plays an important role in the clearance of immune complexes by binding to C3b or C4b present on the complexes, and it acts as a cofactor in the cleavage of C3b or C4b by factor I; it also accelerates the decay of the C3 convertases.

There are four genetic variants of human CR1 which differ in apparent molecular weight and gene frequency: CR1-A, 190 kDa (0.83 gene frequency); CR1-B, 220 kDa (0.16); CR1-C, 160 kDa (0.01); and CR1-D, 250 kDa (<0.01). The differences in the apparent molecular weights are due to differences in the lengths of the polypeptide chains rather than post-translational modifications, such as glycosylation, and, to date, no major antigenic or functional differences have been observed between the variants. From protein and cDNA studies of the most common variant[184], the extracellular portion of the molecule was shown to be composed primarily of four tandem long homologous repeating structures (LHRs) each of approximately 450 amino acids. Within each LHR, there are seven SCRs, each of approximately 60 amino acids, of the type found in other members of the RCA cluster. The whole CR1-A chain contains 30 SCRs followed by a membrane-spanning segment of 25 residues, a region of four positively charged residues then a 43-residue C-terminal cytoplasmic tail. The C4b-binding domain has been localized to SCR-1 and/or SCR-2 and a C3b-binding domain has been localized to SCR-8 and/or SCR-9[185]. Protein engineering studies[186] have identified three residues within SCR-2, and a stretch of five residues in SCR-9, which are important for C4b and iC3 binding, respectively. These studies also indicated the necessity for two contiguous SCRs for the interaction of CR1 to take place with its ligands.

The CR1 variants are encoded by a co-dominant allele at a single locus on chromosome 1q32. It seems likely from the cDNA studies that the size polymorphism (~40 kDa) seen between the allotypes is determined at the genomic level by the presence, or absence, of regions encoding an entire LHR and this has been confirmed by genomic studies. The two most common allotypes of CR1 have now been characterized at the genomic level[187,188]. The CR1-B allotype (S allele) is encoded by approximately 158 kb of DNA which includes the coding information for 5 LHRs, each containing 7 SCRs. The coding sequences for the second LHR present in the CR1-B allotype are not present in the CR1-A allotype (F allele), thus accounting for the difference in molecular weight between the two molecules. There are 47 exons in the CR1-B gene and 39 exons in the CR1-A gene. The 5′ untranslated sequence and leader peptide are within 1 exon, and each of the LHRs are encoded by 8 exons. Within each LHR, the SCRs 1, 5 and 7 are each encoded by a single exon, SCRs 2 and 6 are each encoded by 2 exons and SCRs 3 and 4 are encoded within a single exon. The transmembrane region is covered by 2 exons while the cytoplasmic domain and 3′ untranslated region are encoded by separate exons.

No complete deficiency of CR1 has been reported but the number of CR1 molecules on erythrocytes appears to be under genetic control as an autosomal codominately inherited trait which has been linked to an RFLP of the CR1 gene[189]. The CR1 variant associated with this RFLP could be a susceptibility factor in the development of SLE, due to an impaired ability to clear immune complexes, but this is, as yet, unproven.

COMPLEMENT RECEPTOR TYPE 2 (CR2, CD21)

CR2 is a 145 kDa membrane glycoprotein found on B lymphocytes and spleen follicular dendric cells (see Cooper *et al.* (1988) for review[190]). It binds to the C3d fragment of C3 after the C3 has been activated and then processed by selective cleavage by factor I. In addition to recognizing C3d, the CR2 acts as a receptor for the human Epstein–Barr virus by binding to the gp350/220 viral protein. CR2 also appears to play a role in B-cell activation.

The initial cDNA studies showed that the extracellular portion of CR2 was composed of 15 or 16 SCRs. Analysis of the intron–exon boundaries in the CR2 gene has shown that the SCRs within CR2 are encoded by three types of exons: (1) two SCRs encoded by the same exon; (2) single SCRs precisely encoded by single exons; (3) single SCRs encoded by split exons[191]. Thus, SCRs 1 + 2,

5 + 6, 9 + 10 and 13 + 14 are encoded by single exons (a feature not often seen in members of the RCA cluster). Five SCRs, numbers 3, 7, 11, 15 and 16, are encoded by single exons, while three SCRs, numbers 4, 8 and 12, are encoded by split exons (with all the interruptions occurring at the identical position seen in other RCA genes with SCRs encoded by split exons, i.e. within the codon for a glycine residue located 3 amino acids C-terminal to the second conserved cysteine). The reason for the appearance of CR2 cDNA clones with 15 or 16 SCRs can be explained from consideration of the genomic structure which shows that alternative splicing events can eliminate the use of the sequence coding for SCR 11. The two N-terminal SCRs appear to contain the binding sites for C3dg, and also for the viral protein gp 350/220. Protein engineering studies have identified amino acid residues, within these two SCRs, that are involved in both C3dg and gp 350/220 binding[192].

DECAY ACCELERATION FACTOR (DAF) – CD55

DAF is found primarily as a single-chain integral membrane glycoprotein of approximately 70 kDa and contains 35% (w/w) carbohydrate in the form of O-linked sugars. The major form of DAF is linked to membranes, on erythrocytes, platelets, neutrophils, monocytes, granulocytes and leukocytes, by a glycophospholipid (GPI) anchor[193] while a minor (approximately 10%) soluble form is found in plasma, saliva and urine. The membrane-bound DAF interacts with C3b or C4b molecules bound to the same cell as the DAF and thus can prevent assembly of the C3 convertases from either pathway and this may be its major role rather than dissociation of already formed convertases. cDNA clones for DAF have been characterized from Hela and HL-60 cells[194,195]. Two classes of cDNA were obtained which differed by an internal deletion of 118 bp within the C-terminal portion of the coding region. The deleted segment appeared to represent an unspliced intron composed of Alu consensus sequence[194] making it probable that different forms of DAF can be generated by inclusion or exclusion of this intron and this view is supported by the analysis of the gene[196]. The unspliced form of DAF mRNA would encode a 440-amino-acid-long protein (including the 34 residue-long signal peptide) in which residues 328–366 would be derived from the 'intron'. The spliced DAF mRNA yields a shorter protein of 381 amino acids and would have a different C-terminal region which would be hydrophobic in nature while the longer form of DAF would have a hydrophilic C-terminal region. The long form is considered to be the minor soluble form of DAF while the short form, with its hydrophobic tail, may represent the major (90%) form of DAF which is processed further so that it becomes anchored to the membrane by a glycophospholipid tail. The derived amino acid sequence of DAF shows that the protein is composed of four N-terminal SCRs followed by a 70-residue-long region, rich in serine and threonine (which contains all the O-linked carbohydrate) and then the C-terminal hydrophilic or hydrophobic tail. The signal for attachment of the GPI anchor to the DAF molecule appears to lie within the 37-residue-long C-terminal region since attachment of this region to a normally secreted protein was sufficient to target the expressed fusion protein to the plasma membrane via a GPI anchor[194]. Since membrane-bound CD59 appears to play the major regulatory role in prevention of lysis of host cells by autologous complement, it is now not entirely clear whether DAF is required in protection against PNH. However, the wide distribution of DAF on a variety of different types of cells is indicative that it does play an important general protective role. The ability of DAF to protect cells from complement attack has been mimicked by the parasite *Trypanosoma cruzi* which produces a DAF-like protein (gp 160) at the trypomastigote stage[197]. The gp 160 protein is bound to the membrane by a GPI anchor, contains sequences with significant homology to the SCRs in DAF, and restricts complement activation by binding C3b.

The structure of the DAF gene was established by Post *et al.* in 1990[196]. The gene is approximately 40 kb long and contains 11 exons which vary in length from 21 to 956 bp with the intron sizes ranging from 0.5 to 19.8 kb. The SCRs I, II and IV are each precisely encoded by single exons. SCR III is encoded by two exons with there being a splice junction after the second nucleotide of the Gly codon at position 34 in the SCR. A similar situation for SCRs encoded by two exons is also found in CR1, CR2, MCP and mouse factor H. The Ser/Thr rich region is encoded within three separate exons. The finding of an Alu type of sequence within exon 10 is consistent with the finding of two classes of DAF cDNA clones, one of which contains a 118 bp insert near the 3′ region. The internal boundaries of the insert match the intron splice sequences and this confirms the view that the longer soluble minor form of DAF arises by alternative splicing. The final exon, which encodes the hydrophobic carboxyterminal region and 3′ untranslated region, is preceded by the largest (19.8 kb) intron present in the gene. The signal which directs the post-translational attachment of the GPI anchor to DAF appears to be spread over three exons within 20 kb of DNA.

The molecular defect in one case of primary DAF deficiency has been established by analysis of cDNA from a B-cell line derived from the patient[198]. In this case, there was a single base substitution which generated a stop codon at position 53 within the first SCR of DAF.

MEMBRANE COFACTOR PROTEIN (MCP) – CD46

MCP was originally described as gp 45–70 in view of its heterogeneity in SDS–PAGE. It appears mainly as a doublet of 58 kDa and 63 kDa when isolated from a wide variety of cells, including lymphocytes, monocytes, platelets, endothelial cells, epithelial cells and fibroblasts. It has a preferential binding affinity for protein-bound C3b and acts as a cofactor for I in the irreversible activation of C5 convertase[199]. As judged from its derived amino acid sequence[200], MCP is composed of four N-terminal SCRs, followed by an O-glycosylated region (25 residues long and rich in Thr and Ser), a membrane-spanning sequence (23 residues) and a cytoplasmic domain (33 residues). Thus, in its overall structure, the main form of MCP described by Lublin *et al.*[200] is similar to membrane-bound DAF except that it is bound to the membrane via a hydrophobic transmembrane sequence rather than a GPI anchor. Another difference between MCP and DAF is that, although MCP possesses cofactor activity for factor I cleavage of C3b or C4b, it does not possess decay-accelerating activity. More recently, Post *et al.*[201] and Purcel *et al.*[202] have characterized alternatively spliced RNAs which code for several isoforms of MCP. In addition to the original type of cDNA clone described by Lublin *et al.* (1988)[200], four other clones were characterized, all of which contained the four N-terminal SCRs but differed over their C-terminal regions. The four different cDNA isoforms had: (1) a 93 bp exon resulting in a new cytoplasmic tail of 26 amino acids; (2) a 42 bp exon deleted from the Ser/Thr rich region; (3) deletion of 37 bp from an exon which encoded the transmembrane sequence; (4) failure to splice the intron after the four N-terminal SCRs. The originally described form of MCP and forms (1) and (2) were shown to be common in placental mRNA, form (3) was rare and form (4) not seen[202]. These different expressed forms and other possible variants are likely to correlate with the different forms of MCP found in various tissues, tumours and serum.

Studies on deletion mutants of MCP[203] showed that removal of the first SCR had little effect on iC3 binding and cofactor activity but reduced the efficiency of C4b binding. Selective removal of SCRs 2, 3 and 4 had quite marked effects on binding and/or cofactor activity, indicating that these were particularly important for full activity of MCP.

The genomic organization of the MCP gene has been established[204] and the gene mapped to within 100 kb of the 3′ end of the CR1 gene[205]. The MCP gene is approximately 43 kb long and contains 14 exons and 13 introns. Exon 1 encodes the 5′ untranslated region and the signal peptide, exons 2 to 6 encode the four SCRs – with SCRs 1, 3 and 4 each being precisely encoded by a single exon and SCR 2 being encoded by two exons. As in DAF and the other RCA genes containing SCRs encoded by two exons, the split between the two exons is within the Gly codon approximately half-way along the SCR. Exons 7 to 9 encode the Thr/Ser-rich O-glycosylated region. Exons 7 and 8 can be spliced out without interruption of the reading frame; thus alternative splicing events involving these exons can provide different forms of MCP cDNA. Exon 10 encodes for a 13-amino-acid region of unknown function, while exons 11 and 12 encode the hydrophobic transmembrane region. Exon 13 encodes a 93 bp stretch which can code for a cytoplasmic tail and since this exon also shows potential for alternative splicing this can also generate different forms of MCP. Exon 14 also encodes for a cytoplasmic tail (the sequence of the tail depends upon whether exon 13 is utilized or not) and the 3′ untranslated region. Thus, multiple forms of MCP can be generated from the single MCP gene[201] and, from initial analysis of cell lines and peripheral blood cells, there appears to be expression of variable amounts of four primary isoforms with presumably the additional isoforms being expressed in a tissue-specific fashion[201,204].

HOMOLOGOUS RESTRICTION FACTOR AND CD59 IN THE REGULATION OF COMPLEMENT LYSIS

Protection of an animal's cells against attack by its own complement system is largely dependent upon certain specific glycolipid-anchored proteins in the cell membrane. The DAF molecule is a good example of this but its controlling action is directed towards the acceleration of the decay of the C3bBb and C4b2a enzyme complexes rather than against their formation or lytic potential of the terminal complexes. The molecular biology of DAF is covered in the section on the RCA cluster.

CD59 (20 kDa HOMOLOGOUS RESTRICTION FACTOR)

CD59 is a 20 kDa cell surface protein which prevents lysis by homologous complement by inhibiting the formation of the membrane attack complex, probably at the C5b-8 to C5b-9 stages by limiting C9 input into the complex[206]. It was characterized in several laboratories and therefore, besides CD59[207], it has also been described as HRF20[208], MACIF[209], protectin[206], MIRL and MEM-43-Ag. The 103-amino-acid-long sequence of CD59 has been derived by cDNA cloning and been found to show no similarity in sequence to any other complement protein. However, CD59, which is a glycosylphosphatidylinositol- (GPI-) anchored protein, has been shown to have 25% identity to the glycolipid-anchored mouse Ly-6 antigens (T cell activating protein) with 10 out of 11 cysteines being in identical positions[210].

A patient, suffering from paroxysmal nocturnal haemoglobinuria (PNH) has been described who had a genetic deficiency of CD59 but showed no deficiency in the other GPI-anchored proteins[211]. The molecular basis of the defect was established by analysis of mRNA and genomic DNA from an EBV-infected cell line established from the patient's lymphocytes[212]. Northern blot analysis showed that mRNA was transcribed from the patient's CD59 gene but sequencing of cDNA products derived from the cell line showed that there were two single-base deletions within the gene, within the codons for amino acids 16 residues and 96 residues from the N-terminal end of the mature protein. These results were confirmed at the genomic level in the patient and his relatives (who were heterozygous for the defect) showing that the first deletion gave a codon frame shift which prevented the production of intact CD59 in the patient who was homozygous for the defect. These results very clearly show the important protective role which CD59 plays in preventing the destruction of red blood cells by homologous human serum.

S-PROTEIN/VITRONECTIN AND CL1/SP40,40 – REGULATORS OF THE C5b-9 COMPLEX

The isolation of cDNA clones for S-protein from a human liver expression library[213] allowed the complete derivation of the amino acid sequence of the leader peptide (19 residues) and mature chain (459 residues) and showed that S-protein is identical to plasma vitronectin. It appears that S-protein/vitronectin may play a relatively minor role in regulating the C5b-9 complex and that the protein CL1[214], also known as SP40,40[215] could be of more physiological importance in the inhibition of the C5b-9 complex. Isolation of cDNA clones showed that CL1/SP40,40 is synthesized as a single polypeptide chain with a signal peptide (22 amino acids) and a propeptide (427 amino acids) containing the β and α chains (in that order). The CL1/SP40,40 protein is present in both blood plasma and seminal plasma (which is consistent with its extensive 77% sequence identity to the rat sertoli cell glycoprotein, SGP-2). No similarity was seen in amino acid sequence between S-protein and CL1/SP40,40.

References

1. Reid, K. B. M. (1983). Proteins involved in the activation and control of the two pathways of human complement. *Biochem. Soc. Trans.*, **11**, 1–12
2. Knobel, H. R., Villiger, W. and Isliker, H. (1975). Chemical analysis and electron microscopy studies of human C1q prepared by different methods. *Eur. J. Immunol.*, **5**, 78–82
3. Brodsky-Doyle, B., Leonard, K. R. and Reid, K. B. M. (1976). Circular-dichroism and electron-microscopy studies of human subcomponent C1q before and after limited proteolysis by pepsin. *Biochem. J.*, **159**, 279–86
4. Reid, K. B. M. and Thompson, E. O. P. (1978). Amino acid sequence of the N-terminal 108 amino acid residues of the B chain of subcomponent C1q of the first component of human complement. *Biochem. J.*, **173**, 863–8
5. Reid, K. B. M. (1979). Complete amino acid sequences of the three collagen-like regions present in subcomponent C1q of the first component of human complement. *Biochem. J.*, **179**, 367–71
6. Reid, K. B. M., Gagnon, J. and Frampton, J. (1982). Completion of the amino acid sequences of the A and B chains of subcomponent C1q of the first component of human complement. *Biochem. J.*, **203**, 559–69
7. Reid, K. B. M. (1985). Molecular cloning and characterization of the complementary DNA and gene coding for the B-chain of subcomponent C1q of the human complement system. *Biochem. J.*, **231**, 729–35
8. Sellar, G. C., Blake, D. J. and Reid, K. B. M. (1991). Characterization and organization of the genes encoding the A-, B- and C-chains of human complement subcomponent C1q. *Biochem. J.*, **274,** 481–90
9. Sellar, G. C., Goundis, D., McAdam, R. A., Solomon, E. and Reid, K. B. M. (1987). Cloning and chromosomal localisation of the A-chain of human C1q: identification of molecular defect in a C1q-deficient patient. *Complement,* **4**, 225
10. Sellar, G. C., Cockburn, D. and Reid, K. B. M. (1992). Localization of the gene cluster encoding the A, B and C chains of human C1q to 1p34.1–1p36.3. *Immunogenetics*, **35**, 214–16
11. Taylor, M. E., Brickell, P. M., Craig, R. K. and Summerfield, J. A. (1989). Structure and evolutionary origin of the gene encoding a human serum mannose-binding protein. *Biochem. J.*, **262**, 763
12. Lu, J., Thiel, S., Wiedemann, H., Timpl, R. and Reid, K. B. M. (1990). Binding of the pentamer/hexamer forms of mannan-binding protein to zymosan activates the proenzyme $C1r_2C1s_2$ complex, of the classical pathway of complement, without involvement of C1q. *J. Immunol.*, **144**, 2287–94
13. Super, M., Levinsky, R. J. and Turner, M. W. (1990). The level of mannan-binding protein regulates the binding of complement-derived opsonins to mannan and zymosan at low serum concentrations. *Clin. Exp. Immunol.*, **79**, 144–50
14. Petry, F., Reid, K. B. M. and Loos, M. (1989). Molecular cloning and characterization of the complementary DNA coding for the B-chain of murine C1q. *FEBS Lett.*, **258**, 89–93
15. Petry, F., Reid, K. B. M. and Loos, M. (1991). Gene expression of the A- and B-chain of mouse C1q in different tissues and the characterization of the recombinant A-chain. *J. Immunol.*, **147**, 3988–93
16. Bensa, J. C., Reboul, A. and Colomb, M. G. (1983). Biosynthesis in vitro of complement subcomponents C1q, C1s and C1-inhibitor by resting and stimulated human monocytes. *Biochem. J.*, **216**, 385–92
17. Tenner, A. J. and Volkin, D. B. (1986). Complement subcomponent C1q secreted by cultured human monocytes has a subunit structure identical with that of serum C1q. *Biochem. J.*, **233**, 451–8.

18. Loos, M. (1982). The functions of endogenous C1q, a subcomponent of the first component of complement, as a receptor in the membranes of macrophages. *Mol. Immunol.*, **19**, 1229–38
19. McAdam, R. A., Goundis, D. and Reid, K. B. M. (1988). A homozygous point mutation results in a stop codon in the C1q B-chain of a C1q-deficient individual. *Immunogenetics*, **27**, 259–64
20. Leytus, S. P., Kurachi, K., Sakariassen, K. S. and Davie, E. W. (1986). Nucleotide sequence of the cDNA coding for human complement C1r. *Biochemistry*, **25**, 4855–63
21. Journet, A. and Tosi, M. (1986). Cloning and sequencing of full-length cDNA encoding the precursor of human complement component C1r. *Biochem. J.*, **240**, 783–7
22. Tosi, M., Duponchel, C., Meo, T. and Julier, C. (1987). Complete cDNA sequence of human complement C1s and close physical linkage of the homologous genes C1s and C1r. *Biochemistry*, **26**, 8516–24
23. Kusumoto, H., Hirosawa, S., Salier, J. P., Hagen, F. S. and Kurachi, K. (1988). Human genes for complement components C1r and C1s in a close tail-to-tail arrangement. *Proc. Natl. Acad. Sci. USA*, **85**, 7307–11
24. Van Cong, N., Tosi, M., Gross, M. S., Cohen-Haguenauer, O., Jegon-Foubert, C., de Tand, M. F., Meo, T. and Frezal, J. (1988). Assignment of the complement serine protease genes C1r and C1s to chromosome 12 region 12p13. *Hum. Genet.*, **78**, 363–8.
25. Tosi, M., Journet, A., Duponchel, C., Couture-Tosi, E. and Meo, T. (1989). Human complement C1r and C1s proteins and genes: studies with molecular probes. *Behring Inst. Mitt.*, **84**, 65–71
26. Morris, M. K., Colten, H. R. and Bing, D. H. (1978). The first component of complement. A quantitative comparison of its biosynthesis in culture by human epithelial and mesenchymal cells. *J. Exp. Med.*, **148**, 1007–19
27. Drouet, C. and Reboul, A. (1989). Biosynthesis of C1r and C1s subcomponents. *Behring Inst. Mitt.*, **84**, 80–92
28. Reid, K. B. M. and Solomon, E. (1977). Biosynthesis of the first component of human complement by human fibroblasts. *Biochem. J.*, **167**, 647–60
29. Morris, K. M., Goldberger, G. and Colten, H. R. (1982). Biosynthesis and processing of a human precursor complement protein, pro-C3, in a hepatoma-derived cell line. *Science*, **215**, 399–400
30. Gal, P., Sarvari, M., Szillaggi, K., Zavodsky, P. and Schumaker, V. N. (1989). Expression of haemolytically active human complement component C1r proenzyme in insect cells using a baculovirus vector. *Complement Inflamm.*, **6**, 433–41
31. Loos, M. and Heinz, H. (1986). Component deficiencies: The first component: C1q, C1r, C1s. *Prog. Allergy*, **39**, 212–31
32. Carroll, M. C., Campbell, R. D., Bentley, D. R. and Porter, R. R. (1984). A molecular map of the human major histocompatibility complex class III region linking complement genes C4, C2 and factor B. *Nature*, **307,** 237–41
33. Wu, L. C., Morley, B. J. and Campbell, R. D. (1987). Cell-specific expression of the human complement protein factor B gene: evidence for the role of two distinct 5′ flanking elements. *Cell*, **48**, 331–42
34. Carroll, M. C., Belt, K. T., Palsdottir, A. and Porter, R. R. (1984). Structure and organization of C4 genes. *Phil. Trans. R. Soc. Lond. B*, **306**, 379–88
35. Dunham, I., Sargent, C. A., Trowsdale, J. and Campbell, R. D. (1987). Molecular mapping of the human major histocompatibility complex by pulsed-field gel electrophoresis. *Proc. Natl. Acad. Sci. USA*, **84**, 7237–41
36. Carroll, M. C., Campbell, R. D. and Porter, R. R. (1985). The mapping of 21-hydroxylase genes adjacent to complement component C4 genes in HLA, the major histocompatibility complex in man. *Proc. Natl. Acad. Sci. USA*, **82**, 521–5.
37. White, P. C., Grossberger, D., Onufer, B. J., Chaplin, D. D., New, M. I., Dupont, B. and Strominger, J. L. (1985). Two genes encoding steroid 21-hydroxylase are located near the genes encoding the fourth component of complement in man. *Proc. Natl. Acad. Sci. USA*, **82**, 1089–93
38. Higashi, Y., Yoshioka, H., Yamane, M., Gotoh, O. and Fujii-Kuriyama, Y. (1986). Complete nucleotide sequence of two steroid 21-hydroxylase genes tandemly arranged in human chromosome: a pseudogene and a genuine gene. *Proc. Natl. Acad. Sci. USA*, **83**, 2841–5
39. Rodrigues, N. R., Dunham, I., Yu, C. Y., Carroll, M. C., Porter R. R. and Campbell, R. D. (1987). Molecular characterization of the HLA-linked steroid 21-hydroxylase B gene from an individual with congenital adrenal hyperplasia. *EMBO J.*, **6**, 1653–61

40. Levi-Strauss, M., Carroll, M. C., Steinmetz, M. and Meo, T. (1988). A previously undetected MHC gene with an unusual periodic structure. *Science*, **240**, 201–4
41. Sargent, C. A., Durham, I. and Campbell, R. D. (1989). Identification of multiple HTF-island associated genes in the human major histocompatibility complex class III region. *EMBO J.*, **8**, 2305–12
42. Morel, Y., Bristow, J., Gitelman, S. E. and Miller, W. L. (1989). Transcript encoded on the opposite strand of the human steroid 21-hydroxylase/complement component C4 gene locus. *Proc. Natl. Acad. Sci. USA*, **86**, 6582–6
43. Gitelman, S. E., Bristow, J. and Miller, W. L. (1992). Mechanism and consequences of the duplication of the human C4/P450c21/Gene X locus. *Mol. Cell. Biol.*, **12**, 2124–34
44. Matsumoto, K. I., Arai, M., Ishihara, N., Ando, A., Inoko, H. and Ikemura, T. (1992). Cluster of fibronectin type-III repeats found in the human major histocompatibility complex class III region shows the highest homology with the repeats in an extracellular matrix protein, tenascin. *Genomics*, **12**, 485–91
45. Sargent, C. A. (988). Molecular mapping of the HLA class III region. *D. Phil Thesis*, Oxford University
46. Anderson, M. J. (1990). Molecular genetics of the human complement protein C4. *D. Phil Thesis*, Oxford University
47. Sargent, C. A., Dunham, I., Trowsdale, J. and Campbell, R. D. (1989). Human major histocompatibility complex contains genes for the major heat shock protein HSP70. *Proc. Natl. Acad. Sci. USA*, **86**, 1968–72
48. Spies, T., Bresnahan, M. and Strominger, J. L. (1989). Human major histocompatibility complex contains a minimum of 19 genes between the complement cluster and HLA-B. *Proc. Natl. Acad. Sci. USA*, **86**, 8955–8
49. Kendall, E., Sargent, C. A. and Campbell, R. D. (1990). Human major histocompatibility complex contains a new cluster of genes between the HLA-D and complement C4 loci. *Nucleic Acids Res.*, **18**, 7251–7
50. Milner, C. M. and Campbell, R. D. (1990). Structure and expression of the three MHC-linked human HSP70 genes. *Immunogenetics*, **32**, 242–51
51. Hsieh, S. L. and Campbell, R. D. (1991). Evidence that gene G7a in human major histocompatibility complex encodes valyl-tRNA synthetase. *Biochem. J.*, **278**, 809–16
52. Campbell, R. D., Bentley, D. R. and Morley, B. J. (1984). The factor B and C2 genes. *Phil. Trans. R. Soc. Lond. B.*, **306**, 367–78
53. Morley, B. J. and Campbell, R. D. (1984). Internal homologies of the Ba fragment from human complement component factor B, a class III MHC antigen. *EMBO J.*, **3**, 153–7
54. Mancuso, D. J., Tuley, E. A., Westfield, L. A., Worrall, N. K., Shelton-Inloes, B. B., Sorace, J. M., Alevy, Y. G. and Sadler, J. E. (1989). Structure of the gene for human von Willebrand Factor. *J. Biol. Chem.*, **264,** 19514–27
55. Kiss, I., Deak, F., Holloway, R. G. J., Delius, H., Mebust, K. A., Frimberger, E., Argraves, W. S., Tsonis, P. A., Winterbottom, N. and Goetinck, P. F. (1989). Structure of the gene for cartilage matrix protein, a modular protein of the extracellular matrix. Exon/intron organization, unusual splice sites, and relation to α chains of β_2 integrins, von Willebrand factor, complement factors B and C2, and epidermal growth factor. *J. Biol. Chem.*, **264**, 8126–34
56. Corbi, A. L., Garcia-Aguilar, J. and Springer, T. A. (1990). Genomic structure of an integrin α subunit, the leukocyte p150,95 molecule. *J. Biol. Chem.*, **265**, 2782–8
57. Christie, D. L. and Gagnon, J. (1983). Amino acid sequence of the Bb fragment from complement factor B. *Biochem. J.*, **209**, 61–70
58. Campbell, R. D. and Porter R. R. (1983). Molecular cloning and characterisation of the gene coding for human complement protein factor B. *Proc. Natl. Acad. Sci. USA*, **80**, 4464–8
59. Irwin, D. M., Robertson, K. A. and MacGillwray, R. T. A. (1988). Structure and evolution of the bovine prothrombin gene. *J. Mol. Biol.*, **200**, 31–45
60. Ishii, Y., Zhu, Z. B., Macon, K. J. and Volanakis, J. E. (1991). Structure of the gene for human complement component C2. *Complement Inflamm.*, **8**, 167
61. Johnson, C. A., Densen, P., Hurford, R. K., Colten, H. R. and Wetsel, R. A. (1992). Type I human complement C2 deficiency. A 28-base pair gene deletion causes skipping of exon 6 during RNA splicing. *J. Biol. Chem.*, **267**, 9347–53

62. Alper, C. A. (1981). Polymorphism of human complement components C2 and factor B. In Dorf, M. E. (ed.) *The Role of the Major Histocompatibility Complex in Immunobiology*, pp. 173–220. (New York: Garland)
63. Bentley, D. R. and Campbell, R. D. (1986). C2 and factor B: Structure and genetics. *Biochem. Soc. Symp.*, **51**, 7–18
64. Bentley, D. R., Campbell, R. D. and Cross, S. J. (1985). DNA polymorphism of the C2 locus. *Immunogenetics*, **22**, 377–90
65. Zhu, Z. B. and Volanakis, J. E. (1990). Allelic associations of multiple RFLPs of the gene encoding complement protein C2. *Am. J. Hum. Genet.*, **46**, 956–96
66. Ratanachaiyavong, S., Campbell, R. D. and McGregor, A. M. (1989). Enhanced resolution of the SstI polymorphic variants of the C2 locus: description of a new size class. *Hum. Immunol.*, **26**, 310–20
67. Zhu, Z. B., Hsieh, S. L., Bentley, D. R., Campbell, R. D. and Volanakis, J. E. (1992). A variable number of tandem repeats (VNTR) locus within the human complement C2 gene is associated with a retropson derived from a human endogenous retrovirus. *J. Exp. Med.*, **175**, 1783–7
68. Cross, S. J., Edwards, J. H., Bentley, D. R. and Campbell, R. D. (1985). DNA polymorphism of the C2 and factor B genes. *Immunogenetics*, **21**, 39–48
69. Fathallah, D., Abbal, M., Cambon-Thomsen, A., Thomsen, M. and Campbell, R. D. (1986). A DNA restriction fragment length polymorphism in the complement region of the human MHC shows an absolute correlation with polymorphism of complement factor B(Bf) defined by isoelectric focusing. *J. Immunogenet.*, **12**, 321–6
70. Yu, C. Y. (1991). The complete exon–intron structure of a human complement component C4A gene. DNA sequences, polymorphism, and linkage to the 21-hydroxylase gene. *J. Immunol.*, **146**, 1057–66
71. Mauff, G. Brenden, M., Braun-Stilwell, M., Doxiadis, G., Giles, C. M., Hauptmann, G., Rittner, C., Schneider, P. M., Stradmann-Bellinghausen, B. and Uring-Lambert, B. (1990). C4 reference typing report. *Complement Inflamm.*, **7**, 193–212
72. Belt, K. T., Carroll, M. C. and Porter, R. R. (1984). The structural basis of the multiple forms of human complement component C4. *Cell*, **36**, 907–14
73. Belt, K. T. Yu, C. Y., Carroll, M. C. and Porter, R. R. (1985). Polymorphism of human complement component C4. *Immunogenetics*, **21**, 173–80
74. Chakravarti, D. N., Campbell, R. D. and Porter, R. R. (1987). The chemical structure of the C4d fragment of the human complement component C4. *Mol. Immunol.*, **24**, 1187–97
75. Yu, C. Y., Campbell, R. D. and Porter, R. R. (1988). A structural model for the location of the Rodgers and the Chido antigenic determinants and their correlation with the human complement component C4A/C4B isotypes. *Immunogenetics*, **27**, 399–405
76. Yu, C. Y., Belt, K. T., Giles, C. M., Campbell, R. D. and Porter, R. R. (1986). Structural basis of the polymorphism of human complement components C4A and C4B: gene size, reactivity and antigenicity. *EMBO J.*, **5**, 2873–81
77. Dodds, A. W., Law, S. K. A. and Porter R. R. (1985). The origin of the very variable haemolytic activities of the common human complement component C4 allotypes including C4-A6. *EMBO J.*, **4**, 2239–44
78. Schendel, D. J., O'Neill, G. and Wank, R. (1984). MHC-linked Class III genes. Analyses of C4 gene frequencies, complotypes and associations with distinct HLA haplotypes in German Caucasians. *Immunogenetics*, **20**, 23–31
79. Tokunaga, K., Omoto, K., Akaza, T., Akiyama, N., Ameniya, H., Naito, S., Sasazuki, T., Satoh, H. and Juji, T. (1985). Haplotype study of C4 polymorphism in Japanese. Associations with MHC alleles, complotypes, and HLA-complement haplotypes. *Immunogenetics*, **22**, 359–65
80. Carroll, M. C. and Alper, C. A. (1987). Polymorphism and molecular genetics of human C4. *Br. Med. Bull.*, **43**, 50–65
81. Teisberg, P., Olaisen, B., Gedde-Dahl, T., Mevag, B. and Jonassen, R. (1987). Restriction fragment length polymorphism of the complement component C4 loci on chromosome 6. Studies with emphasis on the determination of gene number. *Complement Inflamm.*, **4**, 230
82. Collier, S., Sinnott, P. J., Dyer, P. A., Price, D. A., Harris, R. and Strachan, T. (1989). Pulsed field gel electrophoresis identifies a high degree of variability in the number of tandem 21-hydroxylase and complement C4 gene repeats in 21-hydroxylase deficiency haplotypes. *EMBO J.*, **8**, 1393–1402

83. Dunham, I., Sargent, C. A., Dawkins, R. L. and Campbell, R. D. (1989). Direct observation of the gene organization of the complement C4 and 21-hydroxylase loci by pulsed field gel electrophoresis. *J. Exp. Med.*, **169**, 1803–16
84. Carroll, M. C., Palsdottir, A., Belt, K. T. and Porter, R. R. (1985). Deletion of complement C4 and steroid 21-hydroxylase genes in the HLA class III region. *EMBO J.*, **4**, 2547–52
85. Schneider, P. M., Carroll, M. C., Alper, C. A., Rittner, C., Whitehead, A. S., Yunis, E. J. and Colten, H. R. (1986). Polymorphism of human complement C4 and steroid 21-hydroxylase genes. Restriction fragment length polymorphisms revealing structural deletions, homoduplications, and size variants. *J. Clin. Invest.*, **78**, 650–7
86. Hauptmann, G., Uring-Lambert, B., Vegnaduzzi-Lamouche, N. and Mascart-Lemone, F. (1987). RFLP studies of 3 complete C4 deficient patients. *Complement*, **4**, 166
87. Yu, C. Y. and Campbell, R. D. (1987). Definitive RFLPs to distinguish between the human complement C4A/C4B isotypes and the major Rodgers/Chido determinants. Application to the study of C4 null alleles. *Immunogenetics*, **25**, 383–90
88. Partanen, J. and Campbell, R. D. (1989). Restriction fragment analysis of non-deleted complement C4 null genes suggests point mutations in C4A null alleles, but gene conversions in C4B null alleles. *Immunogenetics*, **30**, 520–3
89. Berg, E. S., Teisberg, P. and Olaisen, B. (1989). Genetic analysis of C4 polymorphism by use of DNA amplification (PCR), allele-specific oligonucleotide probes and allele-specific restriction enzymes. *Ann. Hum. Genet.*, **53**, 221–7
90. Braun, L., Schneider, P. M., Giles, C. M., Bertrams, J. and Rittner, C (1990). Null alleles of human complement C4. Evidence for pseudogenes at the C4A locus and for gene conversion at the C4B locus. *J. Exp. Med.*, **171**, 129–40
91. Palsdottir, A., Fossdal, R., Arnason, A., Edwards, J. H. and Jensson, O. (1987). Heterogeneity of human C4 gene size: a large intron (6.5kb) is present in all C4A genes and some C4B genes. *Immunogenetics*, **25**, 299–304
92. Giles, C. M., Uring-Lambert, B., Boksch, W., Braun, M., Goetz, J., Neumann, R., Mauff, G. and Hauptmann, G. (1987). The study of a French family with two duplicated C4A haplotypes. *Hum. Genet.*,**77**, 359–65
93. Rittner, C., Giles, C. M., Roos, M. L. H., Demant, P. and Mollenhauer, E. (1984). Genetics of human C4 polymorphism: detection and segregation of rare and duplicated haplotypes. *Immunogenetics*, **19**, 321–3
94. Raum, D., Awdeh, Z., Anderson, J., Strong, L., Granados, J., Pevan, L., Giblett, E., Yunis, E. J. and Alper, C. A. (1984). Human C4 haplotypes with duplicated C4A or C4B. *Am. J. Hum. Genet.*, **36**, 72–9
95. McLean, R. H., Giles, C., Yu, C. Y., Campbell, R. D. and Bias, W. B. (1989). Reversed restriction sites for the C4 isotypic and Rodgers(1)/Chido(1) regions on two hybrid C4 genes. *Tissue Antigens*, **35**, 75–81
96. Robson, T., Giles, C. M. and Heard, R. N. S. (1989). An epitope in C4β light (L) chains detected by human anti-Rg: its relationship with β-chain polymorphism and MHC associations. *Immunogenetics*, **30**, 344–9
97. Whitehead, A. S., Woods, D. E., Fleischnick, E., Chin, J. E., Yunis, E. J., Katz, A. J., Gerald, P. S., Alper, C. A. and Colten, H. R. (1984). DNA polymorphism of the C4 genes. A new marker for analysis of the major histocompatibility complex. *N. Engl. J. Med.*, **310**, 88–91
98. Yu, C. Y. and Campbell, R. D. (1987). Sau3A1 polymorphism of human complement component C4 at the C4d region. *Biochem. Soc. Trans.*, **15**, 654–5
99. Palsdottir, A., Cross, S. J., Edwards, J. H. and Carroll, M. C. (1983). Correlation between a DNA restriction fragment length polymorphism and C4A6 protein. *Nature*, **306**, 615–16
100. Palsdottir, A., Arnason, A., Fossdal, R. and Jensson, O. (1987). Gene organization of haplotypes expressing two different C4A allotypes. *Hum. Genet.*, **76**, 220–4
101. Schneider, P. M. and Rittner, C. (1988). Bgl II restriction fragment length polymorphism of human complement C4A gene coincides with BF*F allele of factor B. *Immunogenetics*, **27**, 225–8
102. Uring-Lambert, B., Vegnaduzzi, N., Carroll, M. C., Tongio, M. M., Goetz, J. and Hauptmann, G. (1987). Heterogeneity in the structural basis of the human complement C4A null allele (C4A Q0) as revealed by HindIII restriction fragment length polymorphism analysis. *FEBS Lett.*, **217**, 65–8

103. Johnson, D. M. A., Gagnon, J. and Reid, K. B. M. (1984). Amino acid sequence of human factor D of the complement system. Similarity in sequence between factor D and proteases of non-plasma origin. *FEBS Lett.*, **166**, 347–51
104. Niemann, M. A., Brown, A. S., Bennett, J. C. and Volanakis, J. E. (1984). Amino acid sequence of human D of the alternative complement pathway. *Biochemistry*, **23**, 2482–6
105. White, T., Damm, D., Brown, R., Hancock, N., Rosen, B., Spiegelman, B. M., Lowell, B. and Flier, J. (1989). Isolation and characterization of cDNA clones for human complement factor D. *Complement Inflamm.*, **6**, 415 (Abstract)
106. Young, C. L., Barker, W. C., Tomaselli, C. M. and Dayhoff, M. O. (1978). Serine proteases. In Dayhoff, M. O. (ed.) *Atlas of Protein Sequence and Structure*, pp. 73–93. (Washington DC: National Biomedical Research Foundation)
107. Barnum, S. R. and Volanakis, J. E. (1985). Biosynthesis of complement protein D by HepG2 cells: A comparision of D produced by HepG2 cells, U937 cells and blood monocytes. *Eur. J. Immunol.*, **15**, 1148–51
108. Platt, K. A., Min, H. Y., Ross, S. R. and Spiegelman, B. M. (1989). Obesity-linked regulation of the adipsin gene promotor in transgenic mice. *Proc. Natl. Acad. Sci. USA*, **86**, 7460–94
109. Kluin-Nelemans, H. C., van Velzen-Blad, H., van Helden, H. P. T. and Daha, M. R. (1984). Functional deficiency of complement factor D in a monozygous twin. *Clin. Exp. Immunol.*, **58**, 724–30
110. Hiemstra, P. S., Langeler, E., Compier, B., Keepers, Y., Leijh, P. C., van den Barselaar, M. T., Overbosch, D. and Daha, M. R. (1989). Complete and partial deficiencies of complement factor D in a Dutch family. *J. Clin. Invest.*, **84**, 1957–61
111. Rosen, B. S., Cook, K. S., Yaglon, J., Groves, D. L., Volanakis, J. E., Damm, D., White, T. and Spiegelman, B. M. (1989). Adipsin and complement factor D activity: an immune related defect in obesity. *Science*, **244**, 1483–6
112. Smith, C. A., Pangburn, M. K., Vogel, C. W. and Muller-Eberhard, H. J. (1984). Molecular architecture of human properdin, a positive regulator of the alternative pathway of complement. *J. Biol. Chem.*, **259**, 4582–8
113. Pangburn, M. K. (1989). Analysis of the natural polymeric forms of human properdin and their functions in complement activation. *J. Immunol.*, **142**, 202–7
114. Farries, T. C. and Atkinson, J. P. (1989). Biosynthesis of properdin. *J. Immunol.*, **142**, 842–7
115. Farries, T. C., Lachmann, P. J. and Harrison, R. A. (1988). Analysis of the interaction between properdin and factor B, components of the alternative-pathway C3 convertase of complement. *Biochem. J.*, **253**, 667–75
116. Goundis, D. and Reid, K. B. M. (1988). Properdin, the terminal complement components, thrombospondin and the circumsporozoite protein of malaria parasites contain similar sequence motifs. *Nature*, **335**, 82–5
117. Nolan, K. F., Schwaebel, W., Kaluz, S., Dierich, M. P. and Reid, K. B. M. (1991). Molecular cloning of the cDNA coding for properdin, a positive regulator of the alternative pathway of human complement. *Eur. J. Immunol.*, **21**, 771–6
118. Nolan, K. F., Kaluz, S., Higgins, J. M. G., Goundis, D. and Reid, K. B. M. (1992). Characterisation of the human properdin gene. *Biochem. J.* **287**, 291–7
119. Lawler, J. and Hynes, R. O. (1986). The structure of human thrombospondin, an adhesive glycoprotein with multiple calcium-binding sites and homologies with several different proteins. *J. Cell. Biol.*, **103**, 1635–8
120. Frazier, W. A. (1991). Thrombospondins. *Curr. Opinion Cell Biol.*, **3**, 792–9
121. Patthy, L. (1987). Intron-dependent evolution: preferred types of exons and introns. *FEBS Lett.*, **214**, 1–7
122. Sjoholm, A. G. (1990). Inherited complement deficiency states: implications for immunity and immunological disease. *APMIS*, **98**, 861–74
123. Figueroa, J. E. and Densen, P. (1991). Infectious diseases associated with complement deficiencies. *Clin. Microbiol. Rev.*, **4**, 359–95
124. Coleman, M. P., Murray, J. C., Willard, H. F., Nolan, K. F., Reid, K. B. M., Blake, D. J., Lindsay, S., Bhattacharaya, S. S., Wright, A. and Davies, K. E. (1991). Genetic and physical mapping around the properdin P gene. *Genomics*, **11**, 991–6
125. Goonewardena, P., Sjoholm, A. G., Nilsson, L-Å. and Petterson, U. (1988). Linkage analysis of the properdin deficiency gene: Suggestion of a locus in the proximal part of the short arm of the X chromosome. *Genomics*, **2**, 115–18

126. Kölble, K., Cant, A. J., Fay, A., Whaley, K., Schlesinger, M. and Reid, K. B. M. (1992). Carrier detection in families with properdin deficiency by microsatellite haplotyping. *J. Clin. Invest.* (in press)
127. Catterall, C. F., Lyons, A., Sim, R. B., Day, A. J. and Harris, T. J. R. (1987). Characterization of the primary amino acid sequence of human complement control protein factor I from an analysis of cDNA clones. *Biochem. J.*, **242**, 849–56
128. Goldberger, G., Burns, G. A. P., Rits, M., Edge, M. D. and Kwiatkowski, D. J. (1987). Human complement factor I: analysis of cDNA-derived primary structure. *Biochemistry*, **262**, 10065–71
129. Shiang, R., Murray, J. C., Morton, C. C., Betow, K. H., Wasmuth, J. J., Olney, A. H., Sanger, W. G. and Goldberger, G. (1989). Mapping of the human factor I gene to 4q25. *Genomics*, **4**, 82–6
130. Kölble, K., Buckle, V., Lefranc, G., Halbwachs-Mecarelli, L., Möller-Rasmussen, J., Sim, R. B., Späth, P., Svehag, S. E., Teisner, B. and Wahn, V. (1989). Physical mapping of the complement factor I gene in normal and deficient genomes. *Complement Inflamm.*, **6**, 355 (Abstract)
131. Rasmussen, J. M., Teisner, B., Brandslund, I. and Svehag, S. E. (1987). A family with complement factor I deficiency. *Scand. J. Immunol.*, **23**, 711–15 (Abstract)
132. Whitehead, A. S., Solomon, E., Chambers, S., Bodmer, W. F., Povey, S. and Fey, G. (1982). Assignment of the structural gene for the third component of human complement to chromosome 19. *Proc. Natl. Acad. Sci. USA*, **79**, 5021–5
133. Wetsel, R. A., Lemons, R. S., Le Beau, M. M., Barnum, S. R., Noack, D. and Tack, B. F. (1988). Molecular analysis of human complement component C5: localisation of the structural gene to chromosome 9. *Biochemistry*, **27**, 1474–82
134. Barnum, S. R., Amiguet, P., Amiguet-Barras, F., Fey, G. H. and Tack, B. F. (1989). Complete intron/exon organisation of DNA encoding the alpha chain of human C3. *J. Biol. Chem.*, **264**, 8471–4
135. Fong, K. Y., Botto, M., Walport, M. J. and So, A. K. (1990). Genomic organization of human complement component C3. *Genomics*, **7**, 579–86
136. Vik, D. P., Amiguet, P., Moffat, G. J., Fey, M., Amiguet-Barras, F., Wetsel, R. A. and Tack, B. F. (1991). Structural features of the human C3 gene: intron/exon organization, transcriptional start site, and promoter region sequence. *Biochemistry*, **30**, 1080–5
137. Botto, M., Fong, K. Y., So, A. K., Rudge, A. and Walport, M. J. (1990). Molecular basis of hereditary C3 deficiency. *J. Clin. Invest.*, **86**, 1158–63
138. Botto, M., Fong, K. Y., So, A. K., Barlow, R., Routier, R., Morley, B. J. and Walport, M. J. (1992). Homozygous hereditary C3 deficiency due to a partial gene deletion. *Proc. Natl. Acad. Sci. USA*, **89**, 4957–61
139. Haviland, D. L., Haviland, J. C., Fleischer, D. T., Hunt, A. and Wetsel, R. A. (1991). Complete cDNA sequence of human complement pro-C5. Evidence of truncated transcripts derived from a single copy gene. *J. Immunol.*, **146**, 362–8
140. DiScipio, R. G. and Hugli, T. E. (1989). The molecular architecture of human complement component C6. *J. Biol. Chem.*, **264**, 16197–206
141. Haefliger, J. A., Tschopp, J., Vial, N. and Jenne, D. E. (1989). Complete primary structure and functional characterization of the sixth component of the human complement system. Identification of the C5b-binding domain in complement C6. *J. Biol. Chem.*, **264**, 18041–51
142. DiScipio, R. G., Chakravarti, D. N., Muller-Eberhard, H. J. and Fey, G. H. (1988). The structure of human complement component C7 and the C5b-7 complex. *J. Biol. Chem.*, **263**, 549–60
143. DiScipio, R. G., Gehring, M. R., Podack, E. R., Kan, C. C., Hugli, T. E. and Fey, G. F. (1984). Nucleotide sequence of cDNA and derived amino acid sequence of human complement component C9. *Proc. Natl. Acad. Sci. USA*, **81**, 7298–302
144. Stanley, K. K., Kocher, H. P., Luzio, J. P., Jackson, P. and Tschopp, J. (1985). The sequence and topology of human complement component C9. *EMBO J.*, **4**, 375–82
145. Rao, A. G., Howard, O. M. Z., Ng, S. C., Whitehead, A. S., Colten, H. R. and Sodetz, J. M. (1987). Complementary DNA and derived amino acid sequence for the α subunit of human complement protein C8: evidence for the existence of a separate α subunit mRNA. *Biochemistry*, **26**, 3556–64
146. Haefliger, J. A., Tschopp, J., Naedelli, D., Wahli, W., Kocher, H. P., Tosi, M. and Stanley, K. K. (1987). Complementary DNA cloning of complement C8β and its sequence homology to C9. *Biochemistry*, **26**, 3551–6

147. Howard, O. M. Z., Rao, A. G. and Sodetz, J. M. (1987). Complementary DNA and derived amino acid sequence of the β-subunit of C8: identification of a close structural and ancestral relationship to the α-subunit and C9. *Biochemistry*, **26**, 3565–70
148. Stanley, K. and Luzio, P. (1988). Perforin: A family of killer proteins. *Nature*, **334**, 475–6
149. Shinkai, Y., Takio, K. and Okumura, K. (1988). Homology of perforin to the ninth component of complement (C9). *Nature*, **334**, 525–7
150. Lichtenheld, M. G., Olsen, K. J., Lu, P., Lowry, D. M., Hamed, A., Hengartner, H. and Podack, E. R. (1988). Structure and function of human perforin. *Nature*, **325**, 448–51
151. Hobart, M. J., Fernie, B. A., Lachmann, P. J., Morgan, B. P., Orren, A. and DiScipio, R. (1989). C6 and C7 genes in normal and deficient individuals. *Complement Inflamm.*, **6**, 345 (Abstract)
152. Lachmann, P. J., Hobart, M. J. and Woo, P. (1978). Combined genetic deficiency of C6 and C7 in man. *Clin. Exp. Immunol.*, **75**, 396–401
153. Morgan, B. P., Vora, J. P., Bennett, A. J., Thomas, J. P. and Matthews, N. (1989). A case of hereditary combined deficiency of complement components C6 and C7 in man. *Clin. Exp. Immunol.*, **75**, 396–401
154. Orren, A., Potter, P. C., Cooper, R. C. and du-Toit, E. (1987). Deficiency of the sixth component of complement and susceptibility to Neisseria meningitidis infections: studies in 10 families and five isolated cases. *Immunology*, **62**, 249–53
155. Lim, D., Gewurz, A., Lint, T. F., Ghaze, M., Sepheri, B. and Gewurz, H. (1976). Absence of the sixth component of complement in a patient with repeated episodes of meningococcal meningitis. *J. Pediatr.*, **89**, 42
156. Wurzner, R., Orren, A., Potter, P., Morgan, B. P., Ponard, D., Spath, P., Brai, M., Schulze, M., Happe, L. and Gotze, O. (1991). Functionally active complement proteins C6 and C7 detected in C6- and C7-deficient individuals. *Clin. Exp. Immunol.*, **83**, 430–7
157. Jeremiah, S. J., West, L. F., Abbott, C. M., Murad, Z., Povey, S., Thomas, H. J., Solomon, E., DiScipio, R. and Fey, G. H. (1989). Assignment of the human C6 and C7 genes to chromosome 5q. *Cytogen. Cell Genet.*, **51**, 1019 (Abstract)
158. Kaufman, K. M., Snider, J. V., Spurr, N. K., Schwartz, C. E. and Sodetz, J. M. (1989). Chromosomal assignment of genes encoding the α, β and γ subunits of human complement protein C8: identification of a close physical linkage between the α and the β loci. *Genomics*, **5**, 475–80
159. Tedesco, F. (1986). Component deficiencies. 8 The eighth component. *Prog. Allergy*, **39**, 295–306
160. Tschopp, J., Penea, F., Schifferli, J. and Spath, P. (1986). Dysfunctional C8 beta chain in patients with C8 deficiency. *Scand. J. Immunol.* **24**, 715–20
161. Tedesco, F., Densen, P., Villa, M. A., Petersen, B. H. and Sirchia, G. (1983). Two types of dysfunctional eighth component of complement (C8) molecules in C8 deficiency in man. Reconstitution of normal C8 from the mixture of two abnormal C8 molecules. *J. Clin. Invest.*, **71**, 183–91
162. Warnick, P. R. and Densen, P. (1991). Reduced C8 beta messenger RNA expression in families with hereditary C8 beta deficiency. *J. Immunol.*, **146**, 1052–6
163. Schneider, P. M., Dittmer, B., Tedesco, F., Spath, P. J., Rittner, C. and Sodetz, J. M. (1987). Genomic structure of the complement C8β locus in individuals with inherited C8β deficiency. *Complement*, **4**, 221 (Abstract)
164. Tanaka, S., Suzuki, T., Sakaizumi, M., Harada, Y., Matsushima, Y., Fukumori, Y., Inai, S., Moriveraki, K. and Yonekawa, H. (1991). Gene responsible for deficient activity of the β subunit of C8, the eighth component of complement, is located on mouse chromosome 4. *Immunogenetics*, **33**, 18–23
165. Komatsu, M., Yamamoto, K., Kawashima, T. and Migita, S. (1985). Genetic deficiency of the alpha-gamma-subunit of the eighth complement component in the rabbit. *J. Immunol.*, **134**, 2607–9
166. Marazziti, D., Eggersten, G., Stanley, K. K. and Fey, G (1987). Evolution of the cysteine rich domains of C9. *Complement*, **4**, 189 (Abstract)
167. Abbott, C., West, L., Povey, S., Jeremiah, S., Murad, Z., DiScipio, R. and Fey, G. (1989). The gene for human complement component C9 mapped to chromosome 5 by polymerase chain reaction. *Genomics*, **4**, 606–9
168. Lint, T. F. and Gewurz, H. (1986). Component deficiencies. 9. The ninth component. *Prog. Allergy*, **39**, 307–10

169. Rodriguez de Cordoba, S., Lublin, D. M., Rubinstein, P. and Atkinson, J. P. (1985). Human genes for three complement components that regulate the activation of C3 are tightly linked. *J. Exp. Med.*, **161**, 1189–95
170. Weiss, J. H., Morton, C. C., Bruns, G. A. P., Weiss, J. J., Klickstein, L. B., Wong, W. W. and Fearon, D. T. (1987). A complement receptor locus: genes encoding C3b/C4b receptor and C3d/Epstein Barr virus receptor map to 1q32. *J. Immunol.*, **138**, 312–15
171. Norman, D. G., Barlow, P. N., Baron, M., Day, A. J., Sim, R. B. and Campbell, I. D. (1991). Three-dimensional structure of a complement control protein module in solution. *J. Mol. Biol.*, **219**, 717–25
172. Day, A. J. and Baron, M. (1991). Structure/function inter-relationships of mosaic proteins. *J. Biomed. Sci.*, **1**, 153–63
173. Hourcade, D., Garcia, A. D., Post, T. W., Taillon-Miller, P., Holers, V. M., Wagner, L. M., Bora, N. S. and Atkinson, J. P. (1992). Analysis of the human regulators of complement activation (RCA) gene cluster with yeast artificial chromosomes (YACs). *Genomics*, **12**, 289–300
174. Rey-Campos, J., Rubinstein, P. and Rodriguez de Cordoba, S. (1988). A physical map of the human regulator of complement activation gene cluster linking the complement genes CR1, CR2, DAF, and C4-bp. *J. Exp. Med.*, **167**, 664–9
175. Carroll, M. C., Alicot, E. M., Katzman, P. J., Klickstein, L. B., Smith, J. A. and Fearon, D. T. (1988). Organisation of the genes encoding complement receptors type 1 and 2, decay-accelerating factor, and C4-binding protein in the RCA locus on human chromosome 1. *J. Exp. Med.*, **167**, 1271–80
176. Pardo-Manuel, F., Rey-Campos, J., Hillarp, A., Dahlbäck, B. and Rodriguez de Cordoba, S. (1990). Human genes for the α and β chains of complement C4b-binding protein are closely linked in a head-to-tail arrangement. *Proc. Natl. Acad. Sci, USA*, **87**, 4529–32
177. Hillarp, A., Hessing, M. and Dahlback, B. (1989). Protein S binding in relation to the subunit composition of human C4b-binding protein. *FEBS Lett.*, **259**, 53–6
178. Hillarp, A. and Dahlback, B. (1990). Cloning of cDNA coding for the β chain of human complement component C4b-binding protein. Sequence homology with the α chain. *Proc. Natl. Acad. Sci. USA*, **87**, 1183–7
179. Rodriguez de Cordoba, S., Sanchez-Corral, P. and Rey-Campos, J. (1991). Structure of the gene coding for the α polypeptide chain of the human complement component C4b-binding protein. *J. Exp. Med.*, **173**, 1073–82
180. Ripoche, J., Day, A. J., Harris, T. J. R. and Sim, R. B. (1988). The complete amino acid sequence of human complement factor H. *Biochem. J.*, **249**, 593–602
181. Fontaine, M., Demares, M. J., Koistinen, V., Day, A. J., Davrinche, C., Sim, R. B. and Ripoche, J. (1989). Truncated forms of human complement factor H. *Biochem. J.*, **258**, 927–30
182. Estaller, C., Schwaeble, W., Dierich, M. and Weiss, E. H. (1991). Human complement factor H: two factor H proteins are derived from alternatively spliced transcripts. *Eur. J. Immunol.*, **21**, 799–802
183. Sherka, C., Timmann, C., Horstmann, R. D. and Zipfel, P. F. (1992). Two additional human serum proteins structurally related to complement factor H. *J. Immunol.*, **148**, 3313–18
184. Klickstein, L. B., Wong, W. W., Smith, J. A., Weis, J. H., Wilson, J. G. and Fearon, D. T. (1987). Human C3b/C4b receptor (CR1). Demonstration of long homologous repeating domains that are composed of the short consensus repeats characteristic of C3/C4 binding proteins. *J. Exp. Med.*, **165**, 1095–112
185. Klickstein, L. B., Bartow, T. J., Miletic, V., Rabson, L. D., Smith, J. A. and Fearon, D. T. (1988). Identification of distinct C3b and C4b recognition sites in the human C3b/C4b receptor (CR1, CD35) by deletion mutagenesis. *J. Exp. Med.*, **168**, 1699–717
186. Krych, M., Hourcade, D. and Atkinson, J. P. (1991). Sites within the complement C3b/C4b receptor important for the specificity of ligand biding. *Proc. Natl. Acad. Sci. USA*, **88**, 4353–7
187. Wong, W. W., Cahill, J. M., Rosen, M. D., Kennedy, C. A., Bonaccio, E. T., Morris, M. J., Wilson, J. G., Klickstein, L. B. and Fearon, D. T. (1989). Structure of the human CR1 gene. Molecular basis of the structural and quantitative polymorphisms and identification of a new CR1-like allele. *J. Exp. Med.*, **169**, 847–63
188. Vik. D. P., Tack, B. F. and Wong, W. W. (1991). Structure of the complement receptor type 1 (CR1) gene and sequence of the s allele. *Complement Inflamm.*, **8**, 238 (Abstract)
189. Wilson, J. G., Murphy, E. E., Wong, W. W., Klickstein, L. B., Weis, J. H. and Fearon, D. T. (1986). Identification of a restriction fragment length polymorphism by a CR1 cDNA that correlates with the number of CR1 on erthyrocytes. *J. Exp. Med.*, **164**, 50–62

190. Cooper, N. R., Moore, M. D. and Nemerow, G. R. (1988). Immunobiology of CR2, the B lymphocyte receptor for Epstein–Barr virus and the C3d complement fragment. *Annu. Rev. Immunol.*, **6**, 85–114
191. Fujisaku, A., Harley, J. B., Frank, M. B., Gruner, B. A., Frazier, B. and Holers, V. M. (1989). Genomic organisation and polymorphisms of the human C3d/Epstein–Barr virus receptor. *J. Biol. Chem.*, **264**, 2118–25
192. Martin, D. R., Yuryev, A., Kalli, K. R., Fearon, D. T. and Ahearn, J. M. (1991). Determination of the structural basis for selective binding of Epstein–Barr virus to human complement receptor type 2. *J. Exp. Med.*, **174**, 1299–311
193. Davitz, M. A., Low, M. G. and Nussenzweig, V. (1986). Release of decay-accelerating factor (DAF) from the cell membrane by phosphatidylinositol-specific phospholipase (PIPLC). *J. Exp. Med.*, **163**, 1150–61
194. Caras, I. W., Davitz, M. A., Rhee, L., Weddell, G., Martin, D. W. and Nussenzweig, V. (1987). Cloning of decay-accelerating factor suggests novel sue of splicing to generate two proteins. *Nature*, **325**, 545–9
195. Medof, M. E., Lublin, D. M., Holers, V. M., Ayers, D. J., Getty, R. R., Leykam, J. K., Atkinson, J. P. and Tykocinski, M. L. (1987). Cloning and characterization of cDNAs encoding the complete sequence of decay-accelerating factor of human complement. *Proc. Natl. Acad. Sci, USA*, **84**, 2007–11
196. Post, T. W., Arce, M. A., Liszewski, M. K., Thompson, E. S., Atkinson, J. P. and Lublin, D. M. (1990). Structure of the gene for human complement protein decay accelerating factor. *J. Immunol.*, **144**, 740–4
197. Norris, K. A., Bradt, B., Cooper, N. R. and So, M. (1991). Characterization of a *Trypanosoma cruzi* C3 binding protein with functional and genetic similarities to the human complement regulatory protein, decay-accelerating factor. *J. Immunol.*, **147**, 2240–7
198. Mallinson, G., Tanner, M. J. A., Thompson, E. S., Telen, M. J. and Lublin, D. M. (1991). Sequence analysis of decay accelerating factor (DAF) cDNA and gene in original propositus of DAF-negative Inab phenotype. *Complement Inflamm.* **8**, 189 (Abstract)
199. Seya, T., Okada, M., Matsumoto, M., Hong, K. S., Kinoshita, T. and Atkinson, J. P. (1991). Preferential inactivation of the C5 convertase of the alternative complement pathway by factor I and membrane cofactor protein (MCP). *Mol. Immunol.*, **28**, 1137–47
200. Lublin, D. M., Liszewski, M. K., Post, T. W., Arce, M. A., Le Beau, M. M., Rebentisch, M. B., Lemons, L. S., Seya, T. and Atkinson, J. P. (1988). Molecular cloning and chromosomal localization of the human membrane cofactor protein (MCP). Evidence for inclusion in the multi-gene family of complement-regulatory proteins. *J. Exp. Med.*, **168**, 181–94
201. Post, T. W., Liszewski, M. K., Adams, E. M., Tedja, I., Miller, E. A. and Atkinson, J. P. (1991). Membrane cofactor protein of the complement system: alternative splicing of serine/threonine/proline-rich exons and cytoplasmic tails produces multiple isoforms that correlate with protein phenotype. *J. Exp. Med.*, **174**, 93–102.
202. Purcell, D. F. J., Russell, S. M., Deacon, N. J., Brown, M. A., Hooker, D. J. and McKenzie, I. F. (1991). Alternatively spliced RNAs encode several isoforms of CD46(MCP), a regulator of complement activation. *Immunogenetics*, **33**, 335–44
203. Adams, E. M., Brown, M. C., Nunge, M., Krych, M. and Atkinson, J. P. (1991). Contribution of the repeating domains of membrane cofactor protein (CD46) of the complement system to ligand binding and cofactor activity. *J. Immunol.*, **147**, 3005–11
204. Liszewski, M. K., Post, T. W. and Atkinson, J. P. (1991). Membrane cofactor protein (MCP or CD46): newest member of the regulators of complement activation gene cluster. *Annu. Rev. Immunol.*, **9**, 431–55
205. Bora, N. S., Lublin, D. M., Kumar, B. V., Hockett, R. D., Holers, V. M. and Atkinson, J. P. (1989). Structural gene for human membrane cofactor protein (MCP) of complement maps to within 100 kb of the 3′ end of the C3b/C4b receptor gene. *J. Exp. Med.*, **169**, 597–602
206. Meri, S., Morgan, B. P., Davies, A., Daniels, R. H., Olavesen, M. G., Waldmann, H. and Lachmann, P. J. (1990). Human protectin (CD59), an 18,000–20,000 MW complement lysis restricting factor, inhibits C5b–8 catalysed insertion of C9 into lipid bilayers. *Immunology*, **71**, 1–9
207. Davies, A., Simmons, D. L., Hale, G., Harrison, R. A., Tighe, H., Lachmann, P. J. and Waldmann, H. (1989). CD59, an LY-6-like protein expressed in human lymphoid cells,

regulates the action of the complement membrane attack complex on homologous cells. *J. Exp. Med.*, **170**, 637–54
208. Harada, R., Okada, N., Fujita, T. and Okada, H. (1990). Purification of 1F5 antigen that prevents complement attack on homologous cell membranes. *J. Immunol.*, **144**, 1823–8
209. Sugita, Y., Mazda, T. and Tomita, M. (1989). Amino-terminal amino acid sequence and chemical and functional properties of a membrane attack complex-inhibitory factor from human erythrocyte membranes. *J. Biochem. Tokyo*, **106**, 589–92
210. Okada, H., Nagami, Y., Takahashi, K., Okada, N., Hideshima, T., Takizawa, H. and Kondo, J. (1989). 20 kDa homologous restriction factor of complement resembles T cell activating protein. *Biochem. Biophys. Res. Commun.*, **162**, 1553–9
211. Yamashina, M., Ueda, E., Kinoshita, T., Takami, T., Ojima, A., Ono, H., Tanaka, H., Kondo, N., Orii, T. and Okada, N. (1990). Inherited complete deficiency of 20-kilodalton homologous restriction factor (CD59) as a cause of paroxysmal nocturnal hemoglobinuria. *N. Engl. J. Med.*, **323**, 1184–9
212. Motoyama, N., Okada, N., Yamashina, M. and Okada, H. (1992). Paroxysmal nocturnal hemoglobinuria due to hereditary nucleotide deletion in the HRF 20(CD59) gene. *Eur. J. Immunol.*, **22**, 2669–74
213. Jenne, D. and Stanley, K. K. (1985). Molecular cloning of S-protein, a link between complement, coagulation and cell-substrate adhesion. *EMBO J.*, **4**, 3153–7
214. Jenne, D. E. and Tschopp, J. (1989). Molecular structure and functional characterization of a human complement cytolysis inhibitor found in blood and seminal plasma: Identity to sulphated glycoprotein 2, a constituent of rat testis fluid. *Proc. Natl. Acad. Sci. USA*, **86**, 7123–7
215. Kirszbaum, L., Sharpe, J. A., Murphy, B., d'Apice, A. J., Classon, B., Hudson, P. and Walker, I. D. (1989). Molecular cloning and characterization of the novel, human complement-associated protein, SP-40,40: a link between the complement and reproductive systems. *EMBO J.*, **8**, 711–18

4
Synthesis of complement components in liver and at extrahepatic sites

H. R. COLTEN and R. C. STRUNK

INTRODUCTION

Complement protein biosynthesis has been a subject of study for over 100 years. In the 1890s, Metchinoff suggested that leukocytes were a source of complement[1]. Interest in the liver as a site of complement production was first generated by the experiments of Ehrlich and Morgenroth[2], who demonstrated that complement, but not antibody, was depressed in sera of animals poisoned with phosphorus. Shortly thereafter, Muller found that perfusion of liver with serum led to an increase in complement activity in the effluate, and concluded that the liver was the site of complement synthesis[3]. In the late 1960s, Alper and coworkers[4,5] confirmed this observation that the liver was a major site of serum complement synthesis by studying a patient following liver transplantation; the electrophoretic form of C3 shifted from the recipient FS type to the donor SS type. The complete shift of C3 from recipient to donor type indicated that the liver synthesized at least 95% of the C3 found in serum[4,5]. Also in the 1960s, Thorbecke and her colleagues[6–8] suggested that cell types of endodermal, mesodermal and ectodermal origin in several organs were capable of synthesizing proteins of the complement system. Application of modern molecular biological methods has confirmed that complement proteins are synthesized at multiple sites. In addition, studies of complement metabolism and mRNA expression *in vivo*[9–11] and in tissue culture[12,13] indicate a role for complement produced at extrahepatic sites, especially in the immunopathogenesis of autoimmune injury. The functional importance of this extrahepatic complement production is supported by the elaborate tissue-specific and developmentally regulated controls of complement gene expression now recognized in several species.

It is the purpose of this chapter to summarize current information regarding complement biosynthesis and to suggest some of the interesting questions posed by these data. In the first section, we will summarize the information about sites of synthesis, indicating differences in the pattern of synthesis and regulation in liver and the extrahepatic sites. We will then present more detailed information on the known tissue and cellular sites of synthesis for each of the complement proteins, the supporting evidence and the important problems in interpretation and extension of some of these findings. This will include the molecular genetic elements thus far recognized, translational, co- and post-translational and secretory events. Finally, the complex network controlling modulated expression of complement will be discussed. Although several of the complement proteins display extensive polymorphism, conservation of structure within the coding and flanking regions of the few genes for which data are available permits the use of information derived from study of complement genes from several species.

PATTERNS OF SYNTHESIS AND REGULATION OF COMPLEMENT PROTEINS IN LIVER AND AT EXTRAHEPATIC SITES

Liver

The liver is a site of synthesis of almost all the serum complement proteins, with the exception of C1q, factor D and properdin (Table 4.1). Experiments using immunofluorescent staining for complement proteins in liver tissue and study of synthesis of the proteins in primary hepatocyte cultures[14] and in well-differentiated hepatoma-derived cell lines[15] have indicated that the cell of origin of the complement proteins in the liver is the hepatocyte. Kupffer cells are probably a rich source of C4 and C2, and perhaps other complement proteins.

Complement proteins are acute-phase reactants, with serum concentrations increasing with the onset of inflammation by 2–3-fold[16–18]. These findings suggest that synthesis of the proteins in the hepatocytes is regulated by mediators of inflammation. Changes in content of mRNA for the complement proteins

Table 4.1 Sites of complement protein synthesis

	Classical pathway proteins	*Alternative pathway proteins*	*Effector proteins*
Liver (hepatocyte)	C1r, s, C4, C2, C1-inh	C3, B, H, I	C3, C5, C6 C7, C8, C9
Mononuclear phagocytes	C1q, r, s, C4, C2, C1-inh	C3, B, P, D, H, I	C3, C5
Fibroblasts*	C1q, r, s, C4, C2, C1-inh	C3, B, H	C3
Epithelial cells	C1q, r, s	C3, B	C3
Endothelial cells	C1-inh	C3, B, H, I	C3
Alveolar type II epithelial cells	C4, C2	C3, B	C3, C5

*Studies with primary human fibroblast cultures indicated that I, P, C4, and C5 are not synthesized in these cells. Rodent fibroblasts synthesize C4[8]. Studies in a transformed fibroblast line demonstrated synthesis of C5[105]

in liver after induction of inflammation in animals have confirmed the role of the liver in producing these serum changes. Results of experiments with both primary hepatocyte cultures and hepatoma-derived cell lines have demonstrated that these cells are responsive to mediators induced by endotoxin (IL-1, TNF and IL-6), although they are not responsive to endotoxin itself. Like the acute-phase response in serum, the changes in synthesis induced by the cytokines in hepatocytes are modest, with increases between 2- and 3-fold[19–21].

Extrahepatic sites

Complement proteins of the classical and alternative pathways and C5 are synthesized in several cell types in multiple tissues (Table 4.1). Thus, activation of the cascade through C5 can be accomplished by proteins synthesized at the extrahepatic sites without a requirement for liver-derived proteins. The widespread synthesis of C3 and factor B, which have been identified in virtually every cell type studied, suggests that this extrahepatic synthesis provides a source of alternative complement proteins for use in local host defences before influx of serum proteins. The synthesis of two alternative complement proteins, factor D and properdin, only at extrahepatic sites is consistent with this concept and with other potential functions of one or several of these complement proteins. Mononuclear phagocytes provide the single richest source of complement proteins, with synthesis of all the activator and inhibitor proteins in both activation pathways. Fibroblasts are also a rich source of complement proteins, synthesizing at least 7 effectors and inhibitors of the system (Figure 4.1).

Detailed studies in fibroblasts have provided evidence that the pattern of synthesis of the proteins under resting conditions favours inhibition of both the classical and alternative activation pathways. Specifically, synthesis rates for inhibitors (C1-inh and factor H in fibroblasts) are higher than synthesis rates for activators[22,23]. Under conditions of stimulation by mediators of inflammation, this pattern changes, with increases in rates of synthesis for activators greater than the increase for inhibitors[22]. In addition, the mediators of inflammation, such as IL-1, TNF, IL-6 and endotoxin, all stimulate activators of the alternative pathway much more than activators of the classical pathway[19,24–26]. For example, IL-1 and TNF induce large increases in the synthesis of factor B (up to 100-fold) and C3 (approximately 10–20-fold) in human skin-derived fibroblasts[19]. Synthesis of factor H is either unaffected (IL-1) or affected much less (TNF) than synthesis of factor B and C3[22]. In addition, there is no significant stimulation of the synthesis of the classical pathway complement components in these cells: in contrast to the situation in hepatocytes in which synthesis of C1r, C1s, C1 inhibitor[17] and C2 (Y. Katz and R. C. Strunk, unpublished observation) is increased 2–3-fold by TNF (TNF has no effect on C2 expression in hepatocytes (HepG-2)), but which is unaffected by IL-1.

Examples of the role of complement produced at extrahepatic sites

Several cell types synthesize complement proteins in the lung. Bronchoalveolar macrophages synthesize C1q, C2, C4, C3, and factor B[27–29]. Proteins known to

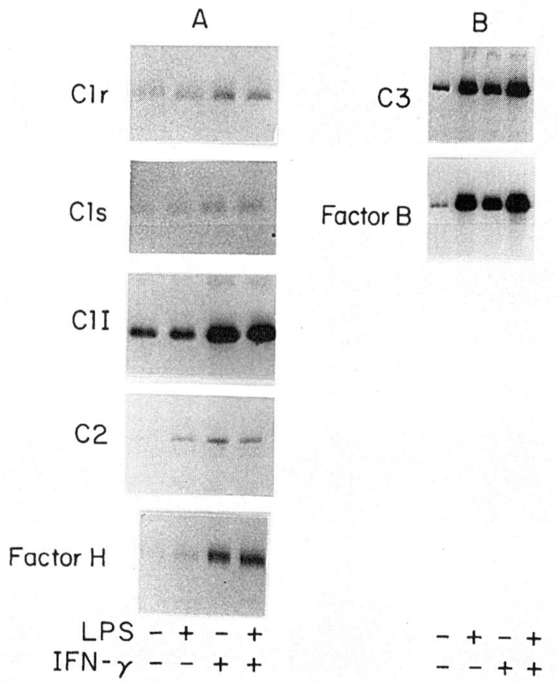

Figure 4.1 SDS-PAGE of ^{35}[S]methionine metabolically labelled cell lysates immunoprecipitated with antisera to complement proteins. Reprinted with permission from Katz, Y., Strunk, R. C. *Arthritis Rheum.*, 1988; **31**: 1365–70

be synthesized in peripheral blood monocytes, C1r, C1s, D, I, and H[30], have not been studied in detail, but may also be synthesized in the bronchoalveolar macrophages. The alveolar type II epithelial cell is another rich source of complement proteins, C2, C4, C3, factor B, and C5[31]. Relative to macrophages, type II cells synthesize much more C3 and C4, but less C2 and factor B. Fibroblasts also represent another source of complement proteins in the lung. Fibroblasts derived specifically from the lung have been shown to synthesize C1q, C1r, C1s[32,33], C1 inhibitor, C2, C3, B, and H (Circolo, Katz and Strunk, unpublished observations). Regulation of synthesis of complement proteins in lung is governed by the same general rules applying to other extrahepatic sites of complement production. For example, interferon-γ increases synthesis of C2 and factor B, but not C3, in both bronchoalveolar macrophages and peripheral blood monocytes (Ref. 34 and Kunke and Strunk, unpublished observations), whereas LPS increases synthesis of B and C3, but not C2[35,36]. Examples of local control of complement synthesis in the lung have been described. For instance, Pennington *et al.*[37] reported specific inhibition of C2 and C4 biosynthesis by guinea pig bronchoalveolar macrophages after intraperitoneal instillation of cortisone acetate or cyclophosphamide, without a corresponding change in serum complement (liver-derived). Conversely, chronic *P. aeruginosa* pneumonia induced by intratracheal instillation of an antigen–agar bead suspension in guinea pigs specifically increases C2 and C4 synthesis by isolated bronchoalveolar macrophages without recruitment of an increased proportion of complement-secreting cells or alteration in serum complement levels[38]. In addition, increased expression of complement in the lung of MRL 1pr/1pr mice, a strain that spontaneously develops systemic lupus erythematosus with lung involvement, exceeds corresponding changes in liver complement gene expression[11].

Previous studies have indicated that cells in the joint might serve as a source of proteins of the complement system. Ruddy and Colten[9] demonstrated synthesis of C2, C3, C4 and C5 in minced synovial tissues obtained from patients with rheumatoid arthritis, but only in a minority of specimens obtained from individuals with degenerative arthritis. De Ceulaer *et al.*[39] established that macrophages obtained by ficoll–hypaque separation of synovial fluids and membranes synthesize complement. These investigators were able to detect functionally active C2, factors B, D, H and I, and properdin. They also demonstrated net increase in protein synthesis by incorporation of radio-labelled amino acids into C3, C4, C5, P, B, H and I. Synovial fibroblasts also synthesize at least 7 proteins of the classical and alternative complement pathways[24]. Identification of complement synthesis in fibroblasts from patients with only minor trauma and no effusion suggests that complement protein synthesis is a constitutive function of cells in the non-rheumatic joint and that the capacity to produce these proteins does not require the presence of inflammation.

Several investigators have suggested that local synthesis of complement proteins might play a role in the evolution of autoimmune disease in various organs. The demonstration that complement gene expression in the liver and extrahepatic sites is under independent regulation is consistent with this

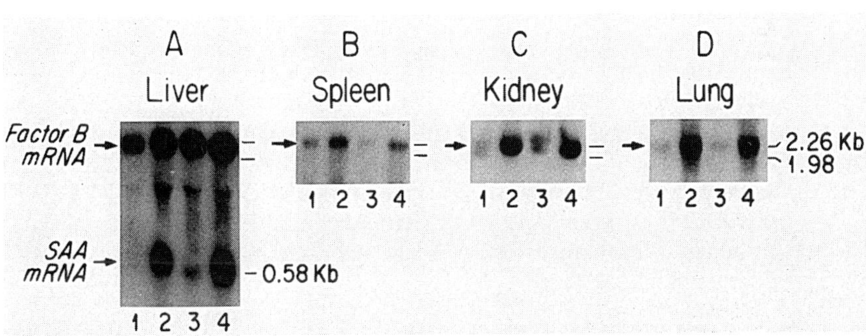

Figure 4.2 Expression of complement factor B and serum amyloid A mRNA in liver, spleen, kidney and lung. For each tissue, lanes 1 and 2 are from B10.AKM (H-2^k) and lanes 3 and 4 are from B10.PL (H-2^u). Lanes 1 and 3 are control and lanes 2 and 4 are IL-1 stimulated. These studies demonstrate tissue- and strain-specific differences in Bf expression. Reprinted with permission from Falus, A., Beuscher, H. U., Auerbach, H. S., Colten, H. R. *J. Immunol.*, 1987; **138**: 856–60

possibility[10,11,40] (Figure 4.2). Passwell *et al.* examined the concentration of mRNA for C3, factor B, C4, and C2 in kidney and other organs of the MRL 1pr/1pr and the congenic MRL +/+ mouse strains at timed intervals to ascertain whether local expression of complement proteins plays a role in immunopathology of lupus nephritis[11]. A marked increase in mRNA for these complement proteins in the 1pr/1pr kidney and in other organs affected by the autoimmune disease was observed to be concomitant with the development of SLE. The increased mRNA content was reflected in increased synthesis of complement in the nephritic kidney. This was the first demonstration of local regulation of complement genes and *in situ* synthesis of complement protein in an organ affected by a naturally evolving autoimmune disease. Interestingly, there was little or no change in C3, C4, C2 and factor B mRNA in the liver, reinforcing the concept of the importance of local production of complement proteins in the evolution of local inflammatory responses.

CELLULAR AND TISSUE SITES OF COMPLEMENT SYNTHESIS

Classical pathway proteins

The first component (C1)

The macromolecular complex, C1, is the product of five genes: three encoding the polypeptides (A, B and C chains) that comprise the C1q component[41,42] and the genes encoding the C1r[43] and C1s[44,45] subcomponents. C1r and C1s are encoded by genes on chromosome 12p within a 10 kb region where they are oriented tail to tail[44,45] and the C1q A, B and C chains are encoded within 24 kb on chromosome 1p (34.1–36.3)[41,46,47]. The chromosomal locations of the genes encoding C1q, C1r and C1s, as well as the known locations of the complement protein genes, are shown in Figure 4.3.

Synthesis of functional C1 or its subcomponents has been demonstrated in epithelial cells of diverse origin (bladder, gastrointestinal tract)[48–50] in mononuclear phagocytes[7,30,51] and fibroblasts[23,32,52]. Of these, the mononuclear phagocyte is a rich source of C1q[53]; epithelia and fibroblasts produce C1r and C1s in large amounts but little or no C1q[54,55]. A well-differentiated hepatoma-derived cell line, HepG-2, also synthesizes C1r and C1s but not C1q[15]. Although direct evidence is lacking, these data suggest that the human hepatocyte is capable of synthesizing at least two of the three C1 subcomponents. These data also suggest that regulation of C1q synthesis and secretion is independent of C1r and C1s synthesis and secretion. In fact, some[55] have provided evidence for cell membrane-bound C1q on macrophages which they suggest play a role as one of the Fc receptors in this cell type.

The A, B and C chains of the C1q subunit of C1 are programmed by separate mRNA species of *c.*2–3 kb[41]. Postsynthetic hydroxylation of proline and lysine residues in the collagen-like domains of the C1q chains is a prerequisite for formation of the native triple helix and secretion of C1q[51,56]. Hence, net production of C1 involves transcriptional and translational events but, most importantly, asssembly of the C1 macromolecule. Details of the sequence of events

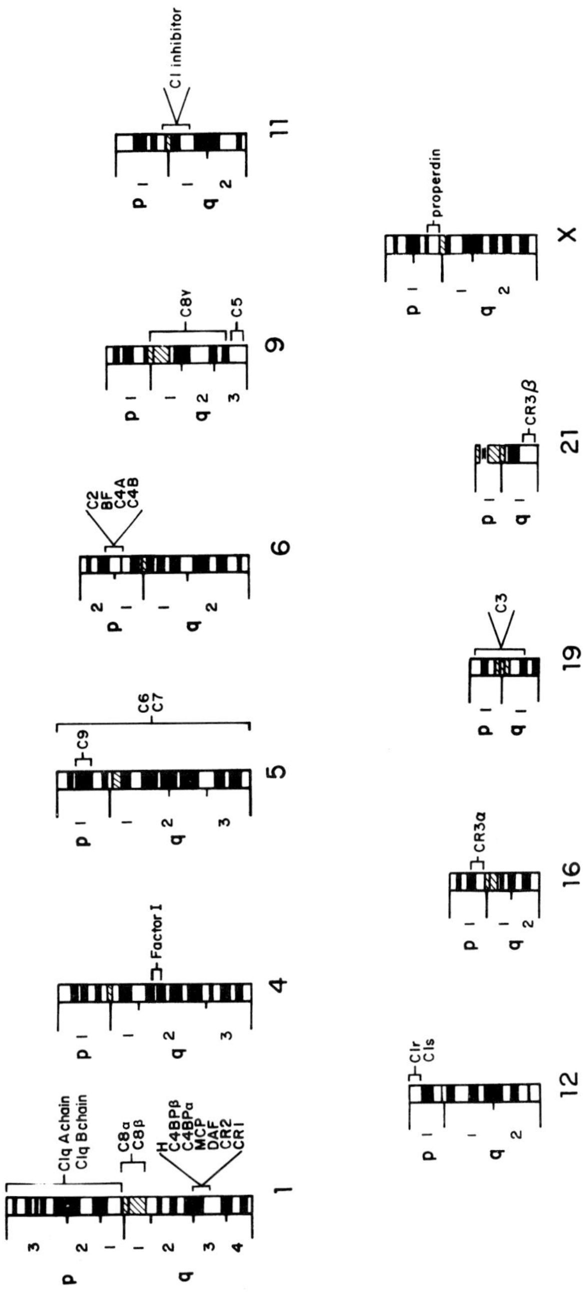

Figure 4.3 Chromosomal localization of genes encoding the complement proteins. Reprinted with permission from Perlmutter, D. P., Colten, H. R. In Gallin, J. L. Goldstein, I. M and Snyderman, R. (eds.) *Inflammation*, 2nd Ed. NY: Raven Press. (In press)

generating precursor protein conversion, disulphide bridge formation, other postsynthetic modifications, and assembly of the intact C1 macromolecule (C1r, C1s dimer association with C1q) are limited to date.

The fourth (C4) and second (C2) components

The constituents of the classical pathway C3 convertase are synthesized in identical cells but the co- and postsynthetic processing of each differs considerably. C2 and C4 are synthesized in hepatocytes[15], fibroblasts (C2)[24,26], (C4)[8], and in mononuclear phagocytes, including several established cell lines[28,30,57–59]. Expression of C2 and C4 in mononuclear phagocytes is a function of cellular maturation. That is, in marrow, only about 10% of the cells produce C4 (no C2 production is detected) whereas 45–50% of tissue macrophages synthesize C4[60]. The proportion of tissue macrophages that synthesize and secrete C2 varies from *c*.2% in bronchoalveolar cells to *c*.45% in breast milk[61], splenic and peritoneal cells[60]. These represent interesting and as yet unexplored developmental and tissue-specific differences in constitutive expression of complement proteins.

C4 is a heterotrimeric glycoprotein[62–64] of approximately 200 kDa. The protein is synthesized as a single precursor (pro-C4) programmed by a 5.5 kb mature mRNA[65]. Precursor product relationships for C4 and several of the other complement proteins are shown in Figure 4.2. In humans, two genes, C4A and C4B, polymorphic in size and fine structure, encode the C4 transcripts[66–70]. Some species, such as guinea pig, express only a single C4 gene. In human populations, a relatively high frequency of duplications and deletions is observed so that the genome of many humans also contains only one C4 gene per haploid[70,71]. The order of the chains in the precursor (NH2-beta-alpha-gamma-COOH) was first suggested by amino acid sequencing of biosynthetically labelled C4[72–74], and later confirmed by nucleotide sequence analysis of C4 cDNA which also reveals a signal peptide[65,75,76]. Processing of prepro-C4 requires proteolytic cleavage by a signal peptidase, excision of two interchain linking peptides, generation of the thiolester bridge, glycosylation of α- and β-chain residues via a dolichol phosphate-dependent intermediate, sulphation and cleavage of a carboxyterminal fragment of a α-chain by an extracellular metalloproteinase[72,73,77–82].

Processing and secretion of C4 occurs with a half-time of about 60–90 minutes[83], a rate similar to the kinetics of synthesis processing and secretion of C3 and C5 in hepatoma HepG-2 cells[15,84,85].

Constitutive expression of C4 is under genetic control and is tissue specific. This phenomenon has been most thoroughly studied in inbred mouse strains, but similar observations have been made in study of human and guinea pig C4 expression as well. The 20-fold difference in plasma C4 concentration among inbred mouse strains of different H-2 haplotypes[86,87] is a reflection of differences in pretranslational (probably transcriptional) regulation of C4 expression[85,88,89]. The tissue specificity of this phenomenon is evidenced by the finding of equal C4 expression (steady-state mRNA and protein) in extrahepatic macrophages from C4-high and C4-low strains[10,85,88,90]. Moreover, the C4-like gene in mouse encoding the sex-limited protein, Slp, is expressed only in liver except in certain strains (e.g. $H\text{-}2^{w-7}$) where extrahepatic expression is observed as well[91,92].

Relevant to these issues (see below), only preliminary data regarding sequences 5′ to the C4/slp genes[93,94] have been obtained and little is known about the transacting elements governing strain- and tissue-specific regulation of constitutive C4 expression[91,95–98]. However, evidence of both H-2-linked[91] and non-H-2 genetic[99] control of C4 constitutive expression has been obtained. The former is almost certainly a consequence of sequences within or flanking the C4 gene, but an impact of other genes within or near the major histocompatibility complex has not been formally excluded. These data should stimulate more detailed studies of the relevant molecular mechanisms.

In tissue culture, C4 expression is particularly unstable in human and, to a lesser extent, murine monocyte/macrophage cultures; i.e. C4 mRNA and synthesis of C4 declines within hours to days[28,83,85]. Maintenance of base-line levels of expression requires exogenous stimuli[28] such as interferon-γ. Moreover, elicited macrophages found in inflammatory exudates produce *less* C4 than resident macrophages[85,88].

C2 is encoded by a gene (15 kb) that is located *c*.400 bp 5′ to the factor B gene. Several C2 primary translation products (84 kDa, 79 kDa, 70 kDa) have been recognized[95]. The largest of these is glycosylated and secreted within about 60 min; the others are also glycosylated but remain cell associated. At least two murine C2 transcripts have been identified[96]; one exhibits a deletion of a seven-amino-acid peptide within the serine proteinase binding pocket. This transcript is expressed at low levels in all tissues thus far examined except in heart where about equal amounts of the two C2 transcripts have been detected. Evidence for multiple human C2 transcripts has also recently been obtained (C. Johnson *et al.*, unpublished). The relationship between these observations and the multiple C2 primary translation products has not been established.

Pretranslational constitutive expression of C2 has been most extensively examined in mice. The extraordinary conservation of overall gene structure, including *c*.65% identity in nucleotide sequence in comparing the human/murine sequences for C2[96–98], suggests that conclusions from these studies may pertain to humans as well. Among inbred mouse strains, marked differences in C2 serum concentrations are paralleled by differences in hepatic mRNA content for each[99]. Constitutive control is tissue specific as indicated by the observation that the relative content of specific C2 mRNA in macrophages is independent of the relative hepatic expression of each gene among the murine strains examined. Another level of control is proposed by Volanakis and his colleagues[100] who suggest that translational control of C2 is due to differences in transcriptional initiation. These generate differences in the 5′ untranslated region, the sequence of which governs the rate of C2 translation. Further analysis of this interesting finding in the context of tissue specificity of C2 expression is warranted.

Alternative pathway proteins

The third (C3) component

Liver is the major site of plasma C3 synthesis[4]. Based on studies of hepatoma cell lines[84] and primary hepatocellular cultures[14], the hepatocyte is thought to be the principal intrahepatic source of C3. However, many other tissues and cells produce biologically active C3; e.g. mononuclear phagocytes[7,30,101], fibroblasts[6,24,26], uterine epithelium[102], astroglia[103], endothelial cells[104], alveolar type II epithelium (primary cells in rat and human[31] and the type II-like line A549[105]), and several cell lines (U-937, the mouse macrophage P388D, etc.)[106,107].

Constitutive expression of C3 as judged by serum concentration and preliminary studies of C3 biosynthesis[108] also varies among inbred mouse strains, but effects of age and sex[109–111] complicate the analysis of the *cis*- and *trans*-acting elements accounting for these differences. Nevertheless, a detailed structural and functional study of the sequences 5′ to the murine and human C3 genes (Kawamura *et al.*, unpublished) and the nucleoproteins that interact with these regions should soon elucidate the pertinent molecular details.

Prepro-C3 is programmed by a ≤5.2 kb mature mRNA derived from a ≥40 kb gene on chromosome 19 in humans[112] and 17 (outside the H-2 complex) in mice[110,111]. Co- and postsynthetic modifications involve cleavage of a signal peptide, excision of a single interchain linking peptide and glycosylation. Generation of the thiolester bridge of C3 probably proceeds via isomerization of a lactam to generate a thiolactone[113], perhaps involving a specific enzyme[114,115]. The hepatic biosynthetic rate, estimated *in vivo* from fractional catabolic rates of ^{125}I-labelled C3[116,117], is 0.45–2.7 mg kg^{-1} h^{-1}, a rate comparable to that observed in HepG-2 hepatoma cells[48].

Factor B

The tissue and cellular distribution of factor B synthesis is also quite broad. Cells of diverse embryological origin are capable of synthesizing factor B though the regulation of its expression varies as a function of developmental factors, for instance well-differentiated intestinal epithelium[118], hepatocytes[119], fibroblasts[26], mononuclear phagocytes[30], alveolar type II epithelial cells (primary cells in rat and human[31] and the type II-like line A549[105]), and astroglia[103]. Tumour cell lines[15,120] representing most of these cellular origins have also been shown to synthesize and secrete factor B. Expression of the factor B gene is regulated independently in hepatic and extrahepatic tissues. Moreover, an alternative upstream start site for transcription is used in specific tissues (kidney and intestine) and during modulated expression[121]. Expression of factor B is regulated by endotoxin[26,35], several growth factors (PDGF, IL-4, etc.)[122,123], and the cytokines, IL-1, IL-6 and IFN-γ (reviewed in Ref. 124).

Factor B is synthesized as an *c*.80 kDa propolypeptide which undergoes signal peptide cleavage, glycosylation and secretion in about 60–90 min. Two factor B transcripts resulting from alternative transcriptional initiation sites have been recognized in studies of murine Bf expression in kidney and intestine[10,11,121]. The larger of the two is expressed in amounts equal to the shorter message only in those two tissues; in liver, the long transcript represents ≤5% of the Bf mRNA[96]. No obvious promoter sequence has been recognized at the upstream initiation site but mutations near this site which parallel differences in expressions of the Bf long transcript in different mouse strains should help in the analysis of the specific sequences essential for upstream transcriptional initiation (Garnier, unpublished).

As with C2, pretranslational constitutive expression of factor B has been most extensively examined in mice, where expression of Bf varies widely among inbred mouse strains (Figure. 4.2). In addition, expression of C2 and expression of Bf in these strains vary independently of one another[99]. As with C2, extraordinary conservation of overall gene structure, including *c*. 65% identity in nucleotide sequence in comparing the human/murine sequences for Bf[96–98], suggests that conclusions from these studies will pertain to humans as well. Constitutive control is tissue specific as indicated by the observation that the relative content of specific B mRNA in macrophages is independent of the relative hepatic expression of each gene among the murine strains examined; i.e. **hepatic** Bf mRNA in H-2^{u} is greater than in H-2^{d} or H-2^{f}, but, in H-2^{d} **macrophages**, Bf mRNA content is greater than in either H-2^{u} or H-2^{f} strains. Recent studies by Garnier *et al.* (unpublished) have begun to identify the *cis*- and *trans*-acting elements responsible for this phenomenon.

Factor D

Adipocytes constitute the quantitatively most important site of factor D synthesis[125]. Schwann cells in peripheral nerve, lung (Nogee and Colten, unpublished) (probably alveolar macrophages), mononuclear phagocytes elsewhere[30,57,126], and monocytic cell lines also produce factor D. The tissue distribution of D synthesis suggests a role in lipid metabolism, perhaps independent of its function as a constituent of the alternative pathway in host defences. The marked variation in expression of factor D in several animal models of obesity has suggested a role of this protein in energy metabolism. The mechanism for this variation is not understood.

Factor D is secreted from human mononuclear phagocyte cell lines (U937) rapidly ($t_{1/2}$ *c*.30–60 min). The human protein is not glycosylated intracellularly, and non-enzymatic glycation extracellularly probably accounts for the carbohydrate moiety observed in the plasma protein[127]. Murine factor D synthesis has been most extensively studied in fat where it was first identified as adipsin and later shown to be identical with the complement protein. Murine D is synthesized, glycosylated and secreted and the intracellular pool is relatively small[125]; i.e. like other secreted complement proteins, little or no intracellular storage is noted so that, in general, secretion rates represent good estimates of synthesis rates. Interestingly, the expression of factor D/adipsin varies markedly as a function of nutritional status of an animal and with fat cell differentiation, but the molecular signals governing this effect are, for the most part, unknown[128–130]. Factor D is apparently secreted as the active enzyme, though, in addition to the signal peptide, a five-residue zymogen peptide is in the primary translation product[131,132]. Factor D is not inhibited to a significant extent by the natural serine proteinase inhibitors.

Properdin

The site(s) of synthesis of properdin are at present not definitively established, but it is clear that mononuclear phagocytes do express properdin mRNA[133].

Although the synthesis of properdin has been studied only to a limited extent, in the few reports available to date, it appears that the properdin protein is synthesized by these cells[30,126]. Farries and Atkinson have documented synthesis of properdin in HL-60 cells differentiated with DMSO, suggesting that granulocytes or granulocyte precursors may also be a source of this protein[134]. Properdin mRNA has not been detected in liver, indicating that this is one of the few complement proteins not synthesized in this organ[134–136].

Terminal components

Complement protein C5

C5 is encoded by a gene of more than 50 kb on chromosome 2 in mouse[137] and chromosome 9q 32–34 in human[138]. A 5.5 kb mature mRNA is the template for prepro-C5, a protein that undergoes co- and postsynthetic cleavage and glycosylation to produce the native C5 disulphide-linked heterodimer. The liver and lung appear to be the major sites of synthesis of C5, as C5 mRNA was found in these but was not detected by Northern blot analysis in other organs[139]. The cells responsible for synthesis in these organs are hepatocytes (Refs. 15, 140, Katz and Strunk, unpublished observations with primary hepatocyte cultures) and alveolar type II epithelial cells (primary cells in rat and human[31] and the type II-like line A549[105]). Mononuclear phagocytes also synthesize C5, as demonstrated in studies of mouse peritoneal macrophages[141,142]. Biosynthetic studies have suggested that human macrophages[143] and monocytes[57] produce C5 protein, although the methods utilized did not allow determination of the size and subunit composition of the protein, and thus do not confirm that the protein was full length and functionally active.

Early studies by Colten[140] and Kohler[144] using fetal tissues indicated that C5 was produced in many other organs, and suggested that human lymphoid cells might synthesize C5. Other reports indicated the presence of C5 on membranes of peripheral blood lymphocytes[145,146]. In a recent report, Reed *et al.* have detected C5 protein by ELISA and C5 mRNA by RNase protection in several human lymphoblastoid cell lines, suggesting that human B- and T-cells may in fact express C5[147]. Evidence for a truncated C5 mRNA[148,149] has stimulated renewed interest in the possibility of C5 protein variants, prompting a search for other cellular sites of C5 expression.

C6–9

In vivo metabolic studies[5] and studies of hepatocellular cell lines[15] provided evidence for liver as an important site of synthesis of the terminal plasma proteins of the lytic complement cascade. Additional support is available in reports demonstrating expression of the mRNA species that programme translation of these proteins in liver: C5[148]; C6[150]; C7[151]; C8[152–155]; C9[156;157]. However, evidence (of variable credibility) for production of these proteins at extrahepatic sites has also been obtained. For instance, mononuclear phagocytes (cell lines and primary cultures)[158] and platelets[159,160] are thought to express at least some of the terminal complement components.

Several interesting cell biological questions may be raised with respect to synthesis of these proteins. For example, C8, like C1, is encoded by separate genes[152–155]. Postsynthetic assembly of the intact C8 protein with its two covalent and one covalently-linked polypeptides represents an interesting cell biological system to test whether the mechanisms responsible for assembly and trafficking of other heteromultimeric secreted proteins (e.g. immunoglobulins) are general or if novel systems are utilized for the complement proteins. Evidence thus far[154] suggests that C8 α–γ chains are synthesized at a more rapid rate than β and that association of α–γ with β-chain is a presecretory event; hence, free α–γ is secreted as well as intact C8. The mechanisms governing this process are unknown.

Isolated rat hepatocytes synthesize C8 from individual propeptides (encoded by genes on chromosome 1p (α, β) and 9q (γ))[161] which undergo co- or postsynthetic assembly, glycosylation and secretion with kinetics similar to C3, C4 and C5[154]. The rates of α- and γ-chain synthesis appear to be approximately equal but greater than the rate of β-chain synthesis. Hence, though intracellular assembly of the heterotrimer represents the dominant secretory pathway, α–γ secretion alone is also observed, accounting for the finding of free α-γ in normal plasma[162].

Soluble regulatory proteins: C1 inhibitor, factor I and the cofactor proteins factor H and C4-bp

Mononuclear phagocytes[30] and hepatocytes[163] are sites of synthesis of factor I. Fibroblasts[22,164], endothelial cells[165], monocytes[166], the promonocyte cell line U937[161,167], and possibly platelets[168] produce factor H, but the full range of cell types capable of synthesizing the regulators of C3b and C4b is not known. C1-inhibitor is synthesized and secreted in liver[140,169] by hepatocytes[15,170] and in monocytes[171,172], platelets[173] and fibroblasts[23] under resting conditions. In the cells that produce proteins active in propagating the complement cascade *and* the soluble regulatory proteins, the latter are generally produced in excess. As noted above, upregulation of the complement genes by proinflammatory stimuli shifts the balance from inhibitor excess to effector excess.

The factor I preproprotein (signal peptide-heavy chain-light chain) is encoded by a single copy gene on chromosome 4, which yields a 2.3 kb mRNA[163,174,175.] Cleavage of the signal peptide, an interchain linking peptide and glycosylation, generates the native heterodimer. In one cell line, the HepG-2 hepatoma, factor I is secreted as its single chain precursor with kinetics similar to that observed in other hepatoma-derived cell lines (e.g. Hep3B) which process the precursor appropriately[163]. The defect in pro-I processing is specific for this protein because pro-C3, pro-C4 and pro-C5 are properly processed in HepG-2. This system offers a model for understanding the cell biology of proprotein cleavage since the primary sequence of prepro-I in HepG-2 is apparently identical to that of liver factor I[174,175]. These data suggest that cleavage of pro I occurs in a compartment distinct from that for pro-C3, pro-C4, etc., or that either a unique enzyme or a dysfunctional enzyme results in a selective failure of pro-I cleavage in HepG-2.

Membrane regulatory proteins and complement receptors

The sites of synthesis of the membrane regulators of complement activation and complement receptors have been inferred from detection of the proteins on the surface of specific cell types. For peripheral blood cells, systematic studies have not yet been undertaken to identify the precursor cells nor the developmental signals for expression and insertion of these membrane proteins. Nevertheless, the data in Table 4.2 give some indication of the precursor and terminally differentiated cells potentially capable of producing the membrane-bound regulators and receptors. Conclusions must be tempered by the recognition that secreted forms of several have been identified; hence, the possible adsorption of soluble proteins to a cell surface must be considered.

Among the membrane-bound complement regulatory proteins anchored by a phosphoinositol linkage, the synthesis and postsynthetic modification of decay accelerating factor (DAF) has been most extensively studied[176]. Two mRNA species differing in size by *c*.0.7 kb programme synthesis of pro-DAF, the 318-amino-acid precursor protein[177–179]. The protein is subjected to glycosylation (both *N*- and *O*-linked)[180], and a carboxyterminal extension peptide is cleaved followed by attachment of the glycophospholipid anchor[181]. The role of the extension peptide in signalling these events has been elegantly established by construction and expression of a chimeric cDNA generated from the 3′ end of DAF joined to sequences encoding another protein[178,182]. A second DAF species is secreted but the details of its synthesis are unknown.

REGULATED COMPLEMENT GENE EXPRESSION

Several of the complement proteins are acute-phase reactants. That is, following tissue injury or an inflammatory stimulus, predictable changes in the plasma concentration of complement are observed in addition to other acute-phase

Table 4.2 Cellular location of complement regulatory proteins

CR1 (CD35)	Haematopoietic cells: granulocytes, mononuclear phagocytes, T cell subsets, B cells at various stages of ontogeny (pre-B and almost all mature B) and erythrocytes (reviewed in Ref. 215); glomerular podocytes; mast cells; Schwann cells in (fetal) peripheral nerve[216]; HSV-infected epidermal and endothelial cells[217].
CR2 (CD21)	Some T cell tumours but not mature T cells[210]; mature and late pre-B cells, but not on others in B cell lineage; follicular dendritic cells[218].
CR3 (CD11b/18)	PMNs (not on granulocyte precursors)[219], monocytes; natural killer cells.
CR4 (CD11c/18)	Polymorphonuclear leukocytes, platelets, B and T cells[220, 221] and hairy cell leukaemia B cells[222].
DAF (CD55)	All circulating cells, except NK cells[223–227]; erythroid and mononuclear progenitors[227]; fibroblasts[228]; endothelium[229]; adult epithelium[227,230]; trophoblast[226].
MCP (CD46) (215)	Parallels DAF, except absent from erythrocytes and present on NK cells[227,231,232]; fibroblast;epithelium, endothelium[228]; sperm; trophoblasts[233].
HRF_{20} (CD59)	Erythrocytes[234,235]; endothelium[236]; platelets[237].

responses (e.g. fever and alterations in fat, protein and trace metal metabolism[13,16,183]). Factor B, C3 and C4 are the quantitatively most prominent of the acute-phase complement proteins, increasing in concentration in plasma 2–3-fold with reproducible kinetics following an acute-phase stimulus. These changes largely reflect an increase in hepatic complement gene expression. Clinical[9,184] and experimental[10,11,13,16] observations established that inflammation and tissue injury also modulate complement gene expression at extrahepatic sites. For some, the magnitude of acute-phase induced changes in extrahepatic complement expression exceed the effects on liver. The acute-phase complement gene response is also affected by genetic background and developmental parameters. In the past few years, efforts have been made to identify the molecular basis of these phenomena. The proximate soluble mediators and their respective receptors, the cell biological events and the *cis*- and *trans*-acting elements that govern regulated complement gene expression, have been examined. In addition, other less well studied modifiers of complement expression, such as sex hormones, corticosteroids and nutrition, offer interesting models for the elucidation of mechanisms by which these influence inflammation in host defences and autoimmune injury.

Endotoxin

Abundant evidence supports the concept that endotoxin, a constituent of the cell wall of gram-negative bacteria, has a direct and derivative effect on regulated complement gene expression. This endotoxin effect is derivative in the sense that many genes upregulated by endotoxin yield products which also regulate complement gene expression. To date, the biochemical mechanisms involved in endotoxin recognition on cell surfaces by lipopolysaccharide (LPS) binding sites and the signal transduction pathways mediating LPS effects are poorly characterized. These constitute problems in the study of LPS effects on complement expression in homogeneous cell populations in culture. Even more complex is the problem of ascertaining which among the LPS-induced effects are of most importance *in vivo*. Nevertheless, it is clear that LPS administration *in vivo* or to cells (mononuclear phagocytes, type II pneumocytes and fibroblasts) in culture results in an increase in net synthesis of several of the complement proteins. This LPS effect is due to the lipid A component[35]. Some cells that express complement genes, such as monocytes[35], type II lung cells[31] and fibroblasts[26], are highly LPS responsive, whereas others, the hepatocyte (HepG-2 hepatoma) and intestinal epithelium ($CaCO_2$ cells), are not.

The LPS effect on C3 and factor B expression serves as a useful model to evaluate this phenomenon because: these have been most well studied; the quantitative effect of LPS on these two genes is substantial; and both gene products are of considerable importance in host defences against gram-negative bacteria. In human peripheral blood monocytes and macrophages, LPS at nanogram concentrations induces a 5–30-fold increase in C3 and Bf synthesis and secretion[26,35,184]. Much of this effect is pretranslational (probably transcriptional), as indicated by corresponding increases in C3 and Bf mRNA. However, two lines of evidence suggest an important translational regulatory effect as well. For example, in adult human fibroblasts, the increased Bf protein synthesis rate following LPS stimulation far exceeds the increase in Bf mRNA[26]. This effect is similar to that observed for LPS induction of TNF synthesis[185].

The second line of evidence depends on the developmental maturation of the LPS effect on C3 and Bf gene expression. St. John Sutton *et al.*[184] noted that lipid A failed to upregulate C3 and Bf synthesis in newborn (umbilical cord) blood monocytes in contrast to its well-recognized effect on adult monocytes. This difference was specific for the complement genes since other LPS-induced phenomena, such as superoxide generation, were equally demonstrable in neonatal and adult cells. Preliminary data suggested that the neonatal cells were unable to process the LPS to its active moieties (e.g. lipid X or lipid Y). The possibility was also suggested that a deficit in arachidonic acid metabolism may account for the developmental differences in response of C3 and Bf to LPS. Further exploration of this phenomenon in fibroblasts permitted evaluation of transcriptional regulation and extension to fetal cells. These data show LPS induction of specific C3 and Bf mRNA in newborn fibroblasts but no increase in C3 or Bf protein synthesis, and, in the fetal cells, no induction of mRNA (Strunk *et al.*, unpublished). Thus, a sequential maturation of transcriptional, then translational, competence from fetal to newborn and adult is suggested. Of importance for future studies of the mechanisms governing this maturation is the stability of the phenomenon during tissue culture.

Significant differences in LPS responsiveness have been observed in comparisons of inbred mouse strains, emphasizing the importance of genetic control of this primordial response. The most extreme example is the LPS-unresponsive strain, C3H/HeJ. This is not a particularly useful model for purposes of elucidating the specific *cis*- and *trans*-acting factors impacting on LPS-induced complement gene regulation because the deficit is rather global. In fact, the interpretation of studies addressing this question is complicated by the effect of LPS on inducing many of the cytokines (IL-1, IL-6, TNF) that have a direct effect on complement gene expression. Accordingly, an extensive evaluation of cytokine-mediated complement gene regulation has been undertaken.

Interleukin-1 (IL-1)

IL-1 is a polypeptide of *c.*17 kDa, first recognized by its manifold biological activities[186]. Mononuclear phagocytes constitute a major source of this cytokine, though other cells produce IL-1 as well. IL-1 is synthesized as a 34 kDa precursor, phosphorylated[187] postsynthetically, and is either membrane associated (mIL-1) or secreted as the 17 kDa peptide[188,189]. Two forms of IL-1, α and β, have been recognized. The mature 17 kDa IL-1 species are each capable of interacting with specific IL-1 receptors which mediate the cell physiological response to this monokine.

Incubation of HepG-2 hepatoma cells or primary murine hepatocyte cultures in IL-1 induces a dose-dependent increase in C3 and Bf synthesis and secretion, but has no effect on C2 or C4 synthesis[20]. This increase in C3 and Bf is due to an increase in transcription, requires specific nucleotide sequences 5′ to the transcriptional initiation site of each of the responsive genes, and is mediated by a signal transduction pathway separable from those for other cytokines[190,191]. IL-1 also regulates complement genes at extrahepatic sites[10,192], but, in these cells, it is more difficult to evaluate whether the effect of IL-1 on C3 and Bf expression is direct or whether the IL-1 effect is on another gene, such as IL-6 or TNF; in that case the latter would also be the proximate mediator of complement gene expression. For instance, both membrane IL-1 and soluble IL-1 induce dose-dependent increases in murine C3 and Bf synthesis in macrophages[192] and human fibroblasts[19], but macrophages and fibroblasts also express IL-6 and/or TNF, both of which could, via a paracrine or autocrine mechanism, induce C3 and Bf. It is probable that, at extrahepatic sites, multiple cytokines are induced by a single stimulus (e.g. IL-1) and that this amplifies the primary event. For example, in a detailed study of regulated C3 and Bf expression in fibroblasts[19], IL-1 increased Bf and C3 expression by 50–100-fold and 10–15-fold respectively, but, in HepG-2, which does not express IL-6, IL-1 increased C3 and Bf only 2–3-fold. The difference in magnitude of the observed induction cannot be compared directly because of differences in constitutive expression in the two cell types but the principle is almost certainly valid. Moreover, the kinetics of induction of IL-6 by IL-1 (2 h) and of Bf (4 h) was consistent with an effect of more than one cytokine[19]. In that set of experiments, the IL-1 effect was modified by dexamethasone (inhibited) and by interferon-γ (enhanced) emphasizing species differences in the modulation of cytokine induction[19]. For instance, several studies suggest that corticosteroids enhance cytokine-mediated upregulation of acute-phase genes in rat[193]. Early experiments showed that hydrocortisone at a concentration of approximately 10^{-6} mol/L stimulated synthesis of C3 and transferrin as judged by semiquantitative methods[8]. In experiments designed to quantitate the magnitude of this effect, incubation of a well-differentiated rat hepatoma with hydrocortisone succinate (4×10^{-7} mol/L) increased rates of C3 production up to 9-fold[194]. However, these findings are not characteristic of the effect of corticosteroid on the same gene(s) in other species, including mice and man.

Within a single species, genetic control of IL-1-regulated C3 and Bf expression has been observed. For example, Falus *et al.*[10] found that, in B10.PL (H-2^u) mice, IL-1 induced a slight increase in hepatic and a marked increase in splenic, kidney and pulmonary C3 mRNA. In contrast, C3 mRNA decreased in liver and spleen of B10.AKM (H-2^k) mice, though the responses to IL-1 in kidney and lung were similar to that observed in the B10.PL. Examination of C3 expression in peritoneal macrophages showed similar strain differences but ruled out an effect closely linked to H-2 since the response of C3 to IL-1 was opposite in two H-2^k strains (B10.AKM, decrease; AKR/J, increase). Recent work by Kawamura *et al.* (unpublished) elucidating the *cis* elements required for the C3 response to IL-1 and IL-6 should be extended since the strain- and tissue-specific differences will make it possible to identify important *trans*-acting regulatory elements as well.

Specific sequences 5′ to the human and mouse Bf gene[191,195] extending into the 3′ untranslated region of the C2 gene confer IL-1 and IL-6 responsiveness to a chimeric gene construct (Bf 5′ flanking sequences – chloramphenicol acetyltransferase gene) when transfected into the HepG-2 hepatoma or L cells (fibroblasts). This intergenic region displays an extraordinary phylogenetic conservation (65% identity between human and mouse) and, within the specific IL-1/IL-6 response elements, even greater sequence identity[96]. Several elements are recognized in C3 as well, but deletion analysis indicates that only some of these structural elements are of functional importance in hepatocytes or fibroblasts. Studies now under way are directed towards identification of the nucleoproteins that mediate the effect of IL-1 and IL-6 on Bf and C3 expression.

Tumour necrosis factor (TNF)

Like IL-1, TNF is a cytokine expressed in mononuclear phagocytes and other cell types[185]. TNF is capable of upregulating expression of several of the complement genes[18,19]. For some, such as C3 and Bf, the kinetics, magnitude and direction of the response to TNF and IL-1 are similar. Factor H, on the other hand, is an example of a complement gene upregulated by TNF, but not by IL-1 or IL-6[22]. Little attention has been given to the molecular mechanisms involved in TNF regulation of complement gene expression, but several obvious areas need further work. For example, the mechanisms involved in the marked effect of starvation on factor D expression and the known effects of TNF on fat cell metabolism[196] certainly should stimulate additional studies of these phenomena. Initial studies demonstrate a profound downregulation of factor D (adipsin) by TNF[196].

Interleukin-6

It has been suggested that the regulation of all acute-phase genes can be explained by converging pathways with IL-6 as the proximate mediator[197,198]. Some genes, such as α_1-antitrypsin and fibrinogen, are clearly only responsive to IL-6 and not at all responsive to IL-1[21], but thus far, it seems that each of the IL-6-responsive complement genes is also IL-1 responsive[19,25]. Others, such as C2 and C4, are responsive to neither IL-1 nor IL-6, but are only regulated by interferon (see below).

At least four lines of evidence indicate that IL-6 is an important mediator of complement gene expression but that other cytokines also exert direct effects on complement genes. First, IL-1 upregulates C3 and Bf in cells (HepG-2) that do not express detectable IL-6 mRNA or protein[19,190]. Another group[199] has reported IL-6 mRNA in HepG-2. These discrepancies may be a result of genetic drift in HepG-2 cell lines. Second, the use of monoclonal antibodies against IL-1 and IL-6 in HepG-2 cultures incubated with IL-1 or IL-6 demonstrated independent quantitatively similar increases in Bf expression with each cytokine and specific inhibition of the effects by the respective monoclonal antibodies[190]. A subclone of HepG-2 provides the third line of evidence. Factor B expression in this subclone, which bears IL-1 receptors in number and affinity similar to the parent cell line, is not increased by IL-1 but is by IL-6[190]. Nevertheless, addition of both IL-1 and IL-6 augments the IL-6 response, suggesting either an effect on IL-6 receptors or common as well as parallel signal transduction pathways for IL-1 and IL-6. Finally, Baumann *et al.*[200] have shown that phorbol ester modulates IL-6 induction of an acute-phase promoter-CAT gene construct by increasing its expression but that the phorbol counter-regulates IL-1 induction. The complexity of this effect is also revealed by the fact that IL-1 and IL-6 together had at least an additive and perhaps a synergistic effect on the chimeric gene in HepG-2.

Growth factor counter-regulation

Selective counter-regulation of cytokine-mediated induction of complement genes has been observed by Strunk and colleagues[122,123] in studying the effect of growth factors on complement genes. They noted that IL-4 (a B-lymphocyte growth factor), platelet-derived growth factor (PDGF), and epidermal growth factor (EGF) abrogated the stimulatory effect of IL-1, IL-6 and TNF on factor B expression in human fibroblasts, but IL-4, in fact, augmented the effect of TNF on C3 expression. That the counter-regulation is also cytokine specific was demonstrated in experiments showing no effect of IL-4 on interferon-dependent upregulation of Bf expression. These counter-regulatory effects of growth factors precede their effect on cellular proliferation. In fact, this may be the principal mechanism by which the complement-dependent inflammatory response is downregulated during tissue repair. Exploration of the molecular mechanisms involved should therefore prove quite fruitful and important.

Interferon

Interferon-γ (IFN-γ), among the well-characterized cytokines that modulate complement gene expression, is the most pluripotent. That is, even those complement genes unresponsive to IL-1, IL-6 and TNF, such as C1r, C1s, C2 and C4, are upregulated by IFN[24,28,34]. In addition, C3 (in some species) and Bf are responsive to IFN-γ in addition to the other cytokines. Moreover, the expression of several inhibitors and cofactors of complement activation, such as C1 inhibitor[23] and factor H[22], is also regulated by IFN-γ. Regulated complement gene expression by IFN-γ has been recognized in different cell types, including hepatocytes[201], mononuclear phagocytes[34], fibroblasts[21,22,26], endothelial cells[202] and epithelial cells[31].

Each of the human class III MHC genes, C2, Bf, C4A and C4B, is upregulated by IFN-γ, but the magnitude and kinetics of the response vary considerably. For example, the response of Bf to IFN-γ is more rapid ($\leq$4 h) and of greater magnitude than the response of C2 ($\geq$10 h)[34]. Likewise, the response of C4A is greater and more prolonged than that of C4B[28]. IFN-γ induces a sustained increase of about 5-fold in C4A mRNA and C4A synthesis in HepG-2 cells and in fibroblasts transfected with the C4A gene, but generates only a transient 1.5–2-fold increase in C4B gene expression[201]. In human monocytes, IFN-γ prevents the rapid extinction of human C4A or C4B expression with time in culture. Surprisingly, this effect of IFN on C4 expression in human monocytes is counter-regulated by exposure of the cells to picogram concentrations of LPS by an as yet uncharacterized mechanism. The LPS inhibitory effect on C4 is not mediated by IL-1, IL-6 or TNF[28]. In contrast[26], LPS synergistically enhances the response of factor B to IFN-γ.

These observations and studies of *cis*-acting elements essential for the IFN-γ response raise several interesting general questions about regulated gene expression. An IFN-γ response element has been identified in sequence analyses of human and murine DNA in the intergenic region between C2 and factor B. Moreover, this element serves as a true enhancer (orientation and position independent) in functional studies of a chimeric gene construct with CAT as the reporter element[96,191,202]. Uncertainty remains about the 5′ boundary of the C2 gene, but thus far an IFN-γ response element has not been recognized 5′ to the C2 gene within a cosmid containing *c.*2 kb of sequences upstream of the C2 coding region. L cells transfected with this cosmid express C2 and its expression is increased by IFN-γ. Taken together, these data suggest the possibility that the same IFN-γ response element is functional for regulating C2 and Bf expression. IL-1/IL-6 response elements are within the 3′ untranslated region of the C2 gene, perhaps accounting for the effect of these cytokines on Bf, not on C2.

IFN-γ upregulates C1s, C1r and C1-inhibitor in cells expressing all three genes[23], but the effect on C1-inhibitor is quantitatively greater than its impact on the effector proteins. Factor H expression is also upregulated by IFN-γ in primary fibroblast[22], and endothelial cell[165] cultures, and in L cells transfected with the H gene[164]. In general, therefore, IFN-γ appears to induce a negative modulatory effect on net complement function, especially in the presence of LPS, though some components that amplify B lymphocyte cell proliferation, such as factor B[203], are increased under these same conditions.

The response of the C3 gene to IFN-γ is less easily understood in this context, however, since the magnitude and even the direction of the IFN effect are species specific. IFN-γ has either no effect, a small negative effect, or a positive regulatory effect on C3 expression in several different human cell types[34, 204]. In contrast, IFN-γ upregulates murine (at least some strains) C3 expression up to 25-fold. This effect on murine C3 is in part transcriptional and is augmented by inhibition of protein synthesis[205]. The differences among mouse strains suggest the possibility of genetic variation in regulation of human C3 by IFN-γ, but thus far the effect of IFN-γ in either direction is small.

Sex hormones

Many historical clinical and experimental observations have suggested a potential role for sex hormones in the regulation of complement protein synthesis. For example, Urbach and Cinader[206] first noted that the concentration of C5 protein in sera of normal male mice was approximately twice that in normal female sera. Churchill *et al.*[207] found that serum concentrations of C6 and C5 in sera from male mice were greater than in females. In humans, it is known that total complement activity[208] and C3[209] are significantly, but modestly, increased late in pregnancy. Lyttle and his colleagues[210,211] noted up to a 25-fold increase in C3 mRNA in uterine luminal and glandular epithelium in response to oestrogen or tamoxifen, a compound that binds to oestrogen receptor and is either antagonist or agonist, depending on the target cell. The oestrogen-stimulated increase in C3 mRNA, which results in increased synthesis and secretion of C3 protein by the uterine epithelium, is counter-regulated by progesterone. Of interest is the unresponsiveness of C3 in liver to oestrogen, i. e. the tissue specificity of this response. Further studies are warranted to define the *cis* and *trans* regulatory mechanisms accounting for the oestrogen effect. Perhaps even more important is the necessity to define the functional role(s) of C3 in uterine biology.

The most androgen-responsive 'complement' gene, the sex-limited protein (Slp), described first by Shreffler and his colleagues [reviewed in Ref. [212]] is the homologue of murine C4. In most inbred mice, Slp is expressed only in liver of males after puberty. Expression of Slp is markedly altered by castration or exogenous hormone administration. Both the coding and 5′ flanking of C4 and Slp are highly homologous[96, 213]. The 5′ regions within 1.9 kb upstream of the transcriptional initiation sites are 95% identical in sequence[97] except for two elements *c*.2.0 and 0.2 kb upstream. Based on functional studies[214], the former seems to the principal androgen enhancer. Based on sequence analysis, this region appears to have derived from the insertion of an ancient pro-virus which conferred androgen responsiveness on the C4 duplication product Slp[96]. In some strains, Slp expression is constitutive[94] and not restricted to hepatocytes. In most of these, Slp gene duplication has been observed. Little information is available regarding the specificity of sex-hormone-modulated transacting elements that influence complement gene expression, but these are under active investigation in several laboratories.

CONCLUSION

In this review, we have exercised selectivity to highlight some of the potentially interesting directions outlined in recent studies of complement gene expression. The broad distribution of cell types and tissues expressing complement effector and regulatory proteins emphasize the importance of local synthesis and consumption of components of the inflammatory response in host defences and in immunopathological events. In addition, unusual tissue distributions, such as that for factor D, or selective responses to specific cytokines (e.g. factor H to TNF) and hormones (e.g. uterine C3 expression and oestrogen), suggest additional functions of the complement proteins unrelated to host defences and inflammation. Nevertheless, the responses of complement genes to bacterial endotoxin, plus the developmental and tissue specificity of this response, re-emphasize the importance of the complement cascade as a primitive first-line defence against bacterial infection. Moreover, these represent models for elucidation of the molecular mechanisms regulating this essential function. Some understanding of these molecular details may permit the design of therapeutic strategies which are more selective in the modulation of disorders of inflammation. Beyond these considerations, extensions of current lines of investigation may yield novel systems for understanding general cell and molecular mechanisms controlling the expression of secreted and integral membrane proteins.

References

1. Mechinoff, E. (1905). *Immunity in Infective Disease*, p. 59. (London–New York: Cambridge University Press)
2. Ehrlich, P. and Morgenroth, J. (1900). Ueber Haemolysine. *Berlin Klin. Wochenschr.*, **37**, 453–8
3. Muller, L. (1911). *Zentralbl. Bacteriol. Parasiter. Infectionshr. Abt* **1**: Orig 57, 577
4. Alper, C. A., Johnson, A. M., Birtch, A. G. and Moore, R. D. (1969). Human C3: Evidence for the liver as the primary site of synthesis. *Science*, **163**, 286–8
5. Alper, C. A., Raum, D., Awdeh, Z., Petersen, B. H., Taylor, P. D. and Starzl, T. E. (1980). Studies of hepatic synthesis *in vivo* of plasma proteins including orosomucoid, transferrin, alpha-1-antitrypsin, C8 and factor B. *Clin. Immunol. Immunopathol.*, **16**, 84–9
6. Thorbecke, G. J., Hochwald, G. M., van Furth, L. R., Muller-Eberhard, H. J. and Jacobson, E. B. (1965). Problems in determining the sites of synthesis of complement components. In Wolstenholme, G. E. W. and Knight, J. (eds.), *CIBA Symposium: Complement*, pp. 99–119. (London: Churchill).
7. Stecher, V. J. and Thorbecke, G. J. (1967). Sites of synthesis of serum proteins. I. Serum proteins produced by macrophages in vitro. *J. Immunol.*, **99**, 643–52
8. Stecher, V. J. and Thorbecke, G. J. (1967). Sites of synthesis of serum proteins. III. Production of beta-1-C, beta-1-E and transferrin by primate and rodent cell lines. *J. Immunol.*, **99**, 660–2
9. Ruddy, S. and Colten, H. R (1974) Rheumatoid arthritis: Biosynthesis of complement proteins by synovial tissues. *N. Engl. J. Med.*, **290**, 1284–8
10. Falus, A., Beuscher, H. U., Auerbach, H. S. and Colten, H. R. (1987). Constitutive and IL-1 regulated murine complement gene expression is strain and tissue specific. *J. Immunol.*, **138**, 856–60
11. Passwell, J., Schreiner, G. F., Nonaka, M., Beuscher, H. U. and Colten, H. R. (1988). Local extrahepatic expression of complement genes C3, factor B, C2 and C4 is increased in murine lupus nephritis. *J. Clin. Invest.*, **82**, 1676–84
12. Colten, H. R. and Gitlin, J. D. (1990). Immunoproteins. In Handin, R. I., Lux, S. E. and Stossel, T. P. (eds.) *Blood: Principles and Practice of Hematology*. (Philadelphia: J. B. Lippincott) (In press)
13. Perlmutter, D. H. and Colten, H. R. (1988). Complement: Molecular genetics. In Gallin, J. I., Goldstein, I. M. and Snyderman, R. (eds.) *Inflammation: Basic Principles and Clinical Correlates*, pp. 75–88. (New York: Raven Press)
14. Ramadori, G., Tedesco, F., Bitter-Suermann, D. and Meyer zum Buschenfelde, K. H. (1985). Biosynthesis of the third (C3), eighth (C8), and ninth (C9) complement components by guinea pig hepatocyte primary cultures. *Immunobiology*, **170**, 203–10
15. Morris, K. M., Aden, D. P., Knowles, B. B. and Colten, H. R. (1982). Complement biosynthesis by the human hepatoma derived cell line HepG2. *J. Clin. Invest.*, **70**, 906–13
16. Manthei, U., Strunk, R. C. and Giclas, P. C. (1984). Acute local inflammation alters synthesis, distribution and catabolism of the third component of complement (C3) in rabbits. *J. Clin. Invest.*, **74**, 424–33
17. Giclas, P. C., Strunk, R. C. and Manthei, U. (1985). The acute phase response of C3, C5, ceruloplasmin and C-reactive protein, induced by turpentine pleurisy in the rabbit. *Am. J. Pathol.*, **120**, 146–56
18. Zahedi, K. and Whitehead, A. S. (1989). Acute phase induction of mouse serum amyloid P component. Correlation with other parameters of inflammation. *J. Immunol.*, **143**, 2880–6
19. Katz, Y. and Strunk, R. C. (1989). IL-1 and tumor necrosis factor. Similarities and differences in stimulation of expression of alternative pathway of complement and IFN-beta 2/IL-6 genes in human fibroblasts. *J. Immunol.*, **142**, 3862–7
20. Perlmutter, D. H., Goldberger, G., Dinarello, C. A., Mizel, S. B. and Colten, H. R. (1986). Regulation of class III major histocompatibility complex (MHC) gene products by interleukin 1. *Science*, **232**, 850–2
21. Perlmutter, D. H., Dinarello, C. A., Punsal, P. I. and Colten, H. R. (1986). Cachectin/tumor necrosis factor regulates hepatic acute phase gene expression. *J. Clin. Invest.*, **78**, 1349–54
22. Katz, Y. and Strunk, R. C. (1988). Synthesis and regulation of complement protein factor H in human fibroblasts. *J. Immunol.*, **141**, 559–63
23. Katz, Y. and Strunk, R. C. (1989). Synthesis and regulation of C1 inhibitor in human skin fibroblasts. *J. Immunol.*, **142**, 2041–5

24. Katz, Y. and Strunk, R. C. (1988). Synovial fibroblast-like cells synthesize seven proteins of the complement system. *Arthritis Rheum.*, **31**, 1365–70
25. Katz, Y., Revel, M. and Strunk, R. C. (1989). Interleukin 6 stimulates synthesis of complement proteins factor B and C3 in human skin fibroblasts. *Eur. J. Immunol.*, **19**, 983–8
26. Katz, Y., Cole, F. S. and Strunk, R. C. (1988). Synergism between interferon-gamma and lipopolysaccharide for synthesis of factor B, but not C2, in human fibroblasts. *J. Exp. Med.*, **167**, 1–14
27. Cole, F. S. and Colten, H. R. (1988). Complement biosynthesis. In Rother, K. and Till, G. O. (eds.), *The Complement System*, pp. 44–70. (Berlin-Heidelberg: Springer-Verlag)
28. Kulics, J., Colten, H. R. and Perlmutter, D. H. (1990). Counter-regulatory effects of interferon-γ and endotoxin on expression of the human C4 genes. *J. Clin. Invest.*, **85**, 943–9
29. Cole, F. S., Matthews, W. J. Jr., Rossing, T. H., Gash, D. J., Lichtenberg, N. A. and Pennington, J. E. (1983). Complement biosynthesis by human bronchoalveolar macrophages. *Clin. Immunol. Immunopathol.*, **27**, 153–9
30. Whaley, K. (1980). Biosynthesis of the complement components and the regulatory proteins of the alternative complement pathway by human peripheral blood monocytes. *J. Exp. Med.*, **151**, 501–16
31. Strunk, R. C., Eidlen, D. M. and Mason, R. J. (1988). Pulmonary alveolar type II epithelial cells synthesize and secrete proteins of the classical and alternative complement pathways. *J. Clin. Invest.*, **81**, 1419–26
32. Al-Adnani, M. S. and McGee, J. O'D. (1976). C1q production and secretion by fibroblasts. *Nature*, **263**, 145–6
33. Reid, K. B. M. and Solomon, E. (1977). Biosynthesis of the first component of complement by human fibroblasts. *Biochem. J.*, **167**, 647–60
34. Strunk, R. C., Cole, F. S., Perlmutter, D. H. and Colten, H. R. (1985). Gamma interferon increases expression of class III complement genes C2 and factor B in human monocytes and in murine fibroblasts transfected with human C2 and factor B genes. *J. Biol. Chem.*, **260**, 15280–5
35. Strunk, R. C., Whitehead, A. S. and Cole, F. S. (1985). Pretranslational regulation of the synthesis of the third component of complement in human mononuclear phagocytes by the lipid A portion of lipopolysaccharide. *J. Clin. Invest.*, **76**, 985–90
36. Barbey-Morel, C., Pierce, J. A., Campbell, E. J. and Perlmutter, D. H. (1987). Lipopolysaccharide modulates the expression of alpha-1-proteinase inhibitor and other serine proteinase inhibitors in human monocytes and macrophages. *J. Exp. Med.*, **166**, 1041–54
37. Pennington, J. E., Matthews, W. J. Jr., Marino, J. T. Jr. and Colten, H. R. (1979). Cyclophosphamide and cortisone acetate inhibit complement biosynthesis by guinea pig bronchoalveolar macrophages. *J. Immunol.*, **123**, 1318–21
38. Alpert, S. E., Pennington, J. E. and Colten, H. R. (1984). Synthesis of complement by guinea pig bronchoalveolar macrophages. Effect of acute and chronic infection with Pseudomonas aeruginosa. *Am. Rev. Respir. Dis.*, **129**, 66–71
39. De Ceulaer, C., Papazoglou, S. and Whaley, K. (1980). Increased biosynthesis of complement components by cultured monocytes, synovial fluid macrophages and synovial membrane cells from patients with rheumatoid arthritis. *Immunology*, **41**, 37–43
40. Ramadori, G., Sipe, J. D. and Colten, H. R. (1985). Expression and regulation of the murine serum amyloid A (SAA) gene in extrahepatic sites. *J. Immunol.*, **135**, 3645–7
41. Reid, K. B. M. (1985). Molecular cloning and characterization of the complementary DNA and gene coding for the B-chain of subcomponent C1q of the human complement system. *Biochem. J.*, **231**, 729–35
42. Sellar, G. C. and Reid, K. B. M. (1990). Molecular cloning and alignment of the genes coding for the A, B, and C chains of human C1q of the serum complement system. *Biochem. J.* (In press)
43. Journet, A. and Tosi, M. (1986). Cloning and sequencing of full-length cDNA encoding the precursor of human complement component C1r. *Biochem. J.*, **240**, 783–7
44. Tosi, M. C., Duponchel, C., Meo, T. and Julier, C. (1987). Complete cDNA sequence of human complement C1s and close physical linkage of the homologous genes C1s and C1r. *Biochemistry*, **26**, 8516–24
45. Kusumoto, H., Hirosawa, S., Salier, J. P., Hagen, F. S. and Kurachi, K. (1988). Human genes for complement components C1r and C1s in a close tail-to-tail arrangement. *Proc. Natl. Acad. Sci. USA*, **85**, 7307–11

46. Sellar, G. C. and Reid, K. B. M. (1990). Molecular cloning and alignment of the genes coding for the A, B and C chains of human C1q of the serum complement system. *Biochem. J.* (In press)
47. Sellar, G. C., Goundis, D., McAdam, R. A., Solomon, E. and Reid, K. B. M. (1987). Cloning and chromosomal localization of human C1q A-chain. Identification of molecular defect in a C1q deficient patient. *Complement*, **4**, 225
48. Morris, K. M., Colten, H. R. and Bing, D. H. (1978). The first component of complement (C1): A quantitative comparison of its biosynthesis in culture by human epithelial and mesenchymal cells. *J. Exp. Med.*, 148, 1007–19
49. Colten, H. R., Borsos, T. and Rapp, H. J. (1966). In vitro synthesis of the first component of complement by guinea pig small intestine. *Proc. Natl. Acad. Sci. USA*, **56**, 1158–63
50. Colten, H. R., Gordon, J. M., Borsos, T. and Rapp, H. J. (1968). Synthesis of the first component of human complement in vitro. *J. Exp. Med.*, **128**, 595–604
51. Loos, M. (1983). Biosynthesis of the collagen-like C1q molecule and its receptor function of Fc and polyanionic molecules on macrophages. *Curr. Top. Microbiol. Immunol.*, **102**, 1–56
52. Al-Adnani, M. S. and McGee, J. O. (1976). C1q production and secretion by fibroblasts. *Nature*, **263**, 145–6
53. Muller, W., Hanauske-Abel, H. and Loos, M. (1978). Biosynthesis of the first component of complement by human and guinea pig peritoneal macrophages. Evidence for an independent production of the C1 subunits. *J. Immunol.*, **121**, 1578–84
54. Bensa, M. C., Reboul, A. and Colomb, M. G. (1983). Biosynthesis in vitro of complement subcomponents C1q, C1s and C1-inhibitor by resting and stimulated human monocytes. *Biochem. J.*, 216, 385–92
55. Loos, M., Martin, H. and Petry, F. (1989). The biosynthesis of C1q, the collagen-like and Fc-recognizing molecule of the complement system. *Behring Inst. Mitt.*, **84**, 32–41
56. Muller, W., Hanauski-Abel, H. and Loos, M. (1978). Reversible inhibition of C1q release from guinea pig macrophages by 2,2′-dipyridyl. *FEBS Lett.*, **90**, 218–22
57. Beatty, D. W., Davis, A. E., Cole, F. S., Einstein, L. P. and Colten, H. R. (1981). Biosynthesis of complement by human monocytes. *Clin. Immunol. Immunopathol.*, **18**, 334–43
58. Einstein, L. P., Schneeberger, E. E. and Colten, H. R. (1976). Synthesis of the second component of complement by long-term primary cultures of human monocytes. *J. Exp. Med.*, **143**, 114–26
59. Littman, B. H., Hall, R. E. and Muchmore, A. V. (1983). Lymphokine and phorbol (PMA) regulation of complement (C2) synthesis using U937. *Cell. Immunol.*, **76**, 189–95
60. Alpert, S. E., Auerbach, H. S., Cole, F. S. and Colten, H. R. (1983). Macrophage maturation: Differences in complement secretion by marrow, monocyte and tissue macrophages detected with an improved hemolytic plaque assay. *J. Immunol.*, **130**, 102–7
61. Cole, F. S., Auerbach, H. S., Goldberger, G. and Colten, H. R. (1985). Tissue specific pretranslational regulation of complement production in human mononuclear phagocytes. *J. Immunol.*, **134**, 2610–16
62. Hall, R. E. and Colten, H. R. (1977). Cell-free synthesis of the fourth component of guinea pig complement (C4): Identification of a precursor of serum C4 (pro-C4). *Proc. Natl. Acad. Sci. USA*, **74**, 1707–10
63. Fey, G., Odink, K. and Chapuis, R. M. (1980). Synthesis of the mouse complement component C4 (Ss-protein) by peritoneal macrophages: Kinetics of secretion and glycosylation of the subunits. *Eur. J. Immunol.*, **10**, 75–82
64. Schreiber, R. D. and Muller-Eberhard, H. J. (1974). Fourth component of human complement: description of a three polypeptide chain structure. *J. Exp. Med.*, **140**, 1324–35
65. Whitehead, A. S., Goldberger, G., Woods, D. E., Markham, A. F. and Colten, H. R. (1983). Use of a cDNA clone for the fourth component of human complement for analysis of a genetic deficiency of C4 in guinea pig. *Proc. Natl. Acad. Sci. USA*, **80**, 5387–91
66. Carroll, M. C., Belt, K. T., Palsdottir, A. and Porter, R. R. (1984). Structure and organization of C4 genes. *Phil. Trans. R. Soc.*, **306**, 379–88
67. Carroll, M. C., Campbell, R. D., Bentley, D. R. and Porter, R. R. (1984). A molecular map of the human MHC complex class III region linking complement genes C4, C2 and factor B. *Nature*, **307**, 237–41
68. Belt, K. T., Carroll, M. C. and Porter, R. R. (1984). The structural basis of the multiple forms of human complement component C4. *Cell*, **36**, 907–14
69. Yu, C. Y., Belt, K. T., Giles, C. M., Campbell, R. D. and Porter, R. R. (1986). Structural basis of the polymorphism of human complement components C4A and C4B gene size, reactivity and antigenicity. *EMBO J.*, **5**, 2873–81

70. Schneider, P. M., Carroll, M. C., Alper, C. A., Rittner, C., Whitehead, A. S., Yunis, E. J. and Colten, H. R. (1986). Polymorphism of the human complement C4 and steroid 21-hydroxylase genes: restriction fragment length polymorphisms revealing structural deletions, homoduplications and size variants. *J. Clin. Invest.*, **78**, 650–7
71. Awdeh, Z. L. and Alper, C. A. (1978). Inherited structural polymorphism of the fourth component of human complement. *Proc. Natl. Acad. Sci. USA*, **77**, 3576–80
72. Goldberger, G., Abraham, G. N., Williams, J. and Colten, H. R. (1980). NH_2-terminal sequence analysis of pro-C4, the precursor of the fourth component of guinea pig complement. *J. Biol. Chem.*, **255**, 7071–4
73. Goldberger, G. and Colten, H. R. (1980). Precursor complement protein (pro-C4) is converted in vitro to native C4 by plasmin. *Nature*, **286**, 514–16
74. Parker, K. L., Capra, J. D. and Shreffler, D. C. (1980). Partial amino acid sequences of the murine fourth component of complement (C4): demonstration of homology with human C4 and identification of amino terminal subunit in pro-C4. *Proc. Natl. Acad. Sci. USA*, **77**, 4275–8
75. Carroll, M. C. and Porter, R. R. (1983). Cloning of a human complement C4 gene. *Proc. Natl. Acad. Sci. USA*, **80**, 264–7
76. Ogata, R. T., Shreffler, D. C., Sepich, D. S. and Lilly, S. P. (1983). cDNA clone spanning the alpha-gamma subunit junction in the precursor of the murine fourth complement component (C4). *Proc. Natl. Acad. Sci. USA*, **80**, 5061–5
77. Karp, D. R. (1983). Post-translational modification of the fourth component of complement. Sulfation of the alpha chain. *J. Biol. Chem.*, **258**, 12745–8
78. Karp, D. R. (1983). Post-translational modification of the fourth component of complement: Effect of tunicamycin and amino acid analogs on the formation of the internal thiol ester and disulfide bonds. *J. Biol. Chem.*, **258**, 14490–5
79. Matthews, W. J., Goldberger, G., Marino, J. T., Einstein, L. P., Gash, D. J. and Colten, H. R. (1982). Complement proteins C2, C4, and factor B: effect of glycosylation on their secretion and catabolism. *Biochem. J.*, **204**, 839–46
80. Roos, M. H., Kornfeld, S. and Shreffler, D. C. (1980). Characterization of the oligosaccharide units of the fourth component of complement (Ss protein) synthesized by murine macrophages. *J. Immunol.*, **124**, 2860–1
81. Chan, A. C., Mitchell, K. R., Munns, T. W., Karp, D. R. and Atkinson, J. P. (1983). Identification and partial characterization of the secreted form of the fourth component of human complement: evidence that it is different from the major plasma form. *Proc. Natl. Acad. Sci. USA*, **80**, 268–72
82. Hortin, G., Chan, A. C., Fok, K. F., Strauss, A. W. and Atkinson, J. P. (1986). Sequence analysis of the COOH terminus of the alpha chain of the fourth component of human complement. Identification of the site of its extracellular cleavage. *J. Biol. Chem.*, **261**, 9065–9
83. Roos, M. H., Atkinson, J. P. and Shreffler, D. C. (1978). Molecular characterization of the Ss and Slp (C4) proteins of the mouse H-2 complex: subunit composition, chain size polymorphism and an intracellular (pro-Ss) precursor. *J. Immunol.*, **121**, 1106–15
84. Morris, K. M., Goldberger, G., Colten, H. R., Aden, D. P. and Knowles, B. B. (1982). Biosynthesis and processing of a human precursor complement protein, pro-C3, in a hepatoma-derived cell line. *Science*, **215**, 399–400
85. Sackstein, R. and Colten, H. R. (1984). Molecular regulation of MHC class III (C4 and factor B) gene expression in mouse peritoneal macrophages. *J. Immunol.*, **133**, 1618–26
86. Shreffler, D. C. (1976). The S region of the mouse major histocompatibility complex (H-2): Genetic variation and functional role in complement system. *Transplant. Rev.*, **32**, 140–67
87. Shreffler, D. C. (1982). MHC-linked complement components. In Parham, P. and Strominger, J. (eds.) *Histocompatibility Antigens: Structure and Function*, pp. 189–219. London: Chapman and Hall
88. Newell, S. L. and Atkinson, J. P. (1983). Biosynthesis of C4 by mouse peritoneal macrophages. II. Comparison of C4 synthesis by resident and elicited cell populations. *J. Immunol.*, **130**, 834–8
89. Rosa, P. A. and Shreffler, D. C. (1983). Cultured hepatocytes from mouse strains expressing high and low levels of the fourth component of complement differ in rate of synthesis of the protein. *Proc. Natl. Acad. Sci. USA*, **80**, 2332–6
90. Cox, B. J. and Robins, D. M. (1988). Tissue-specific variation in C4 and Slp gene regulation. *Nucl. Acids Res.*, **16**, 6857–70
91. Rosa, P. A., Sepich, D. S., Robins, D. M. and Ogata, R. T. (1987). Constitutive expression of Slp genes in mouse strain B10. WR directed by C4 regulatory sequences. *J. Immunol.*, **139**, 1568–77

92. Stavenhagen, J., Loreni, F., Hemenway, C., Kalff, M. and Robins, D. M. (1987). Molecular genetics of androgen-dependent and independent expression of mouse sex-limited protein. *Mol. Cell. Biol.*, **7**, 1716–24
93. Bruisten, S. M., Demant, P. and Robins, D. M. (1989). Trans-regulatory genes affect Slp^a and Slp^o expression and act in a tissue-specific manner. *Immunogenetics*, **29**, 340–5
94. Nakayama, K., Nonaka, M., Yokoyama, S., Yeul, Y. D., Pattanakitsakul, S-N. and Takahashi, M. (1987). Recombination of two homologous MHC class III genes of the mouse (C4 and Slp) that accounts for the loss of testosterone dependence of sex-limited protein expression. *J. Immunol.*, **138**, 620–7
95. Hemenway, C. and Robins, D. M. (1987). DNase I-hypersensitive sites associated with expression and hormonal regulation of mouse C4 and Slp genes. *Proc. Natl. Acad. Sci. USA*, **84**, 4816–20
96. Ishikawa, N., Nonaka, M., Wetsel, R. A. and Colten, H. R. (1990). Murine complement C2 and factor B genomic and cDNA cloning reveals different mechanisms for multiple transcripts of C2 and B. *J. Biol. Chem.*, **265**, 19040–6
97. Bentley, D. R. (1986). Primary structure of human complement component C2: homology to two unrelated protein families. *Biochem. J.*, **239**, 339–45
98. Mole, J. E., Anderson, J. K., Davidson, E. A. and Woods, D. E. (1984). Complete primary structure of the zymogen of human complement factor B. *J. Biol. Chem.*, **259**, 3407–12
99. Falus, A., Wakeland, E. K., McConnell, T. J., Gitlin, J. D., Whitehead, A. S. and Colten, H. R. (1987). DNA polymorphism of MHC III genes in inbred and wild mouse strains. *Immunogenetics*, **25**, 290–8
100. Horiuchi, T., Macon, K. J., Kidd, V. J. and Volanakis, J. E. (1990). Translational regulation of complement protein C2 expression by differential utilization of the 5′-untranslated region of mRNA. *J. Biol. Chem.*, **265**, 6521–4
101. Einstein, L. P., Hansen, P. J., Ballow, M., Davis, A. E., Davis, J. S., Alper, C. A., Rosen, F. S. and Colten, H. R. (1977). Biosynthesis of the third component of complement (C3) in vitro by monocytes from both normal and homozygous C3 deficient humans. *J. Clin Invest.*, **60**, 963–9
102. Sundstrom, S. A., Komm, B. S., Ponce-de-Leon, H., Yi, Z., Teuscher, C. and Lyttle, C. R. (1989). Estrogen regulation of tissue-specific expression of complement C3. *J. Biol. Chem.*, **264**, 16941–7
103. Levi-Strauss, M. and Mallat, M. (1987). Primary cultures of murine astrocytes produce C3 and factor B, two components of the alternative pathway of complement activation. *J. Immunol.*, **139**, 2361–6
104. Warren, H. B., Pantazis, P. and Davies, P. F. (1987). The third component of complement is transcribed and secreted by cultured human endothelial cells. *Am. J. Pathol.*, **129**, 9–13
105. Rothman, B. L., Merrow, M., Bamba, M., Kennedy, T. and Kreutzer, D. L. (1989). Biosynthesis of the third and fifth complement components by isolated human lung cells. *Am. Rev. Respir. Dis.*, **139**, 212–20
106. Nichols, W. K. (1984). LPS stimulation of complement (C3) synthesis by a human monocyte cell line. *Complement*, **1**, 108–15
107. Goodrum, K. J. (1987). Complement component C3 secretion by mouse macrophage-like cell lines. *J. Leukocyte Biol.*, **41**, 295–301
108. Dieli, F., Lio, D., Sireci, G. and Salerno, A. (1988). Genetic control of C3 production by the S region of the mouse MHC. *J. Immunogenet.*, **15**, 339–43
109. Ferreira, A. and Nussenzweig, V. (1975). Genetic linkage between serum levels of the third component of complement and the H-2 complex. *J. Exp. Med.*, **141**, 513–17
110. Natsuume-Sakai, S., Hayarawa, J. I. and Takahashi, M. (1978). Genetic polymorphism of murine C3 controlled by a single codominant locus on chromosome 17. *J. Immunol.*, **121**, 491–8
111. DaSilva, F. P., Hoecker, G. E., Day, N. K., Vienne, D. and Rubinstein, P. (1978). Murine complement component 3: Genetic variation and linkage to H-2. *Proc. Natl. Acad. Sci. USA*, **75**, 963–5
112. Whitehead, A. S., Solomon, E., Chambers, S., Bodmer, W. F., Povey, S. and Fey, G. (1982). Assignment of the structural gene for the third component of human complement to chromosome 19. *Proc. Natl. Acad. Sci. USA*, **79**, 5021–5
113. Khan, S. A. and Erickson, B. W. (1982). An equilibrium model of the metastable binding sites of alpha 2 macroglobulin and complement proteins C3 and C4. *J. Biol. Chem.*, **257**, 11864–7

114. Iijima, M., Tobe, T., Sakamoto, T. and Tomita, M. (1984). Biosynthesis of the internal thioester bond of the third component of complement. *J. Biochem*, **96**, 1539–46
115. Auerbach, H. S., Burger, R., Dodds, A. and Colten, H. R. (1990). Molecular basis of complement C3 deficiency in guinea pigs. *J. Clin, Invest.*, **86**, 96–106
116. Alper, C. A. and Rosen, F. S. (1971). Genetic aspects of the complement system (review). *Adv. Immunol.*, **14**, 251–90
117. Peters, D. K., Martin, A., Weinstein, A., Cameron, J. S., Barratt, T., Ogg, C. S. and Lachmann, P. J. (1972). Complement metabolism in membranoproliferative nephritis. *Clin. Exp. Immunol.*, **11**, 311–20
118. Perlmutter, D. H., Daniels, J. D., Auerbach, H. S., DeSchryver-Kecskemeti, K., Winter, H. S. and Alpers, D. H. (1989). The alpha 1-antitrypsin gene is expressed in a human intestinal epithelial cell line. *J. Biol. Chem.*, **264**, 9485–90
119. Ramadori, G., Sipe, J. D., Dinarello, C. A., Mizel, S. B. and Colten, H. R. (1985). Pretranslational modulation of acute phase hepatic protein synthesis by murine recombinant interleukin 1 (IL-1) and purified human IL-1. *J. Exp. Med.*, **162**, 930–42
120. Minta, J. O. (1988). Synthesis of complement factor B by the human monocyte U-937 cell line. Augmentation by immunostimulatory agents. *J. Immunol.*, **141**, 1636–41
121. Nonaka, M., Ishikawa, N., Passwell, J., Natsuume-Sakai, S. and Colten, H. R. (1989). Tissue specific initiation of murine complement factor B mRNA transcription. *J. Immunol.*, **142**, 1377–82
122. Circolo, A., Pierce, G. F., Katz, Y. and Strunk, R. C. (1990). Anti-inflammatory effects of polypeptide growth factors. Platelet-derived growth factor, epidermal growth factor, and fibroblast growth factor inhibit the cytokine-induced expression of the alternative complement pathway activator factor B in human fibroblasts. *J. Biol. Chem.*, **265**, 5066–71
123. Katz, Y. and Strunk, R. C. (1990). Enhanced synthesis of factor B induced by tumor necrosis factor in human skin fibroblasts is decreased by IL-4. *J. Immunol.*, **144**, 4675–80
124. Perlmutter, D. H. (1989). Distinct mediators and mechanisms regulate human acute phase gene expression. In Purdue, M. L., Feramisco, J. R. and Lindquest, S. (eds.) *Stress Induced Proteins*, pp. 257–74 (New York: Alan R. Liss, Inc.)
125. Cook, K. S., Min, H. Y., Johnson, D., Chaplinsky, R. J., Flier, J. S., Hunt, C. R. and Spiegelman, B. M. (1987). Adipsin: A circulating serine protease homolog secreted by adipose tissue and sciatic nerve. *Science*, **237**, 402–5.
126. Bentley, C., Fries, W. and Brade, V. (1978). Synthesis of factors D, B and P of the alternative pathway of complement activation, as well as of C3, by guinea pig peritoneal macrophages in vitro. *Immunology*, **35**, 971–80
127. Barnum, S. R. and Volanakis, J. E. (1985). In vitro biosynthesis of complement protein D by U937 cells. *J. Immunol.*, **134**, 1799–803
128. Rosen, B. S., Cook, K. S., Yaglom, J., Groves, D. L., Volanakis, J. E., Damm, D., White, T. and Spiegelman, B. M. (1989). Adipsin and complement factor D activity: An immune-related defect in obesity. *Science*, **244**, 1483–7
129. Flier, J. S., Cook, K. S., Usher, P. and Spiegelman, B. M. (1987). Severely impaired adipsin expression in genetic and acquired obesity. *Science*, **237**, 405–8
130. Platt, K. A., Min, H. Y., Ross, S. R. and Spiegelman, B. M. (1989). Obesity-linked regulation of the adipsin gene promoter in transgenic mice. *Proc. Natl. Acad. Sci. USA*, **86**, 7490–4
131. White, T., Damm, D., Brown, R., Hancock, N., Rosen, B., Spiegelman, B. M., Lowell, B. and Flier, J. (1989). Isolation and characterization of cDNA clones for human complement factor D. *Complement Inflamm.*, **6**, 415 (abstract)
132. Barnum, S. R. and Volanakis, J. E. (1985). Biosynthesis of complement protein D by HepG2 cells: A comparison of D produced by HepG2 cells, U937 cells and blood monocytes. *Eur. J. Immunol.*, **15**, 1148–51
133. Reid, K. B. M. unpublished
134. Farries, T. C. and Atkinson, J. P. (1989). Biosynthesis of properdin. *J. Immunol.*, **142**, 842–7
135. Goundis, D, and Reid, K. B. M. (1988). Properdin, the terminal complement components, thrombospondin and circumsporozoite protein of malarial parasites contain similar sequence motifs. *Nature*, **335**, 82–5
136. Goundis, D. and Reid, K. B. M. (1987). Biosynthesis of complement proteins by the U937 cell line. *Biochem. Soc. Trans.*, **15**, 650–1

137. D'Eustachio, P., Kristensen, T., Wetsel, R. A., Riblet, R., Taylor, B. A. and Tack, B. F. (1986). Chromosomal location of the genes encoding complement components C5 and factor H in the mouse. *J. Immunol.*, **137**, 3990–5
138. Wetsel, R. A., Lemons, R. S., LeBeau, M. M., Barnum, S. R., Noack, D. and Tack, B. F. (1988). Molecular analysis of human complement component C5: localization of the structural gene to chromosome 9. *Biochemistry*, **27**, 1474–82
139. Wheat, W. H., Wetsel, R., Falus, A., Tack, B. F. and Strunk, R. C. (1987). The fifth component of complement (C5) in the mouse. Analysis of the molecular basis for deficiency. *J. Exp. Med.*, **165**, 1442–7
140. Colten, H. R. (1972). Ontogeny of the human complement system: In vitro biosynthesis of individual complement components by fetal tissue. *J. Clin. Invest.*, **51**, 725–30
141. Levy, N. L., Snyderman, R., Ladda, R. L. and Lieberman, R. (1973). Cytogenetic engineering in vivo: Restoration of biologic complement activity to C5-deficient mice by intravenous inoculation of hybrid cells. *Proc. Natl. Acad. Sci. USA*, **70**, 3125–9
142. Ooi, Y. M. and Colten, H. R. (1979). Biosynthesis and post-synthetic modification of a precursor (pro-C5) of the fifth component of mouse complement (C5). *J. Immunol.*, **123**, 2494–8
143. Hetland, G., Johnson, E. and Aasebo, U. (1986). Human alveolar macrophages synthesize the functional alternative pathway of complement and active C5 and C9 in vitro. *Scand. J. Immunol.*, **24**, 603–8
144. Kohler, P. F. (1973). Maturation of the human complement system. I. Onset time and sites of fetal C1q, C4, C3, and C5 synthesis. *J. Clin. Invest.*, **52**, 671–7
145. Sundsmo, J. S. and Gotze, O. (1981). Human monocyte spreading by factor Bb of the alternative pathway of complement activation. A possible role for C5 in monocyte spreading. *J. Exp. Med.*, **154**, 763–77
146. Curd, J. G., Sundsmo, J. S., Kolb, W. P., Bluestein, H. G. and Muller-Eberhard, H. J. (1978). Neoantigen of the membrane attack complex of human complement. *Arthritis Rheum.*, **21**, 177–82
147. Reed, W., Roubey, R. A. S., Dalzell, J. G., Matteucci, B. M., Myones, B. L., Hunt, S. W., Kolb, W. P and Ross, G. D. (1990). Synthesis of complement component C5 by human B and T lymphoblastoid cell lines. *Immunogenetics*, **31**, 145–51
148. Lundwall, A. B., Wetsel, R. A., Kristensen, T., Whitehead, A. S., Woods, D. E., Ogden, R. C., Colten, H. R. and Tack, B. F. (1985). Isolation and sequence analysis of a cDNA clone encoding the fifth complement component (C5). *J. Biol. Chem.*, **260**, 2108–12
149. Haviland, D. L., Haviland, J. C., Fleischer, D. T., Hunt, A. and Wetsel, R. A. (1991). Complete cDNA sequence of human complement pro-C5. Evidence of truncated transcripts derived from a single copy gene. *J. Immunol.*, **146**, 362–8
150. Haefliger, J-A., Tschopp, J., Vial, N. and Jenne, D. E. (1989). Complete primary structure and functional characterization of the sixth component of the human complement system. *J. Biol. Chem.*, **264**, 18041–51
151. DiScipio, R. G., Chakravarti, D. N., Muller-Eberhard, H. J. and Fey, G. H. (1988). The structure of human complement component C7 and C5b-7 complex. *J. Biol. Chem.*, **263**, 549–60
152. Rao, A. G., Howard, O. Z. M., Ng, S. C., Whitehead, A. S., Colten, H. R. and Sodetz, J. M. (1987). Complementary DNA and derived amino acid sequence for the α subunit of human complement protein C8: Evidence for the existence of a separate α subunit mRNA. *Biochemistry*, **26**, 3556–64
153. Howard, O. Z. M., Rao, A. G. and Sodetz, J. M. (1987). Complementary DNA and derived amino acid sequence of the β-subunit of C8: identification of a close structural and ancestral relationship to the α-subunit and C9. *Biochemistry*, **26**, 3565–70
154. Ng, S. C. and Sodetz, J. M. (1987). Biosynthesis of C8 by hepatocytes: Differential expression and intracellular association of the α–γ and β subunits. *J. Immunol.*, **139**, 3021–7
155. Ng, S. C., Rao, A. G., Howard, O. M. Z. and Sodetz, J. M. (1987). The eighth component of human complement: Evidence that it is an oligomeric serum protein assembled from products of three different genes. *Biochemistry*, **26**, 5229–33
156. DiScipio, R. G., Gehring, M. R., Podack, E. R., Kan, C. C., Hugli, T. E. and Fey, G. H. (1984). Nucleotide sequence of human complement component C9. *Proc. Natl. Acad. Sci. USA*, **81**, 7298–302
157. Stanley, K. K., Kocher, H. P., Luzio, J. P., Jackson, P. and Tschopp, J. (1985). The sequence and topology of human complement component C9. *EMBO J.*, **4**, 375–83

158. Pettersen, H. B., Johnson, E. and Hetland, G. (1987). Human alveolar macrophages synthesize active complement components C6, C7 and C8 in vitro. *Scand. J. Immunol.*, **25**, 567–70
159. Tedesco, F., Densen, P., Villa, M. A., Presani, G., Roncelli, L. and Rosso Di San Secondo, V. E. M. (1986). Functional C8 associated with human platelets. *Clin. Exp. Immunol.*, **66**, 472–80
160. Houle, J. J., Leddy, J. P. and Rosenfeld, S. I. (1989). Secretion of the terminal complement proteins, C5-C9, by human platelets. *Clin. Immunol. Immunopathol.*, **50**, 385–93
161. Kaufman, K. M., Snider, J. V., Spurr, N. K., Schwartz, C. E. and Sodetz, J. M. (1989). Chromosomal assignment of genes encoding the α, β, and γ subunits of human complement protein C8: Identification of a close physical linkage between the α and the β loci. *Genomics*, **5**, 475–80
162. Densen, P. and McRill, C. M. (1987). Differential expression of C8 subunits: Primary role of C8 beta. *Clin. Res.*, **35**, 613A
163. Goldberger, G., Arnaout, M. A., Aden, D., Kay, R., Rits, M. and Colten, H. R. (1984). Biosynthesis and postsynthetic processing of human C3b/C4b inactivator (factor I) in three hepatoma cell lines. *J. Biol. Chem.*, **259**, 6492–7
164. Munoz-Canoves, P., Tack, B. F. and Vik, D. P. (1989). Analysis of complement factor H mRNA expression: Dexamethasone and IFN-γ increase the level of H in L cells. *Biochemistry*, **28**, 9891–7
165. Brooimans, R. A., Hiemetra, P. S., van der Ark, A. A. J., Sim, R. B., van Es, L. A. and Daha, M. R. (1989). Biosynthesis of complement factor H by human umbilical vein endothelial cells. Regulation by T cell growth factor and IFN-γ. *J. Immunol.*, **142**, 2024–30
166. Lappin, D. F. and Whaley, K. (1990). Interferon-induced transcriptional and post-transcriptional modulation of factor H and C4 binding-protein synthesis in human monocytes. *Biochem. J.*, **271**, 767–72
167. Malhotra, V. and Sim, R. B. (1985). Expression of complement factor H on the cell surface of the human monocytic cell line U937. *Eur. J. Immunol.*, **15**, 935–41
168. Devine, D. V. and Rosse, W. F. (1987). Regulation of the activity of platelet-bound C3 convertase of the alternative pathway of complement by platelet factor H. *Proc. Natl. Acad. Sci USA*, **84**, 5873–7
169. Gitlin, D. and Biasucci, A. (1969). Development of γG, γA, γM, β1C/β1A, C1 esterase inhibitor, ceruloplasmin, transferrin, hemopexin, haptoglobin, fibrinogen, plasminogen, alpha-1-antitrypsin, orosomucoid, beta-lipoprotein, alpha-2-macroglobulin, and prealbumin in the human conceptus. *J. Clin. Invest.*, **48**, 1433–6
170. Johnson, A. M., Alper, C. A., Rosen, R. S. and Graig, J. M. (1971). C1 inhibitor: Evidence for decreased hepatic synthesis in hereditary angioneurotic edema. *Science*, **173**, 553–4
171. Yeung Laiwah, A. C., Jones, L., Hamilton, A. O. and Whaley, K. (1985). Complement subcomponent C1 inhibitor synthesis by human monocytes. *Biochem. J.*, **226**, 199–205
172. Bensa, J. C., Reboul, J. A. and Colomb, M. G. (1983). Biosynthesis *in vitro* of complement subcomponents C1q, C1s and C1-inhibitor by resting and stimulated human monocytes. *Biochem. J.*, **216**, 385–92
173. Schmaier, A. H., Smith, P. M. and Colman, R. W. (1985). Platelet C1 inhibitor. A secreted alpha-granule protein. *J. Clin. Invest.*, **75**, 242–50
174. Goldberger, G., Bruns, G. A. P., Rits, M., Edge, M. D. and Kwiatkowski, D. J. (1987). Human complement factor I: Analysis of cDNA-derived primary structure and assignment of its gene to chromosome 4. *Biochemistry*, **262**, 10065–71
175. Catterall, C. F., Lyons, A., Sim, R. B., Day, A. J. and Harris, T. J. R. (1987). Characterization of the primary amino acid sequence of human complement control protein factor I from an analysis of cDNA clones. *Biochem. J.*, **242**, 849–56
176. Lublin, D. M. and Atkinson, J. P. (1989). Decay-accelerating factor and membrane cofactor protein. *Curr. Top. Microbiol. Immunol.*, **153**, 123–45
177. Bora, N. S., Lublin, D. M., Kumar, B. V., Hockett, R. D., Holers, V. M. and Atkinson, J. P. (1989). Structural gene for human membrane cofactor protein (MCP) of complement maps to within 100 kb of the 3′ end of the C3b/C4b receptor gene. *J. Exp. Med.*, **169**, 597–602
178. Caras, I. W., Weddell, G. N., Davitz, M. A., Nussenzweig, V. and Martin, D. W. (1987). Signal for attachment of a phospholipid membrane anchor in decay-accelerating factor. *Science*, **238**, 1280–3

179. Medof, M. E., Lublin, D. M., Holers, V. M., Ayers, D. J., Getty, R. R., Leykam, J. F., Atkinson, J. P. and Tykocinski, M. L. (1987). Cloning and characterization of cDNAs encoding the complete sequence of decay-accelerating factor of human complement. *Proc. Natl. Acad. Sci. USA*, **84**, 2007–11
180. Lublin, D. M., Krsek-Staples, J., Pangburn, M. K. and Atkinson, J. P. (1986). Biosynthesis and glycosylation of the human complement regulatory protein decay-accelerating factor. *J. Immunol.*, **137**, 1629–35
181. Medof, M. E., Walter, E. I., Roberts, W. L., Haas, R. and Rosenberry, T. L. (1986). Decay accelerating factor of complement is anchored to cells by a C-terminal glycolipid. *Biochemistry*, **25**, 6740–7
182. Tykocinski, M. L., Shu, H. K., Ayers, D. J., Walter, E. I., Getty, R. R., Groger, R. K., Hauer, C. A. and Medof, M. E. (1988). Glycolipid reanchoring of T-lymphocyte surface antigen CD8 using the 3′ end sequence of decay-accelerating factor's mRNA. *Proc. Natl. Acad. Sci. USA*, **85**, 3555–9
183. Kushner, I. (1982). The phenomenon of the acute phase response. (Review). *Ann. NY Acad. Sci.*, **389**, 39–48
184. St. John Sutton, M. B., Strunk, R. C. and Cole, F. S. (1986). Regulation of synthesis of the third component of complement and factor B in cord blood monocytes by lipopolysaccharide. *J. Immunol.*, **136**, 1366–72
185. Beutler, B., Krochin, N., Milsark, I. W., Leudke, C. and Cerami, A. (1986). Control of cachectin (tumor necrosis factor) synthesis: mechanisms of endotoxin resistance. *Science*, **232**, 977–80
186. Dinarello, C. A. (1984). Interleukin 1. *Rev. Infect. Dis.*, **6**, 51–95
187. Beuscher, H. U., Nickells, M. W. and Colten, H. R. (1988). The precursor of interleukin-1α is phosphorylated at residue serine 90. *J. Biol. Chem.*, **263**, 4023–8
188. Kurt-Jones, E. A., Beller, D. I., Mizel, S. B. and Unanue, E. R. (1985). Identification of a membrane-associated interleukin 1 in macrophages. *Proc. Natl. Acad. Sci. USA*, **82**, 1204–8
189. Giri, J. G., Lomedico, P. T. and Mizel, S. B. (1985). Studies on the synthesis and secretion of interleukin 1. I. A 33,000 m.w. precursor for interleukin 1. *J. Immunol.*, **134**, 343–9
190. Perlmutter, D. H., Colten, H. R., Adams, S. P., May, L. T., Sehgal, P. B. and Fallon, R. J. (1989). A cytokine-selective defect in interleukin–1β mediated acute phase gene expression in a subclone of the human hepatoma cell line (HepG2). *J. Biol. Chem.*, **264**, 7669–74
191. Nonaka, M., Gitlin, J. D. and Colten, H. R. (1989). Regulation of human and murine complement: Comparision of 5′ structural and functional elements regulating human and murine complement factor B gene expression. *Mol. Cell. Biochem.*, **89**, 1–14
192. Beuscher, H. U., Fallon, R. J. and Colten, H. R. (1987). Macrophage membrane interleukin 1 regulates the expression of acute phase proteins in human hepatoma Hep3B cells. *J. Immunol.*, **139**, 1896–1901
193. Baumann, H., Onorato, V., Gauldie, J. and Jahreis, G. P. (1987). Distinct sets of acute phase plasma proteins are stimulated by separate human hepatocyte-stimulating factors and monokines in rat hepatoma cells. *J. Biol. Chem.*, **262**, 9756–68
194. Strunk, R. S., Tashjian, A. H. and Colten, H. R. (1975). Complement biosynthesis in vitro by rat hepatoma cell strains. *J. Immunol.*, **114**, 331–5
195. Wu, L-C., Morley, B. J. and Campbell, R. D. (1987). Cell-specific expression of the human complement protein factor B gene: Evidence for the role of two distinct 5′-flanking elements. *Cell*, **48**, 331–42
196. Beutler, B. and Cerami, A. (1989). The biology of cachectin/TNF – a primary mediator of the host response. *Ann. Rev. Immunol.*, **7**, 625–56
197. Gauldie, J., Richards, C., Harnish, D., Landsdorp, P. and Baumann, H. (1987). Interferon beta 2/B-cell stimulatory factor type 2 shares identity with monocyte-derived hepatocyte-stimulating factor and regulates the major acute phase protein response in liver cells. *Proc. Natl. Acad. Sci. USA*, **84**, 7251–5
198. Kishimoto, T. K., Larson, R. S., Corbi, A. L., Dustin, M. L., Stauton, D. E. and Springer, T. A. (1989). The leukocyte integrins. *Adv. Immunol.* **46**, 149–82
199. Akira, S., Hirano, T., Taga, T. and Kishimoto, T. (1990). Biology of multifunctional cytokines: IL 6 and related molecules (IL 1 and TNF). *FASEB J.*, **4**, 2860–7
200. Baumann, H., Isseroff, H., Latimer, J. J. and Jahreis, G. P. (1988). Phorbol ester modulates interleukin 6- and interleukin 1-regulated expression of acute phase plasma proteins in hepatoma cells. *J. Biol. Chem.*, **263**, 17390–6

201. Miura, N., Prentice, H. L., Schneider, P. M. and Perlmutter, D. H. (1987). *J. Biol. Chem.*, **262**, 7298–305
202. Ripoche, J., Mitchell, A., Erdei, A., Madin, C., Moffatt, B., Mokoena, T., Gordon, S. and Sim, R. B. (1988). Interferon gamma induces synthesis of complement alternative pathway proteins by human endothelial cells in culture. *J. Exp. Med.*, **168**, 1917–22
203. Peters, M. G., Ambrus, J. L., Fauci, A. S. and Brown, E. J. (1988). The Bb fragment of complement factor B acts as a cell growth factor. *J. Exp. Med.*, **168**, 1225–35
204. Strunk, R. C. and Colten, H. R. (1985). Regulation of complement synthesis in mononuclear phagocytes. In Filkins, J. P. and Reichard, S. M. (eds.) *The Reticulo-Endothelial System: A Comprehensive Treatise*, pp. 25–46. (New York: Plenum Press)
205. Celada, A., Klemsz, M. J. and Maki, R. A. (1989). Interferon-γ activates multiple pathways to regulate the expression of the genes for major histocompatibility class II I-Aβ, tumour necrosis factor and complement component C3 in mouse macrophages. *Eur. J. Immunol.*, **19**, 1103–9
206. Urbach, G. and Cinader, B. (1966). Hormonal control of MuB1 concentration. *Proc. Soc. Exp. Biol. Med.*, **122**, 779–82
207. Churchill, W. H., Weintraub, R. M., Borsos, T. and Rapp, H. J. (1967). Mouse complement: The effect of sex hormones and castration on two of the late-acting components. *J. Exp. Med.*, **125**, 657–72
208. Ecker, E. E. and Rees, H. M. (1922). Effect of hemorrhage on complement of blood. *J. Infect. Dis.*, **31**, 361–7
209. Alper, C. A. and Propp, R. R. (1968). Genetic polymorphism of the third component of human complement. *J. Clin. Invest.*, **47**, 2181–91
210. Sundstrom, S. A., Komm, B. S., Xu, Q., Boundy, V. and Lyttle, C. R. (1990). The stimulation of uterine complement component C3 gene expression by antiestrogens. *Endocrinology*, **126**, 1449–56
211. Isaacson, K. B., Coutifaris, C., Garcia, C-R. and Lyttle, C. R. (1989). Production and secretion of complement component 3 by endometriotic tissue. *J. Clin. Endocrinol. Metab.*, **69**, 1003–9
212. Shreffler, D. C. and David, C. S. (1975). The H-2 major histocompatibility complex and the I immune response region: Genetic variation, function and organization. *Adv. Immunol.*, **20**, 125–95
213. Levi-Strauss, M., Tosi, M., Steinmetz, M., Klein, J. and Meo, T. (1985). Multiple duplications of complement C4 gene correlate with H-2-controlled testosterone-independent expression of its sex-limited isoform, C4-Slp. *Proc. Natl. Acad. Sci. USA*, **82**, 1746–50
214. Loreni, F., Stavenhagen, J., Kalff, M. and Robins, D. M. (1988). A complex androgen-responsive enhancer resides 2 kilobases upstream of the mouse Slp gene. *Mol. Cell. Biol.*, **8**, 2350–60
215. Hourcade, D., Holers, V. M. and Atkinson, J. P. (1989). The regulators of complement activation (RCA) gene cluster. *Adv. Immunol.*, **45**, 381–416
216. Vedeler, C. A., Scarpini, E., Beretta, S., Doronzo, R. and Matre, R. (1990). The ontogenesis of Fcγ receptors and complement receptors CR1 in human peripheral nerves. *Acta Neuropathol.*, **80**, 35–40
217. Kubota, Y., Gaither, T. A., Cason, J., O'Shea, J. J. and Lawley, T. J. (1987). Characterization of the C3 receptor induced by herpes simplex virus type 1 infection of human epidermal, endothelial, and A431 cells. *J. Immunol.*, **138**, 1137–42
218. Ross, G. D. and Medof, M. E. (1985). Membrane complement receptors specific for bound fragments of C3. *Adv. Immunol.*, **37**, 217–67
219. Todd, R. F. and Schlossman, S. F. (1984). Differential antigens on human monocytes and macrophages defined by monoclonal antibodies. In Volkman, A. (ed.) *Mononuclear Phagocyte Biology*, pp. 129–49. (New York: Marcell Dekker)
220. Schwarting, R., Stein, H. and Wang, C. Y. (1985). The monoclonal antibodies alpha S-HCL 1 (alpha Leu-14) and alpha S-HCL 3 (alpha Leu-M5) allow the diagnosis of hairy cell leukemia. *Blood*, **65**, 974–83
221. LeBien, T. W. and Kersey, J. H. (1980). A monoclonal antibody (TA-1) reactive with human T lymphocytes and monocytes. *J. Immunol.*, **125**, 2208–14
222. Miller, L. J., Schwarting, R. and Springer, T. A. (1986). Regulated expression of the Mac-1, LFA-1, p150,95 glycoprotein family during leukocyte differentiation. *J. Immunol.*, **137**, 2891–900

223. Nicholson-Weller, A., Burge, J., Fearon, D. T., Weller, P. F. and Austen, K. F. (1982). Isolation of a human erythrocyte membrane glycoprotein with decay accelerating activity for C3 convertases of the complement system. *J. Immunol.*, **129**, 184–9
224. Pangburn, M. K., Schreiber, R. D. and Muller-Eberhard, H. J. (1983). Deficiency of an erythrocyte membrane protein with complement regulatory activity in paroxysmal nocturnal hemoglobinuria. *Proc. Natl. Acad. Sci. USA*, **80**, 5430–4
225. Kinoshita, T., Medof, M. E., Silber, R. and Nussenzweig, V. (1985). Distribution of decay-accelerating factor in the peripheral blood of normal individuals and patients with paroxysmal nocturnal hemoglobinuria. *J. Exp. Med.*, **162**, 75–92
226. Nicholson-Weller, A., March, J. P., Rosen, C. E., Spicer, D. B. and Austen, K. F. (1985). Surface membrane expression by human blood leukocytes and platelets of decay-accelerating factor, a regulatory protein of the complement system. *Blood*, **65**, 1237–44
227. Lublin, D. M. and Atkinson, J. P. (1989). Decay-accelerating factor and membrane cofactor protein. *Curr. Top. Microbiol. Immunol.*, **153**, 123–45
228. McNearney, T., Ballard, L., Seya, T. and Atkinson, J. P. (1989). Membrane cofactor protein of complement is present on human fibroblast, epithelial and endothelial cells. *J. Clin. Invest.*, **84**, 538–45
229. Asch, A. S., Kinoshita, T., Jaffe, E. A. and Nussenzweig, V. (1986). Decay-accelerating factor is present on cultured human umbilical vein endothelial cells. *J. Exp. Med.*, **163**, 221–6
230. Medof, M. E., Walter, E. I., Rutgers, J. L., Knowles, D. M. and Nussenzweig, V. (1987). Identification of the complement decay-accelerating factor (DAF) on epithelium and glandular cells and in body fluids. *J. Exp. Med.*, **165**, 848–64
231. Cole, J. L., Housely, G. A., Dykman, T. R., MacDermott, R. P. and Atkinson, J. P. (1985). Identification of an additional class of C3-binding membrane proteins of human peripheral blood leukocytes and cell lines. *Proc. Natl. Acad. Sci. USA*, **82**, 859–63
232. Seya, T., Ballard, L. L., Bora, N. S., Kumar, B. V., Cui, W. and Atkinson, J. P. (1988). Distribution of membrane cofactor protein (MCP) of complement on human peripheral blood cells. *Eur. J. Immunol.*, **18**, 1289–94
233. McIntyre, J. A., Faulk, W. P., Verhulst, S. J. and Colliver, J. A. (1983). Human trophoblast–lymphocyte cross-reactive (TLX) antigens define a new alloantigen system. *Science*, **222**, 1135–7
234. Sugita, Y., Nakano, Y. and Tomita, M. (1988). Isolation from human erythrocytes of a new membrane protein which inhibits the formation of complement transmembrane channels. *J. Biochem. (Tokyo)*, **104**, 633–7
235. Rollins, S. A. and Sims, P. J. (1990). The complement-inhibitory activity of CD59 resides in its capacity to block incorporation of C9 into membrane C5b-9. *J. Immunol.*, **144**, 3478–83
236. Nose, M., Katoh, M., Okada, N., Kyogoku, M. and Okada, H. (1990). Tissue distribution of HRF20, a novel factor preventing the membrane attack of homologous complement, and its predominant expression on endothelial cells *in vivo*. *Immunology*, **70**, 145–9
237. Sims, P. J., Rollins, S. A. and Wiedmer, T. (1989). Regulatory control of complement on blood platelets. Modulation of platelet procoagulant responses by a membrane inhibitor of the C5b-9 complex. *J. Biol. Chem.*, **264**, 19228–35

5 Genetic deficiencies of the complement system: an overview

F. S. ROSEN

Genetically determined deficiencies of the complement system have now been established for almost all the components of the system. Deficiency of the C1-inhibitor results in hereditary angioneurotic oedema; this deficiency is discussed in Chapters 6 and 7. Infectious consequences of complement deficiency are discussed in Chapter 8. The deficiencies can be conveniently grouped according to the most prominent symptoms sustained by affected individuals. A deficiency of the proteins of the classical pathway (C1, C4 and C2) results in immune complex disease, presenting frequently as discoid or systemic lupus erythematosus, which is usually antinuclear antibody negative. Alternative pathway deficiencies (properdin and factor D) are rare; no deficiency of factor B has as yet been described. Deficiency of alternative pathway proteins predisposes to infection with *Neisseria* organisms. This susceptibility is also found in patients with deficiencies of the terminal components (C5, C6, C7 and C8). Patients with deficiencies of C3, factor H and factor I exhibit a broader range of susceptibility to infection, particularly with the pyogenic bacteria, in addition to infections with bacteria of *Neisseria* species. Finally, most individuals with C9 deficiency are asymptomatic although some reports from Japan suggest that C9 deficiency does cause an increased susceptibility to *Neisseria* infections. These distinctions are not firm; patients with early classical component deficiencies also have susceptibility to pyogenic infections and immune complex disease has been observed infrequently in patients with terminal complement defects[1].

C1 DEFICIENCIES

Deficiency of the first component of complement can either be of C1q or C1r together with C1s. The genes for the three chains (A, B and C) of C1q map to the short arm of chromosome 1 at 1p34.1–36.3. They are tandemly arranged in 5′ to 3′ orientation[2] in the order A-C-B and occupy a stretch of 24 kb. On the other hand, the genes encoding C1r and C1s are linked and map[3] to the terminal portion of the short arm of chromosome 12. The genes for C1r and C1s lie within 10 kb of each other and are oriented tail to tail[4].

Reid has recently reviewed C1 deficiency[5]. Two types of C1q deficiency have been reported. In one type, C1q is functionally deficient but is present in normal amounts by immunochemical measurement. In the second type, C1q is functionally and antigenically deficient. In both cases, the defect is inherited phenotypically as an autosomal recessive; it is difficult to identify obligate heterozygotes. The precise molecular basis of C1q deficiency has only been ascertained in one kindred where a premature stop codon in the B chain results in failure of C1q synthesis and assembly. This mutation results in the loss of a Taq 1 cleavage site so that the defect can be detected by restriction fragment length polymorphism (RFLP)[6]. Although more than a dozen kindred with C1r deficiency have been described, the precise basis of the deficiency has not yet been defined. C1r deficiency is almost invariably associated with C1s deficiency. Loos and Heinz have reviewed these patients[7]. Propositi of kindred with C1 deficiency of all types have had severe immune complex disease with lupus symptoms and prominent glomerulonephritis.

C4 DEFICIENCY

C4 is encoded by two genes, C4A and C4B, in the class III region of the major histocompatibility complex on the short arm of chromosome 6. The C4B gene is centromeric (towards HLA-DR) and the C4A gene is telomeric (towards HLA-B)[8]. It is important to note, in the light of their very different biological properties, that C4A and C4B differ by only four amino acid residues in the alpha chain between amino acid residues 1101 and 1106. At these positions, C4A is Pro-Cys-Pro-Val-Leu-Asp and C4B is Leu-Ser-Pro-Val-Ile-His. Despite these small differences, C4A is reactive with amino groups and C4B with hydroxyl side chains. Conversion of the Asp residue at position 1106 to His by site-directed mutagenesis converts C4A functionally into a C4B-like molecule[9]. The presence of two functional C4 alleles is peculiar to humans.

C4A and C4B are highly polymorphic. Although there are six common types of C4A and three common types of C4B, overall as many as 35 different C4 alleles have been discovered. Indeed, C4 is the most polymorphic of all the complement proteins and these variations have been useful markers in immunogenetics[10]. In addition, there may or may not be an extra 6.5 kb intron in the C4B gene giving rise to the so-called 'C4B-long' gene and the 'C4B-short' gene[11]. 1.5 kb 3′ to each C4 gene lies a gene for P-450 21-hydroxylase. In humans, the gene 3′ to C4A is a pseudogene and is not transcribed. Deletion of the gene 3′ to C4B results in congenital adrenal hyperplasia[12].

There is extraordinarily high frequency of C4 null alleles in the population so that approximately 35% of individuals of all races do not express a C4A or C4B gene[13]. Approximately 8–10% do not express two of the four alleles and just under 1% do not express three alleles. Despite this striking non-expression of C4 alleles in the population at large, complete C4 deficiency is very rare. The failure of C4B expression (C4BQO) almost always results from mutations that cause the C4B gene to transcribe a molecule with the properties of C4A. On the other hand, absence of C4A (C4AQO) results from gene deletions, premature stop codons and other mutations that result in the failure of gene transcription[14]. The deletions that have been observed are never long enough to include both the C4A and C4B genes. They are about 28 kb in length (C4A and C4B span a length of 55 kb) and variously include C4A and 21-hydroxylase A, 21-hydroxylase A and C4B, or C4B and 21-hydroxylase B. Thus, the homozygous C4AQO, C4BQO state, resulting in complete C4 deficiency, is very rare[15].

Almost all patients with complete C4 deficiency have systemic or discoid lupus with or without associated glomerulonephritis. The deficiency is frequently fatal from immune complex disease or overwhelming infection[13]. Hauptmann *et al.* reported that, of 12 C4-deficient individuals, 7 were ANA positive and 5 were positive for anti-SSA (Ro) but none had anti-SSB (La).

A female child with lupus and complete C4 deficiency was found to have isodisomy of the short arm of chromosome 6; she was homozygous at the major histocompatibility locus because she had inherited two identical chromosome 6 short arms from her father. The inherited MHC haplotype was HLA-A28, -Cw3, -B40, factor B slow, C4AQO, C4BQO, HLA-DR6. Thus, she was completely C4 deficient although her father was not; his other chromosome 6 expressed C4A and C4B genes[16].

Patients with systemic and discoid lupus erythematosus have a very high incidence of C4AQO on one or both chromosomes, the latter being C4AQO homozygotes[17]. Furthermore, this defect has been found to be striking in SLE patients of all races[18]. On the other hand, C4BQO has been associated with IgA nephropathy[19]. As C4B is the isotype that binds preferentially to carbohydrate antigens, it is perhaps not surprising that there may be a greater than 3.5-fold increase in bacterial meningitis in children who have a C4BQO allele[20].

The class I and class II genes of the major histocompatibility complex are frequently in linkage disequilibrium. C4 null genes are present in at least four common extended haplotypes or supratypes of the MHC. The most common of these, found on 8% of human chromosomes, is HLA-B8, HLA-DR3, the common form of C2 (C2C), the slow form of factor B (BfS), C4AQO, C4B1. This haplotype is associated with several autoimmune diseases, such as gluten-sensitive enteropathy, insulin-dependent diabetes mellitus, dermatitis herpetiformis, as well as with IgA deficiency and common variable immunodeficiency (or acquired a-gamma-globulinaemia). The reasons for these associations are not yet clear. Common variable immunodeficiency has been mapped to a region close to the C4 genes[21].

C2 DEFICIENCY

Unlike C4, C2 exhibits very little genetically determined polymorphism and complete C2 deficiency (C2QO) is relatively common in the Caucasian population. The gene encoding C2 is located in the major histocompatibility complex, telomeric to the genes encoding C4 and factor B[8]. C2 mRNA codes for three distinct polypeptides of Mr 84 kDa, 79 kDa and 70 kDa; only the largest of these is secreted while the other two smaller products remain cell associated[22]. Despite the fact that the C2 protein exhibits very little polymorphism and 96% of the human genome bears the common form of C2 (C2C), there is multiallelic polymorphism in genomic C2[23]. For example, digestion with Sst I gives rise to fragments of 2.4, 2.55, 2.65, 2.7 and 2.75 kb with a 300-base-pair probe for the 5′ end of the C2 genome. All these DNA alleles, with one exception, are associated with C2C. The 2.75 kb allele is associated with the basic form of C2 (C2B) and C2QO. This suggests that C2QO mutated from C2B[24].

C2QO is almost invariably in linkage disequilibrium with slow factor B (BfS), C4A4 and C4B2[25]. In cell cultures from such individuals, no net C2 synthesis can be detected although the C2 mRNA content is normal. There is consistently a 28 base-pair deletion at the 3′ end of exon 6 so that faulty splicing leads to a loss of exon 6, thereby generating a frame shift and stop codon 14 base pairs distal to the end of exon 5 (Johnson and Colten, unpublished observations). In rare cases of C2 deficiency not associated with the usual haplotype (approximately 7% of affected kindred), intracellular C2 synthesis is normal but the C2 is not secreted for unknown reasons (Johnson and Colten, unpublished observations).

Homozygous C2 deficiency was first discovered serendipitously by immunologists who attempted to use their own sera as a source of haemolytic complement[26,27]. One in 100 Caucasians bears the C2QO gene so that 1 in 10 000 is completely C2 deficient. Probably close to half these individuals are perfectly healthy. The others present with lupus-like disease and/or severe bacterial infections, polymyositis, Henoch–Schonlein purpura and other forms of vasculitis. Heterozygous C2 deficiency is present with increased frequency in patients with systemic lupus erythematosus and juvenile rheumatoid arthritis[28].

C3 DEFICIENCY

C3 has a well-defined polymorphism and two common alleles are recognized; they are designated S and F for slow or fast electrophoretic mobility. Several rare variants are also known. On the basis of the ability to detect this polymorphism, C3 deficiency was first found in heterozygotes who had informative inheritance of a null allele[29]. These findings predicted the existence of complete C3 deficiency. Then a hypomorphic variant of C3F was discovered[30]. Complete C3 deficiency was found in an Afrikaaner female who had recurrent pyogenic infection and an immune complex disease of the skin, which resembled Sweet's disease in that the subcutis had sheets of polymorphonuclear leukocytes[31,32]. Subsequently several other kindred have been discovered with complete C3 deficiency in many parts of the world[33–42]. As expected from the biological function of C3, almost all these individuals have recurrent pyogenic infections and some element of immune complex disease, particularly membranoproliferative glomerulonephritis.

C3 deficiency patients have very little or no detectable C3[36]. Although many cell types in culture synthesize C3, *in vivo* C3 appears to be made primarily by hepatocytes[43]. Botto *et al.* found a 61-base-pair deletion in one kindred. This deletion in exon 18 resulted from a faulty 5′ donor splice site in intron 18 that caused a premature stop codon 17 base pairs 3′ to the deletion[44]. These same investigators in studying two further kindred found a 700-base-pair deletion which encompassed exons 22 and 23 and a stop codon 19 base pairs 3′ to the deletion[45]. In surveying an Afrikaaner population, two further propositi were found with the same genetic defect as was found in the original Afrikaaner girl and this strongly suggests a founder effect in the Afrikaaner population where the gene defect has a high incidence[46,47].

DEFICIENCIES OF FACTOR H AND FACTOR I

In 1970, a patient was described who had a history resembling that of a male with X-linked a-gamma-globulinaemia; he had recurrent pyogenic infections. In addition to this, he had recurrent hives following alcohol ingestion or exposure to very hot or cold water[48]. He was found to have decreased amounts of C3 in the circulation, mostly in the form of C3b and absent factor B activity[49]. These defects were found to be due to factor I deficiency[50]. Indeed, the function of factor I was established by studying this patient[51] and infusion of pure factor I corrected all his complement abnormalities[52]. Several further kindred with factor I deficiency were found[53–55]. Although the gene encoding factor I has been cloned and mapped to chromosome 4[56], the molecular basis of factor I deficiency has not yet been ascertained at the DNA level. However, a restriction fragment length polymorphism has been linked to the deficiency in at least four more kindred with factor I deficiency[57].

Factor H deficiency results, not unexpectedly, in the same abnormalities as factor I deficiency, but is a much rarer abnormality[58,59]. It is interesting that the factor H-like activity of CR1 fails to control the positive feedback activation of the alternative pathway in factor H deficiency. The gene encoding factor H is close to the RCA (regulator of complement activity) locus on the short arm of chromosome 1; the molecular basis of factor H deficiency is not known.

PROPERDIN DEFICIENCY

The genetically determined deficiency of properdin is X-linked and this has resulted in mapping the properdin gene[60] to Xp11.23–21.1. Males affected with properdin deficiency have recurrent bacterial infection, particularly with *Neisseria*[61,62]. Since a dysfunctional protein has been found in some patients with this deficiency, a point mutation in the gene may be responsible.

FACTOR D DEFICIENCY

The genetics of factor D deficiency are not clear. As only males have been affected in the few reported cases[63,64], the disorder could be either X-linked or autosomal recessive. The location of the factor D gene has not yet been ascertained. Affected patients appear to have a predisposition to severe *Neisseria* infections.

DEFICIENCIES OF THE TERMINAL COMPLEMENT COMPONENTS

Common to all patients with terminal component deficiencies has been their extraordinary susceptibility to overwhelming infection with *Neisseria meningitidis* and *Neisseria gonorrhoeae*[65]. Surveys in Israel and the Netherlands have shown that there is a high incidence of terminal component deficiencies in older patients (>10 years of age) with meningococcal infections[66,67]. In Israel, 18 of 212 cases of *Neisseria meningitidis* had terminal complement deficiencies and 7 of 43 cases surveyed in the United States had similar findings whereas the incidence of terminal complement deficiencies in similar surveys in Spain and Denmark have shown no cases[68]. Uncommon serotypes of *N. meningitidis* have been cultured from these patients with terminal complement deficiencies[68]. It has been suggested that individuals with terminal complement deficiencies be vaccinated against *N. meningitidis*. Some success has been observed in this regard. Prophylactic antibiotics (particularly penicillin) have been also used in such patients. In rare instances, repeated plasma infusions have been undertaken. Although autoimmune disease is found frequently in patients with classical pathway defects, these diseases have also been seen rarely in patients with terminal complement deficiencies[69–77]. Systemic and discoid lupus have been most frequently encountered but Sjogren's syndrome, glomerulonephritis, Raynaud's phenomenon, rheumatoid arthritis and scleroderma have all been reported in cases of terminal complement deficiencies. There is no evidence that heterozygous relatives of propositi with terminal component deficiencies are at increased risk for autoimmune disease or recurrent *Neisseria* infection.

C5 deficiency is very rare. However, C6 deficiency appears to have a high frequency in the Cape coloureds of South Africa[78]. Lachmann has speculated that there might be a heterozygous advantage to having this deficiency in that it might protect against death from endotoxaemia in infantile gastroenteritis[79]. This suggestion is supported by the difficulty in inducing endotoxaemic shock in C6-deficient rabbits. It has also been suggested that meningococcal infections have a better outcome in those with terminal complement deficiencies.

The genes encoding C6 and C7 are linked on chromosome 5 and no crossover has been found between these two genes[80]. This probably explains the observation of combined C6 and C7 deficiency that has been observed in a few kindred[81–83]. In these cases, the affected are asymptomatic, probably because their serum contains up to 25% of the normal amount of these components. The gene for C9 also maps to the short arm of chromosome 5 and appears linked to the genes for C6 and C7. A physical map of this gene cluster is being made[84].

These authors suggest that the C8α and β genes form one cluster to be called MACI and the C6, 7 and 9 genes another to be designated MACII.

Unlike C5, C6, C7 and C9, which are composed of single polypeptide chains, C8 is a heterotrimer encoded by three separate genes. The genes encoding the alpha and beta chains are linked on the short arm of chromosome 1 whereas the gene encoding the gamma chain is on chromosome 9[85]. The α- and γ-chains are covalently associated after synthesis and the rate of synthesis is more rapid than that of the beta chain, which is not covalently associated with the other chains. This complexity of C8 assembly gives rise to at least three types of genetic deficiency of C8. Deficiency of C8α/γ is found most often in populations of African origin whereas C8β deficiency is more common in Caucasians[86]. When sera from both types of deficients are mixed, C8 functional activity is reconstituted[87]. The third type of C8 deficiency that has been described results from a dysfunctional C8β chain[88]. A recent study has suggested a pretranslational defect in the common form of C8β deficiency where markedly lower C8β mRNA was detected[89].

C9 deficiency has a very high frequency in the Japanese (about 4–10 cases per 10 000[90–92]) but is very rare in Caucasoids[93]. Contrary to previous opinion, patients are susceptible to Neisserial infection[94].

DEFICIENCY OF DECAY ACCELERATING FACTOR (DAF) AND HOMOLOGOUS RESTRICTION FACTOR (CD59)

Recently a 22-year-old Japanese man was described who had a genetically determined deficiency of the homologous restriction factor (CD59). Starting at the age of 13 years, he had recurrent episodes of paroxysmal nocturnal haemoglobulinuria (PNH)[95]. His parents were both heterozygous for the defect, thus demonstrating autosomal recessive inheritance of the defect. It is of great interest that DAF deficiency has been described in two kindred[96,97]. The propositi did not have PNH, thus demonstrating the relative importance of CD59 as opposed to DAF among the proteins that are phosphatidyl inositol linked to the membrane in the pathogenesis of PNH. In one of these kindred, a stop codon has been found[98] in the DAF gene at codon 53.

LEUKOCYTE ADHESION DEFICIENCY (LAD)

Leukocyte adhesion deficiency must be considered among the complement deficiencies because, among other things, it involves a deficiency of the third complement receptor (CR3, CD11b/CD18). LAD results from a genetic defect in the β-chain (CD18) of the β_2 integrin family proteins. Three members of this integrin group have been defined: CR3, LFA-1 and p150,95. All three share a common β-chain whose gene is encoded on chromosome 21. Each of these membrane proteins has a distinct α-chain (CD11a, 11b, 11c) and the group of α-chains is encoded by genes on the short arm of chromosome 16. There are severe phenotypes of LAD where no CD18 can be detected on leukocytes and a mild phenotype in which there is approximately 10% of normal CD18 expression. There is also a difference in clinical severity between the *mild* and *severe* phenotypes.

Children with LAD cannot ingest opsonized organisms via C3bi-CR3 mechanisms. Thus, they are susceptible to recurrent pyogenic infections. Ordinarily, they have a striking leukocytosis because the leukocytes cannot adhere to endothelium and emigrate from blood vessels. Because of this, wound healing is poor and fistulae develop, particularly in the intestinal tract. Delayed separation of the umbilical cord has been noted in affected infants. Fischer *et al.* have reviewed current knowledge about LAD[99]. One of the most striking clinical findings in LAD is severe gingivitis. Successful bone marrow transplantation has been carried out in several patients with LAD.

Kishimoto *et al.* have identified the genetic basis of the CD18 abnormality in several kindred[100]. In summary, undetectable mRNA, decreased levels of mRNA, large precursor mRNA, aberrantly small precursor mRNA and mRNA that cannot undergo post-translational modification have all been found. Splicing errors have also been found by Wright and Law[101]. See Chapter 9 for a full review of CR3 and leukocyte adhesion molecules.

CONCLUSIONS

The first phase of describing the phenotypes of complement deficiencies during the past twenty years has now largely been completed. Extensive polymorphisms of the complement components are well known and this has facilitated the elaboration of the genetics of many of the deficiencies.

Current work is directed towards an understanding of the molecular biology of these defects and several precise examples of these efforts are given in this chapter. More results of this kind should be forthcoming in the near future and will help to clarify the biological functions of the complement system. The study of the complement defects has been heuristic and has provided many unanticipated insights into the functions of complement.

References

1. Colten, H. R. and Rosen, F. S. (1992). Complement deficiencies. *Ann. Rev. Immunol.*, **10**, 809–34
2. Sellar, G. C., Blake, D. J. and Reid, K. B. M. (1991). Characterization and organization of the genes encoding the A-, B- and C-chains of human complement subcomponent C1q. *Biochem. J.*, **272**, 481–90
3. Tosi, M., Duponchel, C., Meo, T. and Julier, C. (1987). Complement C1s sequence and linkage to C1r. *Biochemistry*, **26**, 8516–24
4. Kusumoto, H., Hirosawa, S., Salier, J. P., Hagen, F. S. and Kurachi, K. (1988). Human genes for complement components C1r and C1s in a close tail-to-tail arrangement. *Proc. Natl. Acad. Sci. USA*, **85**, 7307–11
5. Reid, K. B. M. (1988). Deficiency of the first component of human complement. *Immunodefic. Rev.*, **1**, 247–60
6. Reid, K. B. M. and Thompson, R. A. (1983). Characterization of a non-functional form of C1q found in patients with a genetically linked deficiency of C1q activity. *Molec. Immunol.*, **20**, 1117–25

7. Loos, M. and Heinz, H. (1986). Component deficiencies. 1. The first component: C1q, C1r, C1s. *Prog. Allergy*, **39**, 212–31
8. Carroll, M. C., Klatzman, P., Alicot, E. M., Koller, B. H., Geraghty, D. E., Orr, H. T., Strominger, J. L. and Spies, T. (1987). Linkage map of the human major histocompatibility complex including the tumour necrosis factor genes. *Proc. Natl. Acad. Sci. USA*, **84**, 8535–9
9. Carroll, M. C., Fathallah, D. M., Bergamaschini, L., Alicot, E. M. and Isenman, D. E. (1990). Substitution of a single amino acid (aspartic acid for histidine) converts the functional activity of C4B to C4A. *Proc. Natl. Acad. Sci. USA*, **87**, 6868–72
10. Marcus, D. and Alper, C. A. (1986). Methods for allotyping complement proteins. In Rose, N. R., Friedman, H. and Fahey, J. L. (eds.) *Manual of Clinical Laboratory Immunology*, 3rd Edn., pp. 185–96. (Washington: American Society for Microbiology)
11. Palsdottir, A., Fossdal, R., Arnason, A., Edwards, J. H. and Jensson, O. (1987). Heterogeneity of human C4 gene size. *Immunogenetics*, **25**, 299–304
12. Schneider, P. M., Carroll, M. C., Alper, C. A., Rittner, C., Whitehead, A. S., Yunis, E. J. and Colten, H. R. (1986). Polymorphism of the human complement C4 and steroid 21-hydroxylase genes. Restriction fragment length polymorphisms revealing structural deletions, homoduplications and size variants. *J. Clin. Invest.*, **78**, 650–7
13. Hauptmann, G., Tappeiner, G. and Schifferli, J. A. (1988). Inherited deficiency of the fourth component of human complement. *Immunodefic. Rev.*, **1**, 3–22
14. Braun, L., Schneider, P. M., Giles, C. M., Bertrams, J. and Rittner, C. (1990). Null alleles of human complement C4. Evidence for pseudogenes at the C4A locus and gene conversion at the C4B locus. *J. Exp. Med.*, **171**, 129–40
15. Hauptmann, G., Uring-Lambert, B., Vegnaduzzi-Lamouche, N. and Lascart-Lemone, F. (1987). RFLP studies of three complete C4 deficient patients. *Complement*, **4**, 166
16. Welch, T. R., Beischel, L. S., Choi, E., Balakrishnan, K. and Bishof, N. A. (1990). Uniparental isodisomy 6 associated with deficiency of the fourth component of complement. *J. Clin. Invest.*, **86**, 675–8
17. Fielder, A. H. L., Walport, M. J., Batchelor, H. R., Rynes, R. I. and Black, C. M. (1983). Family study of the major histocompatibility complex in patients with systemic lupus erythematosus: Importance of null alleles of C4A and C4B in determining disease susceptibility. *Br. Med. J.*, **286**, 425–8
18. Dunckley, H., Gatenby, P. A., Hawkins, B., Naito, S. and Serjeantson, S. W. (1987). Deficiency of C4A is a genetic determinant of systemic lupus erythematosus in three ethnic groups. *J. Immunogenet.*, **14**, 209–18
19. Welch, T. R., Beischel, L. S. and Choi, E. M. (1989). Molecular genetics of C4B deficiency in IgA nephropathy. *Hum. Immunol.*, **26**, 353–63
20. Rowe, P. C., McLean, R. H., Wood, R. A., Leggiardo, R. J. and Winkelstein, J. A. (1989). Association of homozygous C4B deficiency with bacterial meningitis. *J. Infect. Dis.*, **160**, 448–51
21. Matsumoto, S., Sakiyama, Y., Ariga, T., Gallagher, R. and Taguchi, Y. (1992). Progress in primary immunodeficiency. *Immunol. Today*, **13**, 4–5
22. Perlmutter, D. H., Cole, F. S., Goldberger, G. and Colten, H. R. (1984). Distinct primary translation products of human liver mRNA give rise to secreted and cell associated form of complement C2. *J. Biol. Chem.*, **259**, 10380–5
23. Cross, S. J., Edwards, J. M., Bentley, D. R. and Campbell, R. D. (1985). DNA polymorphism of the C2 and factor B genes. Detection of a restriction fragment length polymorphism which subdivides haplotypes carrying the C2C and factor BF alleles. *Immunogenetics*, **21**, 39–48
24. Simon, S., Awdeh, Z., Campbell, R. D., Ronco, P., Brink, S. J., Eisenbarth, G. S., Yunis, E. J. and Alper, C. A. (1991). A restriction fragment of the C2 gene is a unique marker for C2 deficiency and the uncommon C2 allele $C2^{*}B$ (a marker for type 1 diabetes). *J. Clin. Invest.*, **88**, 2142–5
25. Awdeh, Z. L., Raum, D. D., Glass, D., Agnello, V., Schur, P. H., Johnston, R. B. Jr., Gelfand, E. W., Ballow, M., Yunis, E. and Alper, C. A. (1981). Complement – human histocompatibility antigen haplotypes in C2 deficiency. *J. Clin. Invest.*, **67**, 581–3
26. Klemperer, M. R., Woodworth, H. C., Rosen, F. S. and Austen, K. F. (1966). Hereditary deficiency of the second component of complement in man. *J. Clin. Invest.*, **45**, 880–90
27. Klemperer, M. R., Austen, K. F. and Rosen, F. S. (1967). Hereditary deficiency of the second component of complement (C′2) in man: Further observations on a second kindred. *J. Immunol.*, **98**, 72–8

28. Perlmutter, D. H. and Colten, H. R. (1989). Molecular basis of complement deficiencies. *Immunodefic. Rev.*, **1**, 105–33
29. Alper, C. A., Propp, R. P., Klemperer, M. R. and Rosen, F. S. (1969). Inherited deficiency of the third component of human complement (C'3). *J. Clin. Invest.*, **48**, 553–7
30. Alper, C. A. and Rosen, F. S. (1971). Studies of a hypomorphic variant of human C3. *J. Clin. Invest.*, **50**, 324–6
31. Alper, C. A., Colten, H. R., Rosen, F. S., Rabson, A. R., Macnab, G. M. and Gear, J. S. S. (1972). Homozygous deficiency of C3 in a patient with repeated infections. *Lancet*, **2**, 1179–81
32. Alper, C. A., Colten, H. R., Gear, J. S. S., Rabson, A. R. and Rosen, F. S. (1976). Homozygous human C3 deficiency: The role of C3 in antibody production, C1s-induced vasopermeability, and cobra venom-induced passive hemolysis. *J. Clin. Invest.*, **57**, 222–9
33. Ballow, M., Shira, J. E., Harden, L., Yang, S. Y. and Day, N. K. (1975). Complete absence of the third component of complement in man. *J. Clin. Invest.*, **56**, 703–10
34. Grace, H. J., Brereton-Stiles, G. S., Vos, G. H. and Schonland, M. (1976). A family with partial and total deficiency of complement C3. *S. African Med. J.*, **50**, 139–40
35. Osofsky, S. G., Thompson, B. H., Lint, T. F. and Gewurz, H. (1977). Hereditary deficiency of the third component of complement in a child with fever, skin rash, and arthralgias: response to transfusion of whole blood. *J. Pediatr.*, **90**, 180–6
36. Davis III, A. E., Davis IV, J. S., Rabson, A. R., Osofsky, S. G., Colten, H. R., Rosen, F. S. and Alper, C. A. (1977). Homozygous C3 deficiency. Detection of C3 by radioimmunoassay. *Clin. Immunol. Immunopathol.*, **8**, 543–50
37. Pussell, B. A., Bourke, E., Nayef, M., Morris, S. and Peters, D. K. (1980). Complement deficiency and nephritis. *Lancet*, **1**, 675–7
38. Sano, Y., Nishimukai, H., Kitamura, H., Nagaki, K., Inai, S., Hamasaki, Y., Maruyama, I. and Igata, A. (1981). Hereditary deficiency of the third component in two sisters with systemic lupus erythematosus-like symptoms. *Arthritis Rheum.*, **24**, 1255–60
39. Hsieh, K. H., Lin, C. Y. and Lee, T. C. (1981). Complete absence of the third component of complement in a patient with repeated infections. *Clin. Immunol. Immunopathol.*, **20**, 305–12
40. Roord, J. J., Daha, M., Kuis, W., Verbrugh, H. A., Verhoef, J., Zegers, B. J. M. and Stoop, J. W. (1983). Inherited deficiency of the third component of complement associated with recurrent pyogenic infections, circulating immune complexes, and vasculitis in a Dutch family. *Pediatrics*, **71**, 81–7
41. Berger, M., Balow, J. E., Wilson, C. B. and Frank, M. M. (1983). Circulating immune complexes and glomerulonephritis in a patient with congenital absence of the third component of complement. *N. Engl. J. Med.*, **308**, 1009–12
42. Grumach, A. S., Vilela, M. M. S., Gonzalez, C. H., Starobinas, N., Pereira, A. B., Dias-da-Silva, W. and Carneiro-Sampaio, M. M. S. (1988). Inherited C3 deficiency of the complement system. *Brazilian J. Med. Biol. Res.*, **21**, 247–57
43. Alper, C. A., Johnson, A. M., Birtch, A. G. and Moore, R. D. (1969). Human C3: Evidence for the liver as the primary site of synthesis. *Science*, **163**, 286–8
44. Botto, M., Fong, K. Y., So, A. K., Rudge, A. and Walport, M. J. (1990). Molecular basis of hereditary C3 deficiency. *J. Clin. Invest.*, **86**, 11581–663
45. Botto, M., So, A. K., Fong, K. Y., Barlow, R., Routier, R., Morley, B. J. and Walport, M. J. (1991). Homozygous hereditary C3 deficiency due to a partial gene deletion. Presented at the *XIV International Complement Workshop*, September 15–20, Cambridge, England
46. Botto, M., Fong, K. Y., So, A. K., Rudge, A. and Walport, M. J. (1990). Molecular basis of hereditary C3 deficiency. *J. Clin. Invest.*, **86**, 1158–63
47. Walport, M. J. (1992). Personal communication
48. Alper, C. A., Abramson, N., Johnston, R. B. Jr., Jandl, J. H. and Rosen, F. S. (1970). Increased susceptibility to infection associated with abnormalities of complement-mediated functions and of the third component of complement (C3). *N. Engl. J. Med.*, **282**, 231–6
49. Alper, C. A., Abramson, N., Johnston, R. B. Jr., Jandl, J. H. and Rosen, F. S. (1970). Studies in vivo and in vitro on an abnormality in the metabolism of C3 in a patient with increased susceptibility to infection. *J. Clin. Invest.*, **49**, 1975–85
50. Abramson, N., Alper, C. A., Lachmann, P. J., Rosen, F. S. and Jandl, J. H. (1971). Deficiency of C3 inactivator in man. *J. Immunol.*, **107**, 19–27

51. Alper, C. A., Rosen, F. S. and Lachmann, P. J. (1972). Inactivator of the third component of complement as an inhibitor in the properdin pathway. *Proc. Natl. Acad. Sci.*, **69**, 2910–13
52. Ziegler, J. B., Alper, C. A., Rosen, F. S., Lachmann, P. J. and Sherington, L. (1975). Restoration by purified C3b inactivator of complement-mediated function in vivo in a patient with C3b inactivator deficiency. *J. Clin. Invest.*, **55**, 668–72
53. Thompson, R. A. and Lachmann, P. J. (1977). A second case of human C3b inhibitor (KAF) deficiency. *Clin. Exp. Immunol.*, **27**, 23–9
54. Solal-Celigny, P., Laviolette, M., Herbert, J., Atkins, P. C., Sirois, M., Brun, G., Lehner-Netsch, G. and Delage, J. M. (1982). C3b inactivator deficiency with immune complex manifestations. *Clin. Exp. Immunol.*, **47**, 197–205
55. Teisner, B., Brandslund, I., Folkersen, J., Rasmussen, J. M., Poulsen, L. O. and Svehag, S. E. (1984). Factor I deficiency and C3 nephritic factor: Immunochemical findings and association with Neisseria meningitidis infection in two patients. *Scand. J. Immunol.*, **20**, 291–7
56. Goldberger, G., Bruns, G. A. P., Rits, M., Edge, M. D. and Kwiatkowski, D. J. (1987). Human complement factor I: Analysis of cDNA-derived primary structure and assignment of its gene to chromosome 4. *J. Biol. Chem.*, **262**, 10065–71
57. Kolble, K., Buckle, V., Lefranc, G., Halbwachs-Mecarelli, L., Moller-Rasmussen, J., Sim, R. B., Spath, P., Svehag, S. E., Teisner, B. and Wahn, V. (1989). Physical mapping of complement factor I gene in normal and deficient genomes. *Complement Inflamm.*, **6**, 355
58. Nielsen, H. E., Christensen, K. C., Koch, C., Thomsen, B. S., Heegard, N. H. H. and Tranum-Jensen, J. (1989). Hereditary, complete deficiency of complement factor H associated with recurrent meningococcal disease. *Scand. J. Immunol.*, **30**, 711–18
59. Levy, M., Halbwachs-Mecarelli, L., Gubler, M-C., Kohout, G., Bensenouci, A., Niaudet, P., Hauptmann, G. and Lesavre, P. (1986). H deficiency in two brothers with atypical dense intramembranous deposit disease. *Kidney Int.*, **30**, 949–56
60. Sjoholm, A. G., Kuijper, E. J., Tijssen, C. C., Jansz, A., Bol, P., Spanjaard, L. and Zanen, H. C. (1988). Dysfunctional properdin in a Dutch family with meningococcal disease. *N. Engl. J. Med.*, **319**, 33–7
61. Lambert, B. *et al.* (1989). Familial properdin deficiency associated with chronic discoid lupus erythematosus. *Clin. Exp. Immunol.*, **76**, 76–81
62. Gelfand, E. W., Rao, C. P., Minta, J. O. and Ham, T. (1987). Inherited deficiency of properdin and C2 in a patient with recurrent bacteremia. *Am. J. Med.*, **82**, 671–5
63. Hiemstra, P. S., Langeler, E., Compier, B., Keepers, Y., Leijh, P. C. J., van den Barselaar, M. Th., Overbosch, D. and Daha, M. R. (1989). Complete and partial deficiencies of complement factor D in a Dutch family. *J. Clin. Invest.*, **84**, 1957–61
64. Kluin-Nelemans, H. C., van Velzen-Blad, H., van Helden, H. P. and Daha, M. R. (1984). Functional deficiency of complement factor D in a monozygous twin. *Clin. Exp. Immunol.*, **58**, 724–30
65. Ross, S. C. and Densen, P. (1984). Complement deficiency status and infection: epidemiology, pathogenesis and consequences of Neisserial and other infections in an immune deficiency. *Medicine*, **63**, 243–73
66. Swart, A. G., Fijen, C. A. P., Kuijper, E. J., Daha, M. R. and Dankert, J. (1991). Complement deficiencies in infections with Neisseria meningitidis. Presented at the *XIV International Complement Workshop*, September 15–20, Cambridge, England
67. Schlesinger, M., Nave, Z., Levy, Y., Slater, P. E. and Fishelson, Z. (1990). Prevalence of hereditary properdin, C7 and C8 deficiencies in patients with meningococcal infections. *Clin. Exp. Immunol.*, **81**, 423–7
68. Wurzner, R., Orren, A. and Lachmann, P. J. (1992). Inherited deficiencies of the terminal components of human complement. *Immunodefic. Rev.*, **3**, 123–47
69. Pickering, R. J., Rynes, R. I., LoCascio, N., Monahan, J. B. and Sodetz, J. M. (1982). Identification of the α-γ subunit of the eighth component of complement (C8) in a patient with systemic lupus erythematosus and absence of C8 activity: patient and family studies. *Clin. Immunol. Immunopathol.*, **23**, 323–34
70. Rosenfeld, S. I., Kelly, M. E. and Leddy, J. P. (1976). Hereditary deficiency of the fifth component of complement in man. I. Clinical, immunochemical, and family studies. *J. Clin. Invest.*, **57**, 1626–34

71. Asghar, S. S., Venneker, G. T., van-Meegen, M., Meinardi, M. M., Hulsmans, R. F. and de-Waal, L. P. (1991). Hereditary deficiency of C5 in association with discoid lupus erythematosus. *J. Am. Acad. Dermatol.*, **24**, 376–8
72. Trapp, R. G., Mooney, E., Coleman, T. H., Forristal, J. and Herman, J. H. (1987). Hereditary complement (C6) deficiency associated with systemic lupus erythematosus, Sjogren's syndrome and hyperthyroidism. *J. Rheumatol.*, **14**, 1030–3
73. Zeitz, H. J., Miller, G. W., Lint, T. F., Ali, M. A. and Gewurz, H. (1981). Deficiency of C7 with systemic lupus erythematosus. Solubilization of immune complexes in a complement deficient serum. *Arthritis Rheum.*, **24**, 87–93
74. Kojima, K., Sasaki, A., Yokomatsu, Y., Hiyoshi, M., Tatsumi, N., Okuda, K., Niwa, M., Kitamura, H. and Nagaki, K. (1985). Deficiency of the seventh component of complement with systemic lupus erythematosus. *Osaka City Med. J.*, **31**, 121–8
75. Jasin, H. E. (1977). Absence of the eighth component of complement in association with systemic lupus erythematosus-like disease. *J. Clin. Invest.*, **60**, 709–15
76. Sugimoto, M., Nishikai, M., Sato, A., Suzuki, Y., Nihei, M., Uchida, J. and Mimura, N. (1987). SLE-like and sicca symptoms in late component (C9) complement deficiency. *Ann. Rheum. Dis.*, **46**, 153–5
77. Kawai, T., Katoh, K., Narita, M., Tani, K. and Okubo, T. (1989). Deficiency of the 9th component of complement (C9) in a patient with systemic lupus erythematosus. *J. Rheumatol.*, **16**, 542–3
78. Orren, A., Potter, P. C., Cooper, R. C. and duToit, E. (1987). Deficiency of the sixth component of complement and susceptibility to Neisseria meningitidis infections: Studies in 10 families and five isolated cases. *Immunology*, **62**, 249–53
79. Lachmann, P. J. (1992). Complement deficiencies. In Lachmann, P. J., Peters, D. K., Rosen, F. S. and Walport, M. J. (eds.) *Clinical Aspects of Immunology*, 5th Edn. (Oxford: Blackwell Scientific) (In press)
80. Tokunaga, K. G., Dewald, G., Omoto, K. and Juji, T. (1986). Family study of the polymorphisms of the sixth and seventh components of human complement: linkage and haplotype analysis. *Am. J. Hum. Genet.*, **39**, 414–19
81. Lachmann, P. J., Hobart, M. J. and Woo, P. (1978). Combined genetic deficiency of C6 and C7 in man. *Clin. Exp. Immunol.*, **33**, 193–203
82. Morgan, B. P., Vora, J. P., Bennett, A. J., Thomas, J. P. and Mathews, N. (1989). A case of hereditary combined deficiency of complement components C6 and C7 in man. *Clin. Exp. Immunol.*, **75**, 396–401
83. Wurzner, R., Orren, A., Potter, P., Morgan, B. P., Ponard, D., Spath, P., Brai, M., Schulze, M., Happe, L. and Gotze, O. (1991). Functionally active complement proteins C6 and C7 detected in C6- and C7-deficient individuals. *Clin. Exp. Immunol.*, **83**, 430–7
84. Coto, E., Martinez-Naves, E., Dominguez, O., DiScipio, R. G., *et al.* (1991). DNA polymorphisms and linkage relationship of the human complement component C6, C7 and C9 genes. *Immunogenetics*, **33**, 184–7
85. Howard, O. M. Z., Rao, A. G. and Sodetz, J. M. (1987). Complementary DNA and derived amino acid sequence of the β subunit of human complement protein C8: Identification of a close structural and ancestral relationship to the α subunit and C9. *Biochemistry*, **26**, 3565–70
86. Tedesco, F. (1986). Component deficiencies. The eighth component. *Prog. Allergy*, **39**, 295–306
87. Tedesco, F., Densen, P., Villa, M. A., Petersen, B. H. and Sirchia, G. (1983). Two types of dysfunctional eighth component of complement (C8) molecules in C8 deficiency in man: Reconstitution of normal C8 from the mixture of the two abnormal C8 molecules. *J. Clin. Invest.*, **71**, 183–91
88. Tschopp, J., Penea, F., Schifferli, J. and Spath, P. (1986). Dysfunctional C8 beta chain in patients with C8 deficiency. *Scand. J. Immunol.*, **24**, 715–20
89. Warnick, P. R. and Densen, P. (1991). Reduced messenger RNA expression in families with hereditary C8β deficiency. *J. Immunol.*, **146**, 1052–6
90. Yoshimura, K., Fukumori, Y., Ohnoki, S., O'Kubo, Y. and Yamaguchi, H. (1983). Studies on complement deficiencies in blood donors in Osaka area of Japan. *Jpn. J. Hum. Genet.*, **28**, 120
91. Fukumori, Y., Yoshimura, K., Ohnoki, S., Yamaguchi, H., Akagaki, Y. and Inai, S. (1989). A high incidence of C9 deficiency among healthy blood donors in Osaka, Japan. *Int. Immunol.*, **1**, 85–9

92. Hayama, K., Sugai, N., Tanaka, S., Lee, S., Kikuchi, H., *et al.* (1989). High incidence of C9 deficiency throughout Japan: there are no significant differences in incidence among eight areas of Japan. *Int. Arch. Allergy Appl. Immunol.*, **90**, 400–4
93. Lint, T. F. and Gewurz, H. (1986). Complement deficiencies. The ninth component. *Prog. Allergy*, **39**, 307–10
94. Nagata, M., Hara, T., Aoki, T., Mizuno, Y., Akeda, H., Inaba, S., Tsumoto, K. and Ueda, K. (1989). Inherited deficiency of ninth component of complement: an increased risk of meningococcal meningitis. *J. Pediatr.*, **114**, 260–4
95. Yamashina, M., Ueda, E., Kinoshita, T., Takami, T., Ojima, A., Ono, H., Tanaka, H., Kondo, N., Orii, T., Okada, N., Okada, H., Inoue, K. and Kitani, T. (1990). Inherited complete deficiency of 20-kilodalton homologous restriction factor (CD59) as a cause of paroxysmal nocturnal hemoglobinuria. *N. Engl. J. Med.*, **323**, 1184–9
96. Lin, R. C., Herman, J., Henry, L. and Daniels, G. L. (1988). A family showing inheritance of the Inab phenotype. *Transfusion*, **28**, 427–9
97. Telen, M. J., Hall, S. E., Green, A. M., Moulds, J. J. and Rosse, W. F. (1988). Identification of human erythrocyte blood group antigens on decay accelerating factor (DAF) and an erythrocyte phenotype negative for DAF. *J. Exp. Med.*, **167**, 1993–8
98. Mallinson, G., Tanner, M. J. A., Thompson, E. S., Telen, M. J. and Lublin, D. M. (1991). Sequence analysis of decay accelerating factor (DAF) cDNA and gene in original propositus of DAF-negative Inab phenotype. Presented at the *XIV International Complement Workshop*, September 15-20, Cambridge, England
99. Fischer, A., Lisowska-Grospierre, B., Anderson, D. C. and Springer, T. A. (1988). Leukocyte adhesion deficiency: Molecular basis and functional consequences. *Immunodefic. Rev.*, **1**, 39–54
100. Kishimoto, T. K., Hollander, N., Roberts, T. M., Anderson, D. C. and Springer, T. A. (1987). Heterogeneous mutations in the beta subunit common to the LFA-1, Mac-1 and p150.95 glycoproteins cause leukocyte adhesion deficiency. *Cell*, **50**, 193–202
101. Wright, A. H. and Law, S. K. A. (1991). The leukocyte adhesion deficiency in 5 patients. Presented at the *XIV International Complement Workshop*, September 15–20, Cambridge, England

6
Human complement deficiency states and infection

P. DENSEN

INTRODUCTION

Functional activity convincingly ascribed to the complement cascade was first described by Buchner when he demonstrated the presence of a heat labile serum factor that mediated direct bactericidal activity[1]. Subsequent studies by Bordet resolved this activity into heat-labile (complement) and heat-stable (antibody) components. Both Bordet and Erlich proposed models of serum-mediated immunity involving these components and elements of both theories have stood the test of time. At the turn of the century, studies by Wright and Douglas defined opsonization as an additional important complement-dependent activity. A significant portion of the research effort during the next half century was spent purifying the multiple complement components comprising the fluid-phase cascade and establishing the existence of two activation pathways. Despite these accomplishments, the status of the field in 1970 was such that Nobel laureate, Macfarlane Burnet, stated in his textbook *Cellular Immunology*[2] that 'since the classic studies of Bordet, Erlich and Wassermann, the concept of complement as an essential part of the mechanism of immunity has progressively been replaced by rather uncertain decision that the classic phenomenon of complement lysis of red cells is a laboratory artefact of no real significance for immunity'. This uncertain state of affairs began to resolve itself in the late 1960s with the recognition of both acquired and inherited complement deficiency states. Identification of these individuals permitted detailed comparisons of their response to the associated disease processes with that in normal individuals. These studies convincingly confirmed the previous experimental observations and have yielded fresh insights into the contribution of the complement cascade to normal pathological processes. Examples of this edification process include: delineation of C1-inhibitor (C1-inh) deficiency as the basis for hereditary angio-oedema[3];

recognition of a complement-dependent immunomodulatory effect through studies of C1-, C4-, C2- and C3-deficient individuals[4–8]; establishment of a critical role for complement-dependent bactericidal activity in host defence against meningococcal disease through the close association of this entity with deficiencies of the terminal complement components[9–11]; demonstration of the deficiency of phosphatidyl inositol-linked proteins, such as decay accelerating factor and CD59, as the basis for the clinical manifestations of paroxysmal nocturnal haemoglobinuria[12–14]; and the description of iC3b receptor deficiency (CR3 or CD11/CD18 deficiency) as the basis for leukocyte adhesion deficiency[15–17].

These and other observations have clearly demonstrated the beneficial effects of complement for host defence, modulation of immune responsiveness, initiation of an appropriate inflammatory response and solubilization of immune complexes. As a consequence of these effects, complement-deficient individuals experience a greater susceptibility to infection, exhibit impaired immune responses, manifest abnormal inflammatory processes and have a greater risk of developing certain autoimmune disorders. This chapter focuses on deficiencies of the fluid-phase complement components with the exception of C1-esterase inhibitor deficiency. The latter disorder and disorders of the membrane proteins of the complement system are covered elsewhere.

FREQUENCY OF HEREDITARY COMPLEMENT DEFICIENCY STATES

Disorders affecting the complement cascade constitute a minority (~2%) of the primary immunodeficiency states[18]. Despite this relative infrequency, numerous studies have addressed the prevalence of these disorders, perhaps in part because of the relatively large number of proteins involved in the overall cascade. Analysis of these studies reveals both biological and methodological variables that contribute to the reported frequency of these disorders (Table 6.1). The most important biological variables are the type of population being studied, its genetic composition and, in the case of a targeted population, the disease incidence. The most important methodological considerations are the sample size and the degree of ascertainment. An additional issue is that available studies are limited to countries which possess the financial resources and technology to permit this type of investigation. Consequently, these investigations reflect the ethnic bias of Western Europe, North America and Japan. With this caveat in mind, the overall frequency of inherited complement deficiency states is about 0.03% in Western Europe[19] and 0.11% in Japan[20,21].

Data on the prevalence of individual complement deficiency states are relatively limited, the most complete study being that of Inai *et al.*[21], who examined sera from 145 640 healthy blood donors in Osaka and found that the prevalence of homozygous C5 deficiency was 0.0014%, that of C6 deficiency 0.0027%, C7 deficiency 0.0041%, C8α-γ deficiency 0.0027% and C9 deficiency 0.095%. No individuals were detected with a deficiency of C8β, C3, any of the alternative pathway or early classical pathway components. The absence of these deficiencies probably reflects the genetic composition of the Japanese popu-

Table 6.1 Factors affecting the reported frequency of complement deficiency

Biological variables
- Population
  - Healthy
    - Genetic composition
  - Disease targeted
    - Disease incidence
    - Genetic composition
    - Ethnically determined environmental variables
- Age

Methodological variables
- Sample size
- Degree of ascertainment
- Mode of entry in the study
- Study design – retrospective vs. prospective
- Assay sensitivity

lation. However, the majority (>88%) of individuals with C1, C4, C2 and C3 deficiency present early in life (~2 years of age) with serious and frequently chronic or recurring disease (Table 6.2). These clinical features tend to preclude such patients as blood donors and underscore a limitation of blood-donor-based surveys, that is, that they are generally limited to healthy adults.

Table 6.2 Clinical patterns of disease in complement deficiency states

Clinical variable	*CP (C1, C4, C2)*	*AP (P, D)*	*C3 (C3, H, I)*	*LCCD (C5–C8, C9)*
Functional defect	↓ C′ act. ↓ IC metab. ↓ Imm. resp.	↓ C′ act.	↓ IC metab. ↓ Ops. phag. ↓ Imm. resp. ↓ PMN ↓ CTX ↓ SBA	(↓ CTX) ↓ SBA
Healthy (%)	12	26	0	29
CVD (%)	66	0	79	5
Systemic infection (%)	18	57	78	64†
Median age of first infection (y)	2	14	2	17
Organisms*	S. pn. N. mgc. H. inf.	N. mgc.	N. mgc. S. pn. H. inf.	N. mgc.
Infected patients with infection due to these organisms (%)	40	91	54	99
Recurrent infection with same organism (%)	6.3	3.5	56	50†

CP = classical pathway; AP = alternative pathway; LCCD = late complement component deficiency; IC metab. = immune complex metabolism; C′ act. = complement activation; Imm. resp. = immune response; Ops. phag. = opsonophagocytosis; CTX = chemotaxis; SBA = serum bactericidal activity; CVD = collagen vascular disease; S. pn. = *Streptococcus pneumoniae*; N. mgc. = *Neisseria meningitidis*; H. inf. = *Haemophilus influenzae*; and PMN = polymorphonuclear neutrophils.
*Listed in order of decreasing frequency; †Percentage differs for C9-deficient individuals; see Table 6.3; Adapted from Ref. 11

Unlike the findings in the Japanese population, homozygous C2 deficiency is the most common inherited complement defect affecting Caucasians, occurring in 0.0009% to 0.01% of normal individuals as determined by haplotype analysis or functional studies of normal blood donors, respectively.[22,23] Conversely, C9 deficiency is uncommon in Caucasian populations. Because two structural genes encode distinct but functionally active forms of C4, heterozygous deficiency at one C4 locus is very common, occurring in 15–25% of the Caucasian population.[24,25] Conversely, complete C4 deficiency is quite rare. Deficiencies of C5, C6 and C8α-γ appear to be more common in blacks.[10,11] These contrasting data emphasize the importance of genetic composition in determining the prevalence of the different complement deficiencies.

Since inherited complement deficiency states are uncommon in the general population, screening tests have their greatest utility in populations that display the clinical correlates of abnormal complement inheritance, that is, individuals with rheumatological diseases or recurrent bacterial infections or both. In one such study[26], a single individual with homozygous C2 deficiency and 19 individuals with definite, probable or heterozygous C2 deficiency were detected among 545 patients with rheumatological disorders, whereas only 6 possibly heterozygous C2-deficient individuals were detected among 509 unaffected persons. The frequency of homozygous (0.2%) and heterozygous (3.5%) C2 deficiency in this study is approximately 10 and 3-fold greater, respectively, than that in the general population. Thus, this study provides clear support for the association of complement deficiency states with certain rheumatological disorders, especially systemic lupus erythematosus. Such studies have led to the notion that autoimmune disorders, rather than infection, constitute the predominant clinical manifestations of C1, C4 and C2 deficiency states. However, a recent study of 675 individuals with infections caused by encapsulated bacteria[27] detected two unrelated homozygous C2-deficient individuals. This frequency, 0.3%, is similar to that, 0.2%, noted among individuals with rheumatological disorders. This finding suggests that individuals with a homozygous deficiency of one of the early classical pathway components experience a similar increase in risk for the development of either autoimmune disorders or infection and it underscores the bias inherent in prevalence studies conducted in diseased-based populations.

The recognition of an association between systemic meningococcal and gonococcal infections and an inherited deficiency of one of the terminal-complement components[9,10,28] has led to a number of studies examining the frequency of these defects among patients with these infections[28–40]. In a recent prospective study, we detected seven unrelated complement-deficient individuals among 675 individuals with meningitis or bacteraemia caused by encapsulated bacteria.[27] Six of these seven individuals experienced meningococcal disease whereas the seventh had pneumococcal bacteraemia. The prevalence of complement deficiency states among individuals with meningococcal disease (6 of 85 people, 7%) was significantly greater than that among individuals with pneumococcal or *H. influenzae* infection.

In other studies, the reported frequency of this association ranges between 0 and 50% among individuals presenting with a first episode of documented meningococcal disease. Analysis of these studies[11] reveals an inverse relationship between the prevalence of complement deficiency in persons with meningococcal disease and the incidence of the disease in the general population (Figure 6.1). This relationship suggests that the overall prevalence of complement deficiencies in the general population is relatively constant (0.03–0.11%, see above) but that among populations in which the level of immunity is low and meningococcal disease is epidemic, proportionally more normal than complement-deficient individuals will be infected because there are significantly more of the former than the latter. As the level of immunity in the population increases, the incidence of meningococcal disease falls. However, because the prevalence of complement deficiency in the general population is relatively stable, the frequency of these states among individuals with meningococcal disease increases, and complement deficiency becomes a greater determinant of the risk of infection. As a corollary, this relationship suggests that the determinants of natural immunity to meningococcal disease in the general population are insufficient to provide protection to the complement-deficient patient. This hypothesis has received additional support from other types of studies discussed later.

In summary, the overall frequency of complement deficiencies is relatively constant among different ethnic populations. The genetic composition of these populations is the major determinant of the prevalence of specific complement deficiency states. In contrast, in disease-defined populations, it is the incidence of the targeted disease in the general population that is the main determinant of the frequency of these disorders.

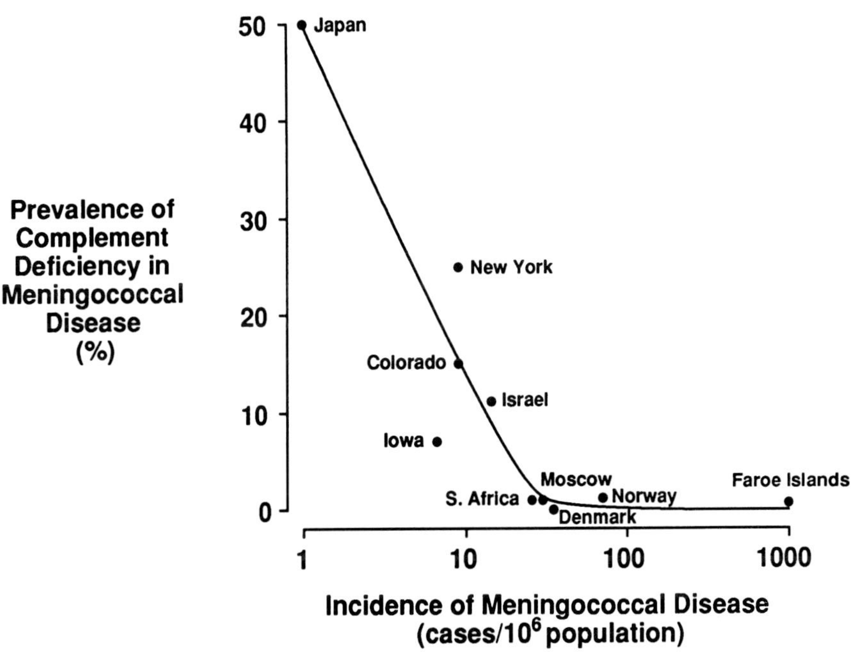

Figure 6.1 Relationship between the prevalence of complement deficiency and the incidence of meningococcal disease. The data were obtained from the literature or by personal communication as described[11] and modified by recent reports from the Faroe Islands[37,38], Norway[39] and Moscow[40]

CLINICAL PATTERNS OF DISEASE

Complement deficiency states can be grouped into four categories based on the phylogeny, sequential organization, and functional activities of the complement cascade (Table 6.2). These categories are: (1) defects involving the early components of the classical pathway, (2) defects affecting alternative pathway proteins, (3) C3 deficiency states, and (4) deficiencies of one of the terminal complement components.

Deficiencies of the classical pathway proteins

Individuals with a deficiency of one of the early components of the classical pathway (C1, C4, C2) exhibit a delay in complement activation, defective immune complex solubilization and impaired immune responsiveness. In addition, their serum concentrations of IgG4 and IgG2 are significantly reduced, the former to a greater extent than the latter[4]. The association of these deficiencies with an increased risk of autoimmune disorders and infection appears to be a direct consequence of the impairment in these functions. Of the reported individuals with these deficiencies, approximately 20% are healthy, 40% have an associated autoimmune disorder, 20% experience significant infections and 20% have both autoimmune disorders and infection[11]. The factors that determine which of these clinical manifestations are observed in a given individual remain enigmatic.

Systemic lupus erythematosus appears to differ slightly in its clinical presentation from that in the general population[41]. In particular, female predominance and severe renal disease are less common, whereas the prevalence of anti-Ro antibodies is increased[42,43]. Although the basis for the development of autoimmune disorders in individuals with these deficiencies has not been delineated precisely, both the defect in immune complex solubilization and the tight genetic linkage of the C2 and C4 loci with the class I and II MHC genes may contribute to this association[44].

Individuals with these deficiencies are also at increased risk of developing systemic infection caused by encapsulated bacteria, particularly *Streptococcus pneumoniae* (Table 6.2). As discussed above, this risk is probably greater than previously believed, although given an intact alternative pathway, the occurrence of infections in these individuals is a bit puzzling. Both the suboptimal modulation of the immune system and the low concentration of IgG2 and IgG4, which play a particularly important role in the response to polysaccharides, probably contribute to this increased susceptibility. The chemical preference of the C4B allotype to form covalent ester linkages with the ubiquitous hydroxyl groups present on polysaccharides has been suggested as an additional risk factor for infections caused by encapsulated bacteria in individuals with homozygous C4B deficiency[45,46]. However, more extensive studies indicate that this is not the case[47,48].

Infections begin early in life and involve the sinopulmonary tree, blood or meninges. Recurrent disease caused by the same organism is uncommon. These features resemble those in individuals with either congenital or physiological hypo-gamma-globulinaemia. Nevertheless, they do distinguish persons with classical pathway defects and infection from those with alternative pathway or late complement component deficiencies in whom the initial infection is almost always caused by the meningococcus and occurs later in life.

The molecular basis of these complement deficiency states remains incompletely delineated but is likely to reflect the entire spectrum of known mechanisms. Gene deletion is a major mechanism accounting for C4A deficiency[49] whereas defective RNA splicing leading to exon deletion and premature cessation of mRNA translation is the most common defect in C2 deficiency[50,51].

Deficiencies of alternative pathway proteins

Inherited deficiencies of the components of the alternative pathway appear less prevalent than those of other complement proteins. The most commonly described defect involves properdin[11,52,53]. In contrast, individuals with homozygous factor B deficiency have yet to be described. Although factors H and I are properly considered as components of the alternative pathway, their absence secondarily leads to C3 consumption and these deficiencies are more appropriately considered in that context.

Defective complement activation is the only recognized functional consequence of properdin and factor D deficiencies. Moreover, this abnormality may be clinically apparent only in the absence of specific antibody which otherwise serves as an effective inhibitor of the classical pathway. Meningococcal disease is the predominant clinical manifestation of these deficiencies. Similar to the clinical picture in the terminal complement deficiencies, 50–60% of affected individuals experience at least one episode of meningococcal disease; typically during their mid-teenage years (Table 6.2). Although this infection may be fulminant and fatal, it does not always carry the poor prognosis reported initially[52–56]. Recurrent infection is uncommon, probably as a consequence of both the ability to utilize the classical pathway once a specific humoral immune response has occurred and the high mortality rate associated with the initial infection in these individuals. These conclusions reflect the great predominance of properdin deficiency as the major disorder in this category. In contrast, recurrent disease has been a characteristic of the infections reported in the few individuals with factor D deficiency[11]. If this trend is supported by observations in additional individuals, the pathophysiological assumptions regarding the above conclusions may require revision.

Properdin deficiency is unique among the inherited complement defects because it is an X-linked trait, which maps near the centromere on the short arm of the X chromosome[57,58]. Three variants have been described, each of which is associated with absent or impaired properdin function. These variants are distinguished largely on the basis of the concentration of antigenically detectable protein. Type I-deficient individuals have extremely low concentrations of properdin (<0.1 μg/ml)[55,56] whereas the concentration of properdin in type II-deficient individuals is approximately 2 μg/ml. Properdin from these individuals has a normal monomeric molecular weight but polymer formation and function are impaired. The defective polymers do not support fluid-phase alternative pathway activation and their function on target particles is abnormal[59]. Type III properdin deficiency is characterized by a normal concentration of antigenically detectable properdin (~25 μg/ml)[60]. The molecular basis for each of these variants as well as that of factor D deficiency remains to be established.

C3 deficiency states

C3 deficiency occurs as both primary and secondary variants. The primary form is an inherited disorder in which an abnormality in the C3 gene results in the synthesis of a defective protein which is catabolized intracellularly. As a result, C3 is absent from the serum of affected individuals. In contrast, in the secondary form of this disorder, C3 synthesis and secretion are normal. C3 deficiency in these individuals is due to uncontrolled consumption. Consequently, their serum contains a markedly depressed concentration of functional C3 (<10%). In addition, antigenic C3 reflecting C3 activation and the presence of typical C3 cleavage products is readily detectable. Secondary C3 deficiency occurs as both an inherited and an acquired disease. The inherited forms are due to factor H or factor I deficiency. The absence of these regulatory proteins results in uncontrolled consumption of C3 via the alternative pathway. The acquired variant reflects the development of an autoantibody, so-called C3 nephritic factor, which stabilizes the alternative pathway C3 convertase thereby circumventing the regulatory effect of factors H and I and leading to C3 consumption[61,62].

The molecular basis for primary C3 deficiency has been characterized in 2 patients. In one instance, a 700-base-pair genomic deletion affecting exons 22 and 23 was responsible for the defect[63], whereas, in the second patient, the defect was due to a splicing abnormality resulting in partial deletion of exon 19[64]. The molecular basis for factor H and factor I deficiency remains to be delineated. Similarly, the mechanisms leading to the production of C3 nephritic factor remain obscure.

With the exception of acquired C3 deficiency, which can present at any age and may be associated with membranoproliferative glomerulonephritis and partial lipodystrophy[65,66], the clinical manifestations of the inherited forms of primary and secondary C3 deficiency are similar. Such individuals exhibit a marked impairment in the solubilization of immune complexes and opsonophagocytosis as well as defective immunomodulation of B cell function. Some individuals with primary C3 deficiency fail to mount a granulocytic response to infection, presumably reflecting the absence of the C3e cleavage product which helps promote this response[67]. As a consequence of the position of C3 at the convergence point of the two activation pathways, as well as its role in initiating activation of C5 and the assembly of the membrane attack complex, C3-deficient individuals have secondary defects in C5a-mediated chemotaxis and complement-dependent bactericidal activity. Given this plethora of immune functions, it is not surprising that all C3-deficient individuals experience significant clinical disease, either autoimmune (79%) or infectious (78%) in nature (Table 6.2). Infection typically occurs early in life, involves the sinopulmonary tree, meninges and bloodstream, and is most often due to encapsulated bacteria, particularly the meningococcus. Recurrent infection is common.

Late complement component deficiencies

With the exception of individuals with C5 deficiency, the sole defect in persons lacking one of the late complement components is the inability to assemble the membrane attack complex and express complement-dependent bactericidal activity. Systemic Neisserial infection, particularly meningococcal disease, is the only clinical manifestation linked with certainty to these deficiencies. Approximately 64% of C5-, C6-, C7- and C8-deficient individuals will experience at least one episode of meningococcal infection and about half of these individuals will experience more than one infection caused by this organism. In contrast to individuals with C3 or classical pathway deficiencies, infection typically occurs in the mid-teenage years as in properdin deficiency (Table 6.2). Despite the chemotactic defect associated with C5 deficiency, the clinical manifestations of meningococcal disease in C5–C8 deficiency are similar (Table 6.3). In C9-deficient persons, meningococcal infection is less common (10%); recurrent meningococcal infection has not been observed and infection has been limited to meningitis.

The molecular basis for these deficiency states remains to be delineated. As with other genetic diseases, heterogeneous mechanisms are likely. For example, the structural genes for C6 and C7 are tightly linked on chromosome 9 yet both combined and individual deficiencies of these proteins have been described[68,69].

In summary, complement deficiency states can be grouped into four categories based on phylogenetic, organizational and functional considerations. Due to the central position of C3 in the complement cascade and its contribution to multiple immune functions, individuals with this deficiency are the most severely affected of any of the persons with these types of defects. Autoimmune

Table 6.3 Comparison of meningococcal (Mgc) disease in late complement component deficiency states

	Deficiency				
	C5	*C6*	*C7*	*C8*	*C9*
Number of individuals	27	77	73	73	165
No. with Mgc disease	19	42	45	40	15
%	70	54	62	55	9.1
No. with recurrent disease	8	23	14	20	0
%	42	55	31	50	0
No. episodes of Mgc disease	30	75	71	69	15
CSF and blood (%)	23(77)	69(92)	56(79)	55(80)	15(100)
Blood (%)	1(3.3)	5(6.6)	5(7.0)	3(4.4)	0
Unspecified (%)	6(20)	1(1.3)	10(14)	11(16)	0
Ratio of CSF:Blood	23:1	14:1	11:1	18:1	15:0

disorders, particularly systemic lupus erythematosus, and infections, especially meningococcal disease, constitute the clinical manifestations that characterize these deficiency states. The former is typically associated with classical pathway defects and C3 deficiency, whereas the latter is most characteristic of alternative pathway, C3 and late complement component deficiencies.

MENINGOCOCCAL DISEASE AND COMPLEMENT DEFICIENCY

Meningococcal disease is the single most common infection sustained by complement-deficient individuals, accounting for 75–85% of the identified systemic infections[10,11]. It is interesting and perhaps a little ironic that the first example of this relationship may have occurred in a prominent microbiologist investigating the bactericidal activity of serum for meningococci and whose own serum lacked this activity[70,71]. In addition to confirming the importance of the complement cascade in protection from meningococcal disease, this striking association suggests that novel insights regarding the pathogenesis of infection may be revealed by the study of meningococcal disease in these individuals.

Consistent with this hypothesis are a number of features, identified originally by Ross and Densen[10], that distinguish meningococcal disease in normal persons from that in individuals with late complement component and properdin deficiency states (Table 6.4). Although the prevalence of meningococcal disease in unselected complement-deficient individuals is largely unknown, these features are unlikely to result solely from ascertainment bias for the following reasons. First, they have been confirmed in multiple studies in different populations around the world. Second, each feature has been borne out by investigations of complement-deficient families following exclusion of the proband from the analysis. Third, at least in the case of the late complement component deficiencies, family studies fail to reveal undiagnosed infections and unexplained or premature deaths. The potential significance of each of these

Table 6.4 Comparison of meningococcal disease in normal, late-complement-component- and properdin-deficient individuals[a]

Parameter	*Normal*	*C5–C8*	*C9*	*Properdin deficient*[b]
No. of homozygotes	—	250	165	54–70
No. with meningococcal disease	—	146	15	25–37
Frequency of infection (%)	0.0072	58	9.1	46–53
Median age (y) at first episode	3	17	16	14–11.5
Recurrence rate (%)	0.34	44	0	2–1.4
Relapse rate (%)	0.6	7.9	0	0
Mortality/100 episodes (%)	19	1.5	0	12–51.4
Infecting serogroup				
No. of isolates	3184	67	2	16
% B	50	19.4	50	18.7
% Y	4.4	32.8	0	37.5

[a]Adapted from Figueroa and Densen[11]
[b]Where a range is given, the first number refers to documented cases and the second number refers to documented plus probable and possible cases

features with respect to the pathogenesis of meningococcal disease is dealt with in the following paragraphs. This discussion is based largely on analysis of meningococcal infection in individuals with C5–C8 deficiency states. Where appropriate, emphasis will also be placed on aspects unique to C9 and properdin deficiency.

Frequency of infection

Approximately 60% of C5–C8-deficient individuals will experience at least one episode of meningococcal disease.[11] This frequency is greater than that noted originally by Ross and Densen[10], presumably due in part to the ascertainment bias created by screening individuals with meningococcal disease and the failure to report incidentally discovered healthy deficient individuals in the literature. Regardless of this, the risk of infection is 6000–9000-fold greater in deficient than in normal individuals. The frequency of infection and the validity of comparing the infection rate with that in normal individuals has been questioned.[21] Nevertheless, detailed epidemiological data concerning the prevalence of C9 and C7 deficiency and the yearly incidence of meningococcal disease in these patients and in the general Japanese population provide firm support for these estimates[34]. These data demonstrate that C7 deficiency is associated with an approximately 5000-fold increase in the risk of developing meningococcal disease compared with that in the general population. This risk is similar to that cited above. In addition, these data clearly establish the increased susceptibility to meningococcal disease of C9-deficient individuals (~700-fold, Table 6.5) relative to the general population although this risk is about 7-fold less than that for C7-deficient individuals[34]. The increased susceptibility of C5–C8-deficient individuals relative to C9-deficient individuals is consistent with *in vitro* studies demonstrating that C9-deficient sera can kill meningococci, albeit at a slower rate[72]. This dose–response relationship, coupled with the fact that the structural genes encoding these proteins are located on multiple chromosomes[11], provides strong evidence for a cause-and-effect relationship between the absence of complement-dependent bactericidal activity and the increased susceptibility of these individuals to meningococcal disease.

An additional point regarding the increased susceptibility of these individuals to meningococcal disease is that, although deficient siblings experience this infection, concurrent infection has not been described despite the increased risk

Table 6.5 Risk of meningococcal disease in C7- and C9-deficient Japanese*

	Prevalence of deficiency (per 10^5 population)	Yearly incidence of of meningococcal disease (%)	Fold increase in risk
Normal Japanese	—	0.00015	1
C9 deficient	36	0.1	667
C7 deficient	5	0.72	4800

*Adapted from Ref. 34

and the established capacity of this organism to cause intrafamilial outbreaks of disease[10]. Thus, the high rate of infection in these individuals is not a quirk of the spread of the disease within families. The absence of concurrent disease in deficient siblings has similar implications regarding the older age of infection and the increased likelihood of recurrent disease.

Age of infection

The initial episode of meningococcal disease in persons with late complement component or properdin deficiency occurs between 14 and 17 years of age. Only 17 (10.4%) of 163 complement-deficient individuals with meningococcal disease were less than 5 years of age. In contrast, the median age of meningococcal infection in the general population is 3 years and 56% of these persons are less than 5 years of age (Figure 6.2)[73,74]. Thus, most deficient individuals pass through the age of life when the deficiency might be expected to maximally increase their susceptibility to meningococcal disease without evincing evidence of that susceptibility. The data in Figure 6.2 also demonstrate that infection in deficient individuals is not evenly distributed by age, rather there is a distinct peak of disease in the mid-teenage years. This finding indicates that considerations, such as: a lifetime of risk; a potential inverse relationship between the age-specific incidence of meningococcal disease and the prevalence of complement deficiencies, analogous to that described above for entire populations; or other stochastic variables, are inadequate to explain the paradoxical difference in the age of first meningococcal infection in deficient and normal individuals. This observation further suggests that unidentified factors may enhance the susceptibility of deficient individuals to infection later in life. The possibility that these factors might also be related to the shift in the age-specific incidence observed during meningococcal epidemics[75,76] and the greater meningococcal carriage rate in 15–19-year-old individuals[77] deserves further consideration.

Infecting serogroup

Meningococcal disease in complement-deficient individuals is caused by uncommon serogroups, particularly groups Y and W135, more often than in normal individuals[10,11]. Conversely, the prevalence of these deficiencies is increased among individuals with meningococcal disease caused by these serogroups[78]. The physiological basis for this observation is not known with certainty. Factors that may be important include:

(1) The critical requirement for anticapsular antibody for prevention of disease in deficient compared with normal individuals (see below).
(2) Group B isolates are more readily eliminated by phagocytic cells in the absence of anticapsular antibody than meningococci belonging to the other serogroups[79].

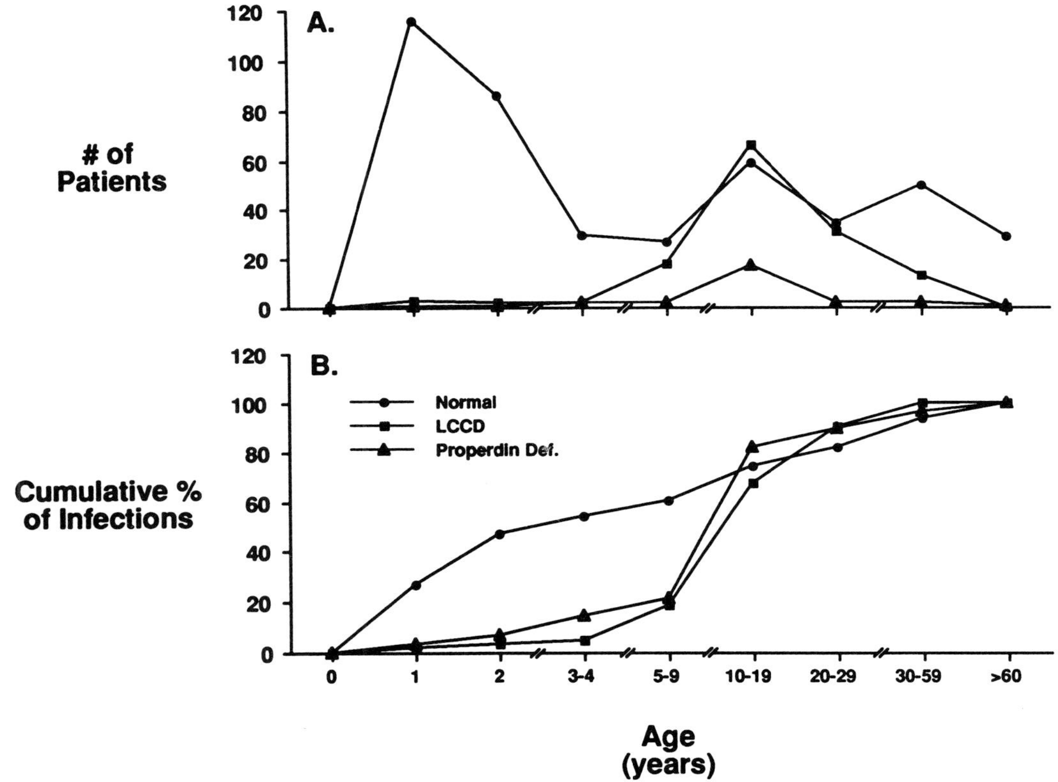

Figure 6.2 The age of first meningococcal infection in normal and complement-deficient individuals. Data for normal individuals (solid circles) were provided by Dr. J. Wenger from the Centers for Disease Control, Atlanta, Georgia, as published[74]. Data for late complement-component-deficient individuals (LCCD, solid squares) and properdin-deficient patients (Properdin Def., solid triangles) are from the literature[10,11]. Results are expressed as the number of infected patients (panel A) or as the cumulative percentage of infections (panel B) by age of infection. Hatches in the horizontal axis indicate discontinuity in the age scale

(3) The propensity for uncommon meningococcal serogroup organisms to cause disease in older individuals[80] who, as discussed above, are relatively more likely to be complement deficient.

Meningococci and gonococci isolated from complement-deficient individuals with systemic Neisserial infection do not differ significantly in their biological properties compared with the same organisms isolated from complement-sufficient individuals[81]. Thus, the absence of complement-dependent bactericidal activity does not automatically provide access to the bloodstream by less virulent serum-sensitive organisms. This observation suggests that serum-sensitive organisms, which predominate on mucosal surfaces, lack determinants in addition to serum resistance (e.g. invasins) that contribute to the pathogenesis of infection.

Recurrent disease

Recurrent meningococcal disease, defined as a new infection occurring more than one month following a previous episode, occurs in about 40–45% of C5–C8-deficient individuals. This recurrence rate is approximately 100–150 times greater than that in the general population.

The overwhelming majority of normal individuals never experience an episode of meningococcal disease despite the fact that 20% of the population carries this organism each year[77,82]. Moreover, normal individuals, who have the misfortune to sustain one of these infections, rarely experience a recurrence. Substantial evidence indicates that protection in normal individuals is afforded by crossreactive antibody to subcapsular meningococcal antigens, particularly lipopolysaccharide[83–85]. Anticapsular antibody is also protective but, in the absence of infection or vaccination, the concentration of these antibodies in serum is low[86,87].

The fact that complement-deficient individuals experience recurrent disease suggests that neither natural antibody nor that developing following an episode of meningococcal infection affords protection to these individuals. This hypothesis is supported by the observation that the prevalence of complement deficiency among individuals with meningococcal disease increases with the level of natural immunity in the population as discussed above. In addition, statistical analysis of the number of individuals with a specified number of episodes of meningococcal disease is consistent with the interpretation that the risk of meningococcal disease in the complement-deficient individuals is independent of prior infection[11]. That is, prior disease does not reduce the risk of subsequent meningococcal infection in these individuals. In this study, the estimated probability of each infection was 0.39[11]. A similar analysis, utilizing a slightly different statistical approach, arrived at an identical conclusion and resulted in an estimate of the probability of infection of 0.6[40,88]. In addition, the latter analysis demonstrated that the interval between infections (4–5 years) did not differ, again suggesting that prior disease does not reduce the risk of subsequent meningococcal infection.

Possible explanations to account for this observation include that the absence of one of the late complement components is associated with an inadequate humoral immune response to meningococci. Alternatively, complement-dependent bactericidal activity might be an absolute requirement for protection from meningococcal disease even though complement-dependent opsonophagocytic mechanisms remain intact in these individuals.

Regarding the first possibility, we have demonstrated that complement-deficient and sufficient individuals do not differ in their response to meningococcal capsular polysaccharides following infection or vaccination and exhibit an enhanced response to subcapsular antigens, particularly lipopolysaccharide[89,90]. Of particular note was our observation that, in general, natural infection constitutes a poor stimulus for the production of anticapsular antibody in both groups, resulting in a median concentration of specific antibody of ~1.0 μg/ml. With respect to the second possibility, we have quantitated antibodies to subcapsular and capsular antigens in an individual with recurrent disease despite prior administration of the tetravalent meningococcal vaccine[90]. The concentration of antibody to subcapsular antigens was maintained throughout 4 years of observation. In contrast, following an initially adequate response to the vaccine, antibody to the group C capsular polysaccharide declined to prevaccination levels over a 2-year period. This decline was temporarily associated with the development of group C meningococcal disease. In subsequent studies, we demonstrated that antibody to both subcapsular and capsular antigens promotes effective complement-dependent bactericidal activity but only the latter antibody promotes efficient opsonophagocytic killing of meningococci[90].

In summary, these observations strongly suggest that: adequate amounts of anticapsular antibody are critical for protection against recurrent disease in complement-deficient individuals; meningococcal disease does not provide protective immunity in C5–C8-deficient individuals because the resulting anticapsular antibody concentrations are low and limited to the serogroup of the infecting strain; and, as in the general population, some deficient individuals will exhibit a limited response to the vaccine and fail to maintain protective levels of anticapsular antibody, resulting in a return of susceptibility and potential vaccine failure.

Disease relapse

Relapse of meningococcal disease, defined as infection with the same serogroup occurring less than one month following the initial infection, occurs in 7.6% of the C5–C8-deficient individuals with meningococcal disease reported in the literature. This frequency is approximately 10 times greater than that in the general population and suggests that meningococci may be sequestered intracellularly where they may be relatively protected from antibiotics. This hypothesis implies that the terminal complement components may contribute to intracellular killing, a possibility that is supported by recent investigations[91,92].

Mortality

One of the most striking aspects of meningococcal disease in late complement component-deficient individuals is that, despite a several-thousand-fold increase in the risk of infection, they experience a 5–10-fold reduction in the chance of dying from the disease compared with normal persons. This reduction is evident regardless of whether the mortality rate is expressed per initial infection or per hundred episodes of infection. Moreover, family studies, in which the proband has been excluded from the analysis, confirm this relationship and fail to reveal unexplained deaths in potentially susceptible individuals, thereby lending further credence to the validity of this observation. Thus, the identical defect that predisposes to infection appears to provide protection from the lethal consequences of the disease. This remarkable observation suggests that the host's exuberant response to the organism is as much responsible for the clinical manifestations and outcome as the organism itself. This deduction is supported by Brandtzaeg's report of a close correlation between the extent of complement activation and mortality in meningococcal disease[93] and suggests that the latter is in part dependent on the assembly of the membrane attack complex.

Several factors may contribute to the lower mortality in late complement component-deficient persons including:

(1) Milder disease;
(2) Fewer organisms required for infection;
(3) Lower endotoxin concentrations; and
(4) Less host cell injury.

The possibility that milder disease may account for the lower mortality in late complement component deficiency is difficult to assess from the reported literature due to the variability in the clinical information provided. However, hypotension, disseminated intravascular coagulopathy and shock have occurred in individual cases[10,11]. Nevertheless, support for this hypothesis has been provided by Platonov and Beloborodov[40,88] who utilized both a grading system based on clinical variables and quantitation of complement consumption to demonstrate that disease severity was less in 17 complement-deficient than in 12 age-matched normal individuals with meningococcal infection. In addition, their analysis demonstrated that the severity of disease in the complement-deficient individuals was independent of the number of episodes of recurrence[40,88]; that is, milder disease was not observed in individuals with prior infection. This finding is consistent with the apparent lack of effect of the immune response on recurrent disease, as discussed above, and the fact that there is no relationship between death and the number of infections in the few deficient individuals with fatal infection.

Meningococcaemia in the absence of meningitis occurs in about 5–10% of late complement deficient individuals infected with this organism (Table 3)[10,11,40,88]. This observation contrasts with the reported frequency of meningococcaemia in the general population (21–31%) and tends to refute the notion that chronic meningococcaemia is common in these persons. Rather meningitis, which has a lower case fatality rate[73], may be more common in deficient than normal individuals.

The possibility that fewer organisms may be required to establish systemic meningococcal disease in deficient than normal individuals is attractive, although data addressing this point are conspicuously absent in the literature. Such an effect would account for the increased number of infections as well as milder disease and the decreased case fatality rate since mortality is directly related to the number of organisms in the blood stream[94,95]. A reduction in the organism load might translate into a lower concentration of circulating endotoxin and less systemic inflammation.

Complement deficient individuals may also be better able to tolerate a given organism load than complement sufficient persons. Support for this possibility comes from the experiments of Brown and Lachmann[96] who injected normal and C6 deficient rabbits with a potentially lethal dose of endotoxin resulting in the death of all the normal but only a portion of the deficient animals. In additional experiments, normal rabbits depleted of C3–C9 through the action of cobra venom factor survived the injection of endotoxin. Survival was inversely correlated with the extent of platelet activation and the release of platelet activating factor.

The ability to tolerate a given organism load or endotoxin dose could be related to either organism or host-related variables that contribute to the severity of meningococcal disease. With respect to organism factors, the insertion of the membrane attack complex into the outer membrane of Gram negative organisms has been shown to disrupt the outer membrane and release free endotoxin[97–101]. Thus, endotoxin release should be less during meningococcal infection in late complement component deficient individuals. This in turn might lead to a reduction in the extent of ongoing complement activation and decreased secretion of various macrophage-derived cytokines that have been linked to development of septic shock in meningococcal disease[93,102–109]. Support for this possibility stems from a preliminary report[110] in which a C6-deficient individual received fresh frozen plasma for treatment of disseminated intravascular coagulopathy in association with meningococcal disease. Circulating endotoxin was undetectable in the fresh frozen plasma or in the patient's serum prior to infusion whereas substantial lipopolysaccharide appeared following infusion. Thus, this case report provides evidence for role of the membrane attack complex in releasing endotoxin *in vivo*.

Support for a role for host-related factors in this process derives from a number of *in vitro* observations. Insertion of the membrane attack complex into the membrane of host cells, while not lethal, has been associated with profound effects[111,112]; for example, leucocyte activation with the resultant release of a plethora of potentially noxious mediators[113] and the increased expression of procoagulant molecules on the surface of endothelial cells[114]. Insertion of the membrane attack complex into host cell membranes might occur *in vivo* as a consequence of exuberant complement activation in the vicinity of innocent bystander cells or as a consequence of endotoxin binding to these cells and subsequent complement activation on their surfaces. These processes would be interrupted in the late complement component deficient individual and potentially could result in an improved ability to tolerate a given load of organisms and endotoxin.

In summary, meningococcal disease in late complement component deficient individuals exhibits a number of unique features which distinguish it from that in complement sufficient persons. On the one hand, these features are valuable for the clinical clues they provide with respect to identifying complement deficient individuals and maximizing the yield of screening programmes. On the other hand, these features have provided novel insights into the pathogenesis of the clinical manifestations of meningococcal disease and have opened the door for both potential therapeutic and preventive strategies.

DIAGNOSIS OF COMPLEMENT DEFICIENCY AND PREVENTION OF MENINGOCOCCAL DISEASE

The possibility of an underlying complement deficiency disorder should be considered in any individual with systemic lupus erythematosus or recurrent infection caused by encapsulated organisms, particularly the meningococcus, or if there is a family history of systemic neisserial infection. Routine screening of individuals with meningococcal infection is probably justified in countries in which the disease is endemic or hypoendemic, that is, the incidence is less than 10–15 cases per million population. In this situation the prevalence of complement deficiency can be expected to be at least 5–10% (Figure 6.1). The probability of detecting complement deficiency states among individuals with meningococcal disease can be further increased by limiting screening to individuals over 10 years of age or to infections caused by unusual serogroups[78]. This approach may have its greatest utility in populations where the incidence of meningococcal disease is high (> 15 cases/10^6 population).

Initial screening tests should assess the functional activity of both the entire classical and alternative pathway sequences. Since alternative pathway assays are less readily available and since properdin deficiency accounts for the overwhelming majority of the defects affecting this pathway, it may be reasonable to limit the use of this assay to males or to unusual clinical circumstances (e.g. recurrent disease) in individuals whose classical pathway is normal. The presence of significantly reduced but not absent complement activity in sera obtained from individuals with meningococcal infection when they are healthy should alert the clinician to the possibility of either C9 deficiency or C3 consumption disorders. The latter diagnosis can be established by quantitation of C3 antigen, detection of C3 cleavage products by serum electrophoresis, and quantitation of factors H and I.

All complement deficient individuals should receive the tetravalent meningococcal vaccine. Individuals with classical pathway deficiencies should also receive the pneumococcal and conjugated *Haemophilus influenzae* vaccines. Data cited above and reported in the literature convincingly support the principle that anticapsular antibodies will facilitate utilization of the alternative pathway in classical pathway deficient individuals; the classical pathway in alternative pathway deficient individuals; and promote opsonophagocytic elimination of meningococci in individuals with C5–C9 deficiency[55,79,90,115,116]. No data are available regarding the utility of vaccination in C3 deficient individuals but the possibility of facilitating antibody-mediated complement-independent clearance of encapsulated organisms, coupled with the safety of these vaccines, probably justifies their use in these patients. Recommendations regarding the utility of quantitating pre- and post-vaccination antibody responses to capsular polysaccharides or routinely employing these assays as a guide to revaccination are highly subjective and should probably be limited by the cost and availability of the assays. However, our experience clearly supports revaccination in the event of recurrent disease caused by a serogroup represented in the vaccine[90].

An alternative strategy for the prevention of meningococcal disease in complement deficient individuals is the employment of prophylactic antibiotics. This approach significantly reduces the frequency of infection in these individuals and has its greatest utility in populations in which group B meningococcal disease is highly prevalent[117]. It is unclear whether prophylaxis should be lifelong or whether the development of antibiotic resistance by meningococci will limit the efficacy of this approach.

Although fresh frozen plasma has been employed as replacement therapy for complement deficient individuals its use has been shown to be beneficial only in the various forms of C3 deficiency[10,118] and perhaps C1 deficiency. The recent experience of Lehner *et al.*[110] in which the administration of fresh frozen plasma to a C6-deficient individual with meningococcal disease was associated with the appearance of free endotoxin in the patient's plasma and the subsequent development of anti-C6 antibodies constitute dramatic testimony to the potential hazards of this approach.

In conclusion, the study of complement deficient individuals has provided a wealth of pathophysiological insight into collagen vascular disorders, host defence mechanisms, meningococcal disease, and the molecular basis for these genetic disorders. More importantly these studies have provided a rationale for the use of vaccines as an immunological mechanism for bypassing the genetic deficiency by recruiting additional host defence mechanisms to aid in the prevention of infection. These insights should encourage all physicians and investigators to continue making clinical observations, pursuing them in the laboratory and reporting them in the literature.

ACKNOWLEDGEMENTS

I gratefully acknowledge productive discussions with Anders G. Sjöholm and Alexander E. Platonov, the constructive suggestions of Robert A. Clark; and the secretarial assistance of Naomi Erickson. This work was supported in part by a Merit Review Award from the Department of Veterans Affairs.

References

1. Ross, G. D. (1986). Introduction and history of complement research. In Ross, G. D. (ed.) *Immunobiology of the Complement System*, pp. 1–20. (Orlando, FL: Academic Press)
2. Burnet, S. M. (1970). *Cellular Immunology*, p. 160. (Melbourne University Press; Cambridge University Press)
3. Donaldson, V. H. and Evans, R. R. (1963) A biochemical abnormality in hereditary angioneurotic edema: absence of serum inhibitor of C′1-esterase. *Am. J. Med.* **35**, 37–44
4. Bird, P. and Lachmann, P. J. (1988). The regulation of IgG subclass production in man: low serum IgG4 in inherited deficiencies of the classical pathway of C3 activation *Eur. J. Immunol.*, **18**, 1217–22
5. Bottger, E. C. and Bitter-Suermann, D. (1987). Complement and the regulation of humoral immune responses. *Immunol. Today*, **8**, 261–4

6. Laham, M. N., Caldwell, J. R. and Panush, R. S. (1982). Modulation of lymphocyte proliferative response to mitogens and antigens by complement components C1, C4 and C2. *J. Clin. Lab. Immunol.*, **9**, 39–47
7. Ochs, H. D., Wedgwood, R. J., Frank, M. M., Heller, S. R. and Hosea, S. W. (1983). The role of complement in the induction of antibody responses. *Clin. Exp. Immunol.*, **53**, 208–16
8. O'Neil, K. M., Ochs, H. D., Heller, S. R., Cork, L. C., Morris, J. M. and Winkelstein, J. A. (1988). Role of C3 in humoral immunity. Defective antibody production in C3-deficient dogs. *J. Immunol.*, **140**, 1939–45
9. Petersen, B. H., Lee, T. J., Snyderman, R. and Brooks, G. F. (1979). *Neisseria meningitidis* and *Neisseria gonorrhoeae* bacteremia associated with C6, C7, or C8-deficiency. *Ann. Intern. Med.*, **90**, 917–20
10. Ross, S. C. and Densen, P. (1984). Complement deficiency states and infection: epidemiology, pathogenesis and consequences of *Neisseria* and other infections in an immune deficiency. *Medicine (Baltimore)*, **63**, 243–73
11. Figueroa, J. E. and Densen, P. (1991). Infectious diseases associated with complement deficiences. *Clin. Microbiol. Rev.*, **4**, 359–95
12. Nicholson-Weller, A., March, J. P., Rosenfeld, S. I. and Austen, K. F. (1983). Affected erythrocytes of patients with paroxysmal nocturnal hemoglobinuria are deficient in the complement regulatory protein, decay accelerating factor. *Proc. Natl. Acad. Sci. USA*, **80**, 5066–70
13. Pangburn, M. K., Schreiber, R. D. and Muller-Eberhard, H. J. (1983). Deficiency of an erythrocyte membrane protein with complement regulatory activity in paroxysmal nocturnal hemoglobinuria. *Proc. Natl. Acad. Sci. USA*, **80**, 5430–4
14. Rosse, W. F. (1990). Phosphatidylinositol-linked proteins and paroxysmal nocturnal hemoglobinuria. *Blood*, **75**, 1595–1601
15. Sanchez-Madrid, F., Nagy, J. A., Robbins, E., Simon, P. and Springer, T. A. (1983). A human leukocyte differentiation antigen family with distinct α-subunits and a common β-subunit: the lymphocyte function-associated antigen (LFA-1), the iC3b complement receptor (OKM1/Mac-1), and the p150,95 molecule. *J. Exp. Med.*, **158**, 1785–95
16. Arnaout, M. A., Spits, H., Terhorst, C., Pitt, J and Todd, R. F. III. (1984). Deficiency of a leukocyte surface glycoprotein (LFA-1) in two patients with Mo1 deficiency. *J. Clin. Invest.*, **74**, 1291–1300
17. Anderson, D. C., Schmalsteig, F. C., Finegold, M. J., Hughes, B. J., Rothlein, R., Miller, L. J., Kohl, S., Tosi, M. F., Jacobs, R. L. and Waldrop, T. C. (1985). The severe and moderate phenotypes of heritable Mac-1, LFA-1 deficiency: their quantitative definition and relation to leukocyte dysfunction and clinical features. *J. Infect. Dis.*, **152**, 668–89
18. Stiehm, E. R., Chin, T. W., Haas, A. and Peerless, A. G. (1986). Infectious complications of the primary immunodeficiencies. *Clin. Immunol. Immunopathol.*, **40**, 69–86
19. Hassig, A., Borel, J. F. and Ammann, P. (1964). Essentialle hypokomplementamie. *Pathol. Microbiol. (Basel)*, **27**, 542–7
20. Fukomori, Y., Yoshimura, K., Ohnoki, S., Yamaguchi, H., Akagaki, Y and Inai, S. (1989). A high incidence of C9 deficiency among healthy blood donors in Osaka, Japan. *Int. Immunol.*, **1**, 85–9
21. Inai, S., Akagaki, Y., Moriyama, T., Fukumori, Y., Yoshimura, K., Ohnoki, S. and Yamaguchi, H. (1989). Inherited deficiencies of the late-acting complement components other than C9 among healthy blood donors. *Int. Arch. Allergy Appl. Immunol.*, **90**, 274–9
22. Lachmann, P. J. (1974). Genetic deficiencies of the complement system. *Boll. First Sierotes Milanese*, **53**, 195–207
23. Alper, C. A., Awdeh, Z. and Yunis, E. J. (1987). Frequency of the C2 deficiency gene among normal Caucasians. *Complement*, **4**, 125(Abstract)
24. Baur, M. P., Neugebauer, M., Deppe, H., Sigmund, H., Luton, T., Mayr, W. R. and Albert, E. D. (1984). Population analysis on the basis of deduced haplotypes from random families. In Albert, E. D., Baur, M. P. and Mayr, W. R. (eds.). *Histocompatibility Testing*, p. 333. (Berlin: Springer-Verlag)
25. Hauptmann, G., Goetz, J., Uring-Lambert, B. and Grosshans, E. (1986). Component deficiencies. 2. The fourth component. *Prog. Allergy*, **39**, 232–49
26. Glass, D., Raum, D., Gibson, D., Stillman, J. S. and Schur, P. H. (1976). Inherited deficiency of the second component of complement: rheumatic disease association *J. Clin. Invest.*, **58**, 853

27. Densen, P., Sanford, M., Burke, T., Densen, E. and Wintermeyer, L. (1990). Prospective study of the prevalence of complement deficiency in meningitis. In *Program and Abstracts of the 30th Interscience Congress for Antimicrobial Agents*, p. 140. (Abstract)
28. Ellison, R. T. III, Curd, J. G., Kohler, P. F., Reller, L. B. and Judson, F. N. (1987). Underlying complement deficiency in patients with disseminated gonococcal infection. *Sex. Transm. Dis.*, **14**, 201–4
29. Eng, R. H. K. (1980). Bactericidal screening test for late complement component deficiencies or defects. *J. Clin. Microbiol.*, **11**, 631–4
30. Ellison, R. T. III, Kohler, P. F., Curd, J. G., Judson, F. N. and Reller, L. B. (1983). Prevalence of congenital or acquired complement deficiency in patients with sporadic meningococcal disease. *N. Engl. J. Med.*, **308**, 913–16
31. Beatty, D. W., Ryder, C. R. and Heese, H. D. (1986). Complement abnormalities during an epidemic of group B meningococcal infection in children. *Clin. Exp. Immunol.*, **64**, 465–70
32. Leggiadro, R. J. and Winkelstein, J. A. (1987). Prevalence of complement deficiencies in children with systemic meningococcal infections. *Pediatr. Infect. Dis. J.*, **6**, 75–6
33. Rasmussen, J. M., Brandslund, I., Teisner, B., Isager, H., Svehag, S. E. and Maarup, L. (1987). Screening for complement deficiencies in unselected patients with meningitis. *Clin. Exp. Immunol.*, **68**, 437–45
34. Nagata, M., Hara, T., Aoki, T., Mizuno, Y., Akeda, H., Inaba, S., Tsumoto, K. and Ueda, K. (1989). Inherited deficiency of ninth component of complement: an increased risk of meningococcal meningitis. *J. Pediatr.*, **114**, 260–4
35. Nielsen, H. E., Christensen, K. C., Koch, C., Thomsen, B. S., Heegaard, N. H. and Tranum-Jensen, J. (1989). Hereditary, complete deficiency of complement factor H associated with recurrent meningococcal disease. *Scand. J. Immunol.*, **30**, 711–18
36. Schlesinger, M., Nave, Z., Levy, Y., Slater, P. E. and Fishelson, Z. (1990). Prevalence of hereditary properdin, C7 and C8 deficiencies in patients with meningococcal infections. *Clin. Exp. Immunol.*, **81**, 423–7
37. Rasmussen, J. M., Teisner, B., Weihe, P., Mathiassen, B., Petersen, T. and Isager, H. (1988). Screening for complement deficiencies in patients surviving from epidemic meningococcal disease. *J. Clin. Lab. Immunol.*, **25**, 161–5
38. Weihe, P., Mathiassen, B., Rasmussen, J. M., Petersen, T. and Isager, H. (1988). An epidemic outbreak of group B meningococcal disease on the Faroe Islands. *Scand. J. Infect. Dis.*, **20**, 291–6
39. Rogde, S., Hoiby, E. A., Teisberg, P. and Olaisen, B. (1990). Genetic aspects of complement component C8 in Norwegian meningococcal disease patients. *Scand. J. Infect. Dis.*, **22**, 673–9
40. Beloborodov, V. B. and Platonov, A. E. (1991). Meningococcal disease in the USSR in patients with deficiencies in late complement components. In Achtman, M., Kohl, P., Marchal, C., Morelli, G., Seiler, A. and Thiesen, B. (eds). *Neisseriae 1990*, pp. 659–63. (Berlin: Walter de Gruyter & Co.)
41. Agnello, V. (1978). Complement deficiency states. *Medicine (Baltimore)*, **57**, 1–23
42. Provost, T. T., Arnett, F. C. and Reichlin, M. (1983). Homozygous C2–deficiency, lupus erythematosus, and anti-Ro (SSA) antibodies. *Arthritis Rheum.*, **26**, 1279–82
43. Meyer, O., Hauptmann, G., Tappeiner, G., Ochs, H. D. and Mascart-Lemone, F. (1985). Genetic deficiency of C4, C2 or C1q and lupus syndromes. Association with anti-Ro (SS-A) antibodies. *Clin. Exp. Immunol.*, **62**, 678–84
44. Davis, A. E. III (1983). The efficiency of complement activation in MHC-linked diseases. *Immunol. Today*, **4**, 250–2
45. Rowe, P. C., McLean, R. H., Wood, R. A., Leggiadro, R. J. and Windelstein, J. A. (1989). Association of homozygous C4B deficiency with bacterial meningitis. *J. Infect. Dis.*, **160**, 448–51
46. Bishof, N. A., Welch, T. R. and Beischel, L. S. (1990). C4B deficiency: a risk factor for bacteremia with encapsulated organisms. *J. Infect. Dis.*, **162**, 248–50
47. Fasano, M. B., Densen, P., McLean, R. H. and Windelstein, J. A. (1990). Prevalence of homozygous C4B deficiency in patients with deficiencies of terminal complement components and meningococcemia. *J. Infect. Dis.*, **162**, 1220–1
48. Cates, K. L., Dodds, A. W., Lockman, J., Densen, P. and Levine, R. P. (1990). C4B deficiency is not associated with meningitis or bacteremia with encapsulated bacteria. *FASEB J.*, **4**, A2089 (Abstract)

49. Kemp, M. E., Atkinson, J. P., Skanes, V. M., Levine, R. P. and Chaplin, D. D. (1987). Deletion of C4A genes in patients with systemic lupus erythematosus. *Arthritis Rheum.*, **30**, 1015–22
50. Johnson, C., Densen, P., Cole, F. S., Wetsel, R. and Colten, H. R. (1989). Molecular heterogeneity of human C2 deficiency. *Complement*, **6**, 351–2 (Abstract)
51. Johnson, C. A., Densen, P., Hurford, R., Colten, H. R. and Wetsel, R. A. (1991). Deficiency of human complement C2, Type I: A 28BP gene deletion leads to a splicing defect. *Clin. Res.*, **39**, 304A (Abstract)
52. Sjöholm, A. G. (1989). Absence and dysfunction of properdin as a basis for susceptibility to meningococcal disease. *Immunopathol. Immunother. Forum*, **4**, 3–12
53. Sjöholm, A. G. (1990). Inherited complement deficiency states: implications for immunity and immunological disease. *Acta Pathol. Microbiol. Immunol. Scand.* [c], **98**, 861–74
54. Braconier, J. H., Sjöholm, A. G. and Söderstrom, C. (1983). Fulminant meningococcal infections in a family with inherited deficiency of properdin. *Scand. J. Infect. Dis.*, **15**, 339–45
55. Densen, P., Weiler, J. M., Griffiss, J. M. and Hoffman, L. G. (1987). Familial properdin deficiency and fatal meningococcemia: correction of the bactericidal defect by vaccination. *N. Engl. J. Med.*, **316**, 922–6
56. Sjöholm, A. G., Braconier, J. H. and Söderstrom, C. (1982). Properdin deficiency in a family with fulminant meningococcal infections. *Clin. Exp. Immunol.*, **50**, 291–7
57. Goonewardena, P., Sjöholm, A. G., Nilsson, L. A. and Pettersson, U. (1988). Linkage analysis of the properdin deficiency gene: suggestion of a locus in the proximal part of the short arm of the X chromosome. *Genomics*, **2**, 115–18
58. Goundis, D., Holt, S. M., Boyd, Y. and Reid, K. B. (1989). Localization of the properdin structural locus to Xp11.23–Xp21.1. *Genomics*, **5**, 56–60
59. Sjöholm, A. G., Söderstrom, C. and Nilsson, L. A. (1988). A second variant of properdin deficiency: the detection of properdin at low concentrations in affected males. *Complement*, **5**, 130–40
60. Sjöholm, A. G., Kuijper, E. J., Tijssen, C. C., Jansz, A., Bol, P., Spanjaard, L. and Zanen, H. C. (1988). Dysfunctional properdin in a Dutch family with meningococcal disease. *N. Engl. J. Med.*, **319**, 33–7
61. Daha, M. R., Fearon, D. T. and Austen, K. F. (1976). C3 nephritic factor (CeNeF): stabilization of fluid phase and cell-bound alternative pathway convertase. *J. Immunol.*, **116**, 1–7
62. Fearon, D. T. (1976). Glomerulonephritis, complement and C3NeF. *N. Engl. J. Med.*, **294**, 495–7
63. Botto, M., So, A. K., Fong, K. Y., Barlow, R., Routier, R., Morley, B. J. and Walport, M. J. (1991). Homozygous hereditary C3 deficiency due to a partial gene deletion. *Complement Inflamm.*, **8**, 130 (Abstract)
64. Botto, M., Fong, K. Y., So, A. E., Rudge, A. and Walport, M. J. (1990). Molecular basis of hereditary C3 deficiency. *J. Clin. Invest.*, **86**, 1158–63
65. Sissons, J. G., West, R. J., Fallows, J., Williams, D. G., Boucher, B. J., Amos, N. and Peters, D. K. (1976). The complement abnormalities of lipodystrophy. *N. Engl. J. Med.*, **294**, 461–5
66. Ipp, M. M., Minta, J. O. and Gelfand, E. W. (1977). Disorders of the complement system in lipodystrophy. *Clin. Immunol. Immunopathol.*, **7**, 281–7
67. Fearon, D. T. (1983). Complement. *J. Allergy Clin. Immunol.*, **71**, 520–9
68. Morgan, B., Vora, J., Bennett, A., Thomas, J. and Matthews, N. (1989). A case of hereditary combined deficiency of complement components C6 and C7 in man. *Clin. Exp. Immunol.*, **75**, 396–401
69. Hobart, M. J., Fernie, B. A., Lachmann, P. J., Morgan, B. P., Orren, A. and DiScipio, R. G. (1989). C6 and C7 in normal and deficient individuals. *Complement*, **6**, 345 (Abstract)
70. Schifferli, J. A. and Hirschel, B. (1985). Meningococcal meningitis in the first case of complement deficiency. *Lancet*, **2**, 1240
71. Heist, G. D., Solis-Cohen, S. and Solis-Cohen, M. (1921). A study of the virulence of meningococci for man and of human susceptibility to meningococcic infection. *J. Immunol.*, **7**, 1–33
72. Harriman, G. R., Esser, A. F., Podack, E. R., Wunderlich, A. C., Braude, A. I., Lint, T. F. and Curd, J. G. (1981). The role of C9 in complement-mediated killing of *Neisseria*. *J. Immunol.*, **127**, 2386–90

73. Anonymous (1979). Bacterial meningitis and meningococcemia – United States, 1978. *MMWR*, **28**, 277–9
74. Wenger, J. D., Hightower, A. W., Facklam, R. R., Gaventa, S. and Broome, C. V. (1990). Bacterial meningitis in the United States, 1986: report of multistate surveillance study. *J. Infect. Dis.*, **162**, 1316–23
75. Peltola, H., Kataja, J. M. and Mäkelä, P. H. (1982). Shift in the age-distribution of meningococcal disease as predictor of an epidemic? *Lancet*, **2**, 595–7
76. Caugant, D. A., Froholm, L. O., Sacchi, C. T. and Selander, R. K. (1991). Genetic structure and epidemiology of serogroup B *Neisseria meningitidis*. In Achtman, M., Kohl, P., Marchal, C., Morelli, G., Seiler, A. and Thiesen, B. (eds). *Neisseriae 1990*, pp. 37–42. (Berlin: Walter de Gruyter & Co.)
77. Kuzemenska, P. and Kriz, B. (1987). Epidemiology of meningococcal disease in central and eastern Europe. In Vedros, N. A. (ed.) *Evolution of Meningococcal Disease*, Volume I, pp. 103–37 (Boca Raton, FL: CRC Press)
78. Fijen, C. A., Kuijper, E. J., Hannema, A. J., Sjöholm, A. G. and van Putten, J. P. (1989). Complement deficiencies in patients over ten years old with meningococcal disease due to uncommon serogroups. *Lancet*, **2**, 585–8
79. Ross, S. C., Rosenthal, J., Berberich, H. M. and Densen, P. (1987). Killing of *Neisseria meningitidis* by human neutrophils: implications for normal and complement-deficient individuals. *J. Infect. Dis.* **155**, 1266–75
80. Anonymous (1976). Analysis of endemic meningococcal disease by serogroup and evaluation of chemoprophylaxis. *J. Infect. Dis.* **134**, 201–4
81. Ross, S. C., Berberich, H. M. and Densen, P. (1985). Natural serum bactericidal activity against *Neisseria meningitidis* isolates from disseminated infections in normal and complement-deficient hosts. *J. Infect. Dis.*, **152**, 1332–5
82. Harrison, L. H. and Broome, C. V. (1987). The epidemiology of meningococcal meningitis in the U.S. civilian population. In Vedros, N. A. (ed.) *Evolution of Meningococcal Disease*, Volume I, pp. 27–45. (Boca Raton, FL: CRC Press)
83. Griffiss, J. M. (1982). Epidemic meningococcal disease: synthesis of a hypothetical immunoepidemiologic model. *Rev. Infect. Dis.*, **4**, 159–72
84. Griffiss, J. M., Brandt, B. L., Broud, D. D., Goroff, D. K. and Baker, C. J. (1984). Immune response of infants and children to disseminated infections with *Neisseria meningitidis*. *J. Infect. Dis.*, **150**, 71–9
85. Kim, J. J., Mandrell, R. E. and Griffiss, J. M. (1989). *Neisseria lactamica* and *Neisseria meningitidis* share lipooligosaccharide epitopes but lack common capsular and class 1, 2, and 3 protein epitopes. *Infect. Immun.*, **57**, 602–8
86. Goldschneider, I., Gotschlich, E. C. and Artenstein, M. S. (1969). Human immunity to the meningococcus. I. The role of humoral antibodies. *J. Exp. Med.*, **129**, 1307–26
87. Goldschneider, I., Gotschlich, E. C. and Artenstein, M. S. (1969). Human immunity to the meningococcus. II. Development of natural immunity. *J. Exp. Med.*, **129**, 1327–48
88. Platonov, A. E. and Beloborodov, V. B. (1991). Late complement component deficiency (LCCD) in the USSR: The situation in 1991. *Complement Inflamm.*, **8**, 211 (Abstract)
89. Densen, P., Zaleski, A., Sanford, M. and Frasch, C. (1991). Antibody response to meningococcal infection in late complement component deficient individuals. In Achtman, M., Kohl, P., Marchal, C., Morelli, G., Seiler, A. and Thiesen, B. (eds). *Neisseriae 1990*, pp. 671–7. (Berlin: Walter de Gruyter & Co.)
90. Andreoni, J., Kähty, H., Bruch, B. and Densen, P. (1991). Basis for recurrent meningococcal disease in complement deficiency. In *Program and Abstracts of the 31st Interscience Conference on Antimicrobial Agents and Chemotherapy*, p. 149 (Abstract)
91. Mannion, B. A., Weiss, J. and Elsbach, P. (1990). Separation of sublethal and lethal effects of polymorphonuclear leukocytes on *Escherichia coli*. *J. Clin. Invest.*, **86**, 631–41
92. Tedesco, F., Rottini, G. and Patriarca, P. (1981). Modulating effect of the late-acting components of the complement system on the bactericidal activity of human polymorphonuclear leukocytes on *E. coli* 0111:B4. *J. Immunol.*, **127**, 1910–15
93. Brandtzaeg, P., Mollnes, T. E. and Kierulf, P. (1989). Complement activation and endotoxin levels in systemic meningococcal disease. *J. Infect. Dis.*, **160**, 58–65

94. Zwahlen, A. and Waldvogel, F. A. (1984). Magnitude of bacteremia and complement activation during *Neisseria meningitidis* infection: study of two co-primary cases with different clinical presentations. *Eur. J. Clin. Microbiol.*, **3**, 439–41
95. Sullivan, T. D. and LaScolea, L. J. Jr. (1987). *Neisseria meningitidis* bacteremia in children: Quantitation of bacteremia and spontaneous clinical recovery without antibiotic therapy. *Pediatrics*, **80**, 63–7
96. Brown, D. L. and Lachmann, P. J. (1973). The behaviour of complement and platelets in lethal endotoxin shock in rabbits. *Int. Arch. Allergy*, **45**, 193–205
97. Densen, P., McRill, C. M. and Ross, S. C. (1988). Assembly of the membrane attack complex promotes decay of the alternative pathway C3 convertase on *Neisseria gonorrhoeae*. *J. Immunol.*, **141**, 3902–9
98. Swanson, J. and Goldschneider, I. (1969). The serum bactericidal system: ultrastructural changes in *Neisseria meningitidis* exposed to normal rat serum. *J. Exp. Med.*, **129**, 51–79
99. Wilson, L. A. and Spitznagel, J. K. (1968). Molecular and structural damage to *Escherichia coli* produced by antibody, complement, and lysozyme systems. *J. Bacteriol.*, **96**, 1339–48
100. Wilson, L. A. and Spitznagel, J. K. (1971). Characteristics of complement-dependent release of phospholipid from *Escherichia coli*. *Infect. Immun.*, **4**, 23–8
101. Tesh, V. L., Duncan, R. L. Jr and Morrison, D. C. (1986). The interaction of *Escherichia coli* with normal human serum: The kinetics of serum-mediated lipopolysaccharide release and its dissociation from bacterial killing. *J. Immunol.*, **137**, 1329–35
102. Brandtzaeg, P., Kierulf, P., Gaustad, P., Skulberg, A., Bruun, J. N., Halvorsen, S. and Sorensen, E. (1989). Plasma endotoxin as a predictor of multiple organ failure and death in systemic meningococcal disease. *J. Infect. Dis.*, **159**, 195–204
103. Brandtzaeg, P., Joo, G. B., Brusletto, B. and Kierulf, P. (1990). Plasminogen activator inhibitor 1 and 2, alpha-2-antiplasmin, plasminogen, and endotoxin levels in systemic meningococcal disease. *Thromb. Res.*, **57**, 271–8
104. Brandtzaeg, P., Sandset, P. M., Joo, G. B., Ovsteb, R., Abildgaard, U. and Kierulf, P. (1989). The quantitative association of plasma endotoxin, antithrombin, protein C, extrinsic pathway inhibitor and fibrinopeptide A in systemic meningococcal disease. *Thromb. Res.*, **55**, 459–70
105. Waage, A., Brandtzaeg, P., Halstensen, A., Kierulf, P. and Espevik, T. (1989). The complex pattern of cytokines in serum from patients with meningococcal septic shock. Association between interleukin 6, interleukin 1, and fatal outcome. *J. Exp. Med.*, **169**, 333–8
106. Girardin, E., Grau, G. E., Dayer, J. M., Roux-Lombard, P. and Lambert, P. H. (1988). Tumor necrosis factor and interleukin-1 in the serum of children with severe infectious purpura. *N. Engl. J. Med.*, **319**, 397–400
107. Waage, A., Halstensen, A. and Espevik, T. (1987). Association between tumour necrosis factor in serum and fatal outcome in patients with meningococcal disease. *Lancet*, **1**, 355–7
108. Engebretsen, L. F., Kierulf, P. and Brandtzaeg, P. (1986). Extreme plasminogen activator inhibitor and endotoxin values in patients with meningococcal disease. *Thromb. Res.*, **42**, 713–16
109. Waage, A., Halstensen, A., Shalaby, R., Brandtzaeg, P., Kierulf, P. and Espevik, T. (1989). Local production of tumor necrosis factor a, interleukin 1, and interleukin 6 in meningococcal meningitis: relation to the inflammatory response. *J. Exp. Med.*, **170**, 1859–67
110. Lehner, P. J., Davies, K. A., Walport, M. J., Oshisanya, D., Cope, A. P., Orren, A., Morgan, B. P. and Cohen, J. (1991). Impaired lipopolysaccharide release in a C6 deficient patient with meningococcal septicaemia; the effects of plasma transfusion and generation of anti-C6 antibody. *Clin. Exp. Immunol.* (Suppl. 1), **86**, 13–14 (Abstract)
111. Morgan, B. P. (1989). Mechanisms of tissue damage by the membrane attack complex of complement. *Complement Inflamm.*, **6**, 104–111
112. Sims, P. J. and Wiedmer, T. (1991). The response of human platelets to activated components of the complement system. *Immunol. Today*, **12**, 338–42
113. Platonov, A. E. and Gracheva, A. M. (1991). Effects of lipopolysaccharide from *N. meningitidis* on human granulocyte lysis and chemiluminescence. In Achtman, M., Kohl, P., Marchal, C., Morelli, G., Seiler, A. and Thiesen, B. (eds). *Neisseriae 1990*, pp. 627–31. (Berlin: Walter de Gruyter)
114. Hamilton, K. K., Hattori, R., Esmon, C. T. and Sims, P. J. (1990). Complement proteins C5b-9 induce vesiculation of the endothelial plasma membrane and expose catalytic surface for assembly of the prothrombinase enzyme complex. *J. Biol. Chem.*, **265**, 3809–14

115. Söderstrom, C., Braconier, J. H., Danielsson, D. and Sjöholm, A. G. (1987). Bactericidal activity for *Neisseria meningitidis* in properdin-deficient sera. *J. Infect. Dis.*, **156**, 107–12
116. Söderstrom, C., Braconier, J. H., Käthy, H., Sjöholm, A. G. and Thuresson, B. (1989). Immune response to tetravalent meningococcal vaccine: opsonic and bactericidal functions of normal and properdin deficient sera. *Eur. J. Clin. Microbiol. Infect. Dis.*, **8**, 220–4
117. Potter, P. C., Frasch, C. E., van der Sande, W. J., Cooper, R. C., Patel, Y. and Orren, A. (1990). Prophylaxis against *Neisseria meningitidis* infections and antibody responses in patients with deficiency of the sixth component of complement. *J. Infect. Dis.*, **161**, 932–7
118. Alper, C. A., Abramson, N., Johnston, R. B. Jr., Jandl, J. H. and Rosen, F. S. (1970). Increased susceptibility to infection associated with abnormalities of complement-mediated functions and of the third component of complement (C3). *N. Engl. J. Med.*, **282**, 350–4

7
Complement, immune complexes and immune complex disease

Y. C. NG and J. A. SCHIFFERLI

INTRODUCTION

Formation of immune complexes is a physiological process and an essential part of humoral immunity. Complement plays a major role in the normal processing of these complexes so that they are efficiently and safely disposed of in the reticuloendothelial system. In certain situations, however, immune aggregates come to be situated outside the reticuloendothelial system where they serve as a focus for the inflammatory response. Tissue injury ensues and is expressed by the clinical manifestations of immune complex disease.

Complement plays an important role in the inflammatory response, and its contribution to host defence mechanisms against microorganisms and other foreign bodies was the first of its functions to be recognized. Its interactions with soluble immune complexes were, however, less easy to observe. Heidelberger, in 1941[1], was first to observe that the presence of complement was associated with inhibition of immune precipitation. These observations were, however, overlooked in the succeeding two decades when significant advances were made in the understanding of the pathological effects of immune complexes in animal models of immune complex disease, such as serum sickness. At this time, interest in the biological effects of complement on immune complexes was focused on the generation of the inflammatory response and mediation of tissue injury. In the last few years, interest has turned to the effects of complement on immune complexes which might have a role in the prevention of their deposition in tissues and in their efficient removal. These reactions of complement include inhibition of immune precipitation, solubilization of immune aggregates and binding of immune complexes to erythrocyte CR1 (complement receptor type 1, C3b receptor, CD35). It has also been recognized that complement plays a role in the afferent limb of the immune response; the mechanisms for this function have yet to be elucidated but may well involve CR2 (complement receptor type 2, CD21); this receptor binds C3dg and is found on B lymphocytes.

In this chapter, we shall first describe the reactions between complement and immune complexes with particular reference to their biological consequences, namely inflammation, immune complex processing and clearance, and the immune response. This is followed by a discussion of the contribution of these reactions to the pathogenesis of immune complex disease culled from a combination of studies in animals and humans and studies performed *in vitro*.

PROCESSING OF IMMUNE COMPLEXES BY COMPLEMENT

As previously mentioned, the interactions of complement with immune complexes may result, on the one hand, in tissue injury and, on the other, in prevention of such injury. The precise factors that determine which of these effects predominate will be discussed later. The evidence that complement plays an important role in the prevention of tissue damage by immune complexes comes from the observation that subjects with genetic deficiency of complement components have a markedly increased susceptibility to immune complex disease with glomerulonephritis and SLE-like symptoms[2]. Susceptibility is greatest for those with deficiency of classical pathway components, C4, C1q, C1r or C1s, but is also increased in those with deficiency of C2 or C3. Since C4 and C2 are encoded within the major histocompatibility complex on the short arm of chromosome 6, it has been suggested that the association of deficiencies of C2 and C4 with immune complex diseases is due to the genetic linkage of those abnormalities with an immune-response gene. However, this reasoning does not explain the association of similar diseases with deficiencies in C1q, C1r, C1s or C3, since the genes encoding these proteins are located outside the major histocompatibility complex. This suggests that the susceptibility of these individuals to immune complex disease is likely to reflect a deficiency of complement function.

The protective role of complement is probably related to the prevention of deposition and aggregation of immune complexes in tissues[2]. Additional functions of complement that may contribute to susceptibility to immune complex diseases include the contribution of C3 to the localization of antigen/antibody complexes in the germinal centres of lymph nodes, an effect that may be important in the generation of B-cell memory[3]. Complement also appears to have a role in the induction of some immune responses: guinea-pigs genetically deficient in C2 or C4 have an abnormal antibody response to low doses of a T-dependent antigen, phage X174[4,5]. The antibody level is low with a decreased primary peak response. There is a weak secondary response with no amplification and no switch from IgM to IgG. The abnormal secondary response is partially corrected by injection of normal guinea-pig serum which contains complement. Further evidence comes from the demonstration of impaired immune responses in a subject with total C4 deficiency[6], and of defective immune responsiveness to hepatitis B surface antigen in subjects with partial C4 deficiency[7]. Such effects of complement on the antibody response may in turn affect susceptibility to immune complex disease. Finally complement, together with C-reactive protein, is involved in the disposal of DNA released by cell death[8].

Complement reacts with immune complexes to inhibit immune precipitation, solubilize immune aggregates and bind immune complexes to erythrocyte CR1. These reactions serve to prevent local accumulation of immune complexes in tissues outside the reticuloendothelial system by producing soluble complexes which are removed not only by simple diffusion away from the site of formation but also by interactions with complement receptors. CR1 acts both as a transport mechanism and as a mechanism for decreasing the phlogistic potential of immune complexes.

The covalent binding of C4b and C3b to immune complexes is critical to the efficacy of their processing by complement. This focuses complement activation to the biological surface and provides the ligand for interactions with complement receptors. C4 exists as two isotypes, C4A and C4B, encoded by two separate genes. Structural differences between the two isotypes reside in a small number of amino acid differences that are clustered around the thiolester region and are expressed functionally by a difference in affinity for acceptor amino and hydroxyl groups. C4A binds preferentially to amino groups and so interacts more efficiently with immune complexes, whereas C4B binds preferentially to hydroxyl groups and so is more efficient in haemolysis[9–12].

Historical background

The significance of the role of complement in prevention of immune complex diseases has been recognized only relatively recently. However, descriptions of these various interactions between complement and immune complexes have a much longer history.

Incorporation of complement proteins (or fragments) into antigen–antibody aggregates was recognized decades ago when it was shown that immune precipitates formed in normal serum, contained more measurable NH_2 than those formed in heated serum. Heidelberger observed that the presence of complement reduced the rate of immune precipitation[1]. This phenomenon was described again twenty years later by investigators who were developing radioimmunoassays and who observed that complement interfered with the precipitation reaction[13–15]. In 1975, Miller and Nussenzweig described a new function of complement – solubilization of immune precipitates – a reaction which required mainly alternative pathway function[16]. This was followed by the elucidation of the role of the classical pathway in complement-mediated inhibition of immune precipitation[17].

The complement-mediated immune adherence reaction similarly has a very long history (reviewed in Ref. 18). In 1915, Bull described binding reactions of microorganisms to murine platelets in the presence of serum; this binding was shown later to be abolished by heating the serum (which removed functional complement). Adherence of microorganisms to human erythrocytes was described in 1930 and the role of complement in this reaction was clearly demonstrated by Nelson in 1953[19]. He observed similar reactions in a rhesus monkey injected with pneumococci coated with specific antibodies; these bacteria bound rapidly to erythrocytes *in vivo*. In 1980, Fearon isolated the molecule involved in the adherence reactions of human erythrocytes, the C3b receptor (complement receptor type 1, CR1, CD35)[20]. This receptor bound large immune complexes and its role in the transport of immune complexes in primates was demonstrated by Hebert and collaborators (reviewed in Ref. 21). It also functions in the catabolism of C3b bound to immune complexes[22].

The immune complex lattice

When antigen meets antibody at equivalence or in antibody excess, rapid precipitation occurs. This reaction requires intact IgG molecules as distinct from $F(ab')_2$ fragments suggesting that Fc–Fc interactions are more important in catalysing the reaction[23,24]. Within seconds of the antigen–antibody reaction, complexes of various sizes are formed. Initial precipitation is due to secondary forces involving the Fc portions of IgG and various experiments suggest that nucleation phenomena are involved, i.e. large complexes inducing the aggregation of small complexes on their surface[25]. Indeed, these interactions bring the reacting molecules into close proximity which is followed by formation of an infinite lattice of alternating antigen–antibody bonds between antigen that is multivalent and antibody which has at least two combining sites. The ‘infinite lattice’ is responsible for insolubility of immune complexes. Such a lattice can also build up, starting with a ‘planted’ antigen or antibody; such *in-situ* formation of immune complexes has been demonstrated in experimental glomerulonephritis in which planting antigens (or antibodies) is the initial event that, if exposed successively to antibody or antigen, leads to large microscopically visible deposits.

Many immune complex diseases are characterized by continuous antibody overproduction, e.g. SLE and essential mixed cryoglobulinaemia. In such diseases, large immune complexes are formed in antibody excess and are likely to be complement activating. The devastating consequences of ‘immobilization’ of immune complexes in various organs, either because of *in-situ* formation or because of deposition from the blood stream are well recognized. Efficient removal of immune complexes is clearly important. For this to happen efficiently, immune complexes should be soluble and show little tendency for further aggregation. This is achieved by complement-mediated inhibition of immune precipitation.

Inhibition of immune precipitation

The immune precipitation that occurs when radio-labelled antigen is mixed with antibody is inhibited if the reaction occurs in normal human serum[26] incubated at 37°C. This effect is blocked by EDTA or by heating the serum at 56°C for 30 min, both of which abrogate complement function (Figure 7.1). The soluble complexes formed in this way are very large (greater than 19S, i.e. more than

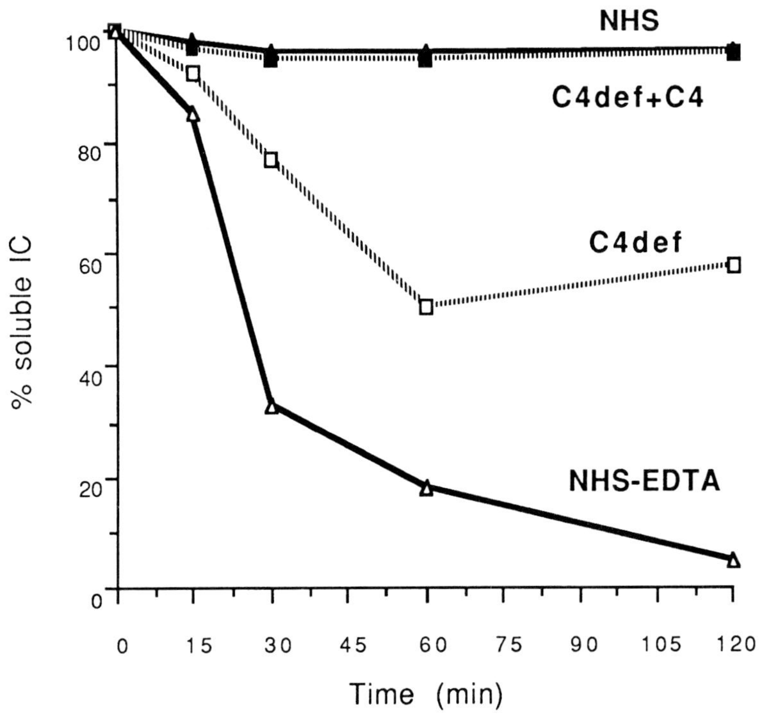

Figure 7.1 Inhibition of immune precipitation by complement at the time of the antigen–antibody reaction. Radio-labelled antigen and specific antibody were added successively into different serum samples that were preincubated at 37°C. The percentage of soluble immune complex (IC) was determined after various time intervals. Immune precipitation was blocked in normal serum (NHS), but proceeded rapidly in the absence of complement function (NHS-EDTA). Note the defective IIP in C4-deficient (C4def) serum which was restored by the addition of purified C4.

1000 kDa) and, besides containing antigen and antibody molecules, they also contain various complement fragments – C1 subcomponents, C4 and C3 fragments; this suggests that complement is incorporated into the immune complex lattice. Binding of C3 fragments appears to be necessary for maintaining the solubility of immune complexes. The binding is covalent and, in one set of circumstances at least (ovalbumin, rabbit anti-ovalbumin immune complexes), involves amide bonds between C3b and the IgG heavy chain[27].

The mechanism by which complement, in particular C3b, modifies immune complex solubility is, however, unclear. Possible explanations are that complement fragments interfere with antigen–antibody bonds, either by changing the antibody valency from 2 to 1[26] or by binding to antigen and masking epitopes, thereby reducing the valency of the antigen. They may also interfere with Fc–Fc interactions that have been shown to catalyse the rapid aggregation of immune complexes[23]. Inhibition of immune precipitation by complement does not, in general, reduce the size of the immune complex – in fact, large soluble tetanus toxoid/anti-tetanus toxoid complexes formed in antibody excess actually increase in size in the presence of complement[28].

Activation of complement during inhibition of immune precipitation results in three major effects which occur in sequence. First, macromolecular C1 delays immune aggregation in a dose-dependent manner in both its activated and non-activated forms[29]. This effect is particularly striking during the initial minutes of the precipitation reaction and is not seen after prolonged antigen–antibody reaction. This suggests that the macromolecular C1 complex reduces the Fc–Fc interactions that are responsible for immediate aggregation of the complex but has little effect on the formation of the infinite lattice which occurs at a slower rate and is associated with redistribution of antigen–antibody bonds. The effect of C1 on inhibition of immune precipitation is relatively transient due to the action of C1-inhibitor; C1-inhibitor disrupts activated C1 to leave only C1q on the complex[30], a molecule that is well known to enhance immune precipitation[31]. This effect of C1-inhibitor occurs rapidly and resembles that of EDTA, a calcium chelator, which prevents assembly of the C1 complex. Thus, under physiological conditions, the effect of C1 on inhibition of immune precipitation is likely to be transient.

The second step occurs with the cleavage of C4 by activated C1. A small fraction of the C4b generated binds covalently to immune complexes – some of this binding occurs to the heavy chain of IgG; using a fluid-phase system, C4A3 was shown to have a greater binding efficiency that C4B1 and to bind IgG predominantly by amide linkage, whereas C4B1 bound to IgG by either amide or ester bonds[32]. Binding of C4b to the immune complex has little effect on solubility of the complex, but it allows assembly of the classical pathway C3 convertase (C4b2a)[30]. This is followed by cleavage of C3 generating C3b, which binds to the immune complex, rendering it soluble. C3 activation is a vital step in inhibition of immune precipitation and C3-deficient serum will not support this reaction. Similarly, sera deficient in C2 or C4 which are unable to form a C3 convertase, are unable to sustain inhibition of immune precipitation[33].

The third step involves amplification of complement activation via the alternative pathway around the C3b molecules deposited on the immune complex. This is associated with the formation of even smaller immune complexes[34] and probably involves the binding of additional C3b molecules.

Thus, there is an absolute requirement for the classical complement pathway in inhibition of immune precipitation. In contrast, the alternative pathway is not essential, but, under normal circumstances, its function is associated with the formation of smaller opsonized immune complexes. Alternative pathway activity is reduced in properdin-deficient sera and absent in factor D-depleted sera. Despite this, soluble immune complexes are formed in these sera.

These results have been confirmed with purified components of both classical and alternative pathways[30,35].

Neither the terminal components of complement (C5, C6, C7, C8 and C9)[36] nor the various cellular receptors for complement that are present on erythrocytes (CR1, decay accelerating factor, DAF) have any measurable effect on inhibition of immune precipitation.

Clearly, the isotypes of the antibody in the immune complex influence inhibition of immune precipitation, since only isotypes that activate the classical pathway will exhibit this activity. Thus, inhibition of immune precipitation occurs with IgG and IgM complexes but not with IgA complexes[37]. Other factors affecting the efficacy of this reaction include the nature of the antigen, the affinity of the antibody, the concentration of the reactants and their relative ratio. Finally, rheumatoid factors have been shown to interfere with inhibition of immune precipitation[38,39]. IgM rheumatoid factor accelerates the formation of large insoluble complexes because it crosslinks the Fc pieces of different IgG antibody molecules in the immune complex. In addition, although it produces efficient C1 activation and C4 cleavage, C3 convertase formation and C3 activation are reduced markedly[40,41]. Reduced convertase formation may occur because of lack of available C4b binding sites on IgM-rheumatoid factor. It has also been shown that DNA/IgM complexes consume more complement but bind less C3 than DNA/IgG complexes[41].

Solubilization of immune aggregates

Failure of inhibition of immune precipitation leads to the formation of insoluble aggregates which can activate the alternative pathway of complement. Miller and Nussenzweig showed that preformed immune aggregates could be dissolved by complement[16]. Solubilization of immune precipitates is associated with covalent binding of C3b to antigen and antibody molecules, which reduces the various forces that hold the aggregate together (reviewed in Ref. 42). A fraction of antibody is released from the complex during solubilization but the mechanism by which bound C3b interferes with primary antigen–antibody bonds is unclear. The solubilization reaction is relatively inefficient and requires a large amount of complement activation. Approximately one molecule of C3b has to bind per antibody molecule in order to produce solubilization. Since probably no

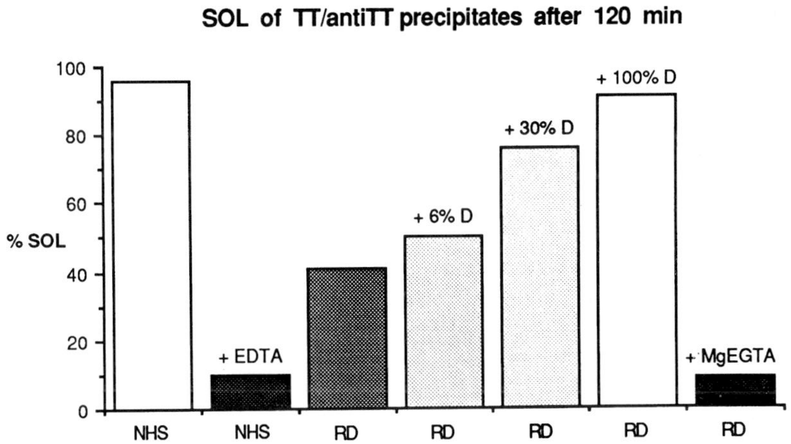

Figure 7.2 Solubilization of immune toxoid (TT)/human anti-tetanus toxoid antibody immune precipitate in various serum samples. The precipitates were incubated for 60 min at 37°C. Solubilization, as observed in normal serum (NHS), is abolished in the absence of complement function (+EDTA). In serum depleted of factor D (RD) of the alternative pathway, the precipitate is partially solubilized, but, when classical pathway function is blocked (RD + MgEGTA), the RD cannot sustain solubilization.

more than 10% of activated C3 binds to the immune aggregate, large quantities of complement are consumed during solubilization. C3b is bound to the Fc piece of the IgG antibody in the immune complex in the form of covalent dimers[43], which is a high-affinity binding site for C5[44]. Thus C5 activation and C5a and C5b-9 membrane attack complex formation occur during solubilization. The massive complement activation required for solubilization can be generated only by alternative pathway amplification; insoluble immune aggregates appear to possess 'protected' surfaces to which factor H has limited access, thereby providing sites where amplification of complement activation is favoured[45]. All six proteins of the alternative pathway, including properdin, are required. Although partial solubilization by classical pathway activation alone has been demonstrated using immune precipitates of human antibodies[46] (Figure 7.2), activation of the classical pathway on its own does not in general suffice. Indeed, the classical pathway does not appear to be necessary for solubilization since serum deficient in C1, C4 or C2 shows no impairment in solubilization except for a slight delay in its initiation, which suggests that the rapid deposition of C3b by classical pathway activation allows early recruitment of the alternative pathway. In the absence of an intact classical pathway, the initial deposition of C3b depends on the efficient fluid-phase alternative pathway turnover and therefore occurs more slowly.

Although the dissociation of Fc–Fc interactions is thought to be important in solubilization, disruption of primary antigen–antibody bonds must occur as the extent of solubilization shows an inverse correlation with the affinity of the antibody in the immune complex[47]. Furthermore, immune complexes in which the antigen and antibody are linked covalently through the antigen binding site cannot be solubilized despite activating complement[48].

Two observations of biological relevance are worth noting: first the capacity for complement to inhibit immune precipitation is ten times greater than its capacity for solubilization reflecting the ease of prevention of Fc–Fc and antigen–antibody interactions compared with disruption of a preformed lattice. Second, the reactions differ in their inflammatory potential since inhibition of immune precipitation generates less of the anaphylatoxins, C3a and C5a, than does solubilization[49]. Thus, solubilization of an immune aggregate is associated with a greater inflammatory response than inhibition of immune precipitation.

Immune adherence receptor on human erythrocytes

Immune complexes coated with C3b (opsonized complexes) bind to CR1 (immune adherence). The majority of circulating CR1 in primates is present on erythrocytes. Erythrocyte CR1 serves two functions: first, it contributes to the catabolism of bound C3b by factor I, thereby reducing the phlogistic potential of immune complexes. Second, it functions as a transport mechanism for opsonized immune complexes to the reticuloendothelial system where the complexes are safely disposed.

The ligands for CR1 are C3b, C4b and iC3b[50]; with C3b having the greatest affinity for the receptor. In humans, CR1 is present on erythrocytes, polymorphonuclear leukocytes, monocytes, B lymphocytes, some T lymphocytes, glomerular podocytes and follicular dendritic cells. On all these cells, monospecific rabbit antibody immunoprecipitates a single membrane protein of apparently identical size[30,51–53]. CR1 is a membrane glycoprotein which exists in 4 allotypic forms, with sizes of 160 kDa, 210 kDa, 250 kDa and 290 kDa[54]. Erythrocyte CR1 also demonstrates numerical polymorphism within the normal population with a range between 200 and 1200 receptors per cell[55,56]; this is associated with two codominant alleles that are identified by restriction fragment length polymorphism analysis and which correspond respectively with high and low CR1 numbers. The molecular basis of the structural and numerical polymorphisms of CR1 has been defined[54].

In vitro studies

Insight into the biological functions of CR1 was first obtained from *in vitro* studies: isolated CR1 was shown to accelerate the decay of the C3 convertases of both the classical and alternative pathways[57,58]. A similar effect on the classical pathway C3 convertase was demonstrated for CR1 that was membrane associated[59].

CR1 was also shown to act as cofactor for factor I in the cleavage of substrate-bound C3b to iC3b and also the cofactor for factor I in the cleavage of iC3b to C3dg which is followed by release of C3c, the C3d remaining bound to substrate[60–63]. CR1 appears to be an obligatory cofactor in the latter reaction. CR1 has an analogous function in the I-mediated cleavage of C4b to iC4b and C4c[57].

Opsonized immune complexes bind to human erythrocyte CR1[64] and undergo processing which alters their biological properties[65]. During processing, bound immune complexes are released from erythrocytes by serum and the released complexes are unable to rebind to erythrocytes as C3b has been degraded to C3dg which has no affinity for CR1. One consequence of this release reaction is that potentially misleading information may be derived from laboratory measurements of circulating immune complexes in serum or plasma samples since the immune complexes detected may have been released from erythrocytes after venesection.

Monomeric C3b has little affinity for CR1 (approximately 10^6 L/mol but the affinity is increased several fold for dimers and trimers of C3b[66]. These observations suggest that the efficient attachment of a ligand bearing C3b is multimeric. Using DNA/anti-DNA complexes, Edberg *et al.*[67] have suggested that CR1 distribution on erythrocytes is not random, but is distributed in small clusters of approximately 10 units which would allow multimeric binding. CR1 was subsequently shown by immunofluorescent and electron microscopic techniques to be distributed in multiple well-defined clusters (8–20 clusters per erythrocyte) (Figure 7.3)[68,69]. Such clustering would allow multimeric binding to opsonized immune complexes and is consistent with the relatively high measured affinity of this interaction[70] of 10^{11} L/mol. Furthermore, clustering of CR1 may represent one mechanism of control of binding opsonized complexes. Polymorphonuclear leukocytes express 2–10-fold more CR1 than erythrocytes. They bind opsonized immune complexes less efficiently, probably because their

Figure 7.3 Localization of CR1 on erythrocytes by electron microscopy, using immunogold. Note the clustered distribution of CR1 (×10 000)

CR1 are not clustered[71]. This mechanism may inhibit activation of polymorphonuclear leukocytes by complexes in the circulation[71].

Activation of complement by the classical pathway is required to coat immune complexes with C3b. This has been demonstrated using purified complement proteins, and sera deficient in or depleted of various complement proteins[28,72]. In the absence of C3, significant binding does not occur, suggesting that C4b is not an important physiological ligand, either because its affinity for CR1 is low or because it is rapidly inactivated in plasma. As with inhibition of immune precipitation, immune adherence does not require alternative pathway activation (Figure 7.4). Indeed, BSA/anti-BSA complexes formed in the presence of serum lacking alternative pathway function due to depletion of factor D, bind more efficiently to human erythrocytes than complexes formed in the presence of normal human serum[73]. The reason for this observation is unclear but one possible explanation is that immune complexes formed in the

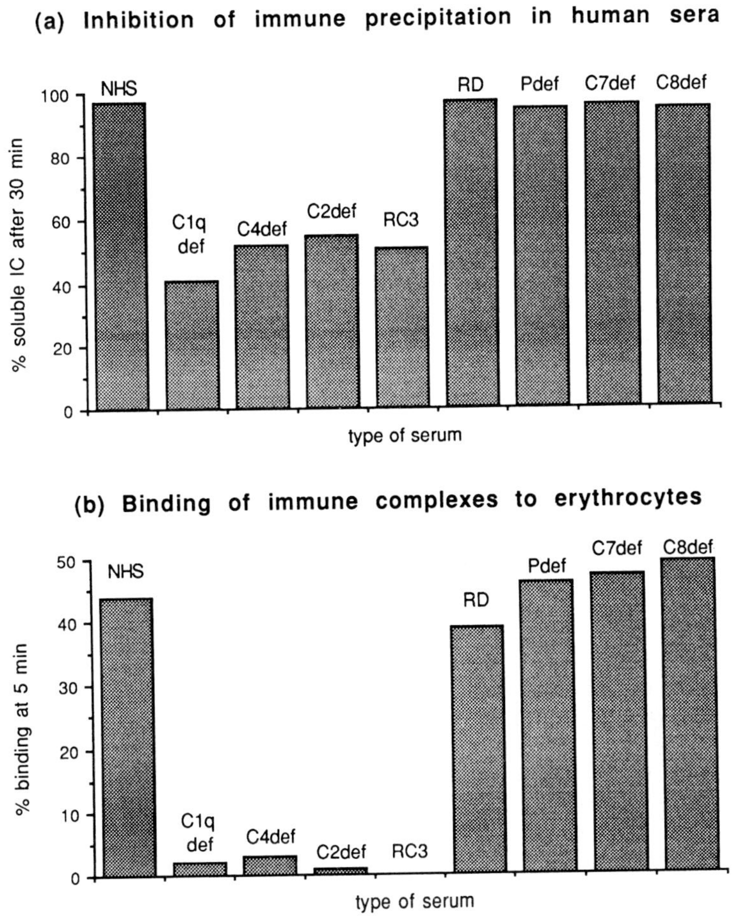

Figure 7.4 Inhibition of immune precipitation (**a**) and immune adherence (**b**) in sera deficient (def) or depleted (R) in different complement proteins. Both functions require classical pathway activity, and are abnormal in sera deficient in C1q, C2 or C4, or depleted in C3

presence of an intact alternative pathway are larger than those formed in its absence and larger complexes, all other factors being equal, have greater binding efficiency for CR1.

The characteristics of immune complexes engaging in immune adherence have been studied using a variety of systems (with varying degrees of potential physiological relevance). These include BSA/rabbit anti-BSA (IgG), tetanus toxoid (TT)/human anti-TT (IgG), human IgG/human IgM rheumatoid factor, DNA/anti-DNA (IgG and IgM), dinitrophenyl (DNP)-BSA/mouse monoclonal anti-DNP (IgG and IgA), hepatitis B surface antigen (HBSAg)/human anti-HSB (IgG) and human IgG/rabbit anti-human IgG (IgG)[28,40,63,74–78]. Clearly the details of binding and release reactions differ with the different systems used; nevertheless, it appears that in each of these systems, efficiency of complement activation and immune complex size are the most important characteristics determining binding to CR1. The effect of size on the efficiency of binding has been clearly demonstrated by Lennek *et al.*[77] who used DNA/anti-DNA complexes which do not precipitate because anti-DNA antibodies do not crosslink DNA strands. Thus, when excess antibodies are used, the final size of the immune complex is directly proportional to the size of antigen. The sizes of the DNA fragments used in this study ranged from 200 paired bases (approximately 140 kDa) to 9000 paired bases (approximately 6000 kDa) and it was shown that the ability of opsonized immune complexes to bind to ECR1 was directly proportional to the size of the complex. Complexes which bound to erythrocytes were larger than 100S (100 000 kDa).

The structure of immune complexes is also affected by the nature of the antigen, as well as the relative concentrations of antigen and antibody.

The isotype of the antibody in an immune complex influences its ability to bind to ECR1. For example, immune complexes formed with murine monoclonal IgA anti-DNP and DNP-BSA do not activate the classical pathway[47] and therefore cannot bind to ECR1[76].

Transport of immune complexes in animal models

The interactions between erythrocyte CR1 and immune complexes *in vivo* were first demonstrated clearly by the experiments of Cornacoff *et al.*[74] Radiolabelled preformed immune complexes were infused into the aorta of baboons and bound rapidly to erythrocytes. Immune complexes were stripped from the erythrocytes during passage through the liver and, to a lesser extent, the spleen, leaving the erythrocytes free to recirculate. There was no evidence of trapping of the erythrocytes which transported the immune complexes. The role of complement in this process was demonstrated using baboons decomplemented with cobra venom factor[75]. In this situation, infused immune complexes were unable to bind to erythrocytes, and were cleared more rapidly from the circulation and deposited in tissues outside the reticuloendothelial system, principally in the kidney and lung. These findings are consistent with previous observations that the deposition of injected soluble immune complexes in the liver of rabbits was significantly reduced if the antibody in the complex was reduced and alkylated so that complement activation did not occur[79]. Similar effects were demonstrated using IgA immune complexes that fixed poorly to erythrocyte CR1[76]. These experiments showed that, in primates, opsonized immune complexes may bind to erythrocyte CR1 and be transported to the reticuloendothelial system for safe removal. Failure of this sytem (either because of decomplementation or because the injected complexes were non-complement fixing) was associated with deposition of immune complexes in tissues with potential to cause tissue injury. Furthermore, binding to erythrocyte CR1 also seems to provide a mechanism for removal of deposited complexes from tissues. It has been demonstrated that DNA–anti-DNA complexes deposited in baboon kidneys are removed from the organ bound to erythrocytes[80].

These experiments provide clear evidence for the existence of an immune complex transport system in the circulation of primates; furthermore, the erythrocyte – the transport vehicle – does not appear to be modified by interactions with the opsonized immune complexes. Rodent models of immune complex handling demonstrate a similar system although, in these animals, the immune adherence receptor is located on platelets. Thus, when poorly soluble immune complexes are injected into mice, they bind rapidly to platelets[81]. Such binding was absent in NZB/W lupus mice that were hypocomplementaemic. Similar binding of injected immune complexes to platelets *in vivo* has been demonstrated in rabbits and guinea-pigs. However, platelets, unlike the erythrocytes in primates, are activated by this binding and aggregate rapidly. This is consistent with the demonstrated role of platelets in inducing or perpetuating vascular injury in the many rodent immune complex models studied to date, so that their relevance to human pathology is doubtful.

The characteristics of immune complexes that evade or engage the transport system have been defined using DNA/human anti-DNA immune complexes[67,82]. Variations in size and complement-activating properties of the complexes have a profound influence on the binding to erythrocytes (or platelets in rodents) and their elimination rate. It has been suggested that the pathogenetic immune complexes are those of intermediate size that are sufficiently large to activate complement but too small to bind efficiently to erythrocytes. Such complexes would have time to circulate freely through the microcirculation where they could be trapped[82].

Binding to erythrocytes also occurs when immune complexes are formed in the presence of complement (nascent immune complexes), a situation more likely than preformed complexes to reflect physiological conditions. Sequential infusion of DNA and anti-DNA resulted in the formation of immune complexes that bound to erythrocytes[83]. Other experiments have shown that little or no binding of nascent immune complexes formed in the presence of complement to erythrocytes, and any binding occurred more slowly than with preformed immune complexes[84–86]. The reasons for these observations are unclear but may include the smaller size of such complexes and inadequate clustering of C3b. These observations suggest that *in vivo* the ECR1 transport mechanism may be required for immune complexes formed with large and perhaps relatively insoluble antigens.

Transport of immune complexes in humans

Processing of preformed immune complexes has been studied in humans by injecting radio-labelled soluble tetanus (TT)/anti-TT immune complexes intravenously as a bolus. Binding to erythrocyte CR1 is rapid with maximum binding occurring within one minute. The proportion of immune complexes bound to erythrocytes at one minute varied between individuals and was directly proportional to the numbers of erythrocyte CR1 (Figure 7.5). In other words, individuals with low erythrocyte CR1 numbers had a smaller proportion of erythrocyte-bound complexes than individuals with high erythrocyte CR1 numbers[70,87]. This finding is consistent with the previously described dynamic nature of the interaction between opsonized immune complexes and CR1. Opsonized immune complexes are released from CR1 by catabolism of C3b to iC3b or C3dg;

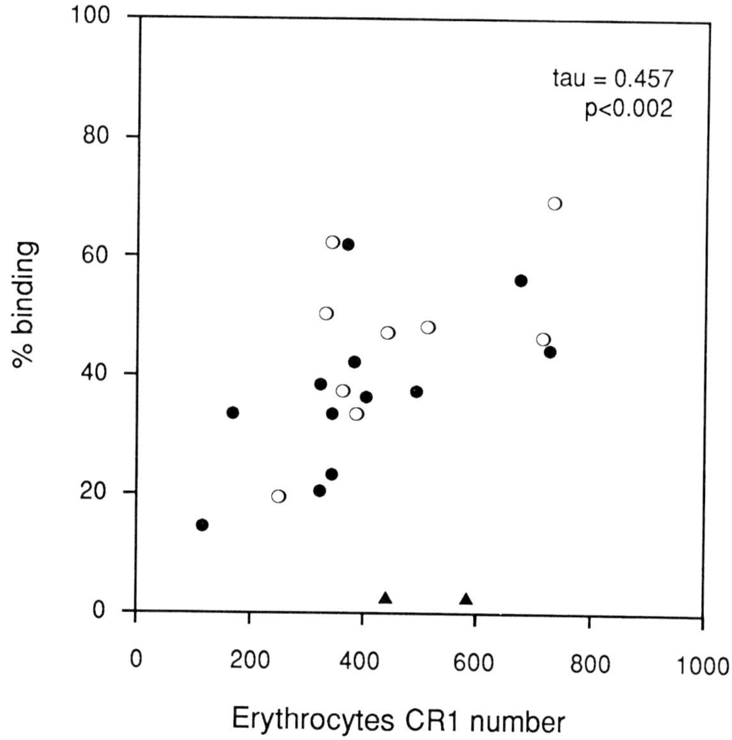

Figure 7.5 Correlation between erythrocyte CR1 number and immune adherence observed *in vivo* 1 min after the injection of ICs in normal individuals (○) and in patients with various diseases (●), excluding the 2 complement-deficient patients (▲). Adapted from Ref. 91

however, rebinding to erythrocytes occurs as further molecules of C3b are bound to the same immune complex. Thus, the proportion of complexes bound at any given time represents an equilibrium between release and rebinding that is determined by the number of erythrocyte CR1, rebinding being favoured by high erythrocyte CR1[88]. It is also consistent with the finding, in the same study, that, when complexes were injected prebound to autologous erythrocytes, they were rapidly released during the first minute in proportions that were inversely proportional to erythrocyte CR1 numbers, i.e. individuals with the lowest erythrocyte CR1 released the highest proportion of prebound complexes[87].

A further effect of decreased erythrocyte CR1 and hypocomplementaemia was demonstrated in the same studies. The elimination rate of TT/anti-TT complexes was best explained by a simple compartmental model: in most normal individuals studied, complexes were rapidly cleared from the circulation in a monoexponential fashion (11% complexes cleared/min)[87], which was similar to clearance kinetics demonstrated in monkeys injected with DNA/anti-DNA complexes[89]. In a significant number of patients, especially those with very low erythrocyte CR1 or those with a genetically determined deficiency of a classical pathway component, a large proportion of injected complexes disappeared from

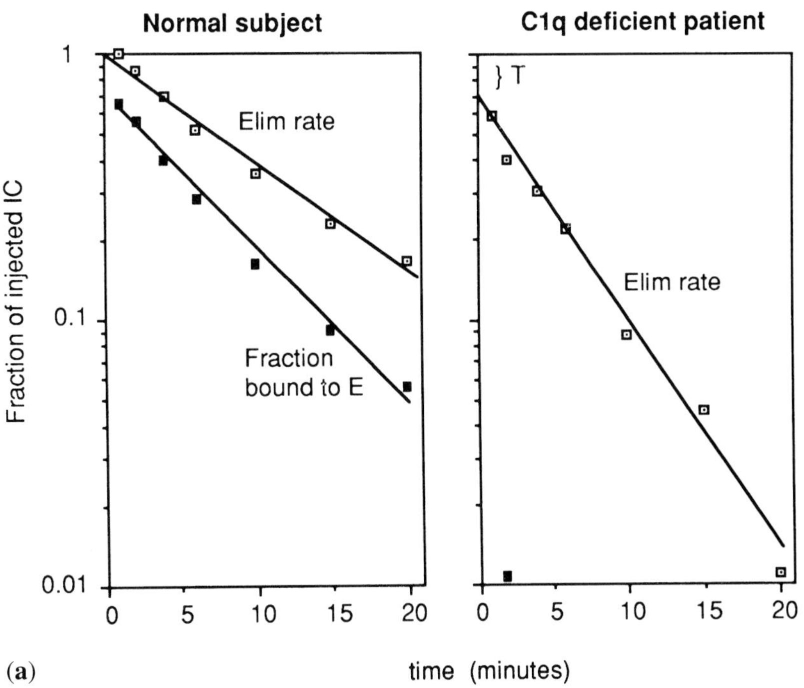

(a)

Figure 7.6 (**a**) Elimination and immune adherence of TT/anti-TT complexes injected into a normal individual. ⊡ Fraction of complexes remaining in whole blood; ■ fraction attached to erythrocytes. Upon i.v. injection, ICs were cleared at a monoexponential rate and a large fraction bound immediately to erythrocytes (in less than 1 min). The same study was performed in a C1q-deficient patient: ICs did not bind to erythrocytes, a fraction of them disappeared almost immediately (trapping: T), and the remainder were cleared at a fast rate.

the circulation within the first minute – this suggested that complexes were rapidly 'trapped' in tissues outside the reticuloendothelial system; however the precise disposition of the complexes could not be demonstrated (Figure 7.6).

Transfer of immune complexes to the reticuloendothelial system

The experiments of Cornacoff *et al.*[74] demonstrated clearly that most of the immune complexes bound to circulating erythrocytes were removed in the liver and spleen. Here, it is assumed that the complexes were transferred to fixed macrophages by which they were phagocytosed. These reactions have been studied in chimpanzees injected with DNA/anti-DNA immune complexes[90]. Erythrocyte-bound complexes were efficiently stripped off erythroyctes in the reticuloendothelial system in a reaction that involved FcγR-III receptors since it was blocked by the appropriate monoclonal antibody.

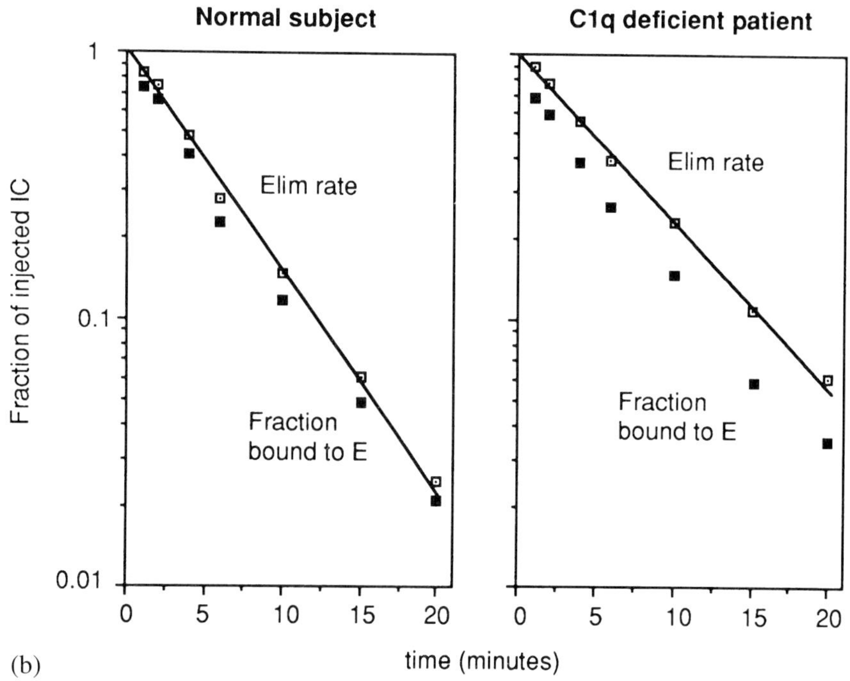

(b)

Figure 7.6 (*contd.*) (**b**) TT/anti-TT complexes bound to autologous erythrocytes were injected in the normal subject. The elimination rate was again monoexponential, and only a few ICs were released from the erythrocytes. The same study performed in the C1q-deficient patient produced a result almost identical to that of the normal subject, indicating that the absence of complement was responsible for the abnormalities observed in (a).

Transfer of immune complexes to monocytes/macrophages has also been studied *in vitro*[91]. In this system, transfer was found to be most efficient in the presence of factor I, suggesting that the catabolism of bound C3b to iC3b or C3dg was an important part of the transfer reaction. This is consistent with the different affinities of iC3b for CR1 and CR3 which are low and high respectively. Since macrophages express CR3, whereas erythrocytes do not, transfer of complexes to macrophages is favoured. This reaction also appears to involve Fc receptors and CR4 since it is inhibited by monoclonal antibodies to each of these entities. In this system, the number of erythrocyte CR1 was decreased following removal of immune complexes by macrophages, suggesting that proteolysis of CR1 had occurred.

PATHOGENESIS OF HUMAN IMMUNE COMPLEX DISEASE

In light of the foregoing account of the various mechanisms by which complement contributes to the normal processing of immune complexes, it is of interest to focus on the ways in which these reactions contribute to the pathogenesis of immune complex disease. In disease involving exogenous antigen, such as subacute bacterial endocarditis, shunt nephritis and serum sickness, excess immune complexes are formed following an appropriate antibody response stimulated by foreign antigens. However, in immune complex diseases that involve endogenous antigens, such as SLE and essential mixed cryoglobulinaemia, the underlying pathogenetic mechanisms are less clear. Recently, interest has centred on complement and its role in immune complex processing.

Systemic lupus erythematosus (SLE)

In SLE, the autoantigens involved are native DNA and a variety of other nuclear antigens[82]. The evidence for a pathogenetic role for immune complexes comes from the demonstration of DNA and specific antibody in affected tissues, in association with C3 and, in some instances, with the membrane attack complex[92,93]. Circulating immune complexes are detectable in patients with SLE; it is frequently associated with hypocomplementaemia which is associated with increased disease activity[94]. However, in most SLE patients, positive C1q binding assays for immune complexes are due to the presence of circulating C1q autoantibodies, which also produce hypocomplementaemia[95].

Perturbations of complement interactions with immune complexes that may contribute to immune complex tissue deposition in SLE include total or partial genetic deficiency of a classical pathway component, acquired hypocomplementaemia secondary to consumption by immune complexes, decreased numbers of erythrocyte CR1 and the presence of various circulating inhibitors that interfere either with complement activation or the interaction between opsonized immune complexes and erythrocyte CR1.

As mentioned previously, genetic deficiency of a classical pathway component represents the strongest identified susceptibility factor for SLE. From the foregoing account of the reactions between complement and immune complexes, it is evident that deficiency of the classical pathway results not only in deficient inhibition of immune precipitation but also in deficient erythrocyte transport of immune complexes.

Partial genetic C4 deficiency is also a susceptibility factor, albeit weaker than complete deficiency. The suggestion that possession of a null allele for C4A could represent a susceptibility factor for SLE first came from the observation by Fielder *et al.*[96] that patients with SLE had an increased incidence of the haplotype A1 B8 C4AQO DR3. In these studies, however, the possibility could not be excluded that the increased susceptibility was due to linkage with an immune response gene. Subsequently, studies in other ethnic groups[97,98] have provided further evidence for the contribution of the C4A null allele *per se* as a susceptibility factor, which is independent of associations with other genes located in the major histocompatibility complex[97–100]. Furthermore, a decreased ability to handle immune complexes in these subjects is consistent with the demonstrated differences in function between C4A and C4B isotypes previously described. Thus C4A is more efficient than C4B in opsonizing immune complexes, so that they may bind to erythrocyte CR1, as well as in inhibiting immune precipitation[101].

Patients with SLE have significantly decreased erythrocyte CR1; whilst there may be a genetic contribution to this decreased CR1[55], there is also undoubtedly an acquired element to the CR1 reduction as demonstrated by family and twin studies[102–105]. Further, CR1 has been shown to be lost from normal erythrocytes transfused into patients with active SLE and haemolytic anaemia[106] and CR1 numbers in SLE vary inversely with disease activity[104,107–109]. Furthermore, erythrocyte CR1 has been shown to decrease following transfer of immune complexes from erythrocytes to monocytes *in vitro*[91] suggesting a mechanism for a relationship between acquired low erythrocyte CR1 and immune complex carriage.

The effects of hypocomplementaemia and erythrocyte CR1 number have been demonstrated using [^{125}I]tetanus toxoid (TT)/anti-TT immune complexes injected intravenously into humans[70,87]. Patients with SLE demonstrated the rapid disappearance of a significant proportion of complexes, occurring within the first minute following injection. Such 'trapping' was associated with low erythrocyte CR1, low serum complement and decreased binding of immune complexes to erythrocytes.

In patients with homozygous deficiency of C1q or C2, clinically expressed as SLE, binding of injected complexes to erythrocytes could not be demonstrated and there was significant trapping of complexes within the first minutes, associated with unusually fast elimination rates[87]. However, when immune complexes were opsonized with normal human serum and bound to autologous erythrocytes *in vitro* prior to injection into the same subjects, trapping did not occur and the elimination rate returned to normal. This suggests that trapping and the unusually fast elimination in these subjects represents abnormal deposition of complexes outside the circulation (Figure 7.7).

A variety of other factors have been detected in sera from patients with SLE that may contribute to defective function of the erythrocyte CR1 system; these include a circulating inhibitor of fluid-phase complement amplification[110]; this is a non-IgG molecule that appears to potentiate the interaction of factor H with C3b, thereby inhibiting opsonization of complexes. A lysine-binding protein has also been described in sera of some patients with SLE that inhibits the binding of normally-opsonized immune complexes to normal erythrocytes[111]. Autoantibodies against erythrocyte CR1 have also been described in patients with SLE[112]; these would inhibit the binding of opsonized complexes to erythrocytes. Thus it can be seen that many factors may contribute to defective immune adherence in SLE; this allows increased tissue deposition of circulating complexes as well as preventing their processing by factor I so that the circulating complexes retain their phlogistic potential. *In vivo* studies of the clearance of injected immune complexes demonstrate that deficiencies of complement and the erythrocyte CR1 system are associated with abnormal disposition of complexes, presumably reflecting their deposition in tissues outside the reticuloendothelial system.

The observation that not all circulating immune complexes detected in patients with SLE are DNA/anti-DNA complexes[113] suggests that other autoantigens or exogenous antigens may present in the immune complexes in this disease. Furthermore, circulating DNA/anti-DNA complexes may localize to tissues by specific mechanisms, e.g. DNA binding sites in the kidney[114,115], where they may serve as a nidus for *in situ* complex enlargement by sequential addition of antigen

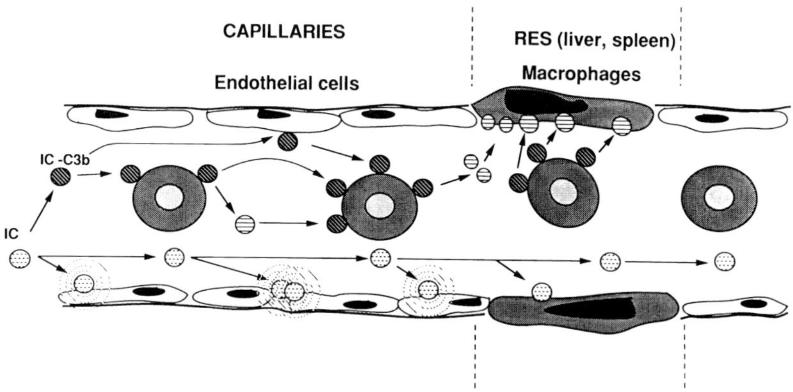

Figure 7.7 Immune complex transport by erythrocytes in the blood stream. The ICs that have fixed C3b remain soluble, bind to erythrocytes, and circulate in the central flow, whereas those which have not fixed complement or have been released are more likely to react with the vessel wall where they might induce inflammation. In the RES, ICs are transferred from the ertythrocytes to the fixed macrophages

and antibody. Their location in these sites not only provides a focus for the inflammatory response, but also results in release of autoantigens that further drive the immune response. An additional mechanism for the perpetuation of antibody generation may arise from the catabolism of such complexes. Immune complexes bearing C3dg (following catabolism of C3b by factor I) arriving at draining lymph nodes may activate B cells; this is suggested by the synergy between surface IgM and CR2 in B cell proliferation demonstrated *in vitro*[116].

Essential mixed cryoglobulinaemia

In essential mixed cryoglobulinaemia, monoclonal rheumatoid factor (usually IgM k) reacts with autologous normal IgG to form the characteristic cryo-precipitate (type II cryoglobulin)[117]. There is widespread vasculitis with purpura, arthralgias, glomerulonephritis and neuropathy; these clinical features are attributable to immune complex deposition since immunoglobulins and C3 have been demonstrated in vessel walls in affected tissues, such as skin[118], nerves[119] and kidney[120–122]. The classes of immunoglobulin found in kidney were identical to those of the associated cryoglobulin[117,123]. Furthermore, using monoclonal anti-idiotypic antibodies raised against rheumatoid factors, it has been shown that circulating cryoglobulin and glomerular deposits in an individual patient share idiotypic determinants[124]. Removal of cryoglobulin may be associated with significant clinical improvement[119,125,126].

It is likely that the monoclonal rheumatoid factor is responsible for the various abnormalities that result in deposition and formation of immune complexes[124]; the monoclonal rheumatoid factor binds to normal autologous IgG to form immune complexes. It will also bind to immune complexes formed with autoantigens or exogenous antigens and alter the physicochemical and biological properties of these complexes so that the processes of complement activation and binding of C3 fragments are perturbed (see above). This interferes with the normal mechanisms of complex transport on erythrocyte CR1 as well as uptake mechanisms of the reticuloendothelial system.

The acquired hypocomplementaemia seen in this disease (especially of early classical pathway components, most notably C4[127]) also reduces inhibition of immune precipitation and opsonization of immune complexes.

The effects of rheumatoid factor on exogenous immune complexes are difficult to unravel, as it has opposing effects on immune complexes; on the one hand, binding of rheumatoid factor to IgG increases lattice size and precipitability of the complex, resulting in increased efficiency of complement activation, while, on the other hand, it interferes with complement activation by the initial complex. Monoclonal IgM rheumatoid factors may or may not activate complement themselves depending on the structure (unique to each) and molecular configuration (only the staple form activates complement[128]). Complement activation by IgM-containing immune complexes also depends on the nature of the antigen, depending on the configuration that is achieved by the IgM when bound to its antigen. Thus, rheumatoid factor may decrease complement activation[129–131], inhibit the binding of C3b and C4b[40,41,132,133] to immune complexes during complement activation despite increased C1 activation and increased fluid-phase C4 turnover[40], or may increase complement activation on the surface of the complex[134,135].

Further insights into immune complex handling in essential mixed cryoglobulinaemia have been derived from *in vivo* studies of both endogenous and exogenous immune complexes. Handling of endogenous immune complexes (monoclonal rheumatoid factor/IgG) has been studied by measuring the turnover of autologous IgG[136,137]; clearance of circulating IgG is very slow, the fastest turnover being 13.4%/day in a patient with active disease. Interestingly, in these studies, one patient with active disease (vasculitis) demonstrated clearance kinetics consistent with the presence of an extravascular pool of non-catabolized IgG, suggesting the accumulation of cryoglobulin in extravascular tissues, where presumably they served as foci initiating tissue injury.

The handling of exogenous immune complexes in patients with essential mixed cryoglobulinaemia has been studied using a bolus intravenous injection of a small amount of soluble ^{125}I-labelled tetanus (TT)/anti-TT immune complexes[138]. There was a rapid disappearance of a significant proportion of these complexes from the circulation within the first minute after injection, which is insufficient time for complexes to be transported to the liver and spleen. These findings were interpreted to indicate deposition of injected complexes outside the reticuloendothelial system although the study could not demonstrate this directly. The mechanisms for this rapid disappearance of complexes are not clear but contributory factors may include increased immune complex size secondary to binding of rheumatoid factor, trapping of exogenous immune complexes in cryoglobulin, or hypocomplementaemia which prevents efficient complement activation and hence binding to erythrocyte CR1. Indeed, the studies performed in these patients suggest that multiple factors are required, including rheumatoid factor and low C4. These observations raise the possibility that abnormal handling of exogenous immune complexes may contribute to some of the tissue damage seen in patients with essential mixed cryoglobulinaemia.

Finally, *in vivo* studies of reticuloendothelial system function in patients with essential mixed cryoglobulinaemia using antibody-coated erythrocytes have shown that splenic extraction was reduced. The defect was corrected by plasma exchange[139]. The role of reduced reticuloendothelial system function in the pathogenesis of immune complex disease is suggested by several animal models – the general thesis being that decreased removal of circulating immune complexes allows them more circulation time to deposit in tissues where they are potentially able to cause injury. In essential mixed cryoglobulinaemia, IgM rheumatoid factor binding to immune complexes may interfere not only with their recognition and uptake by macrophage Fc receptors but also, by decreasing opsonization with C3b. Interaction with complement receptors on phagocytic cells would be impaired.

Thus, it can be seen that tissue damage in essential mixed cryoglobulinaemia may occur secondary to defective clearance of immune complexes. Hypocomplementaemia and the nature of the immune complex which allows only poor fixation of complement may both contribute to decreased binding of immune complexes to erythrocyte CR1 with the potential consequence of increased availability for deposition and decreased processing of immune complexes by factor I. Poor C3 fixation by rheumatoid factor-containing complexes results not only in decreased transport by erythrocytes to the reticuloendothelial system but also in inefficient removal of complexes by phagocytic cells, since the Fc receptor on these cells would be acting alone without the synergy of occupied complement receptors.

Persistence of immune complexes in tissues in these circumstances has two potential consequences. First, the multivalency of IgM may contribute to their enlargement *in situ* by continued trapping of antigen and antibody complexes[131]; a process which may be aided by local factors such as low temperature at the peripheries as well as the increased avidity of rheumatoid factor for surface-bound IgG (as distinct from monomeric IgG). Second, although the resulting complement activation may not allow efficient opsonization of the complex, it is sufficient to allow bystander binding of C3b and C4b to surrounding tissues which act as foci for the inflammatory response.

Other immune complex diseases

SLE and essential mixed cryoglobulinaemia provide examples of immune complex disease where it would appear that malfunction of the complement-mediated handling of immune complexes contributes to pathogenesis of disease. However, tissue-associated immune complexes may arise in the presence of a normal complement system, notably if the immune complexes formed are of an isotype that does not activate the classical pathway, of it tissue-associated complexes are formed *in situ*. Formation of immune complex *in situ* around tissue-associated antigen[140] clearly renders inappropriate clearance mechanisms that involve the generation of soluble complexes.

IgA complexes provide an example of pathogenetic immune complexes arising in the presence of a normal complement system. These arise because IgA is unable to activate the classical pathway, which is required for both inhibition of immune precipitation and opsonization of immune complexes for erythrocyte CR1 binding. The mechanisms underlying increased IgA complex generation in IgA nephropathy are not understood[141,142], but, as complement cannot inhibit their precipitation, large insoluble IgA aggregates are allowed to form which become trapped in the mesangium[143,144]. The aggregates acquire the ability to trigger the alternative pathway of complement which serves to solubilize the complexes but at the price of a powerful inflammatory reaction, resulting in accompanying tissue injury. Furthermore, polymeric IgA and IgA rheumatoid factor have been shown to inhibit complement-mediated processing of immune complexes *in vitro*[145], raising the possibility that unrelated exogenous immune complexes may also be relevant in these conditions.

Local factors contributing to the generation of immune complexes to study so that their contribution to the pathogenesis of immune complex disease tends to be overlooked. Immune complex handling in rheumatoid arthritis is a case in point. It is well recognized that processing of circulating immune complexes is affected by rheumatoid factors and other circulating factors (e.g. inhibitors of inhibition of immune precipitation[146–148]). Clearance of injected immune complexes (heat-aggregated IgG) is decreased in patients with rheumatoid arthritis[149]. However, the contribution of local factors in this condition is suggested by the observed effect of hyaluronic acid on increasing the avidity of IgM rheumatoid factor for IgG which would favour immune complex formation in the joint space[150].

SUMMARY

Complement contributes to the safe and effective elimination of immune complexes in many circumstances (Figure 7.7). When antigen–antibody complexes form in the presence of complement, inhibition of immune precipitation occurs; covalent binding of C3b to immune complex modifies the physico-chemical properties of the complex which remains soluble. In addition, such opsonized (C3b-coated) complexes attach to cells bearing CR1, which, in the primate circulation, is mostly to be found on erythrocytes. This appears to be a physiological system that allows complexes to be transported through the circulation to the reticuloendothelial system, 'buffered' so that they do not deposit in vessel walls on the way. In addition, C3b bound to complexes is catabolized by factor I (with CR1 as cofactor) so that the complement activating properties of the complexes are reduced. Deposition of immune complexes outside the reticuloendothelial system may be considered to be a failure of the system and has been demonstrated in states of hypocomplementaemia and decreased erythrocyte CR1 as well as conditions that generate immune complexes that fix C3 poorly (such as IgM monoclonal rheumatoid factor complexes) or do not activate the classical pathway (such as IgA complexes). The formation of insoluble complexes produces alternative pathway complement activation at the site of the immune aggregate. Such activation, if sufficiently intense, may overwhelm local tissue-associated protective mechanisms against complement activation[151] and allow bystander fixation of C3b that serves as a focus for amplification of complement activation accompanied by the inflammatory reaction.

References

1. Heidelberger, M. (1941). Quantitative chemical studies on complement or alexin. I. A method. *J. Exp. Med.*, **73**, 681–94
2. Schifferli, J. A. and Peters, D. K. (1983). Complement, the immune complex lattice and the pathophysiology of complement-deficient syndromes. *Lancet*, **2**, 957–9
3. Pepys, M. B. (1976). Role of complement in the induction of immunological responses. *Transplant Rev.*, **42**, 93–120
4. Bottger, E. C., Hoffman, T., Hadding, U. and Bitter-Suermann, D. (1985). Influence of genetically inherited complement deficiencies in humoral immune response in guinea pigs. *J. Immunol.*, **135**, 4100–7
5. Bottger, E. C. and Bitter-Suermann, D. (1987). Complement and the regulation of humoral immune responses. *Immunol. Today* **8**, 261–4
6. Jackson, C. G., Ochs, H. D. and Wedgwood, R. J. (1979). Immune response of a patient with deficiency of the fourth component and systemic lupus erythematosus. *N. Engl. J. Med.*, **300**, 1124–9
7. Alper, C. A., Kruskall, M. S., Marcus-Bagley, D., Craven, D. E., Katz, A. J., Brink, S. J., Dinstag, J. L., Awdeh, Z. and Yunis, E. J. (1989). Genetic prediction of nonresponse to hepatitis B vaccine. *N. Engl. J. Med.*, **321**, 708–12
8. Robey, F. A., Jones, K. D. and Steinberg, A. D. (1985). C-reactive protein mediates the solubilization of nuclear DNA by complement *in vitro*. *J. Exp. Med.*, **161**, 1344–56
9. Law, S. K., Dodds, A. W. and Porter, R. R. (1984). A comparison of the properties of two classes C4A, C4B of the human complement component C4. *EMBO J.*, **3**, 1819–23
10. Isenman, D. E. and Young, J. R. (1984). The molecular basis for the difference in immune hemolysis activity of the Chido and Rodgers isotypes of human complement component C4. *J. Immunol.*, **132**, 3019–27
11. Schifferli, J. A., Steiger, G., Paccaud, J. P., Sjoholm, A. G. and Hauptmann, G. (1986). Difference in the biological properties of the two forms of the fourth component of human complement (C4). *Clin. Exp. Immunol.*, **63**, 473–7
12. Schifferli, J. A., Hauptmann, G. and Paccaud, J. P. (1987). Complement mediated adherence of immune complexes to human erythrocytes: difference in the requirements for C4A and C4B. *FEBS Lett.*, **213**, 415–18
13. Utiger, R. D., Parker, M. L. and Daughaday, W. H. (1962). Studies on human growth hormone. I. A radioimmunoassay for human growth hormone. *J. Clin. Invest.*, **41**, 254–61
14. Morgan, C. R., Sorenson, R. L. and Lazarow, A. (1964). Further studies of an inhibitor of the two antibody immunoassay system. *Diabetes*, **13**, 579–84
15. Soeldner, J. S. and Slone, D. (1965). Critical variables in the radioimmunoassay of serum insulin using the double antibody technique. *Diabetes*, **14**, 771–9
16. Miller, G. W. and Nussenzweig, V. (1975). A new complement function: solubilization of antigen–antibody aggregates. *Proc. Natl. Acad. Sci. (USA)*, **72**, 418–22
17. Schifferli, J. A., Bartolotti, S. R. and Peters, D. K. (1980). Inhibition of immune precipitation by complement. *Clin. Exp. Immunol.*, **42**, 387–94
18. Walport, M. J. and Lachmann, P. J. (1988). Erythrocyte complement receptor type 1 (CR1), immune complexes and the rheumatic diseases. *Arthritis Rheum.*, **31**, 153–8
19. Nelson, R. A. (1953). The immune adherence phenomenon: an immunologically specific reaction between micro-organisms and erythrocytes leading to enhanced phagocytosis. *Science*, **118**, 733–7
20. Fearon, D. T. (1980). Identification of the membrane glycoprotein that is the C3b receptor of the human erythrocyte, polymorphonuclear leukocyte, B lymphocyte and monocyte. *J. Exp. Med.*, **152**, 20–30

21. Hebert, L. A. and Cosio, F. G. (1987). The erythrocyte–immune complex–glomerulonephritis connection in man. *Kidney Int.*, **31**, 877–85
22. Medof, M. E. and Prince, G. M. (1983). Immune complex alterations occur on the human red blood cell membrane. *Immunology*, **50**, 11–18
23. Moller, N. P. H. and Steengaard, J. (1979). Fc mediated immune precipitation. I. A new role of the Fc portion of IgG. *Immunology*, **38**, 631–40
24. Rodwell, J. D., Tang, L. H. and Schumaker, V. N. (1980). Antigen valence and Fc-localised secondary forces in antibody precipitation. *Mol. Immunol.*, **17**, 1591–7
25. Moller, N. P. H. and Christiansen, G. (1983). Fc mediated immune precipitation. III. Visualization by electron microscopy. *Immunology*, **48**, 469–76
26. Lachmann, P. J. and Walport, M. J. (1987). Deficiency of the effector mechanisms of the immune response and auto-immunity. In Whelan, J. (ed.) *Autoimmunity and Autoimmune Disease*, pp. 149–71. Ciba Foundation Symposium 129 (Chichester: Wiley)
27. Hong, K., Takata, Y., Sayama, K., Konozo, H., Takeda, J., Nakano, Y., Kinoshita, T. and Inoue, K. (1984). Inhibition of immune precipitation by complement. *J. Immunol.*, **133**, 1464–70
28. Paccaud, J. P., Steiger, G., Sjoholm, A. G., Spath, P. J. and Schifferli, J. A. (1987). Tetanus toxoid–anti-tetanus toxoid complexes: a potential model to study the complement transport system for immune complex in humans. *Clin. Exp. Immunol.*, **69**, 468–76
29. Schifferli, J. A., Steiger, G. and Schapira, M. (1985). The role of C1, C1 inhibitor and C4 in modulating immune precipitation. *Clin. Exp. Immunol.*, **60**, 605–12
30. Naama, J. K., Hamilton, A. O., Yeung-Laiwah, A. C. and Whaley, K. (1984). Prevention of immune precipitation by purified classical pathway complement components. *Clin. Exp. Immunol.*, **58**, 486–92
31. Muller-Eberhard, H. J. and Kunkel, H. G. (1961). Isolation of the thermolabile serum protein which precipitates gammaglobulin aggregates and participates in immune haemolysis. *Proc. Soc. Exp. Biol. Med.*, **106**, 291–5
32. Kishore, N., Shah, D., Skanes, V. M. and Levine, R. P. (1988). The fluid-phase binding of human C4 and its genetic variants, C4A3 and C4B1, to immunoglobulins. *Mol. Immunol.*, **25**, 811–19
33. Schifferli, J. A., Woo, P. and Peters, D. K. (1982). Complement-mediated inhibition of immune precipitation. Role of the classical and alternative pathways. *Clin. Exp. Immunol.*, **47**, 555–62
34. Schifferli, J. A. and Peters, D. K. (1982). Complement-mediated inhibition of immune precipitation. analysis by sucrose density gradient ultracentrifugation. *Clin. Exp. Immunol.*, **47**, 563–9
35. Naama, J. K., Holme, E., Hamilton, E. and Whaley, K. (1985). Prevention of immune precipitation by purified components of the alternative pathway. *Clin. Exp. Immunol.*, **60**, 169–77
36. Schifferli, J. A., Steiger, G., Hauptmann, G., Spath, P. J. and Sjoholm, A. G. (1985). Formation of soluble immune complexes by complement in sera of patients with various hypocomplementemic states. *J. Clin. Invest.*, **74**, 2127–33
37. Johnson, A., Harkin, S., Steward, M. W. and Whaley, K. (1987). The effect of immunoglobulin isotype and antibody affinity on complement-mediated inhibition of immune precipitation and solubilisation. *Mol. Immunol.*, **24**, 1211–17
38. Balestrieri, G., Tincani, A., Migliorini, P., Ferri, C., Cattaneo, R. and Bombardieri, S. (1984). Inhibitory effect of IgM rheumatoid factor on immune complex solubilisation capacity and inhibition of immune precipitation. *Arthritis Rheum.*, **27**, 1130–6
39. Mitchell, W. S., Naama, J. K., Veitch, J. and Whaley, K. (1984). IgM-RF prevents complement mediated inhibition of immune precipitation. *Immunology*, **52**, 445–8
40. Ng, Y. C., Peters, D. K. and Walport, M. J. (1988). Monoclonal rheumatoid factor-IgG immune complexes. Poor fixation of opsonic C4 and C3 despite efficient complement activation. *Arthritis Rheum.*, **31**, 88–107
41. Taylor, R. P., Wright, E. L. and Pocanic, F. (1989). Quantitative analyses of C3b capture and immune adherence of IgM antibody/dsDNA complexes. *J. Immunol.*, **143**, 3626–31
42. Takahashi, M. and Takahashi, S. (1981). Complement-dependent solubilisation of immune complexes. *Clin. Immunol. Allergy*, **1**, 261–79
43. Barrio, E., Anton, L. C., Marques, G., Sanchez, A. and Vivanco, F. (1991). Formation of covalently linked C3–C3 dimers on IgG immune aggregates. *Eur. J. Immunol.*, **21**, 343–9
44. Kinoshita, T., Takata, Y., Kozono, H., Takeda, J., Tanaka, E., Hong, K. and Inoue, K. (1988). C5 convertase of the alternative complement pathway: covalent linkage between two C3b molecules with the trimolecular complex enzyme. *J. Immunol.*, **141**, 3895–901

45. Fries, L. F., Gaither, T. A., Hammer, C. H. and Frank, M. M. (1984). C3b covalently bound to IgG demonstrates a reduced rate of inactivation by factor H and I. *J. Exp. Med.*, **160**, 1640–55
46. Spath, P. J., Pascual, M., Meyer-Hanni, L., Schaad, U. B. and Schifferli, J. A. (1988). Solubilisation of immune precipitates by complement in the absence of properdin or factor D. *FEBS Lett.*, **234**, 131–4
47. Johnson, A., Harkin, S., Steward, M. W. and Whaley, K. (1987). The effects of immunoglobulin isotype and antibody affinity on complement-mediated inhibition of immune precipitation and solubilisation. *Mol. Immunol.*, **24**, 1211–17
48. Whaley, K., Johnson, A., Steward, M. W. and Kerr, M. A. (1989). Dissociation of primary antigen–antibody bonds is essential for complement-mediated solubilization of immune complexes. *Complement Inflamm.*, **6**, 415 (abstract)
49. Schifferli, J. A., Steiger, G. and Paccaud, J. P. (1986). Complement mediated inhibition of immune precipitation and solubilisation generate different concentrations of complement anaphylatoxins (C4a, C3a, C5a). *Clin. Exp. Immunol.*, **64**, 407–14
50. Fearon, D. T. (1984). Cellular receptors for fragments of the third component of complement. *Immunol. Today*, **5**, 105–10
51. Wilson, J. G., Tedder, T. F. and Fearon, D. T. (1983). Characterisation of human T lymphocytes that express the C3b receptor. *J. Immunol.*, **131**, 684–9
52. Kazatchkine, M. D., Fearon, D. T., Appay, M. D., Mandet, C. and Bariety, J. (1982). Immunohistochemical study of the human glomerular C3b receptor in normal kidney and in seventy-five cases of renal diseases. *J. Clin. Invest.*, **69**, 900–12
53. Fischer, E., Appay, M. D., Cook, J. and Kazatchkine, M. D. (1986). Characterisation of the human glomerular C3b receptor as the C3b/C4b complement type one (CR1) receptor. *J. Immunol.*, **136**, 1373–7
54. Wong, W. W., Cahill, J. M., Rosen, M. D., Kennedy, C. A., Bonaccio, E. T., Morris, M. J., Wilson, J. G., Klickstein, L. B. and Fearon, D. T. (1989). Structure of the human CR1 gene. Molecular basis of the structural and quantitative polymorphisms and identification of a new CR1-like allele. *J. Exp. Med.*, **169**, 847–63
55. Wilson, J. G., Wong, W., Schur, P. H. and Fearon, D. T. (1982). Mode of inheritance of decreased C3b receptor on red cells of patients with systemic lupus erythematosus. *N. Engl. J. Med.*, **307**, 981–6
56. Wilson, J. G. and Fearon, D. T. (1984). Altered expression of complement receptors as a pathogenic factor in systemic lupus erythematosus. *Arthritis Rheum.*, **27**, 1321–8
57. Iida, K. and Nussenzweig, V. (1981). Complement receptor is an inhibitor of the complement cascade. *J. Exp. Med.*, **153**, 1138–50
58. Gigli, I. and Fearon, D. T. (1981). Regulation of the classical pathway convertase of human complement by the C3b receptor from human erythrocyte. *Fed. Proc.*, **40**, 1172 (abstract)
59. Iida, K. and Nussenzweig, V. (1983). Functional properties of membrane-associated complement receptor CR1. *J. Immunol.*, **130**, 1876–80
60. Fearon, D. T. (1979). Regulation of the amplification C3 convertase of human complement by an inhibitory protein isolated from human erythrocyte membrane. *Proc. Natl. Acad. Sci. USA*, **76**, 5867–80
61. Medof, M. E., Iida, K., Mold, C. and Nussenzweig, V. (1982). Unique role of the complement receptor CR1 in the degradation of C3b associated with immune complexes. *J. Exp. Med.*, **156**, 1739–54
62. Ros, G. D., Lambris, J. D., Cain, J. S. and Newman, S. L. (1982). Generation of three different fragments of bound C3 with purified factor I or serum. Requirements for factor H vs CR1 cofactor activity. *J. Immunol.*, **129**, 2051–60
63. Medicus, R. G., Melamed, J. and Arnaout, M. A. (1983). Role of human factor I and C3b receptor in the cleavage of surface-bound C3b molecules. *Eur. J. Immunol.*, **13**, 465–70
64. Medof, M. E. and Oger, J. J. F. (1982). Competition for immune complexes by red cells in human blood. *J. Clin. Lab. Immunol.*, **7**, 7–13
65. Medof, M. E., Prince, G. M. and Oger, J. J. F. (1982). Kinetics of interactions of immune complexes with complement receptors on human blood cells: modification of complexes during interaction with red cells. *Clin. Exp. Immunol.*, **48**, 715–25
66. Arnaout, M. A., Dana, N., Melamed, J., Medicus, R. and Colten, H. R. (1983). Low ionic strength or chemical cross-linking of monomeric C3b increases its binding affinity to the human complement C3b receptor. *Immunology*, **48**, 229–37

67. Edberg, J. C., Wright, E. and Taylor, R. P. (1987). Quantitative analyses of the binding of soluble complement-fixing antibody/dsDNA immune complexes to CR1 on human red blood cells. *J. Immunol.*, **139**, 3739–47
68. Paccaud, J. P., Carpentier, J. L. and Schifferli, J. A. (1988). Direct evidence for the clustered nature of complement receptors type 1 on the erythrocyte membrane. *J. Immunol.*, **141**, 3899–94
69. Chevalier, J. and Kazatchkine, M. D. (1989). Distribution in clusters of complement receptor type one (CR1) on human erythrocytes. *J. Immunol.*, **142**, 2031–6
70. Schifferli, J. A., Ng, Y. C., Estreicher, J. and Walport, M. J. (1988). The clearance of tetanus toxoid/anti-tetanus toxoid immune complexes from the circulation of humans. Complement and erythrocyte complement receptor 1-dependent mechanisms. *J. Immunol.*, **140**, 899–904
71. Paccaud, J. P., Carpentier, J. L. and Schifferli, J. A. (1990). Difference in the clustering of complement receptor type I (CR1) on polymorphonuclear leukocytes and erythrocytes: effect on immune adherence. *Eur. J. Immunol.*, **20**, 283–9
72. Taylor, R. P., Burge, J., Horgan, C. and Shasby, D. M. (1983). The complement-mediated binding of soluble antibody/dsDNA immune complexes to human neutrophils. *J. Immunol.*, **130**, 2656–62
73. Schifferli, J. A. and Peters, D. K. (1983). Immune adherence and staphylococcus protein. A binding of soluble immune complexes produced by complement activation. *Clin. Exp. Immunol.*, **54**, 827–33
74. Cornacoff, J. B., Hebert, L. A., Smead, W. L., Van Aman, M. E., Birmingham, D. J. and Waxman, F. J. (1983). Primate erythrocyte immune complex-clearing mechanism. *J. Clin. Invest.*, **71**, 236–47
75. Waxman, F. J., Hebert, L. A., Cornacoff, J. B., Van Aman, M. E., Smead, W. L., Kraut, E. H., Birmingham, D. J. and Taguiam, J. M. (1984). Complement depletion accelerates the clearance of immune complexes from the circulation of primates. *J. Clin. Invest.*, **74**, 1329–40
76. Waxman, F. J., Hebert, L. A., Cosio, F. G., Smead, W. L., Van Aman, M. E., Taguiam, J. M. and Birmingham, D. J. (1986). Differential binding of immunoglobulin A and immunoglobulin G1 immune complexes to primate erythrocytes in vivo: immunoglobulin A immune complexes bind less well to erythrocytes and are preferentially deposited in glomeruli. *J. Clin. Invest.*, **77**, 82–9
77. Lennek, R., Baldwin, A. S., Waller, S. J., Morley, K. W. and Taylor, R. P. (1981). Studies of the physical biochemistry and complement-fixing properties of DNA/anti-DNA immune complexes. *J. Immunol.*, **127**, 602–8
78. Horgan, C. and Taylor, R. P. (1984). Quantitative analysis of complement fixation in three immune complex systems. *Immunology*, **52**, 753–9
79. Cochrane, C. G. and Koffler, D. (1973). Immune complex disease in experimental animals and man. *Adv. Immunol.*, **16**, 185–265
80. Hebert, L. A., Cosio, F. G. and Taylor, R. P. (1986). Clearance of human antibody/DNA immune complexes (DNA-IC) and free DNA from the circulation of nonhuman primates. *Kidney Int.*, **29**, 277 (abstract)
81. Miller, G. W., Steinberg, V., Green, I. and Nussenzweig, V. (1975). Complement-dependent alterations in the handling of immune complexes by NZB/W mice. *J. Immunol.*, **114**, 1166–70
82. Emlen, W., Pisetsky, D. S. and Taylor, R. P. (1986). Antibodies to DNA. *Arthritis Rheum.*, **29**, 1417–26
83. Edberg, J. C., Kujala, G. A. and Taylor, R. P. (1987). Rapid immune adherence reactivity of nascent, soluble antibody/DNA immune complexes in the circulation. *J. Immunol.*, **139**, 1240–4
84. Madi, N., Paccaud, J. P., Steiger, G. and Schifferli, J. A. (1989). Immune adherence of nascent hepatitis B surface antigen–antibody complexes *in vivo* in humans. *Clin. Exp. Immunol.*, **78**, 201–6
85. Paccaud, J. P., Steiger, G. and Schifferli, J. A. (1989). Reduced immune adherence of antigen/antibody complexes formed in the presence of complement *in vivo* and *in vitro*. *Complement Inflamm.*, **6**, 470–9
86. Edberg, J. C., Tosic, L. and Taylor, R. P. (1989). Immune adherence and the processing of soluble complement-fixing antibody/DNA immune complexes in mice. *Clin. Immunol. Immunopathol.*, **51**, 118–32
87. Schifferli, J. A., Ng. Y. C., Paccaud, J. P. and Walport, M. J. (1989). The role of hypocomplementaemia and low erythrocyte complement receptor type 1 numbers in determining abnormal immune complex clearance in humans. *Clin. Exp. Immunol.*, **75**, 329–35

88. Ng, Y. C., Schifferli, J. A. and Walport, M. J. (1988). Immune complexes and erythrocyte CR1 (complement receptor type 1): effect of CR1 numbers on binding and release reactions. *Clin. Exp. Immunol.*, **71**, 481–5
89. Cosio, F. G., Hebert, L. A., Birmingham, J., Dorval, B. L., Bakaletz, A. P., Kujala, G. A., Edberg, J. C. and Taylor, R. P. (1987). Clearance of human antibody/DNA immune complexes and free DNA from the circulation of the nonhuman primate. *Clin. Immunol. Immunopathol.*, **42**, 1–9
90. Kimberly, R., Edberg, J. C., Merriam, L. T., Clarkson, S. B., Unkeless, J. C. and Taylor, R. P. (1989). In vivo handling of soluble complement fixing Ab/dsDNA immune complexes in chimpanzees. *J. Clin. Invest.*, **84**, 962–70
91. Davies, K. A., Savill, J. and Walport, M. J. (1989). In vitro transfer of immune complexes from erythrocytes to monocytes and macrophages. *Complement Inflamm.*, **6**, 328 (abstract)
92. Biesecker, G., Katz, S. and Koffler, D. (1981). Renal localisation of the membrane attack complex in systemic lupus erythematosus nephritis. *J. Exp. Med.*, **154**, 1779–94
93. Biesecker, G., Lavin, L., Ziskind, M. and Koffler, D. (1982). Cutaneous localisation of the membrane attack complex in discoid and systemic lupus erythematosus. *N. Engl. J. Med.*, **306**, 264–70
94. Schur, P. H. and Sandson, J. (1968). Immunologic factors and clinical activity in systemic lupus erythematosus. *N. Engl. J. Med.*, **278**, 533–8
95. Antes, U., Heinz, H-P. and Loos, M. (1988). Evidence for the presence of autoantibodies to the collagen-like portion of C1q in systemic lupus erythematosus. *Arthritis Rheum.*, **31**, 457–64
96. Fielder, A. H. L., Walport, M. J., Batchelor, J. R., Rynes, R. I., Black, C. M., Dodi, A. I. and Hughes, G. R. V. (1983). Family study of the major histocompatibility complex in patients with systemic lupus erythematosus: importance of null alleles of C4A and C4b in determining disease susceptibility. *Br. Med. J.*, **286**, 425–8
97. Dunckley, H., Gatenby, P. A., Hawkins, B., Baito, S. and Serjeantson S. W. (1987). Deficiency of C4A is a genetic determinant of systemic lupus erythematosus in three ethnic groups. *J. Immunogenet.*, **14**, 209–18
98. Howard, P. F., Hochberg, M. C., Bias, W. B., Arnett, F. C. and McLean, R. H. (1986). Relationship between C4 null genes, HLA-D region antigens and genetic susceptibility to systemic lupus erythematosus in Caucasian and black Americans. *Am. J. Med.*, **81**, 187–93
99. Kemp, M. E., Atkinson, J. P., Skanes, V. M., Levine, R. P. and Chaplin, D. D. (1987). Deletion of C4 genes in patients with systemic lupus erythematosus. *Arthritis Rheum.*, **30**, 1015–22
100. Goldestein, R., Arnett, F. C., McLean, R. H., Bias, W. B. and Duvic, M. (1988). Molecular heterogeneity of complement component C4-null and 21-hydroxylase genes in systemic lupus erythematosus. *Arthritis Rheum.*, **31**, 736–44
101. Gatenby, P. A., Barbosa, J. E. and Lachmann, P. J. (1990). Differences between C4A and C4B in the handling of immune complexes: the enhancement of CR1 binding is more important than the inhibition of immunoprecipitation. *Clin. Exp. Immunol.*, **79**, 158–63
102. Moldenhauer, F., David, J., Fielder, A. H., Lachmann, P. J. and Walport, M. J. (1987). Inherited deficiency of erythrocyte complement receptor type 1 does not cause susceptibility to systemic lupus erythematosus. *Arthritis Rheum.*, **30**, 961–6
103. Walport, M. J., Ross, G. D., Mackworth-Young, C. G., Watson, J. V., Hogg, N. and Lachmann, P. J. (1985). Family studies of erythrocyte complement receptor type 1 levels: reduced levels in patients with SLE are acquired, not inherited. *Clin. Exp. Immunol.*, **59**, 547–54
104. Holme, E. R., Fyfe, A., Zoma, A., Veitch, J., Hunter, J. and Whaley, K. (1985). Decreased C3b receptors (CR1) on erythrocytes of patients with systemic lupus erythematosus. *Clin. Exp. Immunol.*, **63**, 41–8
105. Holme, E. R., Fyfe, A., Zoma, A., Veitch, J., Hunter, J. and Whaley, K. (1987). The relative roles of genetic and environmental factors in the regulation of erythrocyte C3b receptor (CR1) numbers in normal individuals. *Clin. Exp. Immunol.*, **70**, 231–7
106. Walport, M. J., Ng, Y. C. and Lachmann, P. J. (1987). Erythrocytes transfused into patients with SLE and haemolytic anaemia lose complement receptor type 1 from their cell surface. *Clin. Exp. Immunol.*, **69**, 501–7
107. Ross, G. D., Yount, W. J., Walport, M. J., Winfield, J. B., Parker, C. J., Randall Fuller, C., Taylor, R. P., Myones, B. L. and Lachmann, P. J. (1985). Disease-associated loss of

erythrocyte complement receptor (CR1, C3b receptor) in patients with systemic lupus erythematosus and other diseases involving autoantibodies and/or complement activation. *J. Immunol.*, **135**, 2005–14

108. Iida, K., Mornaghi, R. and Nussenzweig, V. (1982). CR1 deficiency in red cells from patients with systemic lupus erythematosus. *J. Exp. Med.*, **155**, 1427–38
109. Inada, Y., Kamiyama, M., Kanemitsu, I. and Clark, W. S. (1983). Studies on immune adherence (C3b) receptor activity of human erythrocytes: relationship between receptor activity and membrane osmotic fragility. *J. Clin. Lab. Immunol.*, **12**, 97–103
110. Waldo, F. B., Forristal, J., Beischel, L. and West, C. D. (1985). Circulating inhibitor of fluid-phase amplification. *J. Clin. Invest.*, **75**, 1786–95
111. Ng, Y. C., Peters, D. K., Cederholm-Williams, S. A. and Walport, M. J. (1987). A lysine-binding protein in SLE sera inhibits the binding of immune complexes to normal erythrocyte CR1 (complement receptor type 1). *Clin. Exp. Immunol.*, **69**, 89–97
112. Cook, J. M., Kazatchkine, M. D., Bourgeois, P., Mignon, F., Mery, J. P. and Kahn, M. F. (1986) Anti-C3b receptor (CR1) antibodies in patients with systemic lupus erythematosus. *Clin. Immunol. Immunopathol.*, **38**, 135–8
113. Izui, S., Lambert, P. H. and Miescher, P. A. (1977). Failure to detect circulating DNA:anti-DNA complexes in systemic lupus erythematosus. *Clin. Exp. Immunol.*, **30**, 384–92
114. Horgan, C., Johnson, R., Mannik, M. and Emlen, W. (1988). Binding of dsDNA to glomeruli in vivo. *Arthritis Rheum.*, **31**, S108 (abstract)
115. Izui, S., Lambert, P. H. and Miescher, P. A. (1976). In vitro demonstration of a particular affinity of glomerular basement membrane and collagen for DNA. *J. Exp. Med.*, **144**, 428–43
116. Carter, R. H., Spycher, M. O., Ng, Y. C. and Fearon, D. T. (1988). Synergistic interaction between complement receptor type 2 and membrane IgM on B lymphocytes. *J. Immunol.*, **141**, 457–63
117. Brouet, J. G., Clauvel, J. P., Davon, F., Klein, M. and Seligmann, M. (1974). Biologic and clinical significance of cryoglobulins. A report of 86 cases. *Am. J. Med.*, **57**, 775–88
118. Mathison, D. A., Condemi, J. J., Leddy, J. P., Callerame, M., Panner, B. J. and Vaughan, J. H. (1971). Purpura, arthralgia, IgM-IgG cryoglobulinaemia with rheumatoid factor activity. Response to cyclophosphamide and splenectomy. *Ann. Intern. Med.*, **74**, 383–90
119. Chad, D., Pariser, K., Bradley, W. G., Adeklman, L. S. and Pinn, V. W. (1982). The pathogenesis of cryoglobulinemic neuropathy. *Neurology*, **32**, 725–9
120. D'Amico, G., Colasanti, G., Ferrario, F. and Sinico, R. A. (1989). Renal involvement in essential mixed cryoglobulinaemia. *Kidney Int.*, **35**, 1004–14
121. Druet, P., Leton Turier, L., Contet, A. and Mandet, C. (1973). Cryoglobulinaemia in human renal diseases. A study of seventy six cases. *Clin. Exp. Immunol.*, **15**, 483–96
122. Monga, G., Mazzucco, G., Coppo, R., Piccoli, G. and Coda, R. (1976). Glomerular findings in mixed IgG-IgM cryoglobulinemia. Light, electron microscopic, immunofluorescence and histochemical correlations. *Virchows Arch. [Cell. Pathol.]*, **20**, 185–96
123. Morel-Morger, L. and Verroust, P. (1974). Glomerular lesions in dysproteinemias. *Kidney Int.*, **5**, 249–52
124. Sinico, R. A., Winearls, C. G., Sabadini, E., Fornasieri, A., Castiglione, A. and D'Amico, G. (1987). Identification of glomerular immune deposits in cryoglobulinaemia glomerulonephritis. *Kidney Int.*, **34**, 109–16
125. Germain, M. J., Anderson, R. W. and Kaene, W. F. (1982). Renal disease in cryoglobulinaemia type II; response to therapy. A case report and review of the literature. *Am. J. Nephrol.*, **2**, 221–6
126. Pusey, C. D., Schifferli, J. A., Lockwood, C. M. and Peters, D. K. (1981). Use of plasma exchange in the management of mixed essential cryoglobulinaemia. *Artif. Organs*, **5**, 183s–7s
127. Gigli, L. (1986). Complement activation in patients with mixed cryoglobulinaemia. In Ponticelli, C., Minielli, L. and D'Amico, G. (Eds.) *Antiglobulins, Cryoglobulins and Glomerulonephritis*, pp. 135–46. (Dordrecht, Boston, Lancaster: Martinus Nijhoff)
128. Feinstein, A., Richardson, N. E., Gorick, B. D. and Hughes-Jones, N. C. (1983). Immunoglobulin M conformational change is a signal for complement activation. In Celeda, F., Schumaker, V. N. and Sercarz, E. E. (Eds.) *Protein Conformation as an Immunological Signal*, p. 47. (New York, Plenum Press)

129. Bolton, W. K., Schrock, J. H. and Davis, J. S. (1982). Rheumatoid factor inhibits in vitro binding of IgG complexes in the human glomerulus. *Arthritis Rheum.*, **25**, 297–303
130. Doekes, G., Shcouten, J., Cats, A. and Daha, M. R. (1985). Reduction of the complement activation capacity of soluble IgG aggregates and immune complexes by IgM-rheumatoid factor. *Immunology*, **55**, 555–64
131. Ford, P. M. and Kosatka, I. (1983). In situ immune complex formation in the mouse glomerulus: reactivity with human IgM rheumatoid factor and the effect on subsequent immune complex depositions. *Clin. Exp. Immunol.*, **51**, 285–91
132. Jarvis, J. N. and Levine, P. (1989). Inhibition of C4 binding to immune complexes by IgM-rheumatoid factor. *Complement Inflamm.*, **6**, 351 (Abstract)
133. Kavai, M., Rasmussen, J. M., Baatrup, G., Zsindely, A. and Svehag, S. E. (1988). Inefficient binding of IgM immune complexes to erythrocyte C3b-C4b receptors (CR1) and weak incoporation of C3b-iC3b into the complexes. *Scand. J. Immunol.*, **28**, 123–8
134. Birchmore, D. A., Taylor, R. P., Walker, S. J., Davis, J. S. IV and Morley, K. W. (1981). Interaction between rheumatoid factor and antibody/DNA complexes. *Arthritis Rheum.*, **24**, 527–33
135. Tesar, J. T. and Schmid, F. R. (1970). Conversion of soluble immune complexes into complement-fixing aggregates by IgM rheumatoid factor. *J. Immunol.*, **105**, 1206–14
136. Waldmann, T. A., Johnson, J. S. and Talal, N. (1971). Hypogammaglobulinaemia associated with accelerated catabolism of IgG secondary to its interaction with an IgG-reactive monoclonal IgM. *J. Clin. Invest.*, **50**, 951–9
137. Schifferli, J. A., Amos, N., Pusey, C. D., Sissons, J. G. P. and Peters, D. K. (1983). Metabolism of IgG in type II mixed essential cryoglobulinaemia – autologous cryoprecipitated and normal homologous IgG are incorporated into complexes and metabolised in vivo at similar rates. *Clin. Exp. Immunol.*, **51**, 305–16
138. Madi, N. and Schifferli, J. (1990). Clearance of immune complexes in cryoglobulinaemia. In Dammacco, F. (ed.) *Immunological Aspects of Malignant Lymphomas and Cryoglobulinaemia*, pp. 235–53. (Milano: Edi-Ermes)
139. Walport, M. J., Peters, A. M., Elkon, K. B., Pusey, C. D., Lavender, J. P. and Hughes, G. R. V. (1985). The splenic extraction ratio of antibody-coated erythrocytes and its response to plasma exchange and pulse methylprednisolone. *Clin. Exp. Immunol.*, **60**, 465–73
140. Cosio, F. G., Mahan, J. D. and Sedmark, D. D. (1990). Experimental glomerulonephritis induced by antigen that binds to glomerular fibronectin. *Am. J. Kidney Dis.*, **15**, 160–8
141. Van den Wall-Bake, A. W., Beyer, W. E., Evers-Schouten, J. H., Hermans, J., Daha, M. R., Masurel, N. and van Es, L. A. (1989). Humoral immune response to influenza vaccination in patients with primary immunoglobulin A nephropathy. An analysis of isotype distribution and the size of the influenza-specific antibodies. *J. Clin. Invest.*, **84**, 1070–5
142. Van den Wall-Bake, A. W., Daha, M. R., Haaijman, J. J., Radl, J., van der Ark, A. and van Es, L. A. (1989). Elevated production of polymeric and monomeric IgA1 by the bone marrow in IgA nephropathy. *Kidney Int.*, **35**, 1400–4
143. Cameron, J. S. and Clark, W. F. (1982). A role for insoluble antibody–antigen complexes in glomerulonephritis? *Clin. Nephrol.*, **18**, 55–61
144. Emancipator, S. N., Gallo, G. R. and Lamm, M. E. (1985). IgA nephropathy: perspectives on pathogenesis and classification. *Clin. Nephrol.*, **24**, 161–79
145. Schena, P. F., Pastore, A., Sinico, R. A., Montinaro, V. and Fornasieri, A. (1988). Polymeric IgA and IgA rheumatoid factor decrease the capacity of serum to solubilise circulating immune complexes in patients with primary IgA nephropathy. *J. Immunol.*, **141**, 125–31
146. Whaley, K. and Ahmed, A. E. (1989). Control of immune complexes by the classical pathway. *Behring Inst. Mitt.*, **84**, 111–20
147. Ahmed, A. E., Veitch, J. and Whaley, K. (1990). Mechanism of action of an inhibitor of complement-mediated prevention of immune precipitation. *Immunology*, **70**, 139–44
148. Sandilands, G. P., Ahmed, A. E., Griffiths, M. R. and Whaley, K. (1990). Immunohistochemical localisation of a plasma protein (glycoprotein 60) which inhibits complement-mediated prevention of immune precipitation. *Immunology*, **70**, 303–8
149. Lobatto, S., Daha, M. R., Westedt, M. L., Pauwels, E. K., Evers-Schouten, J. H., Voetman, A. A., Cats, A. and van Es, L. A. (1989). Diminished clearance of soluble aggregates of human immunoglobulin G in patients with rheumatoid arthritis. *Scand. J. Rheumatol.*, **18**, 89–96

150. Faaber, P., van der Rersselaar, L. A. M., van de Putte, L. B. A. and van den Berg, W. B. (1989). Immune complex formation between IgM rheumatoid factor and IgG generated by hyaluronic acid. *Arthritis Rheum.*, **32**, 1521–7
151. Cosio, F. G., Sedmak, D. D., Mahan, J. D. and Nahman, N. S. Jr (1989). Localisation of decay accelerating factor in normal and diseased kidneys. *Kidney Int.*, **36**, 100–7

8
Hereditary angio-oedema

M. M. FRANK

Hereditary angio-oedema is defined clinically by episodic attacks of painless non-pruritic swelling of the external surfaces of the body (Figure 8.1) and/or the gastrointestinal tract that affects multiple generations of a family[1–4]. In the American literature, credit for the original description is often given to William Osler who described a family with the disease affecting members of four generations[5]. The autosomal dominant nature of the inheritance pattern (Figure 8.2) was remarked upon in this early study. In fact, the initial observations of this disease are older; in Europe, the disease is often known as Quincke's oedema[6] and there are older descriptions. As originally noted, the disease is defined by episodic attacks of non-pruritic oedema that affect any external surface of the body as well as by attacks of severe abdominal pain[1–4]. The attacks usually have a duration of one to three days, occurring with no clear pattern. Although clinically the disease is characterized by the occurrence of episodes of oedema of the deeper tissues of the dermis leading to marked local swelling, other organs can be affected. The older literature suggests that many organs can be so affected and there are reported cases of angio-oedema of cerebral tissue leading to episodic hemiparesis as well as angio-oedema of many other organs leading to dysfunction[3]. The original description of Quincke includes such an attack[6]. In fact, those who have followed large numbers of patients with biochemically proven hereditary angio-oedema have not been struck by the frequent attacks of angio-oedema of internal organs with the single exception of the gastrointestinal tract.

It is now known that patients with herediatry angio-oedema have episodic attacks of swelling involving portions of the gastrointestinal submucosa[7,8]. This swelling leads to stretching of the submucosa ultimately producing exquisite pain (Figure 8.3). In some cases, this swelling also leads to partial or complete bowel obstructions. Depending on the location of the oedema, this may lead to constipation with lower gastrointestinal tract involvement or upper bowel obstruction with vomiting. Occasionally, attacks of angio-oedema involve structures of the posterior pharynx, larynx or trachea. In these cases, oedema may

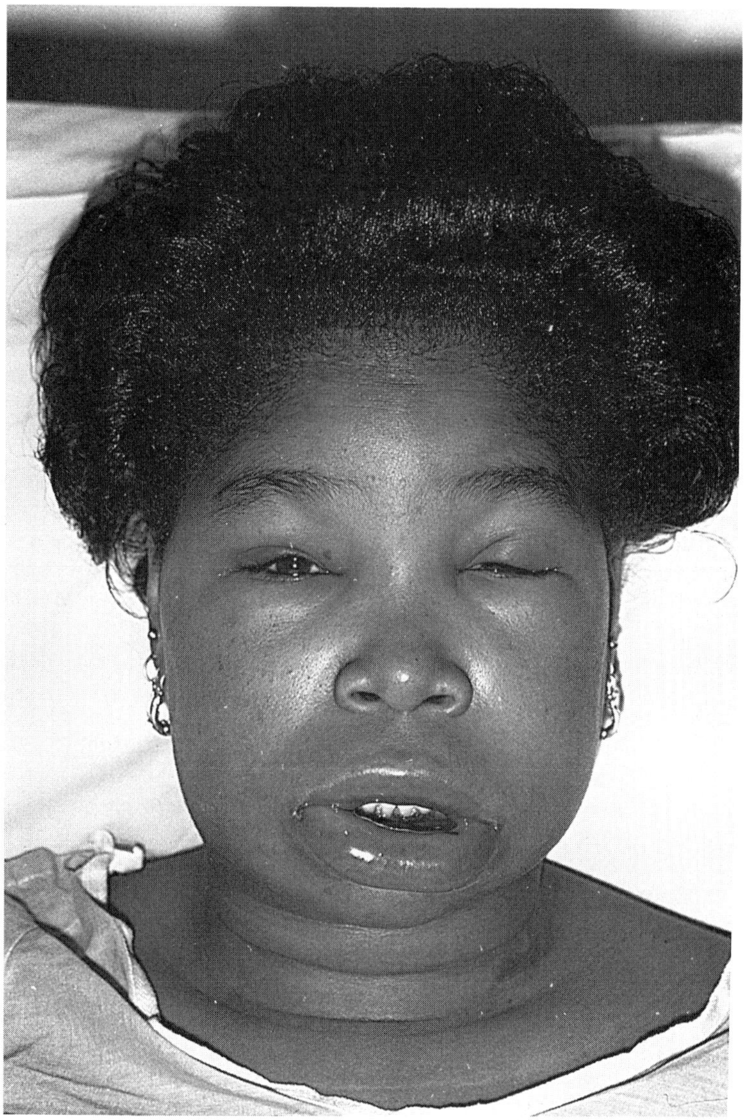

Figure 8.1 Typical attack of facial oedema in a patient with inherited C1-inhibitor deficiency

become so severe or the point of obstruction so critical that asphyxia can result. Thus, in all published series[1–4] of patients with hereditary angio-oedema, family members in whom the appropriate diagnosis was not made, but who had the disease by history, have an incidence of death from asphyxiation of approximately 25%. Typically, attacks of hereditary angio-oedema become increasingly severe for a day and a half and then progressively improve. However,

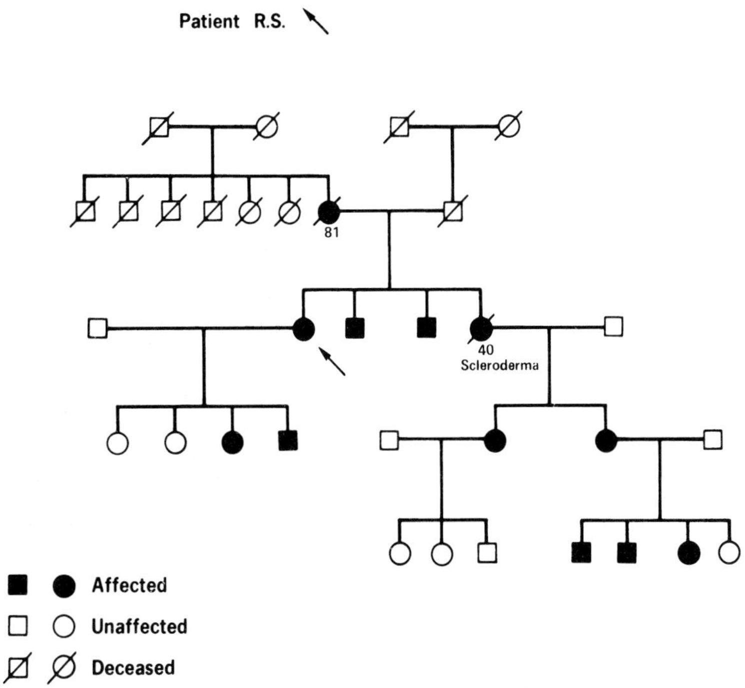

Figure 8.2 Inheritance of C1-inhibitor deficiency through four generations. The level of transmission and the equal involvement of males and females shows an autosomal dominant mode of inheritance

this may not always be the case and occasional attacks may progress slowly moving from one part of the body to another, travelling from hand to foot, ultimately lasting four or five days. Unlike most types of allergic oedema, hereditary angio-oedema attacks do not respond well to epinephrine, antihistamines or steroids. Thus, these can represent true medical emergencies and must be treated in that context.

CLINICAL PRESENTATION

Attacks of hereditary angio-oedema can begin at any time in life. The biochemical abnormality associated with the disease, depressed function of C1-inhibitor, is present from the time of birth and the diagnosis can be made on umbilical cord blood. Nevertheless, first attacks may not occur until the patient reaches the age of 70. The reasons for this are unknown, but are in keeping with the observation that the frequency and severity of clinical symptomatology are not associated with the level of C1-inhibitor[1]. Patients with very low levels of C1-inhibitor do not have more severe disease than patients with levels just below the normal range. Attacks usually begin in infancy or young childhood, but often are not severe and frequently the diagnosis is not established at the

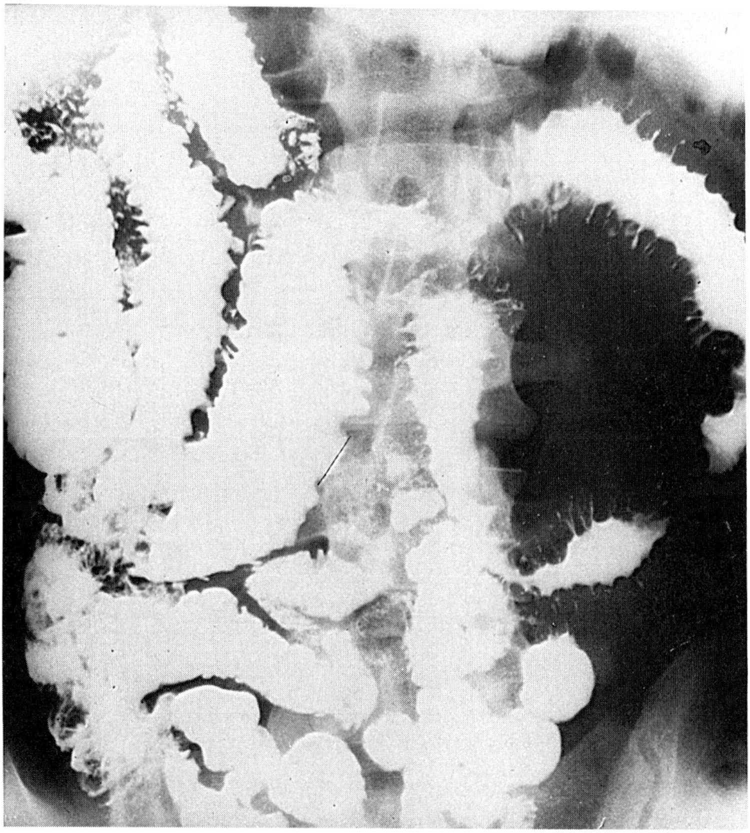

Figure 8.3 Small bowel barium enema of a patient with inherited C1-inhibitor deficiency experiencing an episode of acute abdominal pain. The mucosa is oedematous

time[1–4]. The fact that clinical illness began in childhood is often only recognized retrospectively. Attacks occur with equal frequency in males and females and show a clear autosomal dominant inheritance pattern (Figure 8.2). The NIH experience has been heavily weighted toward females, raising the possibility that attacks are more frequent in females. However, this may simply reflect referral patterns and ascertainment bias, as well as the difficulty in therapy of females leading to referral. This point has not been evaluated carefully. In general, attacks are mild until the time of puberty in both males and females when they become more severe. Hormonal influences on this disease are great and are discussed later. No one has studied carefully the frequency of attacks in the ageing individual. It is my general feeling that attacks often become milder with advancing age, but this has not been proven. Many of our older patients are now on chronic therapy and new patients tend to be in the younger age bracket. Thus, a formal study will be required to determine whether this general impression reflects the true situation.

DESCRIPTION OF ATTACKS

Attacks tend to begin with a prodrome of discomfort lasting minutes to hours before initiation of oedema formation[1-4]. Patients who will have an attack of oedema of a hand will relate that they feel a tingling or 'funny' sensation in the tissue that presages an attack. Similarly, patients who will have an attack of abdominal pain notice a feeling of abdominal discomfort hours before the pain begins. One must assume that this represents initiation of formation of the mediators that will lead ultimately to oedema formation. Attacks may be heralded by the appearance of erythema marginatum at any place on the body surface, particularly on the trunk[9]. These lesions are perceived by the patient as erythematous circles on the skin that are flat and non-pruritic. As mentioned, they often herald an attack but may be unassociated with the formation of peripheral oedema. These last from minutes to hours and disappear without sequelae. Their cause is unknown, but certainly one would like to link them to mediator formation associated with the initiation of the attack. Attacks may be accompanied by a feeling of marked malaise out of keeping with the degree of oedema; malaise, particularly early in the attack, can be quite striking. With the onset of swelling near a joint the patient may notice a limitation of movement or feeling of discomfort in that joint, but there is no true pain or effusion. Oedema formation typically increases over a period of about 36 hours and then decreases over a similar period. Placing a constricting band around the swollen area on a limb will often prevent oedema extension past the point of constriction, once again, suggesting that a mediator must diffuse into the area that is to swell. Unlike true IgE-mediated allergic oedema, urticarial lesions are never associated with the oedema formation of hereditary angio-oedema attacks. Like attacks of peripheral swelling, attacks of abdominal pain are usually increasingly severe for about one and a half days, then improve over a similar period. Although attacks are episodic, in about half of the patients there are identifiable precipitating causes associated with some of the attacks. About half of the patients notice that, in times of anxiety or stress, attack frequency increases markedly[1]. Students will notice increased attacks at the time of an examination. Problems at work lead to a marked exacerbation of attack frequency. Similarly, in about half of patients, trauma, particularly repetitive pressure trauma, will precipitate an attack[1]. Patients will note that standing in one place for a long time may precipitate an attack in the feet; use of a power lawn mower or scissors for a period of time may precipitate attacks in the hands, etc. Nonetheless, in half of patients, this association is not noted, and, even in those patients who have this association, the majority of attacks occur without known cause.

Hormonal influences are clearly important. In a fraction of women, attacks may be linked to the time of menses, and, rarely, attacks only occur at the time of menses. As mentioned earlier, attack frequency increases in both men and women at the time of puberty. Attacks tend to become progressively less severe during pregnancy and women often state that the third trimester of pregnancy is the best period that they have ever had and they are free from attacks completely. Although trauma may precipitate attacks, this author is unaware of any situation in which attacks have occurred during delivery, even if the labour is prolonged. Moreover, attack frequency commonly increases after delivery.

The administration of exogenous oestrogens can strikingly increase attack frequency and severity. The discontinuation of birth control pills may cause striking clinical improvement in some women. The most impressive evidence for the hormonal influence on attacks is the prevention of attacks during androgen therapy in both males and females.

In evaluating attacks of abdominal pain in patients with hereditary angio-oedema, we have been struck by the high frequency of gastric erosions noted on endoscopy[10]. Hyper-acidity is also noted in some patients. Thus, we have tended to treat patients with these symptoms with ranitidine, an H-2 receptor-specific antihistamine, and often see partial relief of symptoms[10]. A host of autoimmune diseases have been described in patients with hereditary angio-oedema. These are described below.

PATHOPHYSIOLOGY

During normal classical pathway activation, C1, composed of three subunits, C1q, C1r and C1s, is activated with the generation of enzymatic esterase activity on both the C1r and C1s subunits[11]. C1-inhibitor binds to activated C1r and C1s to destroy their esterolytic activity. There are two active C1r and two active C1s esterolytic sites in each molecule of C1 and four molecules of C1 inhibitor bind to each molecule of activated C1. The mechanism of action of C1-inhibitor has been under intense study for the last several years. The inhibitor is a member of a family of serine protease inhibitors termed serpins. These proteins present the enzyme to be inhibited with a bait sequence that is cleaved by the target enzyme[12]. Upon cleavage, the inhibitor undergoes a marked conformational change exposing a reactive group that attacks and binds covalently at or near the active enzymatic site. These inhibitors are characterized by the amino acid sequence of the active site. In the case of C1-inhibitor, the critical amino acid at the point of cleavage that determines the enzymatic specificity of the inhibitor is arginine at position 444 linked to threonine at position 445[13]. A second site (P12) is also thought to be critically important[14]. Evidence suggests that C1-inhibitor is a rod-shaped molecule of molecular mass 105 000 containing 478 amino acid residues composed of two domains[15]. The carboxy terminal domain is similar to other serpins. The amino terminal domain is unique[16]. The molecule has an unusually high carbohydrate content (26%) and contains 7 O-linked and 6 N-linked oligosaccharide moieties. It is reported that the carbohydrate is not essential for C1-INH function[15,16]. On cleavage, a major fragment of 96 000 molecular mass is generated[17]. Upon interaction of C1-inhibitor with activated C1, dissociation of the C1 subunits is observed with the generation of free C1q and 2 molecules of $(C1\text{-INH})_2$-C1r-C1s[18–20].

C1-inhibitor is the only circulating inhibitor of activated C1. It is capable of inhibiting activated Hageman factor and its fragments as well as kallikrein, activated factor XI of the intrinsic clotting cascade and plasmin of the fibrinolytic system (Figure 8.4). It is thought to be the principal inhibitor of the plasma kinin generating cascade[21].

Of critical importance in our understanding of hereditary angio-oedema was the demonstration that patients have low functional levels of C1-inhibitor[22].

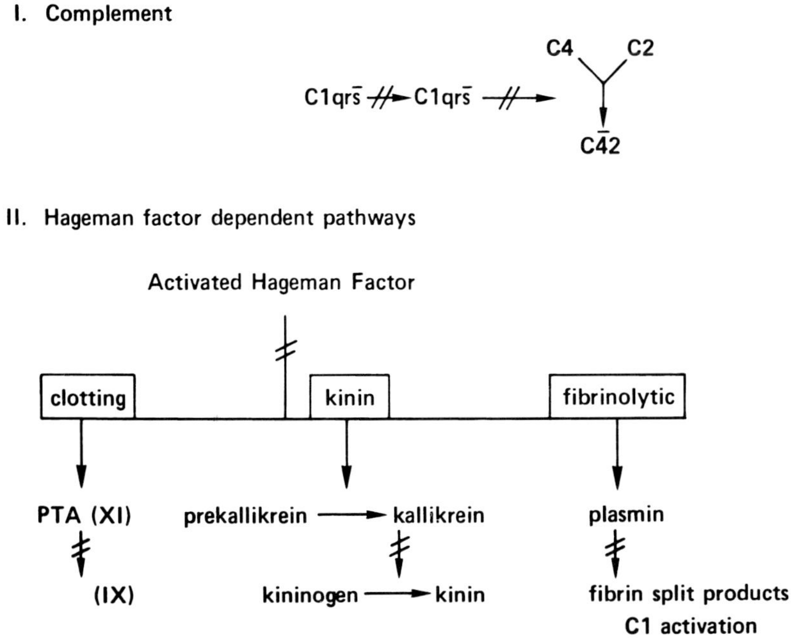

Figure 8.4 Role of C1-inhibitor in the regulation of the plasma mediator systems

Patients either have low levels of circulating protein (about 85% of patients) or have normal or elevated levels of primarily non-functioning protein (about 15%)[23]. The remarkable expansion in our understanding of the structure of the C1-inhibitor gene and the genetic abnormalities that lead to the disease is discussed in detail elsewhere (Chapter 9).

Turnover studies have clearly demonstrated that C1-inhibitor has a modest increase in catabolism (0.035% of plasma pool/h; normal 0.025%) and decreased synthesis in patients with hereditary angio-oedema. In patients with acquired C1-INH deficiency, the fractional catabolic rate is quite rapid (0.353% of plasma pool/h)[24].

Patients with hereditary angio-oedema typically have normal circulating levels of C1 and markedly depressed levels of C4 and C2, reflecting the failure of C1-inhibitor to destroy C1 enzymatic activity and, therefore, the continued cleavage of the natural substrates of activated C1, C4 and C2. On rare occasions, an unusual patient may have normal levels of C4 and C2 between attacks, but these levels are never normal during attacks[1]. As discussed in greater detail below, the presence of a normal C1 level and depressed levels of C4 and C2 helps establish the diagnosis of hereditary angio-oedema, even when confronted with a patient whose disease presumably represents a new mutation and who thus lacks a positive family history. In my experience, in a referral hospital, such patients are common. As discussed below, a number of syndromes have been described with an acquired loss of C1-inhibitor function. Patients with acquired C1-inhibitor deficiency from whatever cause have very low or absent C1 activity, suggesting that the C1-inhibitor deficiency occurs secondary to consumption by large amounts of activated C1.

The factors responsible for oedema formation have never been fully described. A group of investigators[25–27] believe that fragments of C2 formed during complement activation are subsequently cleaved by plasma proteases like plasmin and the small peptides generated from this further cleavage are vasoactive and are responsible for oedema formation (Figure 8.5). This group have formally shown that synthetic peptides derived from the COOH terminus of C2b increase vascular permeability in human and guinea pig skin and induce smooth muscle contraction in rat uterus. There was a direct correlation between peptide length and activity between 5 and 25 amino acid residues, although peptides of larger than 25 residues were not tested[25–27]. One of these peptides (residues 207–223), was not tachyphylactic to itself, or to C3a or C5a. It must therefore have a receptor which is distinct from those of the anaphylatoxins. The anti-

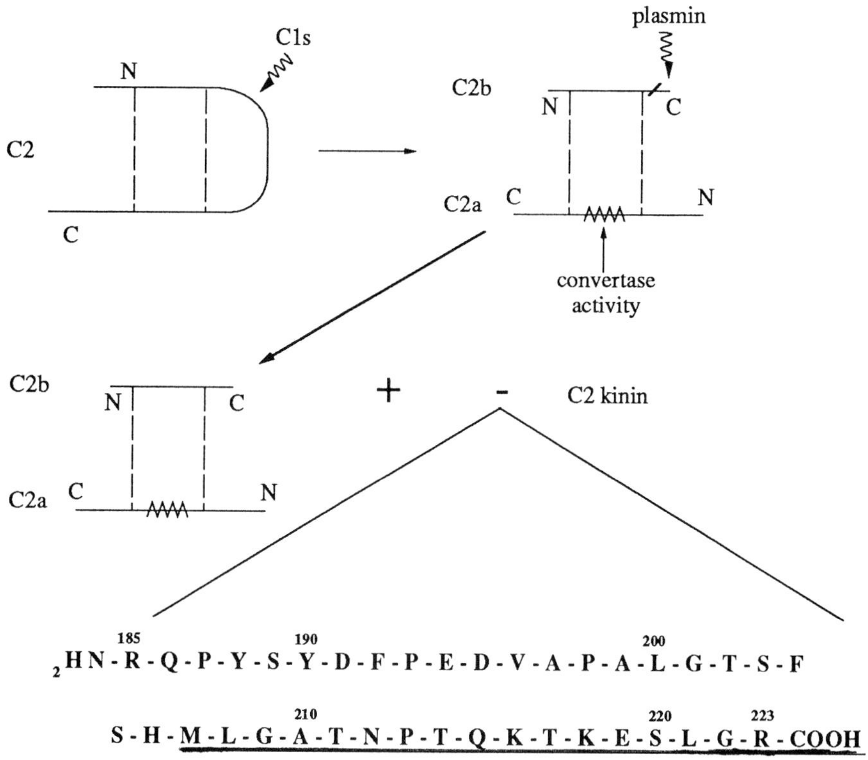

Figure 8.5 Activation of C2 by C1s and the possible generation of C2-kinin from the C-terminus of the C2b fragment by enzymes such as plasmin. Peptides of 5 to 25 residues length from the C-terminus show increasing anaphylatoxic activity. It is possible that the peptide 186–223 could be released as the arginine residue present at position 185 would provide a site for protease cleavage

histamine pyralamine maleate (H1 blocker) was unable to prevent the ability of this peptide to induce angio-oedema or smooth muscle contraction in guinea-pig lung tissue, suggesting that it does not act by stimulating histamine secretion from mast cells. Furthermore, as indomethacin (a cyclooxygenase inhibitor) did not prevent its effects on smooth muscle contraction, the signal used by C2 207–223 is distinct from that used by C3a[28]. These authors believe that the depressed level of C2 reflects its activation and the generation of the pathophysiologically important vasoactive peptide. There is a problem with this formulation as currently understood in that the quantity of peptide required to induce oedema formation in the models thus far studied would appear to be greater than the amount likely to be available in tissue sites. Nevertheless, we know little about tissue levels of relevant mediators and this and related peptides are viable candidates for the cause of angio-oedema. A second group are committed to the idea that bradykinin generated during attacks of angio-oedema by the cleavage of high-molecular-weight kininogen is responsible for oedema formation[29–32]. In keeping with this finding is the fact that angiotensin converting enzyme inhibitors, like captopril, when used to control hypertension in patients with hereditary angio-oedema, have been observed to make attacks more severe[33]. In general, injection of bradykinin subcutaneously into normal individuals causes oedema, but also severe local pain. Pain is completely absent in patients with hereditary angio-oedema, raising a question as to whether bradykinin is the appropriate mediator molecule. Other proteins that interact with both C4 and with molecules of the contact activation cascade are currently being defined and it is possible that fragments derived from one of these other molecules may be the cause of angio-oedema in this disease. It appears that oedema formation is not due to mast cell degranulation with the release of histamine and other intrinsic mast cell mediators as occurs in urticaria and other allergic conditions although the issue is not settled[34–36]. One might have expected histamine to be important since anaphylatoxic peptides can be derived from cleavage of C4 and other proteins of the complement cascade. Such peptides are known to induce mast cell degranulation with release of histamine. Nevertheless, urinary histamine was not elevated in patients having attacks of hereditary angio-oedema[36].

In patients with hereditary angio-oedema, C1 levels are normal and, as mentioned, C4 and C2 are reduced. Presumably, C1 is activated in the normal activation sequence, but activated C1 is not inhibited because of inadequate levels of C1-inhibitor. The activated C1 cleaves and activates both C4 and C2. However, patients with hereditary angio-oedema always have normal levels of C3, suggesting that control mechanisms at this level of the complement cascade are operative. It has been suggested that C4 binding protein is responsible for turning off the cascade at the C2 level and preventing activation of C3[37]. Moreover, as activation in this disease occurs in the fluid phase, the formation of C4b2a, the classical pathway C3 convertase, must be very inefficient. Although serum levels of C3 are normal in patients with hereditary angio-oedema, increased turnover of C3 has been documented; metabolic studies have shown that the fractional catabolic rate of C3 is increased[38] and plasma levels of C3dg are also increased[39]. Components later than C3 are always normal in this disease.

Other diseases are clearly associated with hereditary angio-oedema[40–44]. There are a number of possible reasons for this interesting association. It has been recognized for a number of years that patients with hereditary angio-oedema have a tendency to develop autoimmune disease. Detailed studies have suggested that complement activation plays a regulatory role in the afferent limb of the immune response. It is suggested that, in hereditary angio-oedema patients, activation of the early steps of the classical pathway is associated with a relative lymphocytosis with an increased number of circulating CD4-positive helper T lymphocytes[44]. Interestingly, there is an inverse relationship between the degree of complement activation as reflected in the plasma level of C4 and the degree of lymphocytosis. Possibly associated with this observation is the finding that patients with hereditary angio-oedema have associated autoimmune disease, Sjogren's syndrome being the most common in a large series, but systemic lupus erythematosus, thyroiditis, pernicious anaemia, inflammatory bowel disease and chronic inflammatory polyarthritis all being observed. Interestingly, in our patient group, these disorders have, in general, been mild. Others have described glomerulonephritis and rheumatoid arthritis and it appears that any autoimmune disease can appear during the course of this disease[45,46]. Although a disorder in immunoregulation appears to be an attractive possibility to explain this association, there are other possibilities. It is now clear that complement plays an important role in the proper clearances of immune complexes from the circulation[47]. It is possible that low levels of C4 and C2 lead to failure to remove the complexes from the circulation with an increased prevalence of autoimmunity.

Hereditary angio-oedema was orginally termed hereditary angioneurotic oedema because the disorder was thought to involve nervous supply to the local blood vessels leading to oedema. The word neurotic was removed because some patients were offended by the verbal implication of a psychiatric disorder. Interestingly, our careful evaluation of this patient group suggests that they do have a psychiatric disorder with a tendency to impulsive behaviour that far exceeds the norm. Those that deal with these patients on a regular basis are struck by the fact that often there are difficult medical management problems because of major behavioural disorders.

TREATMENT

Details of treatment of this disease are not appropriate here but some general statements are in order. Long-term management of these patients has been revolutionized by the observation that anabolic steroids are markedly effective in disease treatment[48–52]. Androgens with a 17-methyl keto substitution appear to be required for therapeutic effect. Patients before treatment are usually observed to have about one third of the normal level of C1-inhibitor. They are clearly heterozygotes with one normal C1-inhibitor gene coding for synthesis. The fact that C1-inhibitor is consumed during its function in peripheral sites presumably explains the fact that they have less than half normal levels of protein. Treatment of patients with a wide variety of anabolic steroids leads to increased C1-inhibitor levels, apparently reflecting increased synthesis. All androgens are not equal in this regard and some, like danazol, are highly effective in normalizing C1-inhibitor levels[51]. Interestingly, although not formally studied, there is no clear relationship between the efficiency of an androgen in raising C1-inhibitor levels and its efficacy in decreasing symptoms; perhaps reflecting the lack of concordance between levels and symptoms noted earlier.

About 15% of patients have normal or elevated levels of C1-inhibitor, reflecting the presence of one abnormal gene that codes for a defective protein rather than absence of a normal final product as is usually the case[23,53,54]. The patients with an abnormal gene product respond in the same way to treatment with androgens as do the patients with low C1-inhibitor levels. In these patients, the level of normal C1-inhibitor in plasma rises. Interestingly, in a limited number of carefully studied patients, the level of abnormal protein was unchanged or fell.

Epsilon aminocaproic acid (EACA) and related drugs have also proved to be effective in treatment of this disorder[55–60]. Their mechanism of action is less clear. Patients note the occurrence of prodromes of disease suggesting that mediator formation occurs, but do not note the usual frequency of attacks. When attacks occur, they are less severe and usually more prolonged. It would appear that the propagation of attacks is affected rather than the formation of the mediator that initiates attacks. EACA and the related product, tranexamic acid, are plasmin inhibitors and their effectiveness is in keeping with the suggestion that protease acting on C2 peptides induces attacks, but there is no evidence that the levels of drug achieved in treating patients with HAE are sufficient to block plasmin or other protease activity[61].

Purified C1-inhibitor can be used successfully to terminate angio-oedema attacks[59–62]. The rapid turnover of this protein makes simple chronic replacement of the deficient protein impractical, although it has been used successfully[63]. Fresh frozen plasma as a C1-inhibitor source can be used for successful treatment of attacks. However, at the time of attacks, patients are depleted of mediator substrates and may develop more severe oedema before they recover.

ACQUIRED C1-INHIBITOR DEFICIENCY

In 1968, Caldwell *et al.* reported that rare patients with malignancy, often of lymphoid organs, had low levels of C1-inhibitor function and typical symptoms of hereditary angio-oedema[64]. Over the years, a number of such patients have been reported with a variety of malignancies and it was recognized that rare patients with autoimmune disease had similar symptoms[65]. In each case, treatment of the underlying disease led to amelioration of symptoms. It is particularly interesting that all of the patients with acquired C1-inhibitor deficiency have very low levels of C1 as well as C4 and C2. In the autoimmune diseases, it appeared that marked activation of C1 with utilization of C1-inhibitor, for example by antigen–antibody complexes, was responsible for the disease. In the case of malignancy, the situation was more complex. In some cases, it appeared that the tumour secreted a factor that initiated C1 activation and destruction[66]. In other cases, the formulation of antigen–antibody complexes, perhaps by an immune response to tumour antigens, appeared responsible. In all of these cases, activation of C1 and consumption of C1-inhibitor appeared responsible for disease. In one study, it was suggested that myeloma proteins induce anti-idiotype antibodies that activate C1 and consume the inhibitor[67].

In 1987, it was noted that there exist rare patients who form antibody to C1-inhibitor preventing its action[68]. In most cases, this occurred with no additional sign of underlying autoimmune or malignant disease[68–70]. A few such patients have been followed for decades without any sign of underlying disease. Patients with autoantibody to C1-inhibitor have essentially no detectable C1, C4 and C2 and no C1-inhibitor function although antigenic levels may be normal. Studies have shown that the antigenic C1-inhibitor present in the plasma of these patients is cleaved, having a molecular weight of about 96 000 kDa. As discussed, C1-inhibitor is one of the class of molecules termed serpins, offering a bait sequence to the protease to be inhibited and is in turn cleaved. Upon cleavage, a reactive group is uncovered which forms a covalent bond with the protease. Although anti-C1-inhibitor antibody formed in these patients does not appear to bind to the bait sequence, it may interact with the reactive site formed on inhibitor cleavage, thereby preventing its action, or it may act at a number of other steps in this sequence of reactions[70]. Although the antibodies in individual patients may differ in their mode of action, study of one such autoantibody showed that it facilitated the cleavage of normal C1-inhibitor by $C\bar{1}s$ as a consequence of destabilization of the C1s–C1-inhibitor complexes[71]. The reason why this antibody is formed is unknown and the treatment is still uncertain. An occasional patient has been treated successfully with androgens, glucocorticoids or cytotoxic agents but, in general, the treatment of this condition is unsatisfactory. Interestingly, these patients tend to improve clinically with the passage of time, although their antibody does not disappear. It may be that they synthesize anti-idiotype antibody that in turn prevents function of their anti-C1-inhibitor.

References

1. Frank, M. M., Gelfand, J. A. and Atkinson, J. P. (1976). Hereditary angio-oedema: the clinical syndrome and its management. *Ann. Intern. Med.*, **84**, 580–93
2. Agostini, P. (1989). Inherited C1-inhibitor deficiency. *Complement Inflamm.*, **6**, 112–18
3. Landerman, N. S. (1962). Hereditary angioneurotic oedema. *J. Allergy*, **33**, 316–29
4. Donaldson, V. H. and Rosen, F. S. (1966). Hereditary angioneurotic oedema: a clinical survey. *Pediatrics*, **37**, 1017–27
5. Osler, W. (1888). Hereditary angioneurotic oedema. *Am. J. Med. Sci.*, **95**, 362–7
6. Quincke, H. (1882). Uber akutes umschriebenes H autodem. *Monatsschr. Prakt. Dermatol.*, **1**, 129–31
7. Pearson, K. D., Buchignani, J. S. and Shimkin, P. M. (1972). Hereditary angioneurotic oedema of the gastrointestinal tract. *Am. J. Roentgenol. Radium Ther. Nucl. Med.*, **116**, 256–61
8. Johnson, T. H. and Caldwell, K. W. (1971). Angioneurotic oedema of the colon. *Radiology*, **99**, 61–3
9. Starr, J. C. and Brasher, G. W. (1974). Erythema marginatum preceding hereditary angio-oedema. *J. Allergy Clin. Immunol.*, **53**, 352–5
10. Collen, M. J., Brickman, C. M., Lewis, J. H., Deschner, W. K., Ansher, A. F., Zurlo, J. J., Benjamin, S. B. and Frank, M. M. (1989). Abdominal pain in hereditary angio-oedema: the role of acid hypersecretion. *Am. J. Gastroenterol.*, **84**, 873–877, Erratum *ibid.* (1990) **85**, 119
11. Frank, M. M. and Fries, L. F. (1989). Complement. In Paul, W. E. (ed.) *Fundamental Immunology*, 2nd Ed., pp. 679–702. (New York: Raven Press)

12. Loebermann, H., Tokuoka, R., Deisenhofer, J. and Huber, R. (1984). Human alpha 1-proteinase inhibitor. Crystal structure, analysis of crystal modifications, molecular model and preliminary analysis of the implications for function. *J. Mol. Biol.*, **77**, 531–56
13. Salvesan, G. S., Catanese, J. J., Kress, L. F. and Travis, J. (1985). Primary structure of the reactive site of human C1-inhibitor. *J. Biol. Chem.*, **260**, 2432–6
14. Skriver, K., Wikoff, W. R., Patston, P. A., Tausk, F., Schapira, M., Kaplan, A. P. and Bock, S. Q. (1991). Substrate properties of C1-inhibitor Ma (alanine 434 ; glutamic acid). Genetic and structural evidence suggests that the P12-region contains critical determinants of serine protease inhibitor/substrate status. *J. Biol. Chem.*, **266**, 9216–21
15. Perkins, S. J., Smith, K. F., Amatayakul, S., Ashford, D., Rademaches, I. W., Dwek, R. A., Lachmann, P. J. and Harrison, R. A. (1990). Two domain structure of the native and reactive centre cleaved forms of C1 inhibitor of human complement by neutron scattering. *J. Mol. Biol.*, **214**, 751–63
16. Davis, A. E., Whitehead, A. S., Harrison, R. A., Dauphnais, A., Bruns, G. A. P., Cicardi, M. and Rosen, F. S. (1986). Human C1-inhibitor of the first component of complement, C1: characterization of the cDNA clones and localization of the gene to chromosome 11. *Proc. Natl. Acad. Sci. USA*, **83**, 3161–5
17. Davis, A. E. (1989). Hereditary and acquired deficiencies of C1-inhibitor. *Immunodefic. Rev.*, **1**, 207–26
18. Sim, P. B., Arlaud, G. J. and Colomb, M. G. (1979). Cl-inhibitor dependent dissociation of human complement C1 bound to immune complexes. *Biochem. J.*, **179**, 449
19. Ziccardi, R. J. and Cooper, N. R. (1979). Active disassembly of the first complement component C1 by C1-inactivator. *J. Immuol.*, **123**, 788
20. Schapira, M., de Agostini, A., Schifferli, J. A. and Colman R. W. (1986). Biochemistry and pathophysiology of human C1-inhibitor: Current issues. *Complement*, **2**, 111
21. Ratnoff, O. D., Pensky, J. and Ogston, D. (1969). The inhibition of plasmin, plasma kallikrein, plasma permeability factor and the C′1r subcomponent of the first component of complement by serum C′1 esterase inhibitor. *J. Exp. Med.*, **129**, 315–31
22. Donaldson, V. H. and Evans, R. R. (1963). A biochemical abnormality in hereditary angioneurotic oedema. *Am. J. Med.*, **35**, 37–44
23. Rosen, F. S., Alper, C. A., Pensky, J. and Donaldson, V. (1965). Hereditary angioneurotic oedema: two genetic variants. *Science*, **148**, 957–8
24. Woo, P., Lachmann, P. J., Harrison, R. A., Amos, N., Cooper, C. and Rosen, F. S. (1985) Simultaneous turnover of normal and dysfunctional C1-inhibitor as a probe of in vivo activation of C1 and contact activatable proteases.
25. Strang, C. J., Spragg, J. J., Cholin, S. and Davis, A. E. (1987). Kinin-like activity from a peptide derived from complement component C2. *Fed. Proc.*, **46**, 1196 (abstract)
26. Cholin, S., Strang, C. J., Spragg, J. J., Rosen, F. S. and Davis, A. E. (1988). Synthetic peptides derived from the second component of complement: spasmogenicity and enhanced vasopermeability. *FASEB* J., 2871 (abstract)
27. Strang, C. J., Cholin, S., Spragg, J., Davis, A. E., Schneeberger, E. E., Donaldson, V. H. and Rosen, F. S. (1988). Angio-oedema induced by a peptide derived from complement component C2. *J. Exp. Med.*, **168**, 1685–98
28. Cholin, S., Gerard, N. P., Strang, C. J. and Davis, A. E. (1989). Biologic activity of a C2-derived peptide: demonstration of a specific interaction with guinea pig lung tissues. *J. Immunol.*, **142**, 2401–4
29. Curd, J. G., Prograis, L. J. and Cochrane, C. G. (1980). Detection of active kallikrein in induced blister fluids of hereditary angio-oedema patients. *J. Exp. Med.*, **152**, 742
30. Schapira, M., Silver, L. D. and Scott, C. F. (1983). Pre-kallikrein activation and high molecular weight kininogen consumption in hereditary angio-oedema. *N. Engl.,J. Med.*, **308**, 1050–3
31. Fields, T., Ghebrehiwet, B. and Kaplan, A. P. (1983). Kinin formation in hereditary angio-oedema plasma: evidence against kinin derivation from C2 and in support of "spontaneous" formation of bradykinin. *J. Allergy Clin. Immunol.*, **72**, 54–60
32. Lammle, B., Zuraw, B. L., Haeb, M. J., Schwarz, H. P., Berrettini, M., Curd, J. G. and Griffin, J. H. (1988). Detection and quantitation of cleaved and uncleaved high molecular weight kininogen in plasma by ligand blotting with radiolabelled plasma pre-kallikrein or factor XI. *Thromb. Haemost.*, **59**, 151–61
33. Shepherd, G. M. (1990). Possible contraindication of angiotensin enzyme inhibitors in patients with hereditary angio-oedema. *Am. J. Med.*, **88**, 446

34. Granerus, G., Hallberg, L. and Laurell, A. B. (1967). Studies on the histamine metabolism and the complement system in hereditary angioneurotic oedema. *Acta Med. Scand.*, **185**, 11–22
35. Donaldson, V. H. (1970). Plasma enzymes in inflammation. *Ser. Haematol.*, **3**, 28–95
36. Brickman, C. M., Frank, M. M. and Kaliner, M. (1988). Urine histamine levels in patients with hereditary angio-oedema. *J. Allergy Clin. Immunol.*, **82**, 403–6
37. Gronski, P., Bodenbender, L., Kanzy, E. J. and Seiler, F. R. (1988). C4 binding protein prevents spontaneous cleavage of C3 in sera of patients with hereditary angio-oedema. *Complement*, **5**, 1–12
38. Ruddy, S., Carpenter, C. B., Chin, K. W., Knostman, J. N., Soter, N. A., Gotze, O., Muller-Eberhard, H. J. and Austen, K. F. (1975) Human complement metabolism: and analysis of 144 studies. *Medicine (Baltimore)*, **54**, 165–78
39. Ballogh, Z. and Whaley, K. (1980). Hereditary angio-oedema; problems in diagnosis and management. *Scott. Med. J.*, **25**, 187–95
40. Donaldson, V. A., Hess, E. V. and McAdams, A. J. (1977). Lupus erythematosus-like disease in three unrelated women with hereditary angioneurotic oedema. *Ann. Intern. Med.*, **86**, 312
41. Tuffanelli, D. L. (1977). Discoid lupus erythematosus and the variant form of hereditary angio-oedema. *Arch. Dermatol.*, **113**, 374
42. Seignalet, C., Berthoux, F., Seignalet, J. and Michel, F. B. (1979). Hereditary angio-oedema and C3 nephritic factor-HLA study. *Clin. Allergy*, **9**, 527
43. Brickman, C. M., Tsokos, G. C., Balow, J. E., Lawley, T. J., Santaella, M., Hammer, C. H. and Frank, M. M. (1986). Immunoregulatory disorders associated with hereditary angio-oedema I. Clinical manifestation of autoimmune disease. *J. Allergy Clin. Immunol.*, **77**, 749–57
44. Brickman, C. M., Tsokos, G. C., Chused, T. M., Balow, J. E., Lawley, T. J., Santaella, M., Hammer, C. H., Linton, G. F. and Frank, M. M. (1986). Immunoregulatory disorders associated with hereditary angio-oedema. II. Serologic and cellular abnormalities. *J. Allergy Clin Immunol.*, **77**, 758–67
45. Hory, B. and Haultier, J. J. (1989). Glomerulonephritis and hereditary angio-oedema: A report of two cases. *Clin. Nephrol.* **31**, 259–63
46. Duncan, I. J., Tymms, K. E. and Carney, G. (1989). Rheumatoid arthritis and hereditary angio-oedema. *J. Rheumatol.*, **15**, 700–2
47. Cornacoff, J. B., Hebert, L. A., Smead, W. L., Van Aman, M. E., Birmingham, D. J. and Waxman, F. J. (1983). Primate erythrocyte immune complex-clearance mechanism. *J. Clin. Invest.*, **71**, 236–47
48. Spaulding, W. B. (1960). Methyltestosterone therapy for hereditary episodic oedema (hereditary angioneurotic oedema). *Ann. Intern. Med.*, **53**, 739–45
49. Davis, P. J., Davis, F. B. and Charache, P. (1974). Long-term therapy of hereditary angio-oedema (HAE). Preventive management with fluoxymesterone and oxymetholone in severely affected males and females. *Johns Hopkins Med. J.*, **135**, 391–8
50. Rosse, W. F., Logue, G. W., Silberman, H. R. and Frank, M. M. (1976). The effect of synthetic androgens in hereditary angio-oedema: alteration of C1-inhibitor and C4 levels. *Trans. Assoc. Am. Physicians*, **89**, 122–33
51. Gelfand, J. A., Sherins, R. J., Alling, D. W. and Frank, M. M. (1976). Treatment of hereditary angio-oedema with danazol: reversal of clinical and biochemical abnormalities. *N. Engl. J. Med.*, **295**, 1444–8
52. Sheffer, A. L., Fearon, D. T. and Austen, K. F. (1981). Clinical and biochemical effects of stanozolol therapy for hereditary angio-oedema. *J. Allergy Clin. Immunol.* **68**, 181
53. Rosen, F. S., Alper, C. A., Pensky, J., Klemperer, M. R. and Donaldson, V. H. (1971). Genetically determined heterogeneity of the C1 esterase inhibitor in patients with hereditary angioneurotic oedema. *J. Clin. Invest.*, **50**, 2143–9
54. Gadek, J. E., Hosea, S. W., Gelfand, J. A. and Frank, M. M. (1979). Response of variant hereditary angio-oedema phenotypes to danazol therapy: genetic implications. *J. Clin. Invest.*, **64**, 280–6
55. Nilsson, I. M., Andersson, L. and Bjorkman, S. E. (1966). Epsilon-amino-caproic acid (E-ACA) as a therapeutic agent based on 5 years' clinical experience. *Acta Med. Scand.*, **448** (suppl.), 1–46
56. Lundh, B., Laurell, A. B. and Wetterquist, H. (1968). A case of hereditary angioneurotic oedema successfully treated with epsilon-aminocaproic acid. *Clin. Exp. Immunol.*, **3**, 733–45

57. Gwynn, C. M. (1974). Therapy in hereditary angioneurotic oedema. *Arch. Dis. Child*, **49**, 636–40
58. Blohme, G. (1972). Treatment of hereditary angioneurotic oedema with tranexamic acid. *Acta Med. Scand.*, **192**, 293–8
59. Frank, M. M., Sergent, J. S., Kane, M. A. and Alling, D. W. (1972). Epsilon aminocaproic acid therapy of hereditary angioneurotic oedema: a double-blind study. *N. Engl. J. Med.*, **286**, 808–12
60. Sheffer, A. L., Austen, K. F. and Rosen, F. S. (1972). Tranexamic acid therapy in hereditary angioneurotic oedema. *N. Engl. J. Med.*, **287**, 452–4
61. Soter, N. A., Austen, K. F. and Gigli, I. (1975). Inhibition by epsilon aminocaproic acid of the activation of the first component of the complement system. *J. Immunol.*, **114**, 928–32
62. Gadek, J. E., Hosea, S. W., Gelfand, J. A., Santaella, M., Wickerhauser, M., Triantaphyllopoulos, D. C. and Frank, M. M. (1980). Replacement therapy in hereditary angio-oedema: successful treatment of acute episodes of angio-oedema with partially purified C1-inhibitor. *N. Engl. J. Med.*, **302**, 542–6
63. Bork, K. and Witzka, G. (1989). Long-term prophylaxis with C1-inhibitor (C1-inh) concentrate in patients with recurrent angio-oedema caused by inherited and acquired C1-inhibitor deficiency. *J. Allergy Clin. Immunol.*, **83**, 677–682
64. Caldwell, J. R., Ruddy, S., Schur, P. H. and Austen, K. F. (1972). Acquired C1-inhibitor deficiency in lymphosarcoma. *Clin. Immunol. Immunopathol.*, **1**, 39–52
65. Gelfand, J. A., Boss, G. R., Conley, C. L., Reinhart, R. and Frank, M. M. (1979). Acquired C1 esterase inhibitor deficiency and angio-oedema: a review. *Medicine (Baltimore)*, **58**, 321–8
66. Frank, M. M. (1989). Acquired C1 inhibitor deficiency. *Behring Inst. Mitteilungen*, **84**, 161–4
67. Geha, R. S., Quinti, I., Austen, K. F., Cicardi, M., Scheffer A. and Rosen, F. S. (1985). Acquired C1-inhibitor deficiency associated with anti-idiotypic antibody to monoclonal immunoglobulins. *N. Engl. J. Med.*, **312**, 534–40
68. Alsenz, J., Bork, K. and Loos, M. (1987). Autoantibody-mediated acquired deficiency of C1-inhibitor. *N. Engl. J. Med.*, **316**, 1360–6
69. Jackson, J., Sim, R. B., Whelan, A. and Feighery, C. (1986). An IgG autoantibody which inactivates C1-inhibitor. *Nature*, **323**, 722–4
70. Malbran, A., Hammer, C. H., Frank, M. M. and Fries, L. F. (1988). Acquired angio-oedema: observations on the mechanism of action of autoantibodies directed against C1 esterase inhibitor. *J. Allergy Clin. Immunol.*, **81**, 1199–1204
71. Jackson, J., Sim, R. B., Whaley, K. and Feighery, C. (1989). Autoantibody facilitated cleavage of C1-inhibitor in autoimmune angio-oedema. *J. Clin. Invest.*, **83**, 698–707

9
Molecular genetics of C1-inhibitor and hereditary angio-oedema

M. TOSI

The hereditary transmission of angioneurotic oedema was documented as early as 1888 by the remarkable pedigree investigations of W. Osler[1]. His work and subsequent family studies led to the recognition of the autosomal dominant mode of transmission of the disease[2].

The first biochemical characterization of hereditary angio(neurotic)oedema was provided by the demonstration of a deficit of kallikrein inhibitory activity in the plasma of patients[3]. Shortly after the preliminary characterization[4] of a plasma protein which controls the protease activity of C1, the first component of complement, the hereditary abnormality was related to the function of the complement system by the demonstration that the serum of hereditary angio-oedema patients essentially lacks this inhibitor[5]. A few years later, C1-inhibitor was found to be identical with α_2-neuraminoglycoprotein, a plasma protein which had been previously identified on the basis of its electrophoretic mobility and its relatively high *N*-acetylneuraminate (sialic acid) content[6,7].

Molecular probes for human C1-inhibitor were isolated independently in several laboratories in the form of complementary DNA (cDNA) clones[8–14]. Using these molecular probes and the DNA from suitable somatic cell hybrids, the *C1-inhibitor* (*C1-INH*) gene was mapped[9] to chromosome 11, more specifically[8] to subregions 11p11.2-q13. The regional assignment was subsequently refined down to 11q12-q13.1 (Ref. 15) or 11q11-q13.1 (Ref. 16) by *in situ* hybridization. The exon–intron structure of the normal *C1-INH* gene was elucidated using genomic clones isolated by screening cosmid libraries[12] or libraries constructed in bacteriophage lambda vectors[17]. The complete nucleotide sequence of the normal gene has been established, including the transcription start site and more than 1 kb of 5′ upstream sequences[18].

Our understanding of the C1-inhibitor protein has also improved substantially thanks to the nucleotide sequence data derived from the cDNA clones. Partial peptide sequences were verified and extended. The deduced amino acid sequences[8–13] conclusively demonstrated that C1-inhibitor is a member of the large family of serine protease inhibitors (serpins), although it displays several distinct features, particularly in the N-terminal region, as discussed below. The structural and functional features of serpins are described in Refs. 19 and 20.

C1-inhibitor and hereditary angio-oedema (HAE) have been discussed extensively[21,22]. Recent reviews on HAE[23,24] also give an account of the first insights into the molecular bases of the disease. Here, we examine the latest reported molecular lesions in the *C1-INH* locus, and discuss their implications for diagnostic purposes. Finally, we consider briefly the potential for therapy of studies which are under way on the activity of genetically engineered variants of the C1-inhibitor protein and on the regulation of the expression of the *C1-INH* gene.

THE C1-INHIBITOR PROTEIN

C1-inhibitor is a plasma glycoprotein with a molecular mass of 105 kDa, as determined by SDS–gel electrophoresis[25], although varying amounts of an additional 96 kDa polypeptide have also been observed (cf. Ref. 21). It is synthesized as a precursor protein from which a putative signal peptide consisting of the 22 aminoterminal residues is removed during the initial steps of intracellular maturation. The high degree of glycosylation of C1-inhibitor is readily apparent from a comparison with the estimated mass of only 54 kDa calculated from the size of the 478 amino acids composing the mature protein (see Figure 9.1). It contains, in fact, an unusually high number of potential oligosaccharide attachment sites, of which six are sites of N-linked glycosylation, with the consensus sequence Asn-X-Thr/Ser (boxed in Figure 9.1). Glucosamine-based oligosaccharide groups were indeed found on all of those six asparagine residues[8]. The post-translational modification of these sites of N-linked glycosylation can also be followed *in vitro* using synthetic C1-inhibitor mRNAs and a rabbit reticulocyte lysate supplemented with limiting amounts of microsomal membranes (Meo and Bourgarel, unpublished results). In addition, at least seven O-linked glycosylation sites have been suggested in the C1-inhibitor protein, all located within a stretch of 100 amino acids at the aminoterminal end of the molecule[8]. This number has recently been confirmed[26] and the composition of N-linked and O-linked oligosaccharides has been determined[26,27]. The total mass of oligosaccharides accounts for 26% of the mass of C1-inhibitor, which has been found by neutron scattering to be 76 ± 4 kDa[26]. The much higher apparent size in SDS–PAGE (105 kDa) seems, at least in part, due to the effect of the high proline content of the N-terminal portion of the protein, since the carbohydrate-free protein produced *in vitro* also has an abnormally slow electrophoretic mobility[11]. It is interesting to note that this aminoterminal region represents an extension unique to this member of the serpin family, and that it consists of a long stretch of repetition of the tetrapeptide Gln-Pro-Thr-Thr or a variant thereof (underlined in Figure 9.1).

```
          exon2                                              ↓exon3
                  m a s r l t l l t l l l l l l a g ↓d r a s
    1
    s N P N A T S S S S Q D P E S L Q D R G E G K V A T T V I S
 30 K M L F V E P I L E V S S L P T T N S T T N S A T K I T A N
 60 T T D E P T T Q P T T E P T T Q P T I Q P T Q P T T Q L P T
 90 D S P T Q P T T G S F C P G P V T L C S D L E S H S T E A V
120 L G D A L V D F S L K L Y H A F S A M K K V E T N M A F S P
                          ↓exon4
150 F S I A S L L T Q V L L G A G Q N T K T N L E S I L S Y P K
                                                       ↓exon5
180 D F T C V H Q A L K G F T T K G V T S V S Q I F H S P D L A
210 I R D T F V N A S R T L Y S S S P R V L S N N S D A N L E L
240 I N T W V A K N T N N K I S R L L D S L P S D T R L V L L N
              ↓exon6
270 A I Y L S A ↓K W K T T F D P K K T R M E P F H F K N S V I K
                                                 ↓exon7
300 V P M M N S K K Y P V A H F I D Q T L K A K V ↓G Q L Q L S H
330 N L S L V I L V P Q N L K H R L E D M E Q A L S P S V F K A
360 I M E K L E M S K F Q P T L L T L P R I K V T T S Q D M L S
              ↓exon8
390 I M E K L E F F D F S Y D L N L C G L T E D P D L Q V S A M
                                                  444
420 Q H Q T V L E L T E T G V E A A A A S A I S V A R T L L V F
450 E V Q Q P F L F V L W D Q Q H K F P V F M G R V Y D P R A
                      M
```

Figure 9.1 Sequence of the C1-inhibitor precursor protein, deduced from cDNA clones[8–13]. The putative leader peptide is in lower-case letters. Circles mark the four cysteine residues and arginine-444 of the reactive site. N-linked glycosylation sites are boxed, and the repeated tetrapeptide, glutamine-proline-threonine-threonine (QPTT), or its variants are underlined. Arrows mark the position of introns in the *C1-INH* gene (cf. Figure 9.2). They occur either between codons (arrows separating amino acid residues) or after the first nucleotide of a codon (arrows above an amino acid residue)[12]. Note that the translation initiation site is within exon 2. The one-letter amino acid code is used: A = alanine; C = cysteine; D = aspartic acid; E = glutamic acid; F = phenylalanine; G = glycine; H = histidine; I = isoleucine; K = lysine; L = leucine; M = methionine; N = asparagine; P = proline; Q = glutamine; R = arginine; S = serine; T = threonine; V = valine; W = tryptophan; Y = tyrosine

These threonines repeated in a particular context provide a partial explanation for the unusually high density of O-linked glycosylation sites. The presence of a proline residue within this tetrapeptide repeat also accounts for the high proline content of this aminoterminal extension, which probably plays a role in determining the elongated overall shape of the aminoterminal portion of C1-inhibitor[26,28]. It has been suggested, based on molecular models for C1q, C1r, C1s and C1-inhibitor, that the N-terminal domain reduces the affinity of binding to C1q of inhibited C1r and C1s because it masks the non-protease domains of the latter proteins[26]. The unusually high oligosaccharide content of C1-inhibitor may also play a role in the catabolism of the protein.

The reactive site, which presents a substrate-like structure to the target proteases, features an arginine residue at the crucial P1 position of C1-inhibitor (Arg-444, Figures 9.1 and 9.7). This residue forms a heat- and denaturant-stable complex with target proteases. The reaction mechanism leading to the formation of this complex is not known with precision. At a later step of the reaction, the peptide bond between the P1 and the P1′ residue (Thr-445 in C1-inhibitor; cf. Figures 9.1 and 9.7) is often cleaved. Enzymatic or chemical removal of oligosaccharides does not abolish the *in vitro* inhibitory activity of C1-inhibitor towards serine proteases[29]. Furthermore, *in vitro* synthesized polypeptides which lack the 93 aminoterminal residues still retain the ability to form complexes with activated C1s (our unpublished data). These observations confirm and extend previous data on the natural protein, which showed that the 40 aminoterminal residues can be removed without affecting protein activity or heat stability[30]. Taken together, these data indicate the presence in C1-inhibitor of two structurally and functionally distinct domains: a 'serpin' domain, which positions the reactive site for recognition and irreversible binding of the target proteases, and a 'glyco' domain[13], whose function is still a matter of speculation[26].

Also marked in Figure 9.1 are the four cysteine residues, which form the two disulphide bridges[8], Cys-101 to Cys-406 and Cys-108 to Cys-183, and the only position where a protein polymorphism, which apparently affects neither the inhibitory functions nor protein stability, has been observed (valine or methionine residues at position 458)[8]. This polymorphism, detected at the DNA level using the restriction enzyme *Hgi* AI, is one of two DNA polymorphisms known in the *C1-INH* locus, the other being a *Kpn* I site which, however, lies in the 3′ flanking region of the gene[31].

Superimposed on the protein sequence is the distribution of the coding sequences among the seven coding exons of the gene (cf. Figure 9.2). One should note that introns occur either between codons (arrows separating amino acid residues) or within codons (arrows on top of an amino acid residue). Thus, the effect of internal deletions of the gene on the reading frame of the residual protein product will depend on the particular exons which are deleted, as discussed below.

TYPE I AND TYPE II HAE: ORIGINAL BASIS OF THE CLASSIFICATION

By determining the plasma levels of C1-inhibitor using conventional antisera, two distinct forms of HAE were defined. The more common one (type I HAE) results from a quantitative defect, with low or trace amounts of C1-inhibitor protein, which only in a few cases reach 30% of the normal level (20 mg/100 ml; see e.g. Refs. 32 and 23). On the other hand, in approximately 15–24% of affected families, normal or even greater than normal amounts of a dysfunc-

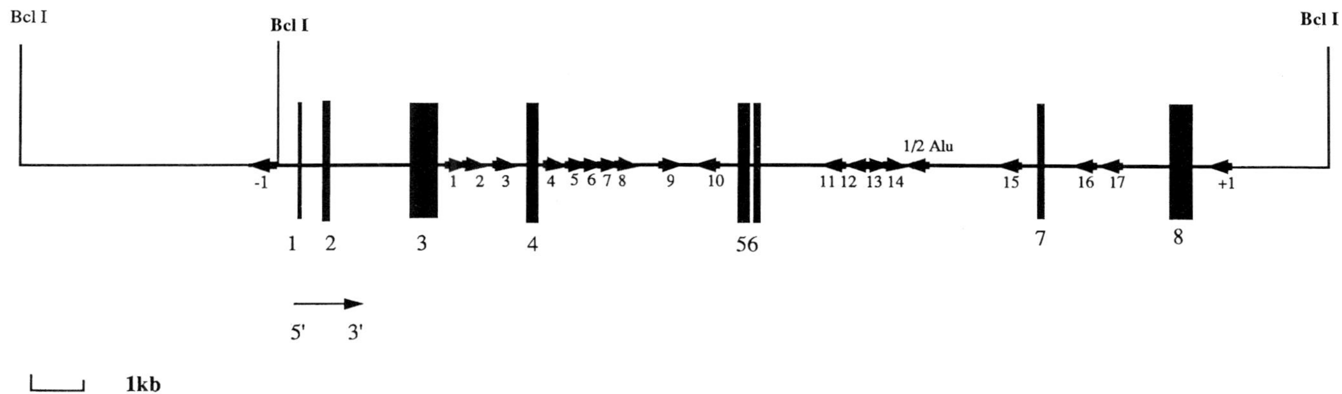

Figure 9.2 Structure of the normal *C1-INH* gene. Exons are shown as full boxes. Arrows mark the position and orientation of repetitive *Alu* sequences[18]. Note that, among *Alu* repeats lying outside the gene, only the most proximal ones are shown (–1 and +1, respectively), and that only the *Bcl* I restriction endonuclease sites are indicated. Adapted from Ref. 18

tional protein were found (type II HAE)[23,32,33]. For type II HAE, it was straightforward to postulate a change at the essential P1 residue Arg-444, or at a nearby location, to explain the lack of inhibitory activity. When the reactivity of several type II proteins was examined with serine proteases recognized by C1-inhibitor (activated C1s, activated plasminogen, plasma kallikrein, activated Hageman factor), shifts in the spectrum of inhibitory activity towards these proteases were indeed observed[34].

For the more common form of the disorder, it was, however, difficult to reconcile a low C1-inhibitor plasma level with the dominant mode of transmission of the disease. From the heterozygous genotype of the patients, one would have in fact predicted the presence of about 50% of the normal levels of C1-inhibitor. To resolve this inconsistency, it was proposed that the defect in type I HAE could be at the level of regulation of expression of the *C1-INH* locus, rather than in the structural *C1-INH* gene, and that, for example, a defective regulatory protein could reduce the expression of both allelic *C1-INH* gene copies[35].

These speculations about the molecular basis of type I HAE persisted until the *C1-INH* locus and its expression at the mRNA level were examined using cDNA probes. The lack of useful genetic markers of the *C1-INH* locus or of the protein itself had, in fact, prevented segregation studies in affected families. Shortly after the description of the first cDNA clones, the detection in a large multi-generation family of variant C1-inhibitor restriction fragments made it possible to demonstrate their strict cosegregation with the disease[36]. These altered restriction fragments turned out to result from a major change in the *C1-INH* gene, as discussed below. Indeed, several affected families were found, each characterized by cosegregation of the disease with a readily detectable and family-specific gene alteration[36]. On the other hand, in contrast to the plasma level of the protein, C1-inhibitor mRNA was indeed found at about 50% of normal levels in monocytes from type I HAE patients[37,38]. The former study[37] also reported a patient whose cultured monocytes produced a shorter C1-inhibitor mRNA in addition to the normal one. A preliminary report suggested that skin fibroblast lines developed from type I HAE patients also produce about 50% of normal amounts of C1-inhibitor[39]. However, a re-examination of C1-inhibitor mRNA and protein produced by cultured fibroblasts from four unrelated type I and two unrelated type II patients indicated that, in type I fibroblasts, both the intracellular C1-inhibitor and the secreted protein are present at levels significantly and consistently below the 50% value[40]. The same study also suggested that the reduced expression of the normal allele may be determined at a pretranslational level because the amounts of C1-inhibitor mRNA in type I fibroblasts were estimated to correspond to about one third of the mRNA levels in normal fibroblasts. Additional experiments are needed to demonstrate the molecular basis of this interesting 'trans-inhibition' effect (discussed below).

However, an adequate explanation of the discrepancy between the heterozygous genotype of HAE patients and the observation of plasma protein levels much lower than the expected 50% was brought forth by studies of the C1-inhibitor catabolism, along the lines proposed by Quastel and colleagues[41] and Lachman and Rosen[42]. Both the lower than expected amount of C1-inhibitor in type I patients and the vanishingly low amounts of functional activity in type II patients result from hypercatabolism determined by the formation of complexes with target proteases. A recent examination of the composition of these complexes supports the notion that consumption of C1-inhibitor by activated uncontrolled C1s contributes in a significant way to the increased catabolism[43].

MAJOR C1-INH GENE ALTERATIONS OBSERVED IN ALMOST 20% OF TYPE I HAE FAMILIES

Initial attempts to detect structural abnormalities in the *C1-INH* locus of type I patients[8,36,44,45] were based on DNA blot analyses, i.e. digestion of leukocyte DNA with various restriction endonucleases, followed by gel electrophoresis, transfer of the DNA fragments onto a membrane and hybridization with cDNA probes of various length. Because the organization of the normal *C1-INH* gene was not known, various sets of randomly chosen restriction endonucleases were used in different laboratories. Although they were successful in several cases, such early studies failed to detect some gene alterations[36,44]; this became apparent only upon re-examination using additional restriction enzymes and/or different cDNA probes[46-48]. Subsequently, the DNA blot analyses were greatly facilitated by the availability of an essentially full-length cDNA probe[8] and of restriction maps obtained from molecular clones representing the normal gene[12,17]. This information, recently completed by the determination of the entire gene sequence[18], allows one to select restriction endonucleases suitable for a rapid screening of unrelated affected individuals and then to choose additional enzymes in order to examine in detail patients carrying readily-detectable gene alterations. The enzyme *BcI* I proved to be particularly useful[17] because it generates a 20 kb fragment containing the entire gene (see Figure 9.2) and it allows the detection of the major alterations, provided an adequate resolution of the electrophoretic separation.[48]

The normal *C1-INH* gene (Figure 9.2) covers 17 159 bp from the transcription start site to the site of RNA polyadenylation[18]. It is composed of eight exons, of which the first contains only 5′-non-coding sequences. As already noted above (cf. Figure 9.1), introns split the coding sequences either between codons (phase 0) or after the first nucleotide of a triplet (phase 1). Currently, no obvious correlation can be seen between exons and particular structural or functional domains of the protein.

A previously unsuspected feature of the sequence of the normal gene is the presence of an exceptionally high number of repeats of the *Alu* family in various orientations (marked by arrows in Figure 9.2). *Alu* sequences represent the largest class of short interspersed repetitive sequences in the human genome and are found on average every 5–10 kb[49]. They have already been found to be involved in deleterious alterations of several human genes (see e.g. Ref. 50 and the references in 48 and 51). Particularly dense clusters of tandem *Alu* repeats were found around the fourth exon of the *C1-INH* gene (Figure 9.2), a region where several changes had already been mapped roughly[36] before the structure of the normal gene was known. Such clusters of *Alu* repeats represent a major source of genetic instability in the *C1-INH* gene[51], as illustrated by the examples shown in Figure 9.3. The affected gene of several unrelated type I patients revealed, in fact, distinct alterations of the 6.9 kb *Bam* HI fragment containing exons 3–6, betrayed by the presence of additional shorter and family-specific fragments. To determine the precise nature of these alterations, two genomic libraries were prepared from the DNA of an affected member of family F1 and of family F4, respectively, and the family-specific 3.7 kb and 4.3 kb *Bam* HI fragments (Figure 9.3) were isolated. Nucleotide sequence analyses of these fragments yielded the information shown in Figure 9.4. In family F4, the deletion boundaries were found within the first repeat (Alu 1) and within the sixth one (Alu 6). Likewise, the boundaries of the larger deletion of family F1 were found within Alu 1 and Alu 8, respectively.

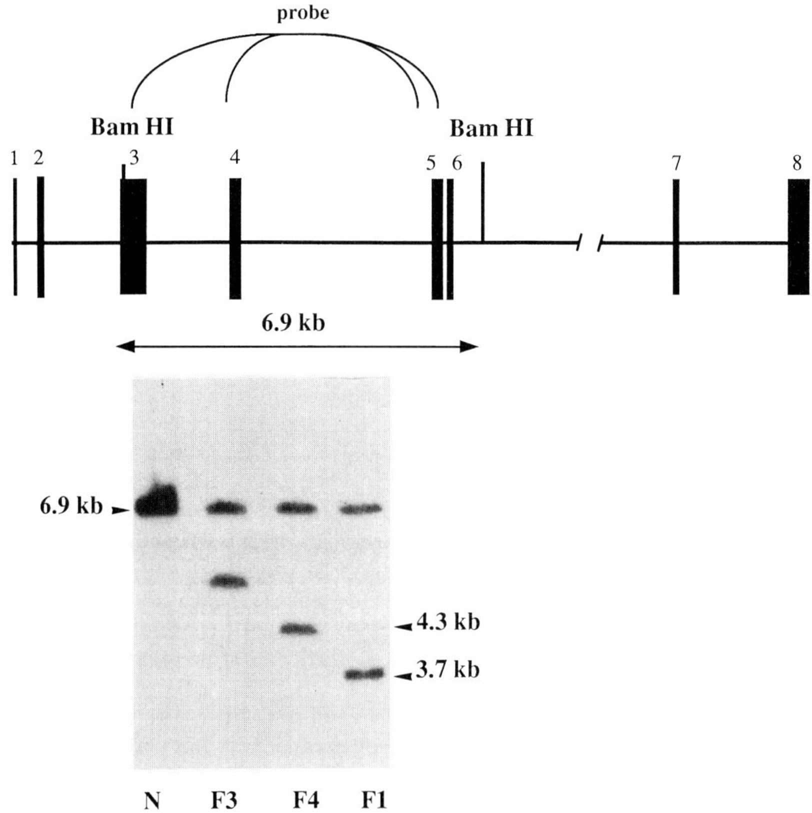

Figure 9.3 Examples of partial deletions detected in the 5′ half of the *C1-INH* gene. DNAs from unrelated HAE patients and from a normal person were digested with the restriction endonuclease *Bam* HI and the DNA blot was hybridized with a cDNA probe covering exons 3–6. Only the *Bam* HI sites delimiting the 6.9 kb fragment are shown in the scheme of the normal gene. Note the presence of a shorter and family-specific *Bam* HI fragment in the affected persons, in addition to the normal one. N = normal; F1, F3, F4 = hereditary HAE patients

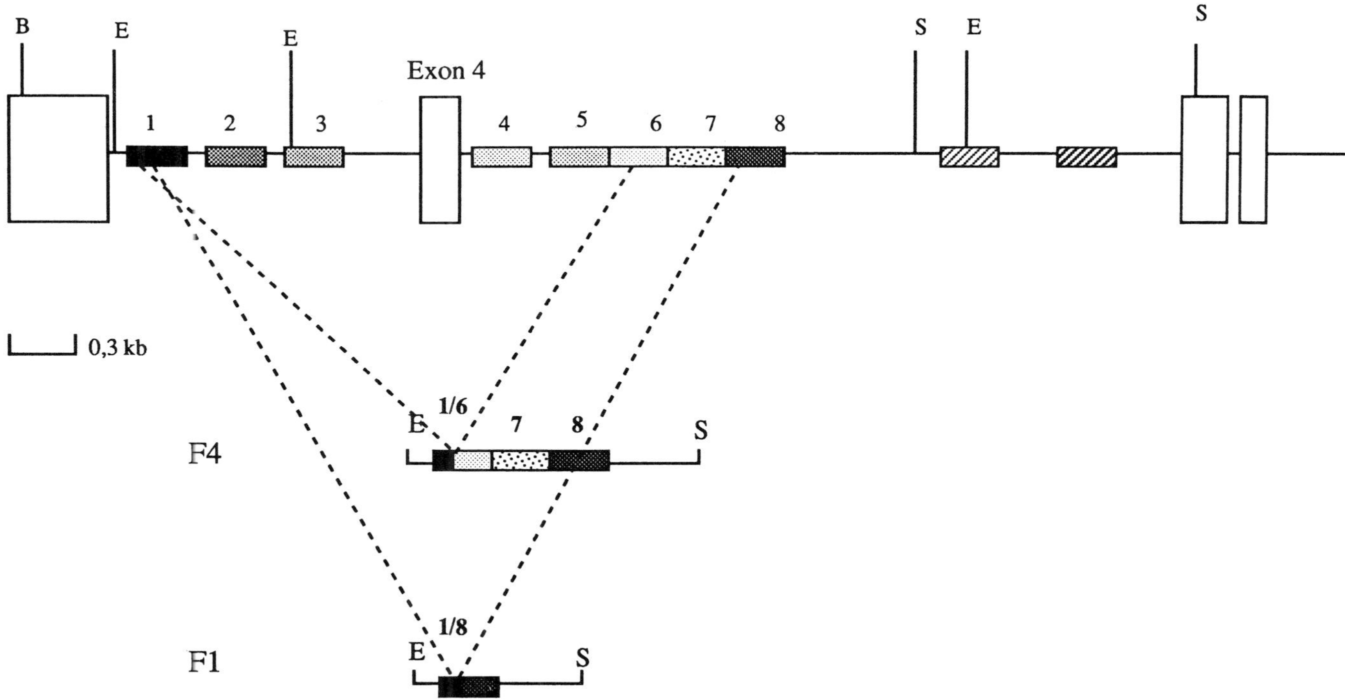

Figure 9.4 Localization of the boundaries of the deletions observed in families F1 and F4. The upper scheme depicts the normal 6.9 kb *Bam* HI (B) fragment with exons shown as open boxes and *Alu* repeats as small rectangles. Both deletions have their 5′ breakpoints within Alu 1 but at different nucleotide positions[51]. The deletion of family F4 joins a 5′ portion of Alu 1 to a 3′ portion of Alu 6, and generates a novel *Alu* repeat. The larger deletion of family F1 joins Alu 1 and Alu 8 sequences. This scheme summarizes data obtained by molecular cloning of the family-specific 4.3 kb and 3.7 kb *Bam* HI fragments shown in Figure 9.3, followed by sequence analyses of the *Eco*RI(E)-*Sac*I(S) fragments containing the deletion boundaries

These are but two examples of a variety of *C1-INH* gene alterations brought about by the presence of dense clusters of intragenic *Alu* repeats. In our study of 46 unrelated kindred, we have, in fact, observed 8 different partial deletions and one example of partial duplication[48,51].

Similar results were obtained by other investigators. Four out of 12 kindred with type I HAE revealed changes of restriction fragments in a study performed with 38 restriction enzymes[45]. Because of the large number of enzymes used in this study, DNA changes were detected in about 30% of the type I kindred examined. However, only two kindred had a partially deleted *C1-INH* gene. In one case, akin to those illustrated in Figure 9.4, the deletion was localized around exon 4 but it extends over only about 1 kb, as opposed to 2.6 kb in the example shown here for family F4. In another kindred, the deletion was localized to about 1.7 kb around exon 7. Although the precise deletion boundaries have not been defined by sequence analysis, the location and orientation of *Alu* repeats in the proximity of these exons (cf. Figure 9.2) suggest that *Alu* sequences may also be involved in these two deletions. In two other kindred described by McPhaden *et al.*[45], a single restriction fragment was altered, suggesting minor changes. The exon 6/intron 6 boundary is modified in one case[52], and, in the other family, the molecular basis of the disease seems to be related to a change at the *BgI* II site within exon 8.

Partial *C1-INH* gene alterations in type I HAE patients were also reported in other studies[46,47] in which the deletion boundaries were sequenced and localized within *Alu* repeats. Interestingly, one of these deletions included a stretch of about 2 kb around exon 7, with boundaries within *Alu* repeats 15 and 17, respectively (cf. family A in Figure 9.6). Affected members of this family were in fact those in which a shorter monocyte mRNA had been detected, in addition to the normal-sized one[37,46]. The other deletion extends from within *Alu* 1 to within *Alu* 14 (cf. family B in Figure 9.6), and thus encompasses exons 4–6.

These results from different laboratories are in keeping with the notion that major structural changes account for almost 20% of the genes affected by type I HAE and that most of them involve *Alu* repeats at their boundaries. Thus, the discovery of an unusually high number of *Alu* repeats in the normal *C1-INH* gene, and their presence at the boundaries of a large number of deletions (cf. also Figure 9.6), have fully confirmed earlier predictions that structural properties of this gene make it prone to undergo occasional rearrangements[36], although the frequency of such major changes turned out to be somewhat lower than could be anticipated from the initial study of seven unrelated kindred. The finding that these deletions are family specific, as documented by their size and location, but are related to the presence of clusters of *Alu* repeats in the normal gene, also rules out the hypothesis that such major alterations might be specific of certain populations[53]. Moreover, no obvious population bias could be discerned in each of the two initial studies[36,44].

Homologous recombination, driven by the similarity of mispaired *Alu* repeats, which amounts to about 80% nucleotide identity, is the most likely explanation for the occurrence of these deletions, and for their length variation. As illustrated in Figure 9.5, unequal crossovers may take place at meiosis between *Alu* sequences mispaired in a variety at registers, particularly around exon 4. In the example shown in this figure, the recombination event would involve *Alu*

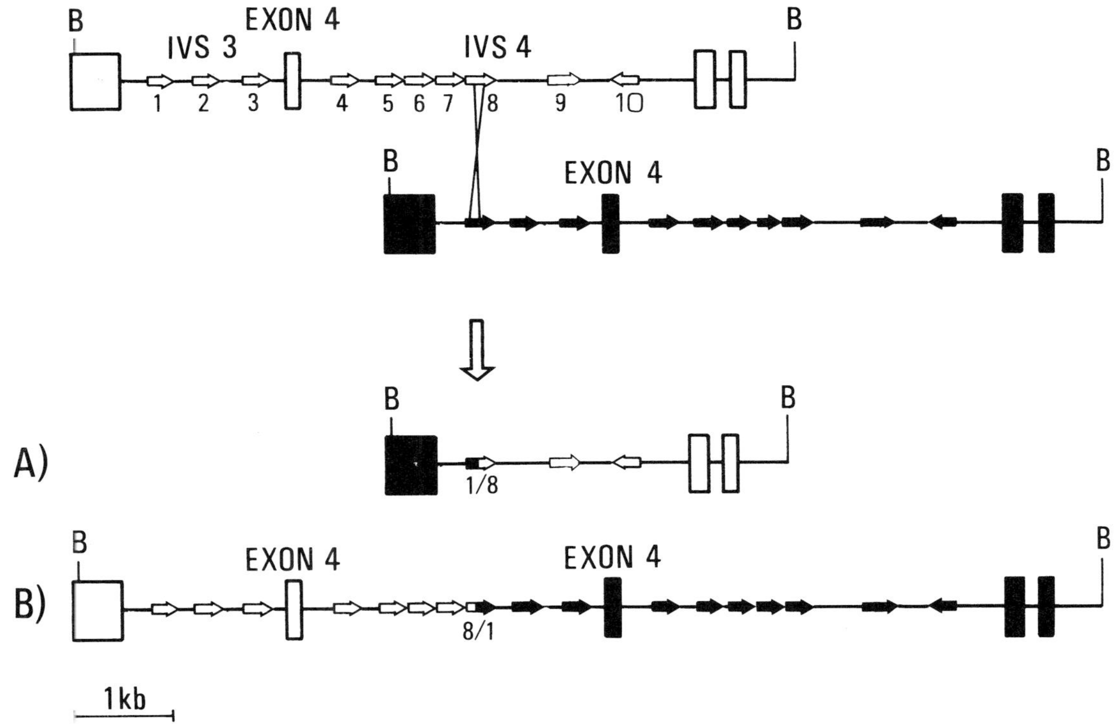

Figure 9.5 Model of meiotic unequal crossover between misaligned *Alu* sequences of normal genes. Only the portion containing exons 3–6, which is delimited by *Bam* HI sites (B), is shown. **A**) shows a deletion around exon 4, as observed in family F1. **B**) shows a partial duplication, as observed in family F5 (cf. Figure 9.6). Adapted from Ref. 51

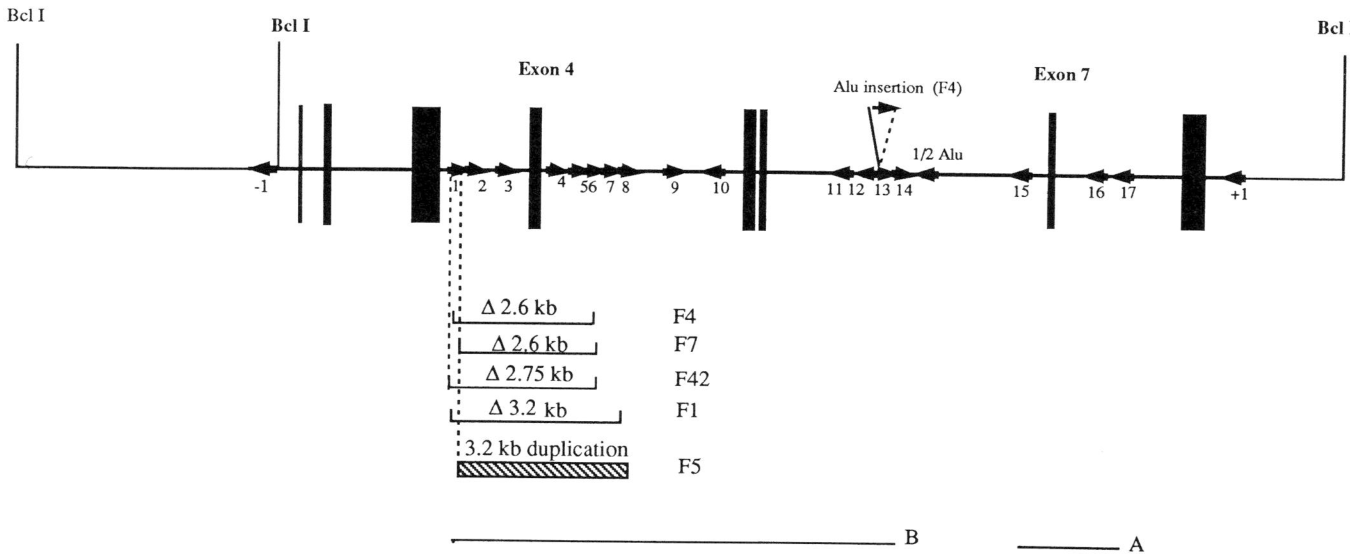

Figure 9.6 Location and extent of gene rearrangements whose boundaries have been defined by nucleotide sequence analysis. Families F1, F4, F5, F7 and F42 were described in Refs. 48 and 51. Families A and B were described in Ref. 47. Note that six rearrangements have their 5′ boundaries within Alu 1, the first intragenic *Alu* repeat. The *Alu* repeat inserted into repeat 13 of family F4 was described in Ref. 51

elements 1 and 8 of genes located on different sister chromatids or homologous chromosomes, and would lead to the production of a gene with a deletion of exon 4, similar to the one observed in family F1 (cf. Figure 9.4). However, the model also predicts the production of a gene with a partial duplication of exon 4, which might be found among type I HAE patients, if such a duplication is deleterious. One of the 46 unrelated families included in our study indeed had a gene with a duplication of exon 4[51]. This finding strongly supports the model of unequal crossover because alternative models, based for example on intra-chromatid recombination, are unable to account for duplications. It is, however, difficult to explain the disproportion between the rather large number of exon 4 deletions and the single exon 4 duplication observed until now if one assumes that all the rearrangements around exon 4 have taken place according to this model.

The propensity of the region around exon 4 to undergo deletions or duplications is underscored by comparisons of all the rearrangements that have been reported. Figure 9.6 includes six deletions and a duplication whose boundaries have been determined by sequence analysis. One should note, however, that three additional large deletions extending into the 5′ flanking regions and a large deletion around exon 8 have been found[48], and that, as already mentioned, an exon 4 and an exon 7 deletion were found, respectively in two of the families studied by McPhaden *et al.*[45] Therefore, out of a total of 13 type I kindred with major gene changes, six rearrangements around exon 4 have been reported. In addition, the deletion of family B (Figure 9.6), although it extends over several exons, also has its 5′ boundary in intron 3. A surprising result of the comparisons shown in Figure 9.6 is, in fact, the disproportionate involvement of the first intragenic *Alu* repeat (Alu 1), which suggests the presence of additional peculiar features, either within this *Alu* repeat or in the upstream regions (see Ref. 48 for a more detailed discussion).

Also shown in Figure 9.6 is an additional *Alu* repeat, inserted in the central portion of Alu 13 of the affected gene of family F4[51]. This gene also has a 2.6 kb deletion around exon 4 as shown above (cf. Figures 9.4 and 9.6). It is therefore unclear whether this insertion of an *Alu* sequence represents an additional accidental modification of an already impaired gene or whether it has preceded, and possibly even favoured, the exon 4 deletion. Nevertheless, it provides a nice example of the potential of *Alu* repeats to vary their number and to invade new chromosomal locations by retroposition[49].

BIOCHEMICAL CONSEQUENCES OF PARTIAL DELETIONS/DUPLICATIONS

In view of the heterogeneity of the defects observed in the *C1-INH* gene, one may wonder whether all type I HAE patients have the same biochemical abnormality and whether they can be distinguished at the protein level. The consequences of large deletions on the expression of the affected gene can be predicted once their boundaries have been defined. Obviously, large deletions spanning the promoter region and extending into the 5′ flanking sequences[48] are expected to prevent the expression of the gene already at the transcriptional level. On the other hand, internal deletions, which represent the largest fraction of the rearrangements, as shown in Figure 9.6, might not prevent the production of an internally truncated or otherwise modified protein. The early observation of a shorter mRNA in one kindred[37], subsequently[46] explained as resulting from the deletion of exon 7 (see family A in Figure 9.6), was already an indication that, in some cases, a rather stable messenger can be produced from a deleted gene, even if the shortened messenger was less abundant than the normal one[46]. However, no translation product of the shorter mRNA could be found in the serum of these patients or as a product of their cultured monocytes[46]. In the shorter mRNA, the nucleotide sequences of exon 8 are joined precisely to those of exon 6, shifting the reading frame, since the introns which flank exon 7 interrupt the coding sequences with different phases. As shown in Figure 9.1, intron 6 is indeed in phase 0, whereas intron 7 is in phase 1. This shift of the reading frame introduces a premature termination codon 14 triplets after the deletion. Failure to detect such polypeptide in cultured monocytes was interpreted as an indication of its rapid intracellular degradation[46]. Reduced levels of this mutant protein were indeed found intracellularly in cultured fibroblasts from a patient with an exon 7 deletion[54] but the intracellular level of the normal protein was also found to be reduced in these fibroblasts (see below).

Deletions of exon 4 (cf. Figure 9.6) call for different predictions of the structure of the putative protein because the boundaries of this exon are in the same phase (cf. Figure 9.1). In the monocytes of patients from families F1 and F4 (cf. Figure 9.4), an internally shortened mRNA was detected at levels similar to those of the normal messenger upon enzymatic amplification using the polymerase chain reaction technique (PCR). Sequence analyses demonstrated that, in the short mRNA, the exon 3 and exon 5 sequences were joined precisely. One therefore expects the production of an internally deleted protein with the same reading frame but lacking the 45 amino acids specified by exon 4. To examine the fate of this C1-inhibitor polypeptide, a plasmid suitable for transfection into COS cells was constructed, in which a full-length C1-inhibitor cDNA[8] was modified and the exon 4 sequences were deleted precisely. Upon transfection of the DNA into cultured COS cells, a shorter and partially glycosylated C1-inhibitor protein was indeed produced, which accumulated intracellularly[55]. It is presently unclear whether lack of secretion is determined primarily by a defective folding, by the loss of a disulphide bridge, since Cys-183 is encoded in exon 4 (cf. Figure 9.1), or simply by the presence of a free cysteine residue.

It is likely, although it remains to be demonstrated directly, that the protein products from deletions encompassing exon 4 also accumulate intracellularly in hepatocytes, monocytes, skin fibroblasts[56], or in other cell-types in which C1-inhibitor is expressed, e.g. endothelial cells[57]. These findings may have practical implications, considering that deletions that allow the production of a grossly altered protein are expected to occur in about 10% of the type I families, as estimated from the combined frequencies of exon 4 and exon 7 deletions (cf. Figure 9.6). Furthermore, a sizeable fraction of point mutations or other minor alterations in exons or exon–intron boundaries may determine the production of C1-inhibitor polypeptides with a variety of impairments in intracellular maturation and/or transport. The probable intracellular accumulation of abnormal proteins in the hepatocyte calls attention to the possibility of hepatic disorders in some HAE patients, particularly under conditions in which the expression of both *C1-INH* gene copies is stimulated, as is probably the case under androgen (e.g. danazol) therapy. However, limited surveys of patients with exon 4 deletion have failed to reveal evidence of such hepatic dysfunctions.

CHANGES NOT AFFECTING THE REACTIVE-SITE RESIDUE Arg-444 BLUR THE BORDERLINE BETWEEN TYPE I AND TYPE II HAE

As already mentioned, type II HAE patients are distinguished because of the presence of normal or even greater than normal serum concentrations of antigenically detectable C1-inhibitor, in spite of the low functional activity. Type II kindred have long been found to be heterogeneous both biochemically and functionally (see e.g. Refs. 23 and 34). Consistent with the essential role of the P1 position of the reactive site, several of these proteins were found to be mutated at the Arg-444 residue[17,58,59]. As shown in Figure 9.7, several examples of arginine-to-cysteine or arginine-to-histidine substitutions have been found at this position, and one serine replacement has been reported[59]. The higher frequency of point mutations yielding a cysteine or a histidine at this position can be explained by the propensity of cytidine residues in the CpG dinucleotide of the Arg-444 codon CGC or in its complement on the opposite DNA strand to undergo spontaneous deamination and conversion to a thymidine[61]. While these changes at the P1 position of the reactive site provide a sufficient explanation for the dysfunctional character of these type II proteins, it was somewhat surprising to find several type II families carrying mutations at a distant location. A valine-to-methionine substitution at position 334 was reported in one patient[23,62], and the deletion of nucleotides encoding the lysine residue at position 251 was described as the most likely cause of type II HAE in another kindred[63]. Interestingly, the latter change generates a new recognition site for N-linked glycosylation (cf. Figure 9.1) by changing the sequence from Asn-Lys-Ile-Ser to Asn-Ile-Ser. Both examples indicate that mutations which affect positions remote from the reactive site on the primary structure interfere with either the initial binding of C1-inhibitor to serine proteases or the function of the reactive site itself. Furthermore, the mutant protein which bears an additional N-linked oligosaccharide may be dysfunctional because it is folded differently or because of a direct effect of the added carbohydrate.

In another mutant[64], also described as type II, a point mutation has converted an alanine into a threonine residue at position 436, eight residues on the aminoterminal side of the P1 position (see Figure 9.7). Since this alanine is rather conserved[19], it is likely that it plays an important role in maintaining a functional conformation of the reactive-centre loop. Thus, it was not surprising to find that mutations at this position affect the inhibitory activity. However, it was quite unexpected to detect lower than normal antigenic levels of plasma C1-inhibitor in some of these patients. In fact, type I HAE had been diagnosed initially in one of two apparently unrelated kindred carrying this point mutation[44,64]. It is possible that this mutant protein is catabolized more rapidly than

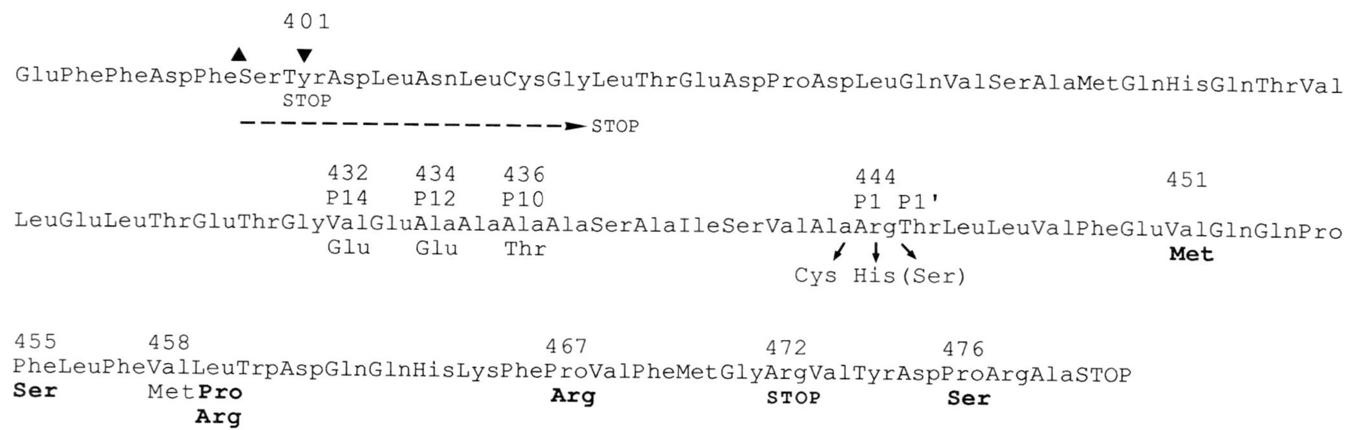

Figure 9.7 Point mutations within exon 8 and the corresponding amino acid changes. The P1 position mutations described in type II patients result in the replacement of arginine-444 by cysteine, histidine or serine, but the latter substitution is rare. Residue 458 is polymorphic[8]. Full triangles at codons 399/400 and at codon 401 denote the deletion and the insertion of a single nucleotide, respectively. The former produces a frame shift and a premature termination of translation and the latter mutation introduces a stop codon[60]. Note that the residues valine-432, alanine-434 and alanine-436 are labelled P14, P12 and P10, respectively, according to the numbering used for other members of the serpin family. Amino acid changes that affect intracellular transport and secretion are shown in boldface letters (Ref. 72 and unpublished data kindly provided by Elisabeth Verpy). References for the P1, P10, P12 and P14 mutations are given in the text

the normal inhibitor, in spite of being dysfunctional. Moreover, this change in a crucial region of the reactive-site loop may not only alter the functional properties, but may also result in a protein which is cleaved by proteases and is poorly recognized by some of the polyclonal antisera used to measure the antigenic levels of C1-inhibitor. However, replacement of alanine at position 436 with threonine does not increase the susceptibility of C1-inhibitor to target proteases, but produces a marked change of the conformation of the reactive-site loop, detected with monoclonal antibodies that recognize neoepitopes[65]. This finding is in sharp contrast with the effect of other mutations in the same region. For example, replacement at position 434 (P12 or serpins; cf. Figure 9.7) of the alanine residue with glutamic acid converts the inhibitor into a substrate for target proteases[66]. A valine-to-glutamic acid substitution has also been described in a type II patient at position 432 (P14)[67]. The properties of this mutant C1-inhibitor are under investigation[67]. Most of these mutants have been characterized by *in vitro* mutagenesis and expression in eucaryotic cells (e.g. COS-1 or COS-7 cells). The same approach has also been followed to study the effects of internal deletions, as already mentioned, and those of mutations at the P1 residue[68]. C1-inhibitor variants which are resistant to neutrophil elastase[69] have also been obtained using this strategy. Interestingly, a combination of substitutions of leucine at position Ile-440 and alanine at position Val-442 has been shown to reduce susceptibility to neutrophil elastase, while maintaining and even improving complex formation with activated C1s[70].

In a systematic search for point mutations in exon 8 of type 1 patients, we were surprised to find a sizeable fraction of changes downstream of the reactive site (Figure 9.7). In fact, different changes were found in this area in 8 out of 36 unrelated patients[71]. The main biochemical consequence of this group of mutations is a marked, and in some cases complete, impairment of intracellular transport and secretion[72].

Precise predictions of the effects of amino acid substitutions await the determination of the three-dimensional structure of C1-inhibitor or at least of another serpin in its uncleaved form, even though interesting indications on the shape of the reactive-site loop can already be deduced from the structure of ovalbumin[73], a member of the serpin family, for which, however, no inhibitory activity against serine proteases is known. Mutations near or within the reactive-site loop may alter the inhibitory function or affect, to varying degrees, the folding of C1-inhibitor and consequently its intracellular or extracellular stability. It may also be of interest to examine these mutant proteins with combinations of antibodies which allow discrimination between the native, the complexed and the cleaved forms of C1-inhibitor[43,69].

REGULATION OF C1-INH GENE EXPRESSION

Physiological or pharmacological mediators of increased C1-inhibitor expression are being studied in several laboratories. While an exhaustive review of this area of intense investigation is outside the scope of this chapter, a few selected aspects will be presented which point to the special interest of studies on the molecular bases of these regulations.

From the data that are currently available, some answers are already emerging to the following questions:

(1) Which cytokines or hormones are most effective in enhancing C1-inhibitor production?
(2) At which level(s) do they modulate the expression of C1-inhibitor?
(3) Will a better understanding of the hormonal modulation of the expression of the *C1-INH* gene allow significant improvements in the treatment of patients?

Interferon-γ (IFN-γ) has a marked effect on C1-inhibitor expression in most cell types which have been studied, including primary hepatocytes and several hepatoma cell lines[74], monocytes[75–77], fibroblasts[56], umbilical vein endothelial cells[78], the monocytic line U937[79] and the erythroleukaemia line HEL[80]. In monocytes, IFN-γ increases steady-state C1-inhibitor mRNA levels by a combination of increased transcription and increased mRNA stability[81,82], but, in other cell types, the effect of IFN-γ on C1-inhibitor mRNA stability is less pronounced[78]. In monocytes, IFN-α and -β seem to act mainly at the level of transcription[82]. IFN-β and TFN-α, but not IL-6 or IL-1, stimulate the expression of C1-inhibitor in skin fibroblasts[56]. IL-6 stimulates C1-inhibitor synthesis in the hepatoma cell lines, HepG2, HepB3 and Alexander PLC, and in primary hepatocyte cultures[74,83]. Besides the effect of several attenuated androgens used in therapy[84], whose mode of action is however unknown, *in vivo* stimulation of C1-inhibitor expression has been observed, at least to our knowledge, only for IFN-γ and for IFN-α. The former has been reported to increase significantly C1-inhibitor plasma levels[80], whereas IFN-α which has a marked effect on mRNA levels in circulating monocytes (Ramadori, Tosi and Duponchel, unpublished), does not seem to affect significantly the plasma level of C1-inhibitor.

A two- to four-fold induction of C1-inhibitor protein and mRNA has been reported, using the androgens, testosterone or dehydroepiandrosterone (DHEA), in HepG2 cells and in the human monocytic cell-line U937[79]. The latter finding is at variance with the results of similar studies on cultured human monocytes, in which no androgen responsiveness was observed[38]. This discrepancy also emphasizes the need for a direct examination of the androgen receptor content in U937 cells and human monocytes.

Other preliminary studies also failed to reveal significant effects of danazol or 17-methyltestosterone[22] on C1-inhibitor expression in hepatoma lines. It is currently unclear whether these inconsistencies are due to the use of different androgenic hormones or to other differences in the experimental conditions. Studies with the cloned *C1-INH* gene[12] or with portions of it containing the putative promoter region[18] should help to define those mediators which act directly on gene transcription.

CONCLUSIONS AND PERSPECTIVES

As suggested by early functional studies and biochemical characterizations of the C1-inhibitor protein of patients[32], HAE turned out to be genetically very heterogeneous. Yet, an unexpected feature of the normal gene, i.e. the high density of repetitive sequences of the *Alu* family within introns, provides a collective explanation for a relevant fraction of type I deficiencies, amounting to almost 20% of the total. On the other hand, in addition to the rather infrequent mutations at the P1 position of the reactive site, which determine the production of a typical type II protein, a sizeable fraction of deficiencies also results from mutations in the last exon of the gene, which, however, do not affect the reactive site P1 residue directly. Most of these amino acid changes were found in type I patients, but mutations in the 'hinge' region of the reactive site loop (residues P14–P10) determine the production of apparently normal amounts of dysfunctional C1-inhibitor proteins that are sometimes highly susceptible to proteolytic cleavage. These findings provide at least an indication of two groups of molecular defects for which systematic searches at the DNA level can easily be performed. Thus, in spite of the genetic heterogeneity of the disease, the chance of detecting the relevant mutation by using Southern blot hybridization on *Bcl* 1 digests combined with sequencing of exon 8 can already be estimated at about 30–40%.

DNA analysis at birth or in young children at risk, which can easily be performed in the increasing fraction of families in which direct DNA markers of the disease are available, has already proven useful because it is more direct and probably more reliable than the quantitative or functional measurements of plasma C1-inhibitor. On the other hand, one occasionally observes cases of angio-oedema without familial history, which cannot be attributed to any of the known acquired forms. Several examples of *de novo* mutations have already been reported[71,72]. Diagnosis at the DNA level provides, in these cases, the only clue to establish the nature of the disease, to re-examine family members and to type the descendants.

The molecular effects of cytokines and hormones will soon be examined in detail at the gene level. There is reasonable hope that a better understanding of the mode of action of these mediators will also contribute to the development of new and better tolerated enhancers of C1-inhibitor expression.

Acknowledgements

I wish to express my gratitude to Tommaso Meo, Dominique Stoppa-Lyonnet, Christiane Duponchel and Pierre Bourgarel for sharing ideas, skills and enthusiasm during the molecular cloning of C1-inhibitor and in our joint effort to understand the molecular bases of HAE. I wish to thank the numerous colleagues who helped to recruit families, and specially Dr. J. Laurent, Prof. G. Lagrue and Prof. A. Sobel for their constant interest in this research. This work was supported in part by grants from the Caisse Nationale d'Assurance Maladie des Travailleurs Salariés.

References

1. Osler, W. (1888). Hereditary angio-neurotic oedema. *Am. J. Med. Sci.*, **95**, 362–7
2. Crowder, J. R. and Crowder, T. R. (1917). Five generations of angioneurotic edema. *Arch. Intern. Med.*, **20**, 840–52

3. Landerman, N. S. (1962). Hereditary angioneurotic edema. II. Deficiency of inhibitor for serum globulin permeability factor and/or plasma kallikrein. *J. Allergy*, **33**, 330–41
4. Pensky, J., Levy, L. and Lepow, I. (1961). Partial purification of a serum inhibitor of C′1 esterase. *J. Biol. Chem.*, **236**, 1674–9
5. Donaldson, V. H. and Evans, R. R. (1963). A biochemical abnormality in hereditary angioneurotic edema. Absence of serum inhibitor of C′1-esterase. *Am. J. Med.*, **35**, 37–44
6. Schultze, H. E., Heide, K. and Haupt, H. (1962). Uber ein bisher unbekanntes saures alpha2-glykoprotein. *Naturwissenschaften*, **49**, 133–4
7. Pensky, J. and Schwick, H. G. (1969). Human serum inhibitor of C′1 esterase: identity with alpha2-neuraminoglycoprotein. *Science*, **163**, 698–9
8. Bock, S. C., Skriver, K., Nielsen, E., Thogersen, H.-C., Wiman, B., Donaldson, V. H., Eddy, R. L., Marrinan, J., Radziejewska, E., Huber, R., Shows, T. B. and Magnusson, S. (1986). Human C1 inhibitor: primary structure, cDNA cloning and chromosomal localization. *Biochemistry*, **25**, 4292–301
9. Davis III, A. E., Whitehead, A. S., Harrison, R. A., Dauphinais, A., Bruns, G. A. P., Cicardi, M. and Rosen, F. S. (1986). Human inhibitor of the first component of complement, C1: characterization of cDNA clones and localization of the gene to chromosome 11. *Proc. Natl. Acad. Sci. USA*, **83**, 3161–5
10. Que, B. G. and Petra, P. H. (1986). Isolation and analysis of a cDNA coding for human C1 inhibitor. *Biochem. Biophys. Res. Commun.*, **137**, 620–5
11. Tosi, M., Duponchel, C., Bourgarel, P., Colomb, M. and Meo, T. (1986). Molecular cloning of human C1 inhibitor: sequence homologies with α1-antitrypsin and other members of the serpins superfamily. *Gene*, **42**, 265–72
12. Carter, P. E., Dunbar, B. and Fothergill, J. E. (1988). Genomic and cDNA cloning of the human C1 inhibitor. *Eur. J. Biochem.*, **173**, 163–9
13. Rauth, G., Schumacher, G., Buckel, P. and Müller-Esterl, W. (1988). Molecular cloning of the cDNA coding for human C1 inhibitor. *Protein Seq. Data Anal.*, **1**, 251–7
14. Eldering, E., Nuijens, J. H. and Hack, C. E. (1988). Expression of functional human C1 inhibitor in COS cells. *J. Biol. Chem.*, **263**, 11776–9
15. Fukushima, Y., Byers, M., Bock, S. and Shows, T. (1987). The human C1 inhibitor gene (C1NH) is located at 11q12–13.1. Ninth International Workshop on Human Gene Mapping (abstract). *Cytogenet. Cell. Genet.*, **45**, 617
16. Theriault, A., Whaley, K., McPhaden, A. R., Boyd, E. and Connor, J. M. (1990). Regional assignment of the human C1 inhibitor gene to 11q11–q13.1. *Hum. Genet.*, **84**, 477–9
17. Skriver, K., Radziejewska, E., Silbermann, J. A., Donaldson, V. H. and Bock, S. C. (1989). Mutations in CpG dinucleotide change reactive site arginine-444 to cysteine in dysfunctional C1 inhibitor Da and histidine in dysfunctional C1 inhibitor Ri. *J. Biol. Chem.*, **264**, 3066–71
18. Carter, P., Duponchel, C., Tosi, M. and Fothergill, J. (1991). Complete nucleotide sequence of the gene for human C1-inhibitor with an unusually high density of Alu elements. *Eur. J. Biochem.*, **197**, 301–8
19. Huber, R. and Carrel, R. (1989). Implications of the three-dimensional structure of α1-antitrypsin for structure and function of serpins. *Biochemistry*, **28**, 8951–66
20. Carrell, R., Aulak, K. and Owen, M. (1989). The molecular pathology of the serpins. *Mol. Biol. Med.*, **6**, 35–42
21. Davis III, A. E. (1988). C1 inhibitor and hereditary angioneurotic edema. *Annu. Rev. Immunol.*, **5**, 595–628
22. Davis, A. (1989). Hereditary and acquired deficiencies of C1 inhibitor. *Immunodefic. Rev.*, **1**, 207–26
23. Donaldson, V. (1989). C1-Inhibitor in hereditary angioneurotic edema: type I and type II. *Behring Inst. Mitt.*, **84**, 151–60
24. Tosi, M., Stoppa-Lyonnet, D., Carter, P. and Meo, T. (1989). Molecular defects of the C1-inhibitor gene in hereditary angio-oedema. *Behring Inst. Mitt.*, **84**, 173–9
25. Harrison, R. A. (1983). Human C1 inhibitor: improved isolation and preliminary structural characterization. *Biochemistry*, **22**, 5001–7
26. Perkins, S., Smith, K., Amatayakul, S., Ashford, D., Rademacher, T., Dwek, R., Lachmann, P. and Harrison, R. (1990). Two-domain structure of the native and reactive centre cleaved forms of C1 inhibitor of human complement by neutron scattering. *J. Mol. Biol.*, **214**, 751–63
27. Strecker, G., Ollier-Hartmann, M.-P., van Halbeek, H., Friederik, J., Vliegenthart, G., Montreuil, J. and Hartmann, L. (1985). Structure primaire des chaînes glycanniques de

l'inhibiteur de C1 esterase normal (C1-INH) aprés I'analyse en RMN á 400 MHz. *C. R. Acad. Sci. Paris*, **301**, 571–6

28. Odermatt, E., Berger, H. and Sano, Y. (1981). Size and shape of human C1-inhibitor. *FEBS Lett.*, **131**, 283–5
29. Reboul, A., Prandini, M.-H. and Colomb, M. G. (1987). Proteolysis and deglycosylation of human C1 inhibitor. Effect on functional properties. *Biochem. J.*, **244**, 117–21
30. Pemberton, P., Harrison, R., Lachmann, P. and Carrell, R. (1989). The structural basis for neutrophil inactivation of C1 inhibitor. *Biochem. J.*, **258**, 193–8
31. McPhaden, A. R. M., Carter, P. E., Birnie, G. D. and Whaley, K. (1989). Kpnl RFLP in the 3′ flanking region of the C1 inhibitor gene. *Nucl. Acids Res.*, **17**, 4912
32. Rosen, F. S., Alper, C. A., Pensky, J., Klemperer, M. R. and Donaldson, V. H. (1971). Genetically determined heterogeneity of the C1 esterase inhibitor in patients with hereditary angioneurotic edema. *J. Clin. Invest.*, **50**, 2143–9
33. Alper, C. A., Rosen, F. S., Pensky, J., Klemperer, M. R. and Donaldson, V. H. (1970). Heterogeneity of genetic variants in hereditary angioneurotic edema. *J. Clin. Invest.*, **49**, 3a (abstract)
34. Donaldson, V. H., Harrison, R. A., Rosen, F. S., Bing, D. H., Kindness, G., Canar, J., Wagner, C. J. and Awad, S. (1985). Variability in purified dysfunctional C1-inhibitor proteins from patients with hereditary angioneurotic edema. *J. Clin. Invest.*, **75**, 124–32
35. Shokeir, M. H. K. (1973). The genetics of hereditary angio-oedema: a hypothesis. *Clin. Genet.*, **4**, 494–9
36. Stoppa-Lyonnet, D., Tosi, M., Laurent, J., Sobel, A., Lagrue, G. and Meo, T. (1987). Altered C1-inhibitor genes in type I hereditary angio-oedema. *N. Engl. J. Med.*, **317**, 1–6
37. Cicardi, M., Igarashi, T., Rosen, F. and Davis III, A. (1987). Molecular basis for the deficiency of complement 1 inhibitor in type I hereditary angioneurotic edema. *J. Clin. Invest.*, **79**, 698–702
38. Lappin, D. F., McPhaden, A. R., Peng-Lee, Y., Carter, P. E., Birnie, G. D., Fothergill, J. E. and Whaley, K. (1989). Monocyte C1-inhibitor synthesis in patients with C1 inhibitor deficiency. *Eur. J. Clin. Invest.*, **19**, 45–52
39. Strunk, R., Rosen, F. and Katz, Y. (1989). Synthesis of C1 inhibitor in fibroblasts in type I and type II hereditary angioneurotic edema. *Compl. Inflamm.*, **6**, 403–4
40. Kramer, J., Katz, Y., Rosen, F. S., Davis A. E. and Strunk, R. C. (1991). Synthesis of C1 inhibitor in fibroblasts from patients with type I and type II hereditary angioneurotic edema. *J. Clin. Invest.*, **87**, 1614–20
41. Quastel, M., Harrison, R., Cicardi, M., Alper, C. A. and Rosen, F. S. (1983). Behaviour in vivo of normal and dysfunctional C1 inhibitor in normal subjects and patients with hereditary angioneurotic edema. *J. Clin. Invest.*, **71**, 1041–6
42. Lachmann, P. J. and Rosen, F. S. (1984). The catabolism of C1-inhibitor and the pathogenesis of hereditary angio-edema. *Acta Pathol. Microbiol. Immunol. Scand.* (*Suppl.*), **284**, 35–9
43. Cugno, M., Nuijens, J., Hack, E., Eerenberg, A., Frangi, D., Agostoni, A. and Cicardi, M. (1990). Plasma levels of C1 inhibitor complexes and cleaved C1 inhibitor in patients with hereditary angioneurotic edema. *J. Clin. Invest.*, **85**, 1215–20
44. Cicardi, M., Igarashi, T., Kim, M. S., Frangi, D., Agostoni, A. and Davis III, A. E. (1987). Restriction fragment length polymorphism of the C1 inhibitor gene in hereditary angioneurotic edema. *J. Clin. Invest.*, **80**, 1640–3
45. McPhaden, A., Birnie, G. and Whaley, K. (1991). Restriction fragment length polymorphism analysis of the C1-inhibitor gene in hereditary C1-inhibitor deficiency. *Clin. Genet.*, **39**, 161–71
46. Ariga, T., Igarashi, T., Ramesh, N., Parad, R., Cicardi, M. and Davis III, A. E. (1989). Type I C1 inhibitor deficiency with a small messenger RNA resulting from deletion of one exon. *J. Clin. Invest.*, **83**, 1888–93
47. Ariga, T., Carter, P. E. and Davis III, A. E. (1990). Recombinations between Alu repeat sequences that result in partial deletions within the C1 inhibitor gene. *Genomics*, **8**, 607–13
48. Stoppa-Lyonnet, D., Duponchel, C., Meo, T., Laurent, J., Arala-Chaves, M., Cohen, J., Dewald, G., Hauptmann, G., Intrator, L., Lagrue, G., Lesavre, P., Lopez-Trescasa, G., Misiano, G., Moraine, C., Sobel, A., Späth, P. and Tosi, M. (1991). Recombinational bias in the rearranged C1-inhibitor genes of hereditary angio-oedema patients. *Am. J. Hum. Genet.*, **49**, 1055–62
49. Weiner, A. M., Deininger, P. L. and Efstratiadis, A. (1986). Nonviral retroposons: genes, pseudogenes, and transposable elements generated by the reverse flow of genetic information. *Ann. Rev. Biochem.*, **55**, 631–61

50. Lehrman, M. A., Goldstein, J. L., Russell, D. W. and Brown, M. S. (1987). Duplication of seven exons in LDL receptor gene caused by Alu-Alu recombination in a subject with familial hypercholesterolemia. *Cell*, **48**, 827–35
51. Stoppa-Lyonnet, D., Carter, P. E., Meo, T. and Tosi, M. (1990). Clusters of intragenic Alu repeats predispose the human C1 inhibitor locus to deleterious rearrangements. *Proc. Natl. Acad. Sci. USA*, **87**, 1551–5
52. Siddique, Z., McPhaden, A. R., Lappin, D. L. and Whaley, K. (1991). An RNA splice site mutation in the C1-inhibitor gene causes type I hereditary angio-oedema. *Hum. Genet.*, **88**, 231–2
53. Colten, H. R. (1987). Hereditary angioneurotic edema 1887 to 1987. *N. Engl. J. Med.*, **317**, 43–5
54. Kramer, J., Rosen, F. S. and Strunk, R. C. (1991). Trans-inhibition of normal C1 inhibitor net synthesis in exon VII deleted type I C1 inhibitor deficiency. *Compl. Inflamm.*, **8**, 177
55. Tosi, M., Bourgarel, P., Bazzali, C., Duponchel, C., Stoppa-Lyonet, D. and Meo, T. (1990). Intracellular retention of C1 inhibitor in two hereditary angio-oedema patients. *Compl. Inflamm.*, **7**, 119
56. Katz, Y. and Strunk, R. C. (1989). Synthesis and regulation of C1 inhibitor in human skin fibroblasts. *J. Immunol.*, **142**, 2041–5
57. Donaldson, V. H., Olivi, L. B., Radziejewska, E., Bock, S. C. and Wagner, C. J. (1989). Human umbilical vein endothelial cells produce C1-inhibitor mRNA and secrete C1-inhibitor. *Behring. Inst. Mitt.*, **84**, 194
58. Aulak, K., Pemberton, P., Rosen, F., Carrell, R., Lachmann, P. and Harrison, R. (1988). Dysfunctional C1-inhibitor (At), isolated from a type II hereditary-angio-oedema plasma, contains a P1 'reactive centre' (Arg444-His) mutation. *Biochem. J.*, **253**, 615–18
59. Aulak, K., Cicardi, M. and Harrison, R. (1990). Identification of a new P1 residue mutation (444Arg-Ser) in a dysfunctional C1-inhibitor protein contained in a type II hereditary angio-oedema plasma. *FEBS Lett.*, **266**, 13–16
60. Frangi, D., Cicardi, M., Sica, A., Colotta, F., Agostoni, A. and Davis III, A. E. (1991). Nonsense mutations affect C1 inhibitor messenger RNA levels in patients with type I hereditary angioneurotic edema. *J. Clin. Invest.*, **88**, 755–9
61. Cooper, D. and Youssoufian, H. (1988). The CpG dinucleotide and human genetic disease. *Hum. Genet.*, **78**, 151–5
62. Aulak, K., Davis, A., Donaldson, V., Lachmann, P., Rosen, F. and Harrison, R. (1988). Analysis of mutant dysfunctional C1-inhibitor proteins isolated from type II hereditary angio-oedema plasmas. *Proceedings of the Ninth European Immunology Meeting, Rome, Italy, September 14–17, 1988* (Abstract)
63. Parad, R., Kramer, J., Strunk, R., Rosen, F. and Davis, A. (1990). Dysfunctional C1 inhibitor Ta: Deletion of Lys-251 results in acquisition of an N-glycosylation site. *Proc. Natl. Acad. Sci. USA*, **87**, 6786–90
64. Levy, N., Ramesh, N., Cicardi, M. and Harrison, R. (1990). Type II hereditary angioneurotic edema that may result from a single nucleotide change in the codon for alanine-436 in the C1 inhibitor gene. *Proc. Natl. Acad. Sci. USA*, **87**, 265–8
65. Eldering, E., Lubbers, Y. T. P., Aulak, K. S., Davis III, A. E., Cicardi, M., Nuijens, J. H. and Hack, C. E. (1992). Analysis of a mutant C1 inhibitor from a type II HAE patient: a novel complex-like conformation in serpins as a result of alanine-436 to threonine (P10) substitution. *Immunobiology*, **184**, 423
66. Skriver, K., Wikoff, W. R., Patston, P. A., Tausk, F., Schapira, M., Kaplan, A. P. and Bock, S. C. (1991). Substrate properties of C1 inhibitor Ma (alanine 434-glutamic acid): genetic and structural evidence suggesting that the P12-region contains critical determinants of serine protease inhibitor/substrate status. *J. Biol. Chem.*, **266**, 9216–21
67. Davis III, A. E., Aulak, K. S., Parad, R. B, Stecklein, H. P., Eldering, E., Hack, C. E., Kramer, J., Strunk, R. C. and Rosen, F. S. (1991). Characterization and expression of C1 inhibitor nonreactive center mutations. *Compl. Inflamm.*, **8**, 138
68. Eldering, E., Huijbregts, C. and Hack, C. (1989). Recombinant C1 inhibitor P1 variants. *Compl. Inflamm.*, **6**, 333
69. Nuijens, J., Eerenberg-Belmer, A., Huijbregts, C., Schreuder, W., Felt-Bersma, R., Abbink, J., Thijs, L. and Hack, C. (1989). Proteolytic inactivation of plasma C1 inhibitor in sepsis. *J. Clin. Invest.*, **84**, 443–50

70. Eldering, E., Huijbregts, C., Nuijens, J. and Hack, C. (1989). C1 inhibitor variants with reduced susceptibility for neutrophil elastase. *Compl. Inflamm.*, **6**, 333
71. Verpy, E., Laurent, J., Späth, P. J., Meo, T. and Tosi, M. (1991). Clustering of point mutations downstream of the C1 inhibitor-reactive site in hereditary angio-oedema patients. *Compl. Inflamm.*, **8**, 238
72. Verpy, E. and Tosi, M. (1992). Detection of point mutations in hereditary angio-oedema patients: impaired intracellular transport and secretion of C1 inhibitor proteins with amino acid changes near the carboxyl-end. *Immunobiology*, **184**, 457
73. Stein, P., Leslie, A., Finch, J., Turnell, W., McLaughlin, P. and Carrell, R. (1990). Crystal structure of ovalbumin as a model for the reactive centre of serpins. *Nature*, **347**, 99–102
74. Zuraw, B. and Lotz, M. (1990). Regulation of the hepatic synthesis of C1 inhibitor by the hepatocyte stimulating factors interleukin 6 and interferon-γ. *J. Biol. Chem.*, **265**, 12664–70
75. Lotz, M. and Zuraw, B. L. (1987). Interferon gamma is a major regulator of C1-inhibitor synthesis by human blood monocytes. *J. Immunol.*, **139**, 3382–7
76. Hamilton, A., Jones, L., Morrison, L. and Whaley, K. (1987). Modulation of monocyte complement synthesis by interferons. *Biochem. J.*, **242**, 809–15
77. Lappin, D., Birnie, G. and Whaley, K. (1990). Modulation by interferons of the expression of monocyte complement genes. *Biochem. J.*, **268**, 387–92
78. Lappin, D. F, Guc, D., Hill, A., McShane, T. and Whaley, K. (1992). Effect of interferon-γ on complement gene expression in different cell types. *Biochem. J.*, **281**, 437–42
79. Falus, A., Fehéer, K. G., Walcz, E., Brozik, M., Fürst, G., Hidvégi, T., Fehér, T. and Merétey, K. (1990). Hormonal regulation of complement biosynthesis in human cell lines. I. Androgens and gamma-interferon stimulate the biosynthesis and gene expression of C1 inhibitor in human cell lines U937 and HepG2. *Mol. Immunol.*, **27**, 191–5
80. Heda, G. D., Mardente, S., Weiner, L. and Schmaier, A. H. (1990). Interferon gamma increases *in vitro* and *in vivo* expression of C1 inhibitor. *Blood*, **75**, 2401–7
81. Lappin, D., Birnie, G. and Whaley, K. (1990). Increased mRNA stability accounts for much of the interferon-gamma mediated stimulation of monocyte C1-Inh and factor B synthesis. *Compl. Inflamm.*, **7**, 160
82. Lappin, D., Birnie, G. and Whaley, K. (1991). Interferon mediated transcriptional and post-transcriptional modulation of complement gene expression in human monocytes. *Eur. J. Biochem.*, **194**, 177–84
83. Falus, A., Rokita, H., Walcz, E., Brozik, M., Hidvégi, T. and Merétey, K. (1990). Hormonal regulation of complement biosynthesis in human cell lines. II. Upregulation of the biosynthesis of complement components C3, factor B and C1 inhibitor by interleukin-6 and interleukin-1 in human hepatoma cell line. *Mol. Immunol.*, **27**, 197–201
84. Gelfand, J. A., Sherins, R. J., Alling, D. W. and Frank, M. M. (1976). Treatment of hereditary angio-oedema with danazol: reversal of clinical and biological abnormalities. *N. Engl. J. Med.*, **295**, 1444–8

10
CR3 and its relationship with other phagocytic receptors

J. B. WEITZMAN and S. K. A. LAW

INTRODUCTION

Complement component C3, when activated on a cell surface via either the classical or the alternative pathway, becomes covalently bound on the cell surface[1] as C3b. C3b serves as a cofactor for the activation of the lytic complement components C5–C9 as well as a ligand for the complement receptor type 1 (CR1). Both activities are terminated by factor I which cleaves C3b at two sites to yield iC3b and C3f. iC3b is subsequently cleaved to C3c and C3dg, which is further degraded to C3d, by serum proteases. iC3b and C3dg (and C3d) remain surface bound and can be recognized by at least two other leukocyte receptors, CR3 and CR2 respectively. iC3b was identified later but is probably the most stable C3 fragment bound to cell surfaces. iC3b is also opsonic and its binding to CR3 is considered to play a major role in the clearance of complement-coated targets. (For a more detailed account on complement and C3 degradation, see Refs. 2 and 3.)

CR3 is a polyspecific receptor and iC3b is only one of its many ligands. In the strictest sense, CR3 may be regarded as a heterogeneous mixture of molecules with the same primary sequence. It is subjected to post-translation modification, including differential glycosylation[4] and phosphorylation[5,6]. It may assume different conformational states when chelated with different divalent cations[7,8]. Its ability to interact with different ligands may depend on these regulated modifications. Finally, its conformation and function may also be affected by its interaction with other protein complexes on the plasma membrane as well as cytoskeletal components. In this chapter, we focus our discussion on CR3 as a complement and phagocytic receptor: how its structure and expression on cell

Footnote: CR, complement receptor when CR1 and CR3 are not distinguished; FcγR, Fc receptor for IgG, class not defined; EIgGC, EIgMC, sheep erythrocytes coated with IgG or IgM and complement. The molecular structure of C3 and C4 fragments on the erythrocytes are not characterized.

surfaces relate to its function to bind and ingest iC3b-, C3b- and IgG-coated targets.

STRUCTURE

CR3, together with the p150,95 antigen and the leukocyte-function-associated antigen-1 (LFA-1), belong to the β2 subgroup of the integrin superfamily. The integrins are heterodimeric surface antigens that are structurally characterized by their composition of an α and a β subunit and functionally by their divalent cation-dependent adhesion properties to the extracellular matrix components and cell surface antigens[9,10]. To date, at least 12 α subunits and 8 β subunits have been described. The αβ combinations are somewhat restricted. Only a fraction of all possible combinations have been identified[10,11]. The known permissible αβ combinations and the general properties of the individual subunits (see later) are listed in Figure 10.1. The members of the β2 subgroup are expressed exclusively on leukocytes and are referred to as the leukocyte integrins[12]. The β2 subunit (designated CD18 in the nomenclature for leukocyte cluster of

				β_1	β_2	β_3	β_4	β_5	β_6	β_7	
				56 C	56 C	56 C	**48** C 1000 cr	56 C	56 C	**54** C	
	(++)	I	P								Ref(α)
α_1	3	+	-	VLA-1							193
α_2	3	+	-	VLA-2							14
α_3	4	-	+	VLA-3							15
α_4	3	-	*	VLA-4						?	16
α_5	4	-	+	VLA-5/FNR							17,18
α_6	3+	-	+	VLA-6			+				19
α_7				+							
α_8	4	-	+	+							194
α_L	3	+	-		LFA-1						20
α_M	3	+	-		CR3/Mac-1						21-23
α_X	3	+	-		p150,95						24
α_{IIb}	4	-	+			gpIIb/IIIa					25
α_V	4	-	+	+		VNR		+	+		18,26
			Ref(β)	17	27,28	29,30	31,32	33-35	36	37,38	

Figure 10.1 Features of the integrin α and β subunits. The references on the primary structures of the human subunits are given except for α1 (rat) and α8 (chicken). The primary structure of the α7 subunit[195] is not available. The number of extracellular cysteine residues for the β subunits is indicated. Note also that the β4 subunit has a relatively large (~1000 residues) cytoplasmic fragment. The number of identifiable divalent cation binding sites, and the presence/absence of the I domain and the proteolytic processing site are indicated for the α subunits. The α4 subunit has an unusual proteolytic cleavage site (*) and the fourth divalent-cation-binding site in the α6 subunit is uncharacteristic of those present in subunits with 4 sites. Known αβ combinations are either marked with a common name or a (+). α4 and β7 may combine with other yet-to-be-defined integrin subunits

differentiation antigens) associates with the αL (CD11a), αM (CD11b) or αX (CD11c) subunit to form the LFA-1, CR3 or p150,95 antigens respectively: the order of CD11 antigens was a reflection on their increasing mobility in SDS–polyacrylamide gels[13]. None of the four subunits is known to interact with other subunits of the integrin superfamily.

The primary structures of most of the integrin subunits have been determined. All the α subunits are similar to each other[14–26] as are all the β subunits[17,27–38]. Hence, it is reasonable to assume that the integrin heterodimers have an overall consensus structure and each is a variant of the consensus. The structure of CR3 is therefore discussed in the context of an integrin heterodimer. Some of the properties described are extrapolations based on studies of other integrins and may require re-evaluation when information specific to CR3 becomes available.

Primary structure

The primary structures of the integrin subunits, both α and β, may be described as simple membrane proteins. Each has an N-terminal extracellular domain, of about 1100 amino acid residues for the α subunits and about 670 for the β subunits, followed by a single classical hydrophobic segment which presumably serves as the transmembrane anchor, and a relatively small cytoplasmic C-terminal segment. An exception is the β4 subunit which has a cytoplasmic segment of about 1000 residues[31,32].

The α subunits have seven repeating elements at the N-terminus. The unit element has not been defined but the repeating structure is about 60 residues apart. Embedded in repeats 5, 6, 7 are stretches of oxygen-rich residues characteristic of the EF-hand loop motifs for divalent cation binding. This motif is also found in repeat 4 of some of the α subunits. It appears that the integrin α subunits may be divided into two groups: they either have an I domain (I for inserted or interactive) of about 200 residues between repeats 2 and 3, or a proteolytic cleavage site C-terminal to the seven repeats. An exception is α4, which does not have an I domain but it is proteolytically modified at a site not characteristic of the other subunits. There are 18 to 22 cysteine residues in the extracellular portion of the α subunits. Although most of the cysteine residues are conserved upon alignment, the remaining ones are aligned in two different patterns which are found to correlate with the presence/absence of I domains[14].

The three α subunits of the leukocyte integrins are more closely related to each other than to the remaining α subunits. αM and αX have a post-alignment identity of 63%, αL is only about 35% identical to either αM or αX whereas all three of them bear approximately 25% identity to the other integrin α subunits. The cDNA sequence of αM has been reported by three groups and differences in the translated sequences are noted: Arnaout *et al.*[21] reported a Pro at position 949 whereas Corbi *et al.*[22] and Hickstein *et al.*[23] reported a Leu; a Glu at position 484 was absent in the sequence of Arnaout *et al.*[21].

The putative divalent cation-binding motifs differ from those found in calmodulin, troponin C and parvalbumin[39] in three aspects.

(1) One of the oxygen-rich residues, a consensus Glu in the intracellular proteins, is absent in the integrin α subunit (Figure 10.2). It has been

```
Consensus sequences of the divalent cation binding sites of:
the integrin a subunits:                  -FG-SI----DIDGDG--DAAA-GAP--
                                              AL       LN       III
                                               V        V       LLL
                                                                VVV

other divalent cation binding proteins    (helix).... D-DGDG-ID--E ....(helix)
                                                                  *
```

Figure 10.2 The consensus sequence of the divalent-cation-binding sites of the integrins α subunits[14–26] and other calcium-binding proteins[39]. The Glu (E) not found in the integrin α subunits is marked (*)

suggested that the extra electron donor may come from the ligand, for example in the Asp in the Arg-Gly-Asp (RGD) tripeptide sequence which has been shown to interact with a number of integrin heterodimers[40].

(2) The flanking sequences on either side of the oxygen-rich residues are of a different type (Figure 10.2). Whereas those of the non-integrin proteins are helices, thus giving an overall structure of the EF-hand helix–loop–helix arrangement[41], those in the integrin α subunits are unlikely to assume helical structures due to the invariable presence of the strong helix breakers Gly, Pro and Tyr[42,43].

(3) The spacings between the divalent cation-binding motifs are significantly larger in the integrins, approximately 60 residues apart in comparison with 40 in the intracellular proteins. This may have functional implications since the spatial arrangement of adjacent motifs may govern the effect of the cations on the overall structure of the proteins[44].

The three points raised may not be independent but may reflect consequence in different usage of the oxygen-rich motifs in the two sets of proteins.

The β subunits are extraordinarily rich in cysteine residues in their extracellular domains with 56 in the β1, β2, β3, β5 and β6 subunits, and 48 and 54 in the β4 and β7 subunits, respectively. Upon alignment, all the cysteine residues appear to be conserved and those absent in the β4 and β7 subunits are replaced by other residues. In one region, the proportion of cysteine is over 20% of the residues. Analysis of the derived protein sequence of any of the β subunits with standard programmes, such as DIAGON[45], suggests the presence of four repeating elements, each with eight cysteine residues. Considering the high scores from matching cysteines in these programmes and the high level of cysteine residues in the region of interest, the standard conclusions drawn are more suggestive than conclusive. Whereas it is likely that each repeating element, if present, contains eight cysteine residues, the boundaries between these elements, and hence their definition, are far from clear. Apart from the β4 subunit, others have relatively short cytoplasmic tails. The cytoplasmic segments of the β1, β2 and β7 subunits are more similar to each other than they are to the other integrin β subunits.

Potential phosphorylation sites are found in the cytoplasmic segments of both α and β subunits of the integrins. The phosphorylation of both subunits, including those of CR3, has been reported[5,6,46,47]. The motif, Asn-Pro-X-

(Tyr/Phe), is also found in the cytoplasmic segment of the integrin β subunits. It is thought to be important in receptor internalization via coated pits[48,49].

Higher-order structure

Information on the higher-order structure of the integrins is rather limited. Except for the short metal-binding motifs and the I domains, other parts of the integrin subunits are not found to match any known motifs. In fact, the metal-binding motifs only match the 'loop' portion of the 'helix–loop–helix' EF-hand structure and the I domains, and their homologous domains on other molecules, are only described at the primary structure level.

Electron microscopy studies of the integrins αIIbβ3 (the platelet glycoprotein gpIIb/IIIa)[50], and α5β1 (the fibronectin receptor)[51], have led to the proposal of a two-pronged plug model. Presumably, the α and β subunits are held together at a site close to the N-terminus and the two hydrophobic segments are separately inserted into the membrane bilayer. The structure of the leukocyte integrins is likely to be similar although allowances must be made for the presence of the I domains and the absence of the proteolytic cleavage site in the α subunit. The suggestion that the transmembrane and cytoplasmic segments of the two subunits are probably not important in the formation of the heterodimer is further strengthened by the expression of a soluble CR3 by transfection into cells of truncated cDNA of both α and β subunits[52]. The CR3 expressed was recognized by specific mAbs and had the capacity to block iC3b–CR3 interactions.

The disulphide bond pattern of αIIb has been determined[53]. The 18 cysteine residues are found to pair with the next available partner along the sequence starting from the N-terminus. Hence, a series of loops may be envisioned. The αIIb subunit lacks the I domain but has a proteolytic processing site, and its cysteine residues are not in complete alignment with those of αM. How these differences would affect the overall structure of the αM subunit is not clear.

Some of the disulphide bonds of the β3 subunit have also been determined[54,55]. Due to the very high cysteine content of the β3 subunit, it is not expected that all the disulphide bonds in the cysteine-rich region could be determined by traditional protein chemistry. Nevertheless, based on the data obtained and the assumptions that all extracellular cysteine residues are engaged in intrachain disulphides and that there are repeating elements in the cysteine-rich region, a model of β3 has been proposed. This model may not be applicable to the β4 and β7 subunits. For example, β7 has only 54 cysteine residues with the two most C-terminal cysteine residues substituted[37,38]. In the model, however, these two cysteine residues are not disulphide bonded to each other. Similar observation can be made with the substituted cysteine residues of β4[31,32]. One possible explanation could be that the assumption that all the cysteine residues are engaged in disulphide bonds is not valid. It is known that cysteine residues, though not engaged in disulphide bonds, are only detectable when reduced; an example would be the cysteine residue found in the A isotype but not the B isotype of the human complement component C4 (Dodds, personal communication; also see Chapter 2). Further work at the protein level is therefore required to resolve this abiguity.

Gene structure

The gene for the β2 subunit (CD18) has been located to chromosome 21 by cell hybrids[56] and to band q22.3 by *in situ* hybridization[57,58]. Using radiation hybridization with PFGE, the location of the gene has been refined to approximately 2000 kb from the q telomere[59]. The gene consists of 16 exons covering approximately 40 kb[60]. The exons encoding the cysteine-rich region do not provide any information regarding the putative repeating elements. The putative promoter region does not have a TATA or a CCAAT box. Using different techniques to determine the 5′ end of the mRNA, it was shown that there are multiple initiation sites[60]. Preliminary results suggest that an upstream region of about 200 bp has promoter activity (Weitzman and Law, unpublished).

The use of *in situ* hybridization has localized the gene for the α subunit of CR3, as well as those of the other leukocyte integrins, LFA-1 and p150,95 to chromosome 16 band p11-13.1[57]. The relative position, orientation and the order of the three genes are not known. The gene structure of the α subunit of p150,95 (CD11c) has been determined[61]. It consists of 31 exons spanning a region of about 25 kb. The first four of the seven repeating elements at the N-terminus of the proteins are split by introns and each of the three repeats containing a divalent cation-binding motif is encoded in a separate exon. The I domain is encoded by four exons. Although somewhat different from the I domains found in other proteins, they do share the common feature of being enclosed by phase-1 introns, suggesting that the I domain may be inserted into or deleted from the genome as a cassette. The first 6 exons of the α subunit of CR3, CD11b, have been determined[62]. They are identical in size and phase to those of the CD11c gene. There are no TATA or CCAAT boxes in the putative promoter regions in both the CD11b and CD11c genes but, unlike that of the β subunit, both genes appear to use a single major initiation site of transcription[62] (Corbi, personal communication). The exonic organization of the gene for the αIIb subunit has also been reported[63]. Although most of the boundaries can be correspondingly mapped to those of the CD11c gene, significant differences are found in the region encoding the divalent cation-binding sites. Specifically, the cation-binding motifs are coded for by split exons.

BIOSYNTHESIS AND REGULATION OF EXPRESSION

Cellular expression of the leukocyte integrins has been studied using subunit-specific monoclonal antibodies. All three heterodimers are expressed on leukocytes and the relative levels of expression differ for different cell types and are regulated during differentiation and cell activation[64–67]. CR3 and p150,95 are expressed primarily on cells of the myeloid lineage[65,68] though their presence has been reported on other cells[69–72]. LFA-1 is expressed on nearly all leukocytes with the exception of some macrophages[73–75]. None of the three leukocyte integrins has been detected on cells other than leukocytes.

Limited results obtained by Northern blot analysis also found the mRNA of the subunits for CR3 only in cells of leukocytic origin[22,76,77]. Steady-state mRNA levels were determined for a number of cell types and they were found, in general, to correlate with the surface expression of the antigen[76,77]. However, the mechanisms for regulating the mRNA level appear to be different for the two subunits. The increase in mRNA level of the β subunit in HL-60 upon stimulation with retinoic acid may be accounted for by the increased rate of transcription as shown in nuclear run-off experiments[76]. The transcription rate of the αM gene, on the other hand, does not appear to be affected by retinoic acid, thus suggesting that the increase in the steady-state mRNA level is regulated post-transcriptionally[77].

Surface expression of CR3 is also regulated at the post-translational level. A high proportion of CR3 and p150,95 is found in intracellular pools of unactivated monocytes and polymorphonuclear leukocytes (PMN)[78–80]. Stimulation with a variety of mediators, including formyl-methionyl-leucyl-phenylalanine (fMLP), C5a, leukotriene B4, tumour necrosis factor and calcium ionophore, leads to the rapid mobilization of CR3 and p150,95 to the cell surface by degranulation[78,79,81,82]. The localization of the intracellular CR3 and p150,95 to peroxidase-negative specific granules suggested their synthesis during the myelocyte stage of maturation when these specific granules form. It is interesting to note that LFA-1 is not localized to the same intracellular vesicles[67,82,83] and that activation results in substantially less enhancement of surface LFA-1[67,82]. Despite the up-modulation in response to many mediators, this burst of surface CR3 does not necessarily correlate with the elevation of functional activities (see later).

The α and β subunits of the leukocyte integrins also serve as expression regulators for each other. This is highlighted in the rare congenital disorder, leukocyte adhesion deficiency (LAD). Patients are defective in their β2 subunit genes and, as a result, fail to express all three leukocyte integrins on their leukocytes, suggesting that the maturation and/or surface expression of the α subunits requires a functional β subunit (for review see Refs. 84 and 85). The requirement of an α subunit for the maturation and expression of the β subunit is less clear. Transfection of K562 cells with β2 cDNA resulted in high levels of β2 mRNA and intracellular protein but surface β2 antigen was not detected[86]. Some, but not all, β2 epitopes, however, may be found on COS cells transfected with the β2 cDNA[87].

LIGANDS OF CR3

CR3 can bind to many ligands; all appear to involve different stages of phagocyte migration from the blood stream towards the site of inflammation and the elimination of the infectious agents. The binding of CR3 to ligands on the endothelium[88–90], which includes ICAM-1[90–91], may be a necessary step in the migration of leukocytes from blood stream into extravascular tissues. The interaction of CR3 with different extracellular matrix molecules, including fibronectin, laminin and collagen[92], may contribute to the mobilization of leukocytes within the tissue structure. The binding of phagocytes to microorganisms, by way of CR3 recognition either of natural microbial surface components, such as β-glucan[93–95], lipopolysaccharide[96], lipophosphoglycan[97] and other undefined structures[94,98], or of iC3b deposited on the surface by activation of the complement pathway[99,100], is the initial event leading to the elimination of microorganisms by ingestion[101]. The binding of CR3 to proteins of the blood clotting system, such as factor X[102,103], fibrinogen[104,105] and fibrin[106], may serve to regulate the clotting process.

CR3 is not unique in most of these binding activities. The binding to endothelial surface is also mediated by the two other leukocyte integrins, LFA-1 and p150,95. CR3 and LFA-1 have different binding sites on the ICAM-1 molecule[107] and LFA-1 also binds ICAM-2[91,108]. It is possible that p150,95 binds to a different ligand on the endothelial surface[89,109]. Binding to extracellular matrix components is also mediated by other integrin molecules, such as the fibronectin receptors[10] or the leukocyte response integrins[110,111]. LFA-1 and p150,95 also bind lipopolysaccharide[96] and lipophosphoglycan[97] though they do not appear to bind β-glucan[95]. It has been reported that p150,95 binds fibrinogen but at a different site from CR3[112]. There are three possible advantages to explain why a leukocyte should employ more than one receptor to mediate similar activities.

(1) The interactions are synergistic in that more than one signal is required to trigger a particular response. This is clearly demonstrated in the case of CR3–iC3b-mediated phagocytosis (see later).
(2) The interactions are complementary such that only one of several is sufficient to bring about an activity. An example would be the binding of leukocytes to microorganisms via the interaction of the leukocyte integrins and microbial surface structures where the contributions of the three leukocyte integrins were demonstrated to be additive[96–98].
(3) The different interactions may provide a method to regulate an activity. For example, both LFA-1 and CR3 on leukocytes bind to ICAM-1 on the endothelium but at different sites on ICAM-1. In addition, the binding of CR3 to ICAM-1 is affected by the glycosylation of ICAM-1. Thus, the adhesion of leukocytes to the endothelium, and hence their migration into tissues, may be regulated via the expression of LFA-1 on lymphocytes, and CR3 on monocytes and neutrophils[107].

As a complement receptor, CR3 binds iC3b. The binding requires both Ca^{2+} and Mg^{2+} and may depend on the activation state of the CR3-bearing cell. Under suitable stimulation, this binding is sufficient to trigger the ingestion process (see later). Since a number of integrins bind to molecules containing the tripeptide sequence, RGD[40], which is found in the primary sequence of C3[113], Wright *et al.*[114] synthesized peptides of C3, inclusive of the RGD sequence, and showed that they inhibit iC3b–CR3 interactions. Peptides homologous to this region of C3 were identified from other CR3 ligands, such as fibrinogen[104] and the gp63 from *Leishmania*[115], and these synthetic peptides were also found to inhibit iC3b binding although they do not necessarily contain the RGD tripeptide. However, conflicting results were obtained from other experiments. Using site-directed mutagenesis, the region containing the RGD tripeptide of human C3 was extensively modified, including the conversion of RGD to AAA, but none of the modifications appeared to affect the interaction between iC3b and CR3[116,117]. On the other hand, the RGD-containing sequence of the filamentous haemagglutinin of *B. pertussis* is absolutely required for its interaction with CR3; the conversion of RGD to RAD in the haemagglutinin abolishes the binding activity[118]. Thus, the CR3 recognition structure on iC3b, as well as its analogues, remains controversial and requires clarification by future work.

p150,95 is very similar to CR3. They have the same β2 subunit[119] and their α subunit has a post-alignment identity of 63%[21–24]. (By contrast, the α subunit of LFA-1 is only about 35% identical to either the α subunit of CR3 or that of p150,95[20].) The binding of p150,95 to iC3b covalently attached to a Sepharose matrix has been demonstrated at low ionic strength[120,121]. It has been the key argument for regarding p150,95 as a complement receptor and it is frequently referred to by some workers as the complement receptor type 4 (CR4). For most easily obtainable p150,95-bearing cells, including peripheral blood monocytes and neutrophils and various cell lines of the myeloid lineage, CR3 is also present in significantly higher quantity[122]. The contribution of p150,95 to the binding of iC3b under physiological conditions has yet to be demonstrated convincingly. In this chapter, p150,95 will not be discussed further.

CR3-, CR1- AND FcγR-MEDIATED PHAGOCYTOSIS

Phagocytosis has long been one of the most fascinating events observable under a light microscope. The involvement of complement proteins as opsonins was described in the early 1900s. The presence of at least two types of complement receptor on leukocytes was first described by Lay and Nussenzweig[123]. Using the rosetting technique, they distinguished the divalent cation-independent and -dependent adhesion of complement-coated targets to leukocytes. These were later correlated to the C3b–CR1 and iC3b–CR3 interactions.

Phagocytosis is a complex phenomenon involving the minimal stages of adhesion, signal transduction and mobilization of cytoskeletal elements to engulf and ingest the opsonized targets. The complexity grows when more than one receptor can trigger the process and ligation of different receptors may be coupled to different cellular events, such as response to cytokines or other stimulants, lysosomal degranulation and the respiratory burst. Since recent findings suggest that CR3 may not only be involved in iC3b–CR3-mediated phagocytosis but may also play a key role in phagocytosis via the C3b–CR1 and IgG–FcγR interactions, we shall describe the basic observations on the phagocytosis mediated by these three types of receptors.

Early work

Early studies on the opsonic receptors of phagocytes differentiated the roles of the complement and Fcγ receptors (CR and FcγR). Using sheep erythrocytes coated with antibodies (EIgG) or with both antibody and complement (EIgGC) as targets, Mantovani *et al.*[124] studied the adhesion and phagocytic activities of mouse peritoneal macrophages. Although the phagocytes bound EIgGC more readily than EIgG, the ingestion of EIgGC was not significantly higher than that of the EIgG targets. In addition, Fab fragments of anti-IgG blocked ingestion of EIgG and EIgGC but only had a marginal effect on the adhesion of EIgGC. These results were interpreted as showing that the two types of receptors were involved in different phases of the phagocytic process: CR in the attachment phase and FcγR in the ingestion phase. The role of CR was thought to be mainly to promote the efficiency of ingestion via FcγR. This view received further support when similar observations were made with other phagocytes, including neutrophils of mouse[125] and man[126,127], and peritoneal macrophages of guinea-pig[128], on targets including opsonized bacteria[126] as well as the standard sheep erythrocytes. Significantly, IgM was used in place of IgG to activate the fixation of complement on the target cell surface[126,129]. Since IgM does not interact with FcγR, more clear-cut results were obtained on the separate effects upon ligation of FcγR and CR by their respective ligands. It was also noted that the IgG–FcγR interaction could also stimulate the phagocytes to release toxic oxygen metabolites and lysosomal contents[127]. However, treatment of neutrophils with cytochalasin B blocked ingestion but not the release of oxygen metabolites, suggesting that the two processes, though triggered by the ligation of FcγR, were not coupled[127].

Peritoneal macrophages from mice sensitized with thioglycollate or *Bacillus Calmette-Guerin* both bound and ingested EIgMC[130,131]. Thus the phagocytes could be 'activated' both to bind and ingest opsonized targets via complement receptors without the participation of FcγR. Subsequently, it was demonstrated that activation could also be induced by the treatment of phagocytes with some undefined lymphokines from T cells[132–134], or simply by prolonged culture *in vitro*, although the level of activation was rather limited[135].

It should be noted that the experiments described so far were carried out before the recognition of the existence of the intermediate iC3b when C3b is cleaved to C3c and C3d. In fact, whereas surface-bound C3b is sensitive to the complement regulatory proteins factors I and H[136,137] which convert C3b into iC3b, surface-bound iC3b is relatively more stable to other serum proteases which ultimately cleave iC3b to C3c and C3d[138]. Using erythrocytes bearing defined C3 fragments, namely C3b, iC3b and C3d, Carlo *et al.*[139] were able to demonstrate the presence of distinct receptors for the three C3 fragments. These receptors were later referred to as CR1, CR3 and CR2, respectively. C4, which resembles C3 in many ways, also binds covalently to the surface of immune complexes when activated to C4b[140,141]. C4b is cleaved by factor I at two sites in the presence of the cofactor C4b-binding protein[142,143]. Although an 'iC4b' intermediate must exist when one of these two sites is cleaved, in practice, the two cleavages take place in quick succession and the conversion to C4c and C4d is invariably completed without a detectable intermediate. C4b is also recognized by CR1, which was demonstrated by the immune adherence reaction between C4b-coated sheep erythrocytes and human erythrocytes[144], which bear CR1 but not CR3 on their cell surface. It was later shown that C4b-coated erythrocytes could be phagocytosed by cultured monocytes via CR1[145].

The ability to prepare sheep erythrocytes with the defined opsonins, IgG, C3b, iC3b and C4b, and advances in the techniques in tissue culture allowed investigators in the 1980s to study phagocytosis under more defined conditions. Furthermore, the availability of monoclonal antibodies not only led to the physical identification and characterization of the FcγR(s) and complement receptors but also provided an independent means to quantitate the expression of these receptors on different cells in response to various stimulants. Mapping of different epitopes also became possible and blocking the binding of different ligands by different sets of mAbs led to the characterization of multiple active sites on the same molecule. Taking the monocyte as a model, the current view on phagocytosis mediated by the three interactions, IgG–FcγR, C3b/C4b–CR1 and iC3b–CR3, is discussed below.

Monocytes

Freshly isolated monocytes have about 25 000 CR1 and about the same number of CR3 on their surface[122]. They bind EIgMC3b and EIgMiC3b but do not ingest them[146]. However, they are phagocytically competent since their ingestion of EIgG, via FcγR, can be readily demonstrated[146]. Culturing of monoctyes leads to a gradual increase in surface CR1 and CR3: CR1 by about 50% and CR3 by about five-fold by day seven[122]. The attachment indices for both EIgMC3b and EIgMiC3b increase by approximately five-fold[146]. The correlation between surface expression of the receptors and the attachment indices is not quantitative and may depend on other parameters, such as distribution/clustering of the receptors on the monocytes and the surface density of the ligands, i.e. C3b and iC3b on the targets (see later). However, their capacity to phagocytose complement-coated targets remains low though detectable after culture for more than 5 days[135] and can be significantly enhanced by the addition of phorbol esters. The stimulatory effect of phorbol esters on complement-mediated phagocytosis is reversible. Monocytes stimulated with soluble phorbol ester progressively lose their phagocytic capacity upon washing but can recover the activity if the phorbol ester is reintroduced[147]. The phagocytic competence of cultured monoctyes can be activated by spreading the cells on surfaces coated with fibronectin[148,149], serum amyloid P component[149] or laminin[145]. In the case of fibronectin, it was demonstrated that the continuous presence of the extracellular matrix protein is required to maintain the monocytes in their activated state[147].

The interactions, C3b–CR1 and iC3b–CR3, can be distinguished by their requirement for divalent cations. Whereas the binding of C3b–CR1 is independent of Ca^{2+} and Mg^{2+}, the phorbol-ester-stimulated ingestion is significantly reduced in the absence of the divalent cations. On the other hand, the interaction between iC3b and CR3 has a strict requirement[146] for both Ca^{2+} and Mg^{2+}.

Phagocytosis via FcγR is coupled with the release of toxic oxygen metabolites[150] which is usually thought to be the means by which the ingested microorganisms are killed. In contrast, complement-receptor-mediated phagocytosis is not coupled to the release of oxygen metabolites; cultured monocytes which were fully capable of binding and ingesting C3b/iC3b/fibronectin-coated erythrocytes released less than 3% of the quantity of hydrogen peroxide which was released by IgG-coated targets[151,152]. It should be noted that phorbol esters can also stimulate the release of toxic oxygen metabolites without the engagement of either FcγR or complement receptors.

A further set of experiments demonstrated that the binding activities of the complement receptors may be down-regulated by the treatment of cultured monocytes with γ-interferon[153]. Neither the number nor the distribution of CR1 or CR3 on the monocytes was affected by exposure to γ-interferon but the adhesion of EIgMC3b or EIgMiC3b, and hence their ingestion, was significantly reduced. This effect was dependent upon both the length of exposure time and the dosage of γ-interferon. Furthermore, adherence activities were recovered upon spreading the γ-interferon-treated monocytes on fibronectin-coated surface but phorbol esters are required to reactivate the ingestion process. Phorbol esters alone cannot restore the binding activity.

The anti-CR3 antibody, anti-Mo1, first described by Todd *et al.*[154], has been studied for its effect on the binding and ingestion of EIgG, EIgMC3b and EIgMiC3b[155]. It inhibited the rosetting of EIgMiC3b but not of EIgGMC3b nor EIgG to PMN and monocytes. In addition, it immunoprecipitated a heterodimeric antigen with subunits of 155 000 and 94 000 daltons[156]. However, the antigen was not identified as CR3 because of the additional observation that anti-Mo1, though not inhibiting EIgG rosetting, inhibits the ingestion of EIgG by PMN. Using a larger panel of anti-CR3 antibodies on PMN, Ross *et al.*[93] showed that there are at least two distinct sites on CR3: one for the recognition of iC3b, and the other for the interaction with an undefined ligand which led to the triggering of ingestion and the respiratory burst.

These observations led Brown *et al.*[157] to reinvestigate the role of CR3 in IgG–FcγR-mediated phagocytosis. Monocytes were allowed to adhere to surfaces coated with the $F(ab')_2$ fragment of anti-CR3 (M1/70) or with bovine serum albumin, and the rosetting of EIgMiC3b and the ingestion of EIgG was studied. The rosetting of EIgMiC3b was lower if the monocytes were adherent to the M1/70-coated surface. The rosetting of EIgG to the monocytes, or their ingestion, however, was the same for both surfaces. This was interpreted as meaning that some of the CR3, but not FcγR, were mobilized from the apical side to the underside of the cell. Upon the addition of extra fluid-phase M1/70 $F(ab')_2$, both the binding and ingestion of EIgG were inhibited. It was therefore concluded that there are two subsets of CR3, one mobile and the other immobile. The immobile subset appears to play an additional role in the phagocytosis of EIgG via FcγR. As the binding of EIgG to monocytes was also inhibited, it was suggested that FcγR and the immobile subset of CR3 might be linked physically. Graham *et al.*[158] extended this study to show that CR3 may play a similar role in C3b/C4b–CR1-mediated phagocytosis. As the binding and phagocytosis of iC3b-coated targets were blocked by two different, though overlapping, sets of anti-CR3 antibodies, these two activities must be mediated by distinct regions of CR3.

Polymorphonuclear leukocytes (neutrophils)

The phagocytosis of IgG-, C3b- and iC3b-coated targets by neutrophils is similar to their phagocytosis by monocytes although there are significant differences in detail. For example:

(1) Both neutrophils and monocytes bind and ingest EIgG, but additional stimulants, such as phorbol esters, are required for the ingestion of complement-coated targets[145,146,148,159,160]. Although monocytes require the continuous presence of phorbol esters for the stimulated activity[147], neutrophils show a biphasic response; the enhancement of binding to and ingestion of the complement-coated targets peaks at 25 min and then declines to below the starting level[160].

(2) Spreading of cultured monocytes on a fibronectin-coated surface is sufficient to activate them to a phagocytically competent state, whereas neutrophils are not 'activated' by fibronectin unless they have been exposed to C5a or f-met-leu-phe previously[159].

(3) FcγR-mediated phagocytosis was not affected by phorbol esters in cultured monocytes[146] but was progressively suppressed in neutrophils[160].

(4) Ligation of FcγR is sufficient to trigger the respiratory burst in monocytes[150] but additional signals are required in the case of neutrophils[161].

(5) $F(ab')_2$ fragments of anti-CR3 antibodies, which inhibit both binding and ingestion of EIgG by monocytes, inhibit only the ingestion but not the adhesion of EIgG by neutrophils[158].

These observations reflect the differences in cell physiology of the two major phagocytic cell types which may be important in the pursuit of their different roles *in vivo*.

DISCUSSION

Figure 10.3 summarizes the basic observations on IgG–FcγR, C3b/C4b–CR1- and iC3b–CR3-mediated phagocytosis by cultured monocytes and neutrophils. There are many unknown effects among these disjointed observations, which are marked in boxes and are discussed separately.

(1) The binding of C3b/C4b to CR1 and iC3b to CR3

Surface expression of CR1 and CR3 does not necessarily correlate with the adherence capacity of the phagocytes to C3b- and iC3b-coated targets. Monoctyes, when cultured in the presence of γ-interferon, have diminished binding activity to EIgMC3b and EIgMiC3b without a corresponding reduction in surface CR1 and CR3[153]. On the other hand, the level of CR1 and CR3 on neutrophils remains high after prolonged treatment with phorbol ester, but the capacity of these cells to bind EIgMC3b and EIgMiC3b is minimal[160]. Treat-

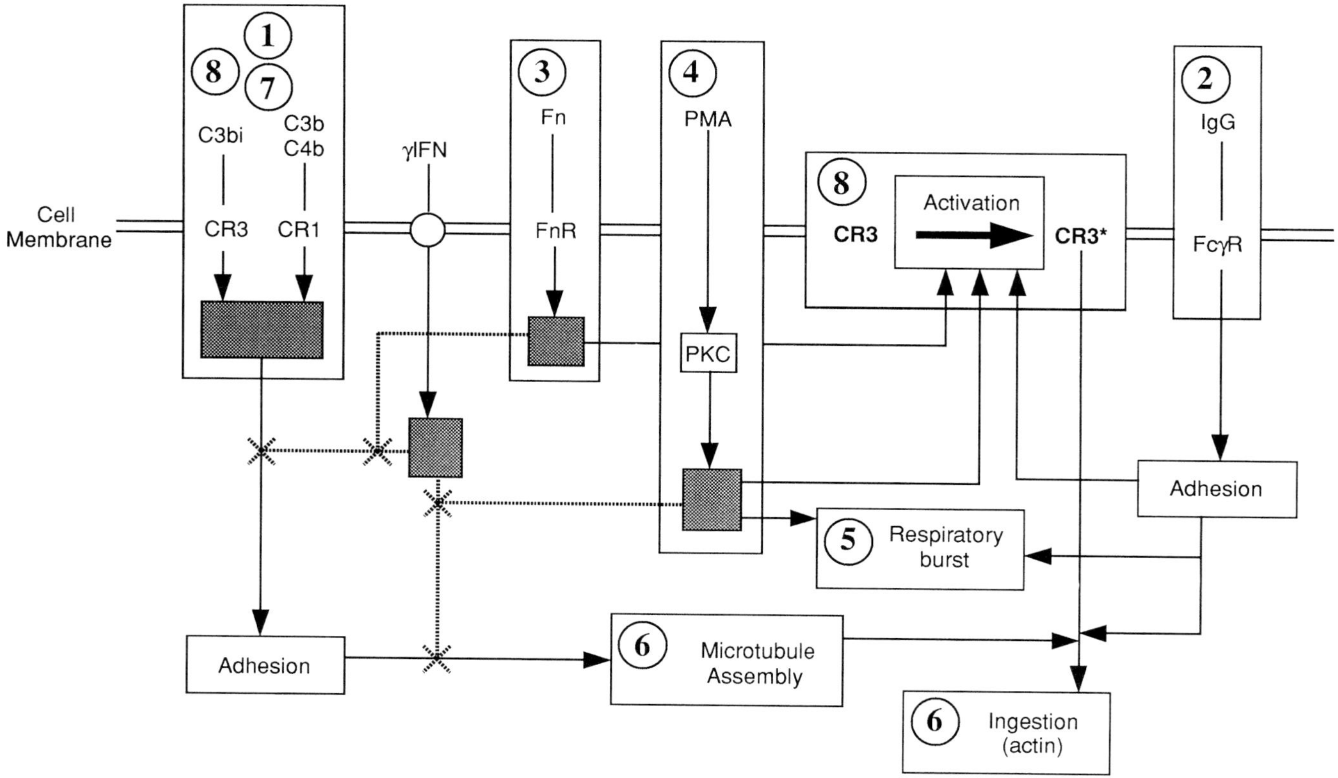

Figure 10.3 CR1-, CR3- and FcγR-mediated phagocytosis by monocytes. See *Discussion* in text for details. Arrow lines represent activating signals, dashed lines inhibitory signals. The different roles of CR3 in iC3b binding (1) and activation of ingestion (8) are stressed by their sensitivity to different mAb's: iC3b–CR3 interaction is blocked by OKM10 but not IB4, whereas the reverse is true for activation of ingestion[100,157,158]

ment of neutrophils with interleukin-8 leads to increased surface expression of CR3 and enhancement of adherence to EIgMiC3b[162]. However, increased adherence can also occur without CR3 up-regulation[162]. In addition, other CR3-mediated adhesion activities, such as homotypic aggregation of neutrophils[163] and adhesion of neutrophils to cultured endothelium[164,165], are not affected by the up-regulation of CR3. Thus, the absolute number of CR3 expressed on neutrophil membranes does not always correlate with adherence to iC3b-coated targets or to other ligands.

It is possible that CR1 and CR3 are both heterogeneous mixtures of binding-competent and the binding-incompetent forms and induction of phagocytes by the different stimulants simply causes a shift in the proportions of these variants on the cell surface. In the case of CR3, there is evidence that its conformation may differ under different conditions. An epitope recognized by the mAb, 24, was found to require Mg^{2+} or Mn^{2+}, but not Ca^{2+}, for expression[7]. In addition, metabolic inhibitors, such as azide and 2-deoxy-D-glucose, abolish the expression of this epitope. Another epitope, 7E3, which is normally associated with the integrin αIIbβ3 (platelet glycoprotein IIb/IIIa)[166], can be expressed on monocyte CR3 upon stimulation with ADP[167]. Furthermore, the appearance of 7E3 may be correlated with the binding of clotting factor X to monocytes, which could be competitively inhibited by soluble iC3b[102]. Graham and Brown[8] studied the effect of divalent cations on CR3. EGTA, a chelator of Ca^{2+} but not of Mg^{2+}, was found to inhibit the adhesion of EIgMiC3b to resting neutrophils but was less effective on the adhesion to phorbol-ester-stimulated neutrophils, suggesting that the conformation of CR3 may be affected by the presence of Ca^{2+}. In addition, IB4, a mAb against the β2 subunit of CR3, blocked the phagocytosis of EIgMC4b, but only in the presence of Ca^{2+}. It could thus be argued that: (1) the immobile subset of CR3, which is involved in the ingestion of IgG- and complement-coated targets, has two different conformations dependent on the presence of Ca^{2+}; and (2) both conformations are active in mediating ingestion[8,158].

The binding of CR1 to C3b, and C4b, is independent of divalent cations but the capacity of phagocytes to bind C3b- and C4b-coated erythrocytes is also affected by various stimulants, such as γ-interferon and phorbol esters[153,160]. However, there is no evidence that these stimuli alter the expression of antigenic epitopes on CR1. Furthermore, the extracellular domain of CR1 is composed of 30 short consensus (SCR) or complement control protein (CCP) repeats[168] with the binding sites of C3b localized to repeats 8 and 9 and 15 and 16 and that of C4b to repeats 1 and 2[169,170]. It is unlikely that these distinct binding sites are affected coordinately. Thus, other mechanisms, distinct from a change in CR1 conformation, are needed to account for the change in binding affinity of stimulated phagocytes for C3b coated targets via CR1. This argument, when extrapolated to CR3, suggests that the changes in conformation do not necessarily correlate with change in affinity for iC3b.

An alternative mechanism may involve changes in the distribution of CR1 and CR3 on the cell surface. CR3, which is dispersed on neutrophils, was shown to cluster upon exposure to phorbol esters but return to a dispersed state on prolonged incubation[171]. The time course follows that of the biphasic pattern of binding and ingestion capacity of complement-coated targets[160]. The correlation between clustering and activity is also observed when neutrophils are treated with f-met-leu-phe, which induces surface mobilization of CR1 and CR3 from the intracellular pool. However, f-met-leu-phe does not induce receptor clustering or the enhancement of binding to iC3b-coated erythrocytes[171]. Although clustering and dispersion may be theoretically attractive in regulation of adhesion to ligand-coated surfaces[172], other properties clearly affect receptor activity. CR3 was found to remain clustered on monocytes upon culture in the presence of γ-interferon although CR3-mediated binding to EIgMiC3b was greatly diminished[153].

(2) IgG–FcγR interactions

There are three major classes of FcγR: FcγRI, FcγRII and FcγRIII. Each has variant forms and possibly plays overlapping roles in different populations of leukocytes[173]. The high-affinity receptor, FcγRI, is probably not involved in phagocytosis since monocytes, when cultured in γ-interferon, have elevated levels of FcγRI[174,175] which only leads to an increase in attachment of EIgG but not their ingestion[153]. Freshly isolated monocytes do not express FcγRIII[176] although they can phagocytose EIgG readily[146]. Cultured monocytes showed a progressive increase in the expression of FcγRIII as well as the attachment and ingestion capacity for EIgG, and a causal relationship can be demonstrated by the inhibition of the enhanced level with 3G8, a monoclonal antibody to FcγRIII[177]. Thus both FcγRII and FcγRIII may be active in phagocytosis. The attachment of EIgG to neutrophils could be completely blocked by 3G8, showing that FcγRIII is the major receptor on neutrophils[158,177]. $F(ab')_2$ fragments of the anti-CR3 monoclonal antibodies, IB4 or Mo-1, partially blocked ingestion of EIgG to both monocyte and neutrophils, thus demonstrating that CR3 plays an active role in the ingestion process[157,158]. However, whereas the binding of EIgG to monocytes can be partially blocked by anti-CR3 monoclonal antibodies, that to neutrophils is not affected[157,158], suggesting that the interaction between FcγRIII and CR3 is different in monoctyes and neutrophils. This may be accounted for by the difference in anchorage of FcγRIII in the two cell types. It has been established that FcγRIII is cell-bound via a phosphatidyl–inositol glycan moiety[178,179], whereas the FcγRIII on cultured monoctyes does not appear to have the same anchor[180]. It remains to be resolved how the signal from the IgG-FcγRIII interaction is transmitted, presumably via different routes, to CR3 and finally to the cytoskeletal apparatus to initiate the ingestion process in neutrophils and monocytes.

(3) Fibronectin and related receptors

Cultured moncoytes bind but do not ingest EIgMC3b and EIgMiC3b unless they are either treated with phorbol esters or spread on a surface coated with fibronectin[148,149], serum amyloid protein[149], or laminin[145]. The effect of fibronectin could be replaced with peptides containing the active sequence

RGD[110,181]. The binding of neutrophils to fibronectin-coated surfaces does not lead to ingestion-competence of EIgMC3b unless they have been pretreated with C5a or f-met-leu-phe[159]. It was later found that more than one integrin can recognize the RGD motif, including the fibronectin receptor, vitronectin receptor and platelet glycoprotein IIb/IIIa[182], the first two of which are known to be expressed on monocytes and neutrophils[83]. It should be noted that the RGD-containing peptide, when coated to a solid support, is able to induce signals to the phagocytes, although the soluble peptides have no effect[181]. Hence, some kind of surface crosslinking of the receptor may be required to generate the necessary signal to promote CR1- and CR3-mediated ingestion. At least two different signals result from ligation of these receptors in monocytes. Monocytes cultured in γ-interferon have diminished binding and ingestion capacity to EIgMC3b and EIgMiC3b and only the spreading of these monocytes on fibronectin can overcome the diminished binding[153]. This signal is therefore distinct from that which promotes the ingestion of EIgMC3b and EIgMiC3b[148,149].

Using RGD-containing peptides crosslinked to a solid-phase support, a new receptor has been purified from neutrophils and two from monocytes. One of the monocyte receptors is identical to the neutrophil receptor[110]. These receptors are integrins which are not members of the β1 or β2 integrin families. It appears that the integrin common to both monocytes and neutrophils is possibly a new member of the β3 integrin subfamily, i.e. it is distinct from the vitronectin receptor and αIIbβ3 (see Figure 10.1), while the second monocyte integrin appears to contain a novel β subunit[110,111], which may be the recently described β7 subunit[37,38]. A monoclonal antibody against the neutrophil receptor, B6H12, was shown to inhibit the fibronectin-stimulated phagocytosis mediated via FcγR[111]. It is not known whether this receptor, called the leukocyte response integrin (LRI), is also responsible for the activation of complement-receptor-mediated phagocytosis.

(4) Phorbol esters and protein kinase C

Treatment of cultured monocytes and neutrophils with phorbol esters converts them from an ingestion-incompetent state to an ingestion-competent state with regard to CR1- and CR3-mediated phagocytosis[146,160]. In the case of monocytes, the maintenance of their activated state requires the continuous presence of phorbol esters[147]. The response of neutrophils to phorbol esters is temporally biphasic. The capacity of neutrophils to ingest both EIgMC3b and EIgMiC3b is greatly elevated in the first 20 minutes followed by a decline to below the level of untreated neutrophils[160]. Phorbol esters are hydrolysis-resistant analogues of diacylglycerol, and act on protein kinase C (PKC) directly without first binding to a receptor. It is therefore reasonable to assume that phorbol esters exert their effects by the phosphorylation of cellular proteins. Indeed, PKC inhibitors were shown to inhibit CR1- and CR3-mediated phagocytosis by neutrophils[183] and monocytes[184]. However, as the PKC inhibitors which inhibit phagocytosis in neutrophils and monocytes are different, the signalling mechanisms may be cell-specific.

Since FcγR-mediated phagocytosis does not require phorbol ester stimulation, it is probable that ligation of the FcγR activates PKC. Indeed, of the proteins in activated mouse peritoneal macrophages which are phosphorylated during phagocytosis of EIgG[185], some are also phosphorylated during EIgMC phagocytosis whereas others are phosphorylated following treatment with phorbol esters. As ligation of FcγR and treatment of phorbol ester also induces the respiratory burst, which does not occur when complement receptors are ligated[151], the patterns of protein phosphorylation under the three different stimulatory conditions allow determination of which proteins are involved in ingestion (phosphorylated during phagocytosis of EIgG and EIgMC but not necessarily when treated with phorbol esters) and which are involved in the triggering of the respiratory burst (phosphorylated during phagocytosis of EIgG and under phorbol ester stimulation but not during phagocytosis of EIgMC)[185]. Although none of these proteins has been identified, it is probable that the set associated with ingestion must contain some of the actin-binding proteins, whose phosphorylation is known to alter the affinity for actin[186]. These may therefore regulate actin polymerization, as a result of which pseudopod formation and the ingestion phase of the phagocytic process are controlled.

CR1 was found to be phosphorylated under the stimulation of phorbol esters in monocytes, neutrophils and eosinophils but not B lymphocytes or erythrocytes[187]. Phosphorylation of CR3 and FcγR was not observed by these authors. Subsequent investigations by others have demonstrated that whereas the α subunit of CR3 is constitutively phosphorylated, the phosphorylation of the β subunit is responsive to stimulation by phorbol ester[5,6]. In the presence of the PKC inhibitor, staurosporine, phorbol-ester-induced phosphorylation of the β subunit of CR3 in neutrophils was inhibited along with the phagocytosis of iC3b-coated erythrocytes[183], although the binding of EiC3b and the phagocytosis of EIgG were not affected. Some PKC inhibitors have been shown to inhibit both FcγR and complement-receptor-mediated phagocytosis by cultured monoctyes while others, including staurosporine, had no effect[184]. It is not known whether staurosporine inhibits the phorbol-ester-stimulated phosphorylation of the complement receptors in cultured monocytes. The results of the above studies do not provide definitive evidence that stimulated phosphorylation of CR1 and CR3 is causally related to their adhesion and phagocytic activities.

(5) The respiratory burst

The respiratory burst includes a complex set of reactions all involving the 'burst' of oxygen consumption leading to the generation of an array of oxidation products. A comprehensive review may be found in Klein[188]. This set of reactions is generally measured as the amount of redox products of hydrogen peroxide or superoxide anion[93,150–152,161]. Many of the products of the respiratory burst are toxic to microorganisms and it has been shown to be the principal means of eliminating pathogens. One major difference between FcγR- and complement-receptor-mediated phagocytosis is the coupling of the former, but not the latter, with the respiratory burst[151,152]. Hence, ingestion may not be an obligatory process to provide the signal to trigger the respiratory burst. Recently, it has been demonstrated that the relationship between FcγR-mediated phagocytosis and the respiratory burst may be more complex. Neutrophils require an additional signal, possibly from cytokines, to stimulate the respiratory burst, the products of which may have a positive feedback effect enhancing FcγR-mediated phagocytosis[161,189]. Although, in monocytes, an exogenous signal is not required, the enhancement of FcγR-mediated phagocytosis by respiratory burst products can only be observed if an exogenous source of lactoferrin is available[161].

(6) Ingestion and involvement of cytoskeletal components

Ingestion involves the mobilization of plasma membrane to engulf the opsonized targets and is driven by the continuous rearrangement of underlying cytoskeletal components towards the final events of membrane fusion and formation of a phagosome. Electron microscopic studies on phagocytosing macrophages of IgG- or complement-coated particles showed the alignment of microfilaments and microtubules around ingested particles[190]. Drugs, such as cytochalasin B which disrupts subplasmalemmal microfilaments, inhibit the ingestion process[191].

Recent work by Newman *et al.*[184] distinguished the phagocytosis of IgG- and complement-coated targets. Drugs that increase the intracellular level of cGMP, such as dibutyryl cGMP, carbachol, bethanechol, as well as phorbol esters, may enhance complement-receptor-mediated phagocytosis by promoting microtubule assembly. In contrast, drugs such as dibutyryl cAMP, epinephrine and isoproterenol, which increase the level of intracellular cAMP, inhibit complement-receptor-mediated phagocytosis by preventing microtubule assembly. These drugs, whether they promote or prevent microtubule assembly, appear not to have any effect on FcγR-mediated phagocytosis. Thus, it may be postulated that microfilaments are involved in the ingestion process in general whereas the communication of the signal from the ligation of complement receptors to the ingestion apparatus requires the assembly of microtubules.

(7) CR1 and CR3

Structurally, CR1 and CR3 are very different. CR1 belongs to the RCA superfamily[192] whereas CR3 belongs to the integrin family (see Figure 10.1). The entire extracellular domain of CR1 is composed of a series of CCP repeats (the most common allotype has 30), followed by a transmembrane and cytoplasmic segment[168] (see Chapter 2). Neither the α nor β subunits of CR3 has CCP repeats. Furthermore, the transmembrane and cytoplasmic segments of CR1 do not bear any similarity to those of either the α or β subunits of CR3 at the primary structural level[21–23,27,28,168]. Although CR1 and CR3 recognize different ligands, CR1 recognizes C3b and C4b in a divalent-cation-independent manner and CR3 recognizes iC3b in a divalent-cation-dependent manner, the processes involved in CR1- and CR3-mediated phagocytosis are remarkably similar. Thus, most of the discussion for phagocytosis by monocytes and neutrophils may be carried out without specifying which of the receptors is involved. For example, both CR1- and CR3-mediated binding can be detected for cultured monocytes but a second signal from phorbol esters or leukocyte response integrin is required to trigger ingestion. The treatment of neutrophils with phorbol esters induces a biphasic response for both CR1- and CR3-mediated adhesion as well as ingestion. Unlike FcγR-mediated phagocytosis, phagocytosis by either complement receptor is not coupled to the respiratory burst.

The entire phagocytic process may be regarded as a series of signals from the initial event of the interaction between the ligands on the target surface and the receptors on the phagocyte. Discovering how the two signals from the ligation of CR1 and CR3 merge to trigger the first identifiable common event, which is the assembly of microtubules, would greatly facilitate our understanding of phagocytosis, as well as the roles of the two structurally very different receptors in the complex process of phagocytosis.

(8) CR3

CR3 is a multifunctional membrane protein complex. Its role(s) in the phagocytic process is perhaps but one of its many functions. Within this context, it mediates at least two activities: (1) the binding of iC3b-coated targets, and (2) the communication of the signals from surface ligation of CR1 and FcγR to the ingestion apparatus. Much needs to be done to define the interaction between iC3b and CR3 as well as to characterize the cellular components, including other membrane proteins and cytoskeletal elements, with which CR3 must interact to serve as a receptor.

Acknowledgement

We would like to thank Professor S. D. Wright for comments on this manuscript.

References

1. Law, S. K. and Levine, R. P. (1977). Interaction between the third complement protein and cell surface macromolecules. *Proc. Natl. Acad. Sci. USA*, **74**, 2701–5
2. Law, S. K. A. and Reid, K. B. M. (1988). *Complement*. (Oxford, UK: IRL Press)
3. Law, S. K. A. (1988). C3 receptors on macrophages. *J. Cell Sci. Suppl.*, **9**, 67–97
4. Skubitz, K. M. and Snook, R. W. II (1987). Monoclonal antibodies that recognize lacto-N-fucopentaose III (CD15) react with the adhesion-promoting glycoprotein family (LFA-1/HMAC-1/GP 150,95) and CR1 on human neutrophils. *J. Immunol.*, **139**, 1631–9
5. Chatila, T. A., Geha, R. S. and Arnaout, M. A. (1989). Constitutive and stimulus-induced phosphorylation of CD11/CD18 leukocyte adhesion molecules. *J. Cell Biol.*, **109**, 3435–44
6. Buyon, J. P., Slade, S. G., Reibman, J., Abramson, S. B., Philips, M. R., Weissmann, G. and Winchester, R. (1990). Constitutive and induced phosphorylation of the a- and b-chains of the CD11/CD18 leukocyte integrin family. *J. Immunol.*, **144**, 191–7

7. Dransfield, I. and Hogg, N. (1989). Regulated expression of Mg2+ binding epitope on leukocyte integrin alpha subunits. *EMBO J.*, **8**, 3759–65
8. Graham, I. L. and Brown, E. J. (1991). Extracellular calcium results in a conformational change in Mac-1 (CD11b/CD18) on neutrophils. Differentiation of adhesion and phagocytosis functions of Mac-1. *J. Immunol.*, **146**, 685–91
9. Hynes, R. O. (1987). Integrins: a family of cell surface receptors. *Cell*, **48**, 549–54
10. Ruoslahti, E. (1991). Integrins. *J. Clin. Invest.*, **87**, 1–5
11. Humphries, M. J. (1990). Molecular basis and specificity of integrin – ligand interactions. *J. Cell Sci.*, **97**, 585–92
12. Larson, R. S. and Springer, T. A. (1990). Structure and function of leukocyte integrins. *Immunol. Rev.*, **114**, 181–217
13. Hogg, N. and Horton, M. A. (1987). Myeloid antigens: new and previously defined clusters. In McMichael, A. J. (ed.) *Leukocyte typing III – White Cell Differentiation Antigens*, pp. 576–602. (Oxford: Oxford University Press)
14. Takada, Y. and Hemler, M. E. (1989). The primary structure of the VLA-2/collagen receptor a2 subunit (platelet GPla): homology to other integrins and the presence of a possible collagen-binding domain. *J. Cell Biol.*, **109**, 397–407
15. Tsuji, T., Hakomori, S. and Osawa, T. (1991). Identification of human galactoprotein b3, an oncogenic transformation-induced membrane glycoprotein, as VLA-3 a subunit: the primary structure of human integrin a3. *J. Biochem.*, **109**, 659–65
16. Takada, Y., Elices, M. J., Crouse, C. and Hemler, M. E. (1989). The primary structure of alpha-4 subunit of VLA-4: homology to other integrins and possible cell–cell adhesion function. *EMBO J.*, **8**, 1361–8
17. Argraves, W. S., Suzuki, S., Arai, H., Thompson, K., Pierschbacher, M. D. and Ruoslahti, E. (1987). Amino acid sequence of the human fibronectin receptor. *J. Cell Biol.*, **105**, 1183–90
18. Fitzgerald, L. A., Poncz, M., Steiner, B., Rall, S. C. Jr., Lo, S. S., Bennett, J. S. and Phillips, D. R. (1987). Comparison of cDNA-derived protein sequences of the human fibronectin and vitronectin receptor a-subunits and platelet glycoprotein IIb. *Biochemistry*, **26**, 8158–65
19. Tamura, R. N., Rozzo, C., Starr, L., Chambers, J., Reichardt, L. F., Cooper, H. M. and Quaranta, V. (1990). Epithelial integrin alpha 6 beta 4: complete primary structure of alpha 6 and variant forms of beta 4. *J. Cell Biol.*, **111**, 1593–604
20. Larson, R. S., Corbi, A. L., Berman, L. and Springer, T. (1989). Primary structure of the leukocyte function-associated molecule-1 a subunit: an integrin with an embedded domain defining a protein superfamily. *J. Cell Biol.*, **108**, 703–12
21. Arnaout, M. A., Gupta, S. K., Pierce, M. W. and Tenen, D. G. (1988). Amino acid sequence of the alpha subunit of human leukocyte adhesion receptor Mo1 (complement receptor type 3). *J. Cell Biol.*, **106**, 2153–8
22. Corbi, A. L., Kishimoto, T. K., Miller, L. J. and Springer, T. A. (1988). The human leukocyte adhesion glycoprotein Mac-1 (complement receptor type 3, CD11b) a subunit: cloning, primary structure, and relation to the integrins, von Willebrand factor and factor B. *J. Biol. Chem.*, **263**, 12403–11
23. Hickstein, D. D., Hickey, M. J., Ozols, J., Baker, D. M., Back, A. L. and Roth, G. J. (1989). cDNA sequence for the alphaM subunit of the human neutrophil adherence receptor indicates homology to integrin a subunits. *Proc. Natl. Acad. Sci. USA*, **86**, 257–61
24. Corbi, A. L., Miller, L. J., O'Connor, K., Larson, R. S. and Springer, T. A. (1987). cDNA cloning and complete primary structure of the alpha subunit of a leukocyte adhesion glycoprotein, p150,95. *EMBO J.*, **6**, 4023–8
25. Poncz, M., Eisman, R., Heidenreich, R., Silver, S. M., Vilaire, G., Surrey, S., Schwartz, E. and Bennett, J. S. (1987). Structure of the platelet membrane glycoprotein IIb. Homology to the alpha subunits of the vitronectin and fibronectin membrane receptors. *J. Biol. Chem.*, **262**, 8476–82
26. Suzuki, S., Argraves, W. S., Arai, H., Languino. L. R., Pierschbacher, M. D. and Ruoslahti, E. (1987). Amino acid sequence of the vitronectin receptor alpha subunit and comparative expression of adhesion receptor mRNAs. *J. Biol. Chem.*, **262**, 327–32
27. Kishimoto, T. K., O'Connor, K., Lee, A., Roberts, T. M. and Springer, T. A. (1987). Cloning of the beta subunit of the leukocyte adhesion proteins: homology to an extracellular matrix receptor defines a novel supergene family. *Cell*, **48**, 681–90
28. Law, S. K. A., Gagnon, J., Hildreth, J. E. K., Wells, C. E., Willis, A. C. and Wong, A. J. (1987). The primary structure of the beta-subunit of the cell surface adhesion glycoproteins LFA-1, CR3 and p150,95 and its relationship to the fibronectin receptor. *EMBO J.*, **6**, 915–19

29. Fitzgerald, L. A., Steiner, B., Rall, S. C. Jr., Lo, S. S. and Phillips, D. R. (1987). Protein sequence of endothelial glycoprotein IIIa derived from a cDNA clone: identity with platelet glycoprotein IIIa and similarity to "integrin". *J. Biol. Chem.*, **262**, 3936–9
30. Zimrin, A. B., Gidwitz, S., Lord, S., Schwartz, E., Bennett, J. S., White, G. C. and Poncz, M. (1990). The genomic organization of platelet glycoprotein IIIa. *J. Biol. Chem.*, **265**, 8590–5
31. Hogervorst, F., Kuikman, I., von dem Borne, A. E. G. Kr. and Sonnenberg, A. (1990). Cloning and sequence analysis of beta-4 cDNA: an integrin subunit that contains a unique 118 kd cytoplasmic domain. *EMBO J.*, **9**, 765–70
32. Suzuki, S. and Naitoh, Y. (1990). Amino acid sequence of a novel integrin b4 subunit and primary expression of the mRNA in epithelial cells. *EMBO J.*, **9**, 757–63
33. McLean, J. W., Vestal, D. J., Cheresh, D. A. and Bodary, S. C. (1990). cDNA sequence of the human integrin b5 subunit. *J. Biol. Chem.*, 265, 17126–31
34. Ramaswamy, H. and Hemler, M. E. (1990). Cloning, primary structure and properties of a novel human integrin b subunit. *EMBO J.*, **9**, 1561–8
35. Suzuki, S., Huang, Z. S. and Tanihara, H. (1990). Cloning of an integrin b subunit exhibiting high homology with integrin b3 subunit. *Proc. Natl. Acad. Sci. USA*, **87**, 5354–8
36. Sheppard, D., Rozzo, C., Starr, L., Quaranta, V., Erle, D. J. and Pytela, R. (1990). Complete amino acid sequence of a novel integrin b subunit (b6) identified in epithelial cells using the polymerase chain reaction. *J. Biol. Chem.*, **265**, 11502–7
37. Yuan, Q., Jiang, W. M., Krissansen, G. W. and Watson, J. D. (1990). Cloning and sequence analysis of a novel beta2-related integrin transcript from T lymphocytes: homology of integrin cysteine-rich repeats to domain III of laminin B chains. *Int. Immunol.*, **2**, 1097–108
38. Erle, D. J., Reugg, C. and Pytela, R. (1991). Complete amino acid sequence of an integrin beta subunit (beta7) identified in leukocytes. *J. Biol. Chem.*, **266**, 11009–16
39. Szebenyi, D. M. E., Obendorf, S. K. and Moffat, K. (1981). Structure of vitamin D-dependent calcium-binding protein from bovine intestine. *Nature*, **294**, 327–32
40. Yamada, K. M. (1991). Adhesive recognition sequences. *J. Biol. Chem.*, **266**, 12809–12
41. Tufty, R. M. and Kretsinger, R. H. (1975). Troponin and parvalbumin calcium binding regions predicted in myosin light chain and T4 lysozyme. *Science*, **187**, 167–9
42. Chou, P. Y. and Fasman, G. D. (1978). Empirical predictions of protein conformation. *Ann. Rev. Biochem.*, **47**, 251–76
43. Garnier, J., Osguthorpe, D. J. and Robson, B. (1978). Analysis of the accuracy and implications of simple methods for predicting the secondary structure of globular proteins. *J. Mol. Biol.*, **120**, 97–120
44. Williams, R. J. P. (1986). The physics and chemistry of the calcium-binding protein. In *Calcium and the Cell. Ciba Foundaiton Symposium*, **122**, 145–61
45. Staden, R. (1982). An interactive graphics program for comparing and aligning nucleic acid and amino acid sequences. *Nucleic Acids Res.*, **10**, 2951–61
46. Golden, A., Brugge, J. S. and Shattil, S. J. (1990). Role of platelet membrane glycoprotein IIb-IIIa in agonist-induced tyrosine phosphorylation of platelet proteins. *J. Cell Biol.*, **111**, 3117–27
47. Shaw, L. M., Messier, J. M. and Mercurio, A. M. (1990). The activation dependent adhesion of macrophages to laminin involves cytoskeletal anchoring and phsophorylation of the alpha 6 beta 1 integrin. *J. Cell Biol.*, **110**, 2167–74
48. Backer, J. M., Kahn, C. R., Cahill, D. A., Ullrich, A. and White, M. F. (1990). Receptor-mediated internalization of insulin requires a 12-amino acid sequence in the juxtamembrane region of the insulin receptor beta-subunit. *J. Biol. Chem.*, **265**, 16450–4
49. Chen, W. J., Goldstein, J. L. and Brown, M. S. (1990). NPXY, a sequence often found in cytoplasmic tails, is required for coated pit-mediated internalization of the low density lipoprotein receptor. *J. Biol. Chem.*, **265**, 3116–23
50. Carrell, N. A., Fitzgerald, L. A., Steiner, B., Erickson, H. P. and Phillips, D. R. (1985). Structure of human platelet membrane glycoproteins IIb and IIIa as determined by electron microscopy. *J. Biol. Chem.*, **260**, 1743–9
51. Nermut, M. V., Green, N. M., Eason, P., Yamada, S. S. and Yamada, K. M. (1988). Electron microscopy and structural model of human fibronectin receptor. *EMBO J.*, **7**, 4093–9
52. Dana, N., Fathallah, D. M. and Arnaout, M. A. (1991). Expression of a soluble and functional form of the human beta 2 integrin CD11b/CD18. *Proc. Natl. Acad. Sci. USA*, **88**, 3106–10

53. Calvete, J. J., Henschen, A. and Gonzalez-Rodriguez, J. (1989). Complete localization of the intrachain disulphide bonds and the N-glycosylation points in the alpha-subunit of human platelet glycoprotein IIb. *Biochem. J.*, **261**, 561–8
54. Beer, J. and Coller, B. S. (1989). Evidence that platelet glycoprotein IIIa has a large disulfide-bonded loop that is susceptible to proteolytic cleavage. *J. Biol. Chem.*, **264**, 17564–73
55. Calvete, J. J., Henschen, A. and González-Rodríguez, J. (1991). Assignment of disulphide bonds in human platelet GPIIIa: a disulphide pattern for the beta-subunits of the integrin family. *Biochem. J.*, **274**, 63–71
56. Marlin, S. D., Morton, C. C., Anderson, D. C. and Springer, T. A. (1986). LFA-1 immunodeficiency disease – definition of the genetic defect and chromosomal mapping of a and b subunits of the lymphocyte function associated antigen 1 (LFA-1) by complementation in hybrid cells. *J. Exp. Med.*, **164**, 855–67
57. Corbi, A. L., Larson, R. S., Kishimoto, T. K., Springer, T. A. and Morton, C. C. (1988). The leukocyte adhesion receptors LFA-1, Mac-1 and p150,95: identification of a gene cluster involved in cell adhesion. *J. Exp. Med.*, **167**, 1597–607
58. Solomon, E., Palmer, R. W., Hing, S. and Law, S. K. A. (1988). Regional localization of CD18, the b-subunit of the cell surface adhesion molecule LFA-1, on human chromosome 21 by in situ hybridization. *Ann. Hum. Genet.*, **52**, 123–8
59. Burmeister, M., Kim, S., Price, R., de Lange, T., Tantravahi, U., Myers, R. M. and Cox, D. R. (1991). A map of the distal region of the long arm of human chromosome 21 constructed by radiation hybrid mapping and pulsed-field gel electrophoresis. *Genomics*, **9**, 19–30
60. Weitzman, J. B., Wells, C. E., Wright, A. H., Clark, P. A. and Law, S. K. A. (1991). The gene organisation of the human β2 integrin subunit (CD18). *FEBS Lett.*, **294**, 97–103
61. Corbi, A. L., Garcia-Aguilar, J. and Springer, T. A. (1990). Genomic structure of an integrin alpha subunit, the leukocyte p150,95 molecule [published erratum appears in J Biol Chem 1990 Jul 25;265(21):12750–1]. *J. Biol. Chem.*, **265**, 2782–8
62. Weitzman, J. B. (1991). Characterisation of the 5′ regions of the leukocyte integrin CD11b/CD18 genes. *D.Phil. thesis*, Oxford University
63. Heidenreich, R., Eisman, R., Surrey, S., Delgrosso, K., Bennett, J.S., Schwartz, E. and Poncz, M. (1990). Organization of the gene for platelet glycoprotein IIb. *Biochemistry*, **29**, 1232–44
64. Miller, B. A., Antognetti, G. and Springer, A. (1985). Identification of cell surface antigens present on murine hematopoietic stem cells. *J. Immunol.*, **134**, 3286–90
65. Miller, L. J., Schwarting, R. and Springer, T. A. (1986). Regulated expression of the Mac-1, LFA-1, p150,95 glycoprotein family during leukocyte differentiation. *J. Immunol.*, **137**, 2891–900
66. Campana, D., Sheridan, B., Tidman, N., Hoffbrand, A. V. and Janossy, G. (1986). Human leukocyte function-associated antigens on lympho-hemopoietic precursor cells. *Eur. J. Immunol.*, **16**, 537–42
67. Freyer, D. R., Morganroth, M. L., Rogers, C. E., Arnaout, M. A. and Todd, R. F. III (1988). Modulation of surface CD11/CD18 glycoproteins (Mo1, LFA-1, p150,95) by human mononuclear phagocytes. *Clin. Immunol. Immunopathol.*, **46**, 272–83
68. Schwarting, R., Stein, H. and Wang, C. Y. (1985). The monoclonal antibodies anti S-HCL 1 (anti Leu 14) and anti S-HCL 3 (anti Leu M5) allow the diagnosis of hairy cell leukemia. *Blood*, **65**, 974–83
69. Ramos, O. F., Kai, C., Yefenov, E. and Klein, E. (1988). The elevated natural killer sensitivity of targets carrying surface-attached C3 fragments require the availability of the iC3b receptor (CR3) on the effectors. *J. Immunol.*, **140**, 1239–43
70. De-la-Hera, A., Alvarez-Mon, M., Sanchez-Madrid, F., Martinez, C. and Durantez, A. (1988). Co-expression of Mac-1 and p150,95 on CD5+ B cells. Structural and functional characterization in a human chronic lymphocytic leukemia. *Eur. J. Immunol.*, **18**, 1131–4
71. Dianzani, U., Zarcone, D., Pistoia, V., Grossi, C. E., Pileri, A., Massaia, M. and Ferrarini, M. (1989). CD8 + CD11b + peripheral blood T lymphocytes contain lymphokine-activated killer cell precursors. *Eur. J. Immunol.*, **19**, 1037–44
72. Keizer, G. D., Borst, J., Visser, W., Schwarting, R., de-Vries, J. E. and Figdor, C. G. (1987). Membrane glycoprotein p150,95 of human cytotoxic T cell clone is involved in conjugate formation with target cells. *J. Immunol.*, **138**, 3130–6

73. Krensky, A. M., Sanchez-Madrid, F., Robbins, E., Nagy, J. A., Springer, T. A. and Burakoff, S. J. (1983). The functional significance, distribution, and structure of LFA-1, LFA-2, and LFA-3: cell surface antigens associated with CTL-target interactions. *J. Immunol.*, **131**, 611–16
74. Strassmann, G., Springer, T. A. and Adams, D. O. (1985). Studies on antigens associated with the activation of murine mononuclear phagocytes: kinetics of and requirements for induction of lymphocyte function-associated (LFA)-1 antigen in vitro. *J. Immunol.*, **135**, 147–51
75. Strassmann, G., Springer, T. A. and Adams, D. O. (1985). Studies on antigens associated with the activation of murine mononuclear phagocytes: kinetics of and requirements for induction of lymphocyte function-associated (LFA)-1 antigen in vitro. *J. Immunol.*, **135**, 147–51
76. Hickstein, D. D., Hickey, M. J. and Collins, S. J. (1988). Transcriptional regulation of the leukocyte adherence protein b subunit during human myeloid cell differentiation. *J. Biol. Chem.*, **263**, 13863–7
77. Hickstein, D. D., Back, A. L. and Collins, S. J. (1989). Regulation of expression of the CD11b and CD18 subunits of the neutrophil adherence receptor during human myeloid differentiation. *J. Biol. Chem.*, **264**, 21812–17
78. Todd, R. F. III, Arnaout, M. A., Rosin, R. E., Crowley, C. A., Peters, W. A. and Babior, B. M. (1984). Subcellular localization of the larger subunit of Mo1 (Mo1-alpha; formerly gp 110), a surface glycoprotein associated with neutrophil adhesion. *J. Clin. Invest.*, **74**, 1280–90
79. Lanier, L. L., Arnaout, M. A., Schwarting, R., Warner, N. L. and Ross, G. D. (1985). p150,95, Third member of the LFA-1/CR3 polypeptide family identified by anti-Leu M5 monoclonal antibody. *Eur. J. Immunol.*, **15**, 713–18
80. Bainton, D. F., Miller, L. J., Kishimoto, T. K. and Springer, T. A. (1987). Leukocyte adhesion receptors are stored in peroxidase-negative granules of human neutrophils. *J. Exp. Med.*, **166**, 1641–53
81. Berger, M., O'Shea, J., Cross, A. S., Folks, T. M., Chused, T. M., Brown, E. J. and Frank, M. M. (1984). Human neutrophils increase expression of iC3b as well as C3b receptors upon activation. *J. Clin. Invest.*, **74**, 1566–71
82. Miller, L. J., Bainton, D. F., Borregaard, N. and Springer, T. A. (1987). Stimulated mobilization of monocyte Mac-1 and p150,95 adhesion proteins from an intracellular vesicular compartment to the cell surface. *J. Clin. Invest.*, **80**, 535–44
83. Singer, I. I., Scott, S., Kawka, D. W. and Kazazis, D. M. (1989). Adhesomes: specific granules containing receptors for laminin, iC3b/fibrinogen fibronectin, and vitronectin in human polymorphonuclear leukocytes and monocytes. *J. Cell Biol.*, **109**, 3169–82
84. Anderson, D. C. and Springer, T. A. (1987). Leukocyte adhesion deficiency: an inherited defect in the Mac-1, LFA-1, and p150,95 glycoproteins. *Annu. Rev. Med.*, **38**, 175–94
85. Arnaout, M. A. (1990). Leukocyte adhesion molecules deficiency: its structural basis, pathophysiology and implications for modulating the inflammatory response. *Immunol. Rev.*, **114**, 145–80
86. Back, A. L., Kwok, W. W., Adam, M., Collins, S. J. and Hickstein, D. (1990). Retroviral-mediated gene transfer of the leukocyte integrin CD18 subunit. *Biochem. Biophys. Res. Commun.*, **171**, 787–95
87. Wardlaw, A. J., Hibbs, M. L., Stacker, S. A. and Springer, T. A. (1990). Distinct mutations in two patients with leukocyte adhesion deficiency and their functional correlates. *J. Exp. Med.*, **172**, 335–45
88. Harlan, J. M. (1985). Leukocyte–endothelial interactions. *Blood,* **65**, 513–25
89. Lo, S. K., Van Seventer, G. A., Levin, S. M. and Wright, S. D. (1989). Two leukocyte receptors (CD11a/CD18 and CD11b/CD18) mediate transient adhesion to endothelium by binding to different ligands. *J. Immunol.*, **143**, 3325–9
90. Smith, C. W., Marlin, S. D., Rothlein, R., Toman, C. and Anderson, D. C. (1989). Cooperative interactions of LFA-1 and Mac-1 with intercellular adhesion molecule-1 in facilitating adherence and transendothelial migration of human neutrophils *in vitro*. *J. Clin. Invest.*, **83**, 2008–17
91. Diamond, M. S., Staunton, D. E., de-Fougerolles, A. R., Stacker, S. A., Garcia-Aguilar, J., Hibbs, M. L. and Springer, T. A. (1990). ICAM-1 (CD54): a counter-receptor for Mac-1 (CD11b/CD18). *J. Cell Biol.*, **111**, 3129–39
92. Bohnsack, J. F., Akiyama, S. K., Damsky, C. H., Knape, W. A. and Zimmerman, G. A. (1990). Human neutrophil adherence to laminin in vitro: evidence for a distinct neutrophil integrin receptor for laminin. *J. Exp. Med.*, **171**, 1221–37

93. Ross, G. D., Cain, J. A. and Lachmann, P. J. (1985). Membrane complement receptor type three (CR3) has lectin-like properties analogous to bovine conglutinin as functions as a receptor for zymosan and rabbit erythrocytes as well as a receptor for iC3b. *J. Immunol.*, **134**, 3307–15
94. Ross, G. D., Thompson, R. A., Walport, M. J., Springer, T. A., Watson, J. V., Ward, R. H., Lida, J., Newman, S. L., Harrison, R. A. and Lachmann, P. J. (1985). Characterization of patients with an increased susceptibility to bacterial infections and a genetic deficiency of leukocyte membrane complement receptor type 3 and the related membrane antigen LFA-1. *Blood*, **66**, 882–90
95. Ross, G. D., Cain, J. A., Myones, B. L., Newman, S. L. and Lachmann, P. J. (1987). Specificity of membrane complement receptor type three (CR3) for beta-glucans. *Complement*, **4**, 61–74
96. Wright, S. D. and Jong, M. T. (1986). Adhesion-promoting receptors on human macrophages recognize Escherichia coli by binding to lipopolysaccharide. *J. Exp. Med.*, **164**, 1876–88
97. Talamas-Rohana, P., Wright, S. D., Lennartz, M. R. and Russell, D.G. (1990). Lipophosphoglycan from Leishmania mexicana promastigotes binds to members of the CR3, p150,95 and LFA-1 family of leukocyte integrins. *J. Immunol.*, **144**, 4817–24
98. Bullock, W. E. and Wright, S. D. (1987). Role of the adherence-promoting receptors, CR3, LFA-1, and p150,95, in binding of Histoplasma capsulatum by human macrophages. *J. Exp. Med.*, **165**, 195–210
99. Beller, D. I., Springer, T. A. and Schreiber, R. D. (1982). Anti-Mac-1 selectively inhibits the mouse and human type three complement receptor. *J. Exp. Med.*, **156**, 1000–9
100. Wright, S. D., Rao, P. E., Van Voorhis, W. C., Craigmyle, L. S., Iida, K., Talle, M. A., Westberg, E. F., Goldstein, G. and Silverstein, S. C. (1983). Identification of the iC3b-receptor of human monocytes and macrophages by using monoclonal antibodies. *Proc. Natl. Acad. Sci. USA*, **80**, 5699–703
101. Newman, S. L., Bucher, C., Rhodes, J. and Bullock, W. E. (1990). Phagocytosis of Histoplasma capsulatum yeasts and microconidia by human cultured macrophages and alveolar macrophages: cellular cytoskeleton requirement for attachment and ingestion. *J. Clin. Invest.*, **85**, 223–30
102. Altieri, D. C. and Edgington, T. S. (1988). The saturable high affinity association of factor X to ADP-stimulated monoctyes defines a novel function of the Mac-1 receptor. *J. Biol. Chem.*, **263**, 7007–15
103. Altieri, D. C., Morrissey, J. H. and Edgington, T. S. (1988). Adhesive receptor Mac-1 coordinates the activation of factor X on stimulated cells of monocytic and myeloid differentiation: an alternative initiation of the coagulation protease cascade. *Proc. Natl. Acad. Sci. USA*, **85**, 7462–6
104. Wright, S. D., Weitz, J. I., Huang, A. J., Levin, S. M., Silverstein, S. C. and Loike, J. D. (1988). Complement receptor type three (CD11b/CD18) of human polymorphonuclear leukocytes recognizes fibrinogen. *Proc. Natl. Acad. Sci. USA*, **85**, 7734–8
105. Altieri, D. C., Bader, R., Mannucci, P. M. and Edgington, T. S. (1988). Oligospecificity of the cellular adhesion receptor MAC-1 encompasses an inducible recognition specificity for fibrinogen. *J. Cell Biol.*, **107**, 1893–900
106. Cooper, J. A., Lo, S. K. and Malik, A. B. (1988). Fibrin is a determinant of neutrophil sequestration in the lung. *Circ. Res.*, **63**, 735–41
107. Diamond, M. S., Staunton, D. E., Marlin, S. D. and Springer, T. A. (1991). Binding of the integrin Mac-1 (CD11b/CD18) to the third immunoglobulin-like domain of ICAM-1 (CD54) and its regulation by glycosylation. *Cell*, **65**, 961–71
108. Staunton, D. E., Dustin, M. L., Erickson, H. P. and Springer, T. A. (1990). The arrangement of the immunoglobulin-like domains of ICAM-1 and the binding sites for LFA-1 and rhinovirus [published erratum appears in Cell 1990 Jun 15; 61(2):1157]. *Cell*, **61**, 243–54
109. Stacker, S. A. and Springer, T. A. (1991). Leukocyte integrin p150,95 (CD11c/CD18) functions as an adhesion molecule binding to a counter-receptor on stimulated endothelium. *J. Immunol.*, **146**, 648–55
110. Brown, E. J. and Goodwin, J. L. (1988). Fibronectin receptors of phagocytes: characterization of the Arg-Gly-Asp binding proteins of human monocytes and polymorphonuclear leukocytes. *J. Exp. Med.*, **167**, 777–93
111. Gresham, H. D., Goodwin, J. L., Allen, P. M., Anderson, D. C. and Brown, E. J. (1989). A novel member of the integrin receptor family mediates Arg-Gly-Asp-stimulated neutrophil phagocytosis. *J. Cell Biol.*, **108**, 1935–43

112. Loike, J. D., Sodeik, B., Cao, L., Leucona, S., Weitz, J. I., Detmers, P. A., Wright, S. D. and Silverstein, S. C. (1991). CD11c/CD18 on neutrophils recognizes a domain at the N terminus of the A alpha chain of fibrinogen. *Proc. Natl. Acad. Sci. USA*, **88**, 1044–8
113. de Bruijn, M. H. L. and Fey, G. H. (1985). Human complement component C3: cDNA coding sequence and derived primary structure. *Proc. Natl. Acad. Sci. USA*, **82**, 708–12
114. Wright, S. D., Reddy, P. A., Jong, M. T. and Erickson, B. W. (1987). iC3b receptor (complement receptor type 3) recognizes a region of complement protein C3 containing the sequence Arg-Gly-Asp. *Proc. Natl. Acad. Sci. USA*, **84**, 1965–8
115. Russell, D. G. and Wright, S. D. (1988). Complement receptor type 3 (CR3) binds to an Arg-Gly-Asp-containing region of the major surface glycoprotein, gp63, of Leishmania promastigotes. *J. Exp. Med.*, **168**, 279–92
116. Taniguchi-Sidle, A. and Isenman, D. E. (1991). Mutagenesis of the Arg-Gly-Asp (RGD) triplet in human complement component C3 does not abolish binding of iC3b to the leukocyte integrin complement receptor type III (CR3, CD11b/CD18). *J. Biol. Chem.* (In press)
117. Taniguchi-Sidle, A. and Isenman, D. E. (1991). Mutagenesis of the Arg-Gly-Asp (RGD) triplet and neighbouring residues of human C3 does not abolish binding of iC3b to CR3. *Complement Inflamm.*, **8**, 229
118. Relman, D., Tuomanen, E., Falkow, S., Golenbock, D. T., Saukkonen, K. and Wright, S. D. (1990). Recognition of a bacterial adhesin by an integrin: macrophage CR3 (aMB2, CD11b/CD18) binds filamentous hemagglutinin of Bordetella pertussis. *Cell*, **61**, 1375–82
119. Sanchez-Madrid, F., Nagy, J. A., Robbins, E., Simon, P. and Springer, T. A. (1983). A human leukocyte differentiation antigen family with distinct alpha-subunits and a common beta-subunit: the lymphocyte function-associated (LFA-1), the iC3b complement receptor (OKM1/Mac-1), and the p150,95 molecule. *J. Exp. Med.*, **158**, 1785–803
120. Malhotra, V., Hogg, N. and Sim, R. B. (1986). Ligand binding by the p150,95 antigen of U937 monocytic cells: properties in common with complement receptor type 3 (CR3). *Eur. J. Immunol.*, **16**, 1117–23
121. Micklem, K. J. and Sim, R. B. (1985). Isolation of complement-fragment-iC3b binding proteins by affinity chromatography: the identification of p150,95 as an iC3b-binding protein. *Biochem. J.*, **231**, 233–6
122. Myones, B. L., Dalzell, J. G., Hogg, N. and Ross, G. D. (1988). Neutrophil and monocyte cell surface p150,95 has iC3b-receptor (CR4) activity resembling CR3. *J. Clin. Invest*, **82**, 640–51
123. Lay, W. H. and Nussenzweig, V. (1968). Receptors for complement on leukocytes. *J. Exp. Med.*, **128**, 991–1010
124. Mantovani, B., Rabinovitch, M. and Nussenzweig, V. (1972). Phagocytosis of immune complexes by macrophages: different roles of the macrophage receptor sites for complement (C3) and for immunoglobulin (IgG). *J. Exp. Med.*, **135**, 780–92
125. Mantovani, B. (1975). Different roles of IgG and complement receptors in phagocytosis by polymorphonuclear leukocykes. *J. Immunol.*, **115**, 15–17
126. Scribner, D. J. and Fahrney, D. (1976). Neutrophil receptors for IgG and complement: their roles in the attachment and ingestion phases of phagocytosis. *J. Immunol.*, **116**, 892–7
127. Newman, S. L. and Johnston, R. B. J. (1979). Role of binding through C3b and IgG in polymorphonuclear neutrophil function: studies with trypsin-generated C3b. *J. Immunol.*, **123**, 1839–46
128. Wellek, B., Hahn, H. and Opferkuch, W. (1975). Quantitative contributions of IgG, IgM and C3 to erythrophagocytosis and rosette formation by peritoneal macrophages, and anti-opsonin activity of dextran sulfate 500. *Eur. J. Immunol.*, **5**, 378-81
129. Griffin, F. M. J., Bianco, C. and Silverstein, S. C. (1975). Characterization of the macrophage receptor for complement and demonstration of its functional independence from the receptor for the Fc portion of immunoglobulin G. *J. Exp. Med.*, **141**, 1269–77
130. Atkinson, J. P. and Frank, M. M. (1974). The effect of bacillus Calmette-Guerin induced macrophage activation on the in vivo clearance of sensitised erythrocytes. *J. Clin. Invest.*, **53**, 1742
131. Bianco, C., Griffin, F. M. and Silverstein, S. C. (1975). Studies of the macrophage complement receptor: alteration of receptor function upon macrophage activation. *J. Exp. Med.*, **141**, 1279–90
132. Griffin, J. A. and Griffin, F. M. J. (1979). Augmentation of macrophage complement receptor function in vitro. I. Characterization of the cellular interactions required for the generation of a T-lymphocyte product that enhances macrophage complement receptor function. *J. Exp. Med.*, **150**, 653–75

133. Griffin, F. M. J. and Griffin, J. A. (1980). Augmentation of macrophage complement receptor function in vitro. II. Characterization of the effects of a unique lymphokine upon the phagocytic capabilities of macrophages. *J. Immunol.*, **125**, 844–9
134. Griffin, F. M. J. and Mullinax, P. J. (1981). Augmentation of macrophage complement receptor function in vitro. III. C3b receptors that promote phagocytosis migrate within the plane of the macrophage plasma membrane. *J. Exp. Med.*, **154**, 291–305
135. Newman, S. L., Musson, R. A. and Henson, P. M. (1980). Development of functional complement receptors during in vitro maturation of human monocytes into macrophages. *J. Immunol.*, **125**, 2236–44
136. Whaley, K. and Ruddy, S. (1976). Modulation of C3b haemolytic activity by a plasma protein distinct from C3b-inactivator. *Science*, **193**, 1011–13
137. Pangburn, M. K., Schreiber, R. D. and Müller-Eberhard, H. J. (1977). Human complement C3b inactivator: isolation, characterization, and demonstration of an absolute requirement for the serum protein B1H for cleavage of C3b and C4b in solution. *J. Exp. Med.*, **146**, 257–70
138. Law, S. K. A., Lichtenberg, N. A. and Levine, R. P. (1979). Evidence for an ester linkage between the labile binding site of C3b and receptive surfaces. *J. Immunol.*, **123**, 1388–94
139. Carlo, J. R., Ruddy, S., Studer, E. J. and Conrad, D. H. (1979). Complement receptor binding of C3b-coated cells treated with C3b inactivator, beta1H globulin and trypsin. *J. Immunol.*, **123**, 523–8
140. Campbell, R. D., Dodds, A. W. and Porter, R. R. (1980). The binding of human complement component C4 to antibody–antigen aggregates. *Biochem. J.*, **189**, 67–80
141. Law, S. K., Lichtenberg, N. A., Holcombe, F. H. and Levine, R. P. (1980). Interaction between the labile binding sites of the fourth (C4) and fifth (C5) human complement proteins and erythrocyte cell membranes. *J. Immunol.*, **125**, 634–9
142. Shiraishi, S. and Stroud, R. M. (1975). Cleavage products of C4b produced by enzymes in human serum. *Immunochemistry*, **12**, 935–9
143. Fujita, T., Gigli, I. and Nussenzweig, V. (1978). Human C4-binding protein. II. Role in proteolysis of C4b by C3b-inactivator. *J. Exp. Med.*, **148**, 1044–51
144. Cooper, N. R. (1969). Immune adherence by the fourth component of complement. *Science*, **165**, 396–8
145. Bohnsack, J. F., O'Shea, J. J., Takahashi, T. and Brown, E. J. (1985). Fibronectin-enhanced phagocytosis of an alternative pathway activator by human culture-derived macrophages is mediated by the C4b/C3b complement receptor (CR1). *J. Immunol.*, **135**, 2680–6
146. Wright, S. D. and Silverstein, S. C. (1982). Tumor-promoting phorbol esters stimulated C3b and C3b′ receptor-mediated phagocytosis in cultured human monocytes. *J. Exp. Med.*, **156**, 1149–64
147. Wright, S. D., Licht, M. R., Craigmyle, L. S. and Silverstein, S. C. (1984). Communication between receptors for different ligands on a single cell: ligation of fibronectin receptors induces a reversible alteration in the function of complement receptors on cultured human monocytes. *J. Cell Biol.*, **99**, 336–9
148. Pommier, C. G., Inada, S., Fries, L. F., Takahashi, T., Frank, M. M. and Brown, E. J. (1983). Plasma fibronectin enhances phagocytosis of opsonized particles by human peripheral blood monocytes. *J. Exp. Med.*, **157**, 1844–54
149. Wright, S. D., Craigmyle, L. S. and Silverstein, S. C. (1983). Fibronectin and serum amyloid P component stimulate C3b- and iC3b-mediated phagocytosis in cultured human monocytes. *J. Exp. Med.*, **158**, 1338–43
150. Johnston, R. B. Jr, Lehmeyer, J. E. and Guthrie, L. A. (1976). Generation of superoxide anion and chemiluminescence by human monocytes during phagocytosis and on contact with surface-bound immunoglobulin G. *J. Exp. Med.*, **143**, 1551–7
151. Wright, S. D. and Silverstein, S. C. (1983). Receptors for C3b and Cb3i promote phagocytosis but not the release of toxic oxygen from human phagocytes. *J. Exp. Med.*, **158**, 2016–23
152. Yamamoto, K. and Johnston, R. B. (1984). Dissociation of phagocytosis from stimulation of the oxidative metabolic burst in macrophages. *J. Exp. Med.*, **159**, 405–16
153. Wright, S. D., Detmers, P. A., Jong, M. T. C. and Meyer, B. C. (1985). Interferon-gamma depresses binding of ligand by C3b and iC3b receptors on cultured human monocytes, an effect reversed by fibronectin. *J. Exp. Med.*, **163**, 1245–59
154. Todd, R. F. III, Nadler, L. M. and Schlossman, S. F. (1981). Antigens on human monocytes identified by monoclonal antibodies. *J. Immunol.*, **126**, 1435–42
155. Arnaout, M. A., Todd, R. F., Dana, N., Melamed, H., Schlossman, S. F. and Colten, H. R. (1983). Inhibition of phagocytosis of complement C3- or immunoglobulin G-coated particles

and of iC3b binding by monoclonal antibodies to a monocyte–granulocyte membrane glycoprotein (Mo1). *J. Clin. Invest.*, **72**, 171–9
156. Todd, R. F. III, van Agthoven, A., Schlossmann, S. F. and Terhorst, C. (1982). Structural analysis of differentiation antigens Mo1 and Mo2 on human monocytes. *Hybridoma*, **1**, 329–37
157. Brown, E. J., Bohnsack, J. F. and Gresham, H. D. (1988). Mechanism of inhibition of immunoglobulin G-mediated phagocytosis by monoclonal antibodies that recognise the Mac-1 antigen. *J. Clin. Invest.*, **81**, 365–75
158. Graham, I. L., Gresham, H. D. and Brown, E. J. (1989). An immobile subset of plasma membrane CD11b/CD18 (Mac-1) is involved in phagocytosis of targets recognised by multiple receptors. *J. Immunol.*, **14**, 2352–8
159. Pommier, C. G., O'Shea, J., Chused, T., Yancey, K., Frank, M. M., Takahashi, T. and Brown, E. J. (1984). Studies on the fibronectin receptors of human peripheral blood leukocytes. Morphologic and functional characterisation. *J. Exp. Med.*, **159**, 137–51
160. Wright, S. D. and Meyer, B. C. (1986). Phorbol esters cause sequential activation and deactivation of complement receptors on polymorphonuclear leukocytes. *J. Immunol.*, **136**, 1759–64
161. Gresham, H. D., McGarr, J. A., Shackelford, P. G. & Brown, E. J. (1988) Studies on the molecular mechanisms of human Fc receptor-mediated phagocytosis. Amplification of ingestion is dependent on the generation of reactive oxygen metabolites and is deficient in polymorphonuclear leukocytes from patients with chronic granulomatous disease. *J. Clin. Invest.*, **82**, 1192–1201
162. Detmers, P. A., Lo, S. K., Olsen-Egbert, E., Walz, A., Baggiolini, M. and Cohn, Z. A. (1990). Neutrophil-activating protein 1/interleukin 8 stimulates the binding activity of the leukocyte adhesion receptor CD11b/CD18 on human neutrophils. *J. Exp. Med.*, **171**, 1155–62
163. Buyon, J. P., Abramson, S. B., Philips, M. R., Slade, S. G., Ross, G. D., Weissmann, G. and Winchester, R. J. (1988). Dissociation between increased surface expression of Gp165/95 and homotypic neutrophil aggregation. *J. Immunol.*, **140**, 3156–60
164. Vedder, N. B. and Harlan, J. M. (1988). Increased surface expression of CD11b/CD18 (Mac-1) is not required for stimulated neutrophil adherence to cultured endothelium. *J. Clin. Invest.*, **81**, 676–82
165. Lo, S. K., Detmers, P. A., Levin, S. M. and Wright, S. D. (1989). Transient adhesion of neutrophil to endothelium. *J. Exp. Med.*, **169**, 1779–93
166. Coller, B. S. (1985). A new murine monoclonal antibody reports an activation-dependent change in the conformation and/or microenvironment of the platelet glycoprotein IIb/IIIa complex. *J. Clin. Invest.*, **76**, 101–8
167. Altieri, D. C. and Edgington, T. S. (1988). A monoclonal antibody reacting with distinct adhesion molecules defines a transition in the functional state of the receptor CD11b/CD18 (Mac-1). *J. Immunol.*, **141**, 2656–60
168. Klickstein, L. B., Wong, W. W., Smith, J. A., Weis, J. H., Wikson, J. G. and Fearon, D. T. (1987). Human C3b/C4b receptor (CR1): demonstration of long homologous repeating domains that are composed of the short consensus repeats characteristic of C3/C4 binding proteins. *J. Exp. Med.*, **165**, 1095–112
169. Klickstein, L. B., Bartow, T. J., Miletic, V., Rabson, L. D., Smith, J. A. and Fearon, D. T. (1988). Identification of distinct C3b and C4b recognition sites in the human C3b/C4b receptor (CR1, CD35) by deletion mutagenesis. *J. Exp. Med.*, **168**, 1699-717
170. Krych, M., Hourcade, D. and Atkinson, J. P. (1991). Sites within the complement C3b/C4b receptor important for the specificity of ligand binding. *Proc. Natl. Acad. Sci. USA*, **88**, 4353–7
171. Detmers, P. A., Wright, S. D., Olsen, E., Kimball, B. and Cohn, Z. A. (1987). Aggregation of complement receptors on human neutrophils in the absence of ligand. *J. Cell Biol.*, **105**, 1137–45
172. Hermanowski-Vosatka, A., Detmers, P. A., Gotze, O., Silverstein, S. C. and Wright, S. D. (1988). Clustering of ligand on the surface of a particle enhances adhesion to receptor-bearing cells. *J. Biol. Chem.*, **263**, 17822–7
173. Unkeless, J. C. (1989). Function and heterogeneity of human Fc receptors for immunoglobulin G. *J. Clin. Invest.*, **83**, 355–61
174. Guyre, P. M., Morganelli, P. M. and Miller, R. (1983). Recombinant immune interferon increases immunoglobulin G Fc receptors on cultured human mononuclear phagocytes. *J. Clin. Invest.*, **72**, 393–7

175. Perussia, B., Dayton, E. T., Lazarus, R., Fanning, V. and Trinchieri, G. (1983). Immune interferon induces the receptor for monomeric IgG1 on human monocytic and myeloid cells. *J. Exp. Med.*, **158**, 1092–113
176. Fleit, H. B., Wright, S. D., Durie, C. J., Valinsky, J. E. and Unkeless, J. C. (1984). Ontogeny of Fc receptors and complement receptor (CR3) during human myeloid differentiation. *J. Clin. Invest.*, **73**, 516–25
177. Fleit, H. B., Wright, S. D. and Unkeless, J. C. (1982). Human neutrophil Fc gamma receptor distribution and structure. *Proc. Natl. Acad. Sci. USA*, **79**, 3275–9
178. Selvaraj, P., Rosse, W. F., Silber, R. and Springer, T. A. (1988). The major Fc receptor in blood has a phosphatidylinositol anchor and is deficient in paroxysmal nocturnal haemoglobinuria. *Nature*, **333**, 565–7
179. Huizinga, T. W., van der Schoot, C. E., Jost, C., Klaassen, R., Kleijer, M., von dem Borne, A. E., Roos, D. and Tetteroo, P. A. (1988). The P1-linked receptor FcRIII is released on stimulation of neutrophils. *Nature*, **333**, 667–9
180. Klaassen, R. J. L., Ouwehand, W. H., Huizinga, T. W. J., Engelfriet, C. P. and Von dem Borne, A. E. G. Kr. (1990). The Fc-receptor III of cultured human monocytes: structural similarity with FcRIII of natural killer cells and role in the extracellular lysis of sensitised erythrocytes. *J. Immunol.*, **144**, 599–606
181. Wright, S. D. and Meyer, B. C. (1985). Fibronectin receptor of human macrophages recognises the sequence of Arg-Gly-Asp-Ser. *J. Exp. Med.*, **162**, 762–7
182. Ruoslahti, E. and Pierschbacher, M. D. (1987). New perspectives in cell adhesion: RGD and integrins. *Science*, **238**, 491–7
183. Roubey, R. A., Ross, G. D., Merrill, J. T., Walton, F., Reed, W., Winchester, R. and Buypn, J. P. (1991). Staurosporine inhibits neutrophil phagocytosis but not iC3b binding mediated by CR3 (CD11b/CD18). *J. Immunol.*, **146**, 3557–62
184. Newman, S. L., Mikus, L. K. and Tucci, M. A. (1991). Differential requirements for cellular cytoskeleton in human macrophage complement receptor- and Fc receptor-mediated phagocytosis. *J. Immunol.*, **146**, 967–74
185. Brozna, J. P., Hauff, N. F., Phillips, W. A. and Johnston, R. B. J. (1988). Activation of the respiratory burst in macrophages. Phosphorylation specifically associated with Fc receptor-mediated stimulation. *J. Immunol.*, **141**, 1642–7
186. Bahler, M. and Greengard, P. (1987). Synapsin I bundles F-actin in a phosphorylation-dependent manner. *Nature*, **326**, 704–7
187. Changelian, P. S. and Fearon, D. T. (1986). Tissue-specific phosphorylation of complement receptors CR1 and CR2. *J. Exp. Med.*, **163**, 101
188. Klein, J. (1990). *Immunology*. Chapter 10: Mediators and messengers, pp. 246–68. (Oxford: Blackwell Scientific Publications Inc.)
189. Gresham, H. D., Zheleznyak, A., Mormol, J. S. and Brown, E. J. (1990). Studies on the molecular mechanisms of human neutrophil Fc receptor-mediated phagocytosis. Evidence that a distinct pathway for activation of the respiratory burst results in reactive oxygen metabolite-dependent amplification of ingestion. *J. Biol. Chem.*, **265**, 7819–26
190. Reaven, E. P. and Axline, S. G. (1973). Subplasmalemmal microfilaments and microtubules in resting and phagocytizing cultivated macrophages. *J. Cell. Biol.*, **59**, 12
191. Axline, S. G. and Raven, E. P. (1974). Inhibition of phagocytosis and plasma membrane mobility of the cultivated macrophage by cytochalasin B: role of subplasmalemmal microfilaments. *J. Cell. Biol.*, **62**, 647–59
192. Reid, K. B. M. and Day, A. J. (1989). Structure–function relationships of the complement components. *Immunol. Today*, **10**, 177–80
193. Ignatius, M. J., Large, T. H., Houde, M., Tawil, J. W., Barton, A., Esch, F., Carbonetto, S. and Reichart, L. F. (1990). Molecular cloning of the rat integrin a1-subunit: a receptor for laminin and collagen. *J. Cell. Biol.*, **111**, 709–20
194. Bossy, B., Bossy-Wetzel, E and Reichardt, L. F. (1991). Characterisation of the integrin a8 subunit: a new integrin b1-associated subunit, which is prominently expressed on exons and on cells in contact with basal laminae in chick embryos. *EMBO J.*, **10**, 2375–85
195. Kramer, R. H., McDonald, K. A. and Vu, M. P. (1989). Human melanoma cells express a novel integrin receptor for laminin. *J. Biol. Chem.*, **264**, 15642–59

11
Anaphylatoxins

J. KÖHL and D. BITTER-SUERMANN

In addition to the basic functions, opsonization and cytolysis, associated with the complement system there are some physiological activities elicited by complement peptides which contribute significantly to antimicrobial defence in infectious diseases and to the physiological and pathological consequences of immune complex formation, in short to the benefit and burden of inflammation. These effects depend on the cleavage of low-molecular-weight activation peptides from C4, C3 and C5: the anaphylatoxic peptides or anaphylatoxins C4a, C3a and C5a. The known primary structures[1] are given in Table 11.1. Generated from the N-termini of the α-chains of C4, C3 or C5 via activation of the classical or alternative pathways of complement, they interact with specific receptors on a number of cell types of the phagocytic system, mainly granulocytes and monocytes/macrophages. In addition, endothelial cells, possibly some T-cell subsets and, in some species, platelets express anaphylatoxin-receptors. Although the C5a receptor is often expressed with the C3a/C4a receptor, they are distinct species. The ligand–receptor interaction triggers G-protein coupled signal transduction pathways and results in a number of cellular responses[2–15], the most significant of which are documented in Table 11.2. Some of these biological effects are in general use as highly sensitive and specific *in vitro* detection systems for anaphylatoxins, e.g. smooth muscle contraction, enzyme release, stimulation of the respiratory burst, histamine release, ATP release, chemotaxis. However, these methods are too laborious for routine use and therefore quantification of anaphylatoxins using ELISA and RIA with monoclonal or polyclonal antibodies has been developed.[16–21] Two natural control mechanisms regulate the biological responses to anaphylatoxins and prevent excessive responses with pathological sequelae. First, a serum carboxypeptidase-N rapidly cleaves off the C-terminal arginine from all three anaphylatoxins and reduces circulating C3a and C4a activities to zero and C5a activity to 1–2%. Nevertheless, this residual C5a des Arg possesses significant biological activity. The second control mechanism works at the level of responder cells. A stimulus-specific receptor-mediated reversible deactivation

Table 11.1 Primary structures of human C3a, C4a and C5a

	1 10 20
Human C3a	NH_2-Ser-Val-Gln-Leu-Thr-Glu-Lys-Arg-Met-Asn-Lys-Val-Gly-Lys-Tyr-Pro-( ) -Lys-Glu-Leu-Arg-Lys-
Human C4a	NH_2-Asn = Asn-Phe-Gln-Lys-Ala-Ile-Asn-Glu = Leu = Gln = Ala-Ser-Pro- Thr-Ala-Lys-Arg-
	1 10 20
Human C5a	NH_2-Thr = Gln-Lys = Ile-Glu-Glu-Ile-Ala-Ala = = Lys-His-Ser- Val-Val-Lys =
	30 40
Human C3a	[Cys-Cys] Glu-Asp-Gly-Met-Arg-Gln-Asn-Pro-Met-Arg-Phe-Ser [Cys] Gln-Arg-Arg-Thr-Arg-Phe- Ile-Ser-
Human C4a	[= =] Gln = = Val-Thr-Arg-Leu- = = Met-Arg = [=] Glu-Gln = Ala- Ala-Arg-Val-Gln-
	30 40
Human C5a	[= =] Tyr = = Ala-Cys-Val = Asn-Asp-Clu-( )- Thr [=] Glu-Gln = Ala-Ala-Arg = =
	50 60
Human C3a	Leu-Gly-Glu-Ala [Cys] Lys-Lys-Val-Phe- Leu-Asp [Cys-Cys] Asn-Tyr-Ile-Thr-Glu-Leu-Arg-Arg-Gln-His-
Human C4a	Gln-() -Pro-Asn [=] Arg-Glu-Pro = = Ser [= =] Cln-Phe-Ala-Glu-Ser = = Lys-Lys-Ser-
	50 60
Human C5a	= = Pro-Arg [=] Ile = Ala = Thr-Glu [= =] Val-Val-Ala-Ser-Gln = = ( )–
	70 77
Human C3a	Ala-Arg-Ala-Ser-His- ( )-Leu-Gly-Leu-Ala-Arg-COOH
	77
Human C4a	Arg-Asp-Lys-Gly-Gln- ( )-Ala = = Gln = COOH
	(CHO) 70 74
Human C5a	= Asn-Ile = = Lys-Asp-Met-Gln = Gly = COOH

Table 11.2 Test systems for biological activities of anaphylatoxins

Cells/organs to be tested	*Products/functions measured*	*C3a*	*C5a*
Rat mast cell	Histamine release	+[2]	+[2]
Guinea pig platelet	Aggregation	+[3]	+[3]
	Serotonine release	+[4]	+[4]
	ATP-release	+[5]	+[5]
Guinea-pig macrophage	Thromboxane A_2 release	+[6]	n.d.
Guinea-pig ileum	Isotonic contraction	+[7]	+[7]
Guinea-pig skin	Vasopermeability	+[8]	+[8]
Human PMNL	Chemotaxis	—	+[9]
	Enzyme release	—	+[10]
	Oxidative burst	—	+[11]
Human monocyte/macrophage	IL-1 release	+[12]	+[13]
Cell line U 937	β-Glucuronidase	n.d	+[129]
Human basophil	Histamine release	+(IL-3)[14]	+[15]
	Leucotriene B4 release	+(IL-3)[14]	+(IL-3)[15]

n.d. = not determined; superior numbers = references; + = active in the test; — = not active in the test

process is effective *in vivo* and *in vitro*[22, 23] and clearly discriminates between C5a and C3a/C4a respectively. This phenomenon is long known as tachyphylaxis.

STRUCTURE–FUNCTION RELATIONSHIPS OF ANAPHYLATOXINS

The information available at the moment on the essential structural features of anaphylatoxins has been obtained from two experimental approaches: synthetic peptides and recombinant peptides. In addition, removal of C-terminal arginine by serum carboxypeptidase-N from these reagents has permitted investigations into the essential role of the C-terminal arginine. The synthetic peptide strategy has been mainly successful for short peptides up to 21 amino acids from the C-terminus of C3a, and has allowed definition of optimal and minimal peptide length and amino acid sequence requirements. In addition, certain amino acids have been substituted by non-peptidic spacer and anchor elements[24,25]. In contrast, until now, the recombinant peptide strategy has been focused exclusively on C5a[26]. Site-directed mutagenesis and expression in *Escherichia coli* has been used to generate mutant peptides with changes of single or multiple amino acids[27]. In summarizing the state of the art, the structural requirements for ligand specificity of C3a are a C-terminal arginine, followed N-terminally by a short group of 4–8 hydrophobic amino acids, which are conserved in all species examined so far.

A non-peptidic N-terminal acyl residue, like the aromatic fluorenylmethoxycarbonyl (FMOC) group, coupled to the aminohexanoyl (Ahx) group potentiates activities of short synthetic peptides 10–50-fold and, in some cases, above that of natural C3a[24,25]. On the other hand, it was possible to shorten the minimal sequence for a specific C3a activity to the tripeptide LAR[28] with this coupling strategy. The C3a peptide 57–77 previously reported to exhibit 100% acitivity[29] recently was shown to exhibit only 10% activity in both guinea-pig ileum contraction assay and in the platelet ATP release assay[30]. The C3a receptor, although until now only characterized from guinea-pig platelets[31,32], can be predicted to have only one binding pocket for properly presented arginine.

On the other hand, the synthetic peptide strategy was not successful for investigation of C5a: even the large C-terminal C5a peptides 55–74 failed to exhibit significant biological activity. Surprisingly, the FMOC membrane anchor and an amino hexanoic spacer (e.g. FMOC–Ahx–KDMQLGR) permit short synthetic C-terminal C5a peptides to trigger the C3a receptor[30]. Thus, site-directed mutagenesis of recombinant C5a has become the method of choice to study the interaction of C5a with the C5a receptor. These experiments have shown that C5a interacts with its receptor by multipoint binding, the crucial amino acid clusters[27,33] being Arg 74, Leu 72, Lys 68, a region around Arg 40 and Arg 37 and possibly His 15. The construction of a recombinant C3a–C5a hybrid peptide (C5a 1–69–LGLAR) representing the five C-terminal C3a amino acids, with both C3a (1%) and C5a (100%) activity, favours the interpretation that the carboxyterminal sequence, LGLAR, is able to bind to two different receptors, the C3a receptor as well as the C5a receptor.[34]

ANAPHYLATOXIN RECEPTORS

Until recently, the knowledge about anaphylatoxin receptors and receptor-mediated events was restricted to binding and crosslinking studies with C5a receptors on human polymorphonuclear leukocytes or macrophage-like cell lines[35,36], guinea-pig platelets[37] and to guinea-pig C3a receptors on platelets[31,32]. In early 1991, the human C5a receptor was finally cloned by an expression cloning strategy and identified as a member of the rhodopsin supergene family[38,39], in line with e.g. the formyl peptide receptor[40] or the β-adrenergic receptor[41]. The common features of this supergene family are seven membrane spanning helices and four short membrane protruding segments. By analogy with the β-adrenergic receptor, where the aspartic acid 82 of the receptor sequence represents a conserved binding site for the ligand, a first binding site for the C5a molecule (Arg 74) was postulated in a hypothetical receptor model (Figure 11.1)[33]. As the Asp 82 is about 20 Å below the outer membrane, not only the Arg 74 but also the adjacent residues, Gly 73 and Leu 72, would have to enter into this pocket. Because of the flexible random coil conformation of the eleven C-terminal amino acids of C5a, this interaction is conceivable. In consequence, the proposed second C5a binding site around Arg 40[27] would find a corresponding counterpart on the receptor at position Glu 179,180.

In the near future, the molecular genetic approaches will elucidate the receptor structure of the ligand binding pockets, the function of the different intra- and extracellular domains, signal transduction and association with regulatory GTP binding proteins, distribution pattern on different cell types and finally

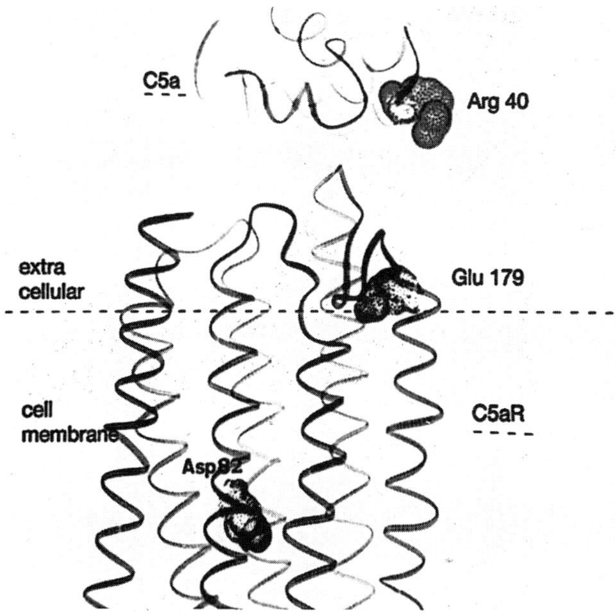

Figure 11.1 Ribbon representation of the C5a receptor model (in violet) viewed in the direction of the membrane plane. The extracellular site is on the top. Helices A–D are in the foreground from left to right, helices E–G in the background from right to left. The side chains of Asp 82 (B) (near the bottom on the left and Glu 180 (DE) (near the top on the right) suggested to bind the functionally essential arginines of C5a (74 and 40, respectively) are shown in dotted surface representation. On top, a ribbon representation of C5a with the side chain of Arg40 is added. (Taken from Grotzinger, J., Engels, M., Jacoby, E. and Wollmer, A. (1991). A model for the C5a receptor and for its interaction with the ligand. *Protein Engineering*, **4**, 767–71)

parallels to the putatively similar C3a receptor. Studies on receptor antagonists and receptor blockade by domain-specific antibodies will influence strategies to cope with the undesirable side-effects of anaphylatoxins (see below).

IN VITRO ASSAYS FOR ANAPHYLATOXINS

Due to the high inflammatory potential of the anaphylatoxins, there are diverse properties which in principle can be determined (see Table 11.2) in an *in vitro* assay. Of the biological activities, enhanced vascular permeability is measured using Evans blue in an *in vivo* skin test in guinea-pigs. Another organ assay using guinea-pigs is the ileum contraction assay. Although these two assays have been used frequently over the last 15 years, the data derived have been limited by the lack of good quantitation, and low sensitivity and considerable variability[30].

For qualitative determination of the biological activities of anaphylatoxins and synthetic anaphylatoxic peptides, new assays have been developed. In general, four homologous and two heterologous cell types have been used for C5a assays: human neutrophils, basophils, monocytes and the promyelotic cell line U937 on the one hand, and the rat mast cell and the guinea-pig platelet on the other. For C3a there exist three heterologous but only two homologous cell types (Table 11.2).

Of these cell assays, only a few can be applied as standard procedures for quantitative estimations. Dose–response curves for C5a activity can be easily obtained with enzyme-release tests from neutrophil[10] and the U937 cell line[42]. Other biological properties of neutrophils can be estimated only semi-quantitatively, e.g. by chemotaxis[9], or display a considerable variability, e.g. the oxidative burst assay using luminol-enhanced chemiluminescence[11]. All assays with human basophils are difficult because of the small number of basophils in peripheral blood[14,15]. An ideal heterologous test system represents the guinea-pig platelet. Cell preparation is easy to perform with a high yield, so that some dose–response curves can be obtained within a day. At least three different reaction types can be measured: ^{3}[H]serotonin release[4], platelet aggregation[3] and ATP-mediated bioluminescence[5]. Each type can be used for determination of C3a and C5a activities since all reactions are mediated by specific receptors which have been described for both anaphylatoxins[31,32,37]. Biological activities of sythetic C3a analogue peptides have been quantitated in this cell assay because of its high sensitivity and reliability[30]. The only reservation to be made is that all data of structural requirements for an ideal C3a peptide are now well adapted to the guinea-pig C3a receptor. Whether these data can be transferred to the human situation remains to be shown with an homologous cell type in which quantitative responses can be obtained.

For the detection of anaphylatoxins in body fluids, two different test principles exist: commercially available radio-immunoassays (RIAs) and different enzyme-linked immunoassays (ELISAs), which differ in the specificity of their monoclonal antibodies. For detection of C3a two different types of antibodies have been described. The first was generated by immunization with intact C3[61] or C3a[16] and reacts with C3a and C3. Therefore, C3 has to be removed by a precipitation step prior to the assay. The second was raised to denatured C3[19] or a synthetic C-terminal C3a octapeptide (69–76)[17] and reacts only with C3a and C3a des Arg, respectively but not with C3. The advantage is obvious as no precipitation step is necessary. The detection limit of these assays is about 1–10 ng/ml. For C5a, the situation is quite similar as monoclonal antibodies which react with both C5a and C5[16] and those which exclusively detect C5a and C5a des Arg, are available[20,21]. The detection limit of these ELISAs is $\leq$ 1 ng/ml.

THE ROLE OF ANAPHYLATOXINS IN THE IMMUNE RESPONSE

Besides the inflammatory potential of the anaphylatoxins, there exist a variety of reports about the immunoregulatory activities of anaphylatoxins[43–49]. In contrast to the similar inflammatory properties of C3a and C5a, they behave in totally different ways in the humoral response. As C3a was found to be a potent supressor of antigen-specific and polyclonal antibody response, C5a was able to augment both *in vitro* humoral and cell-mediated immune response[43]. The suppression of the polyclonal antibody response mediated by C3a seems to depend on the activation of non-specific $CD8^+$ suppressor T cells[44]. In addition, C3a is capable of activating human macrophages to release PGE_2 via the cyclooxygenase pathway of arachidonic acid metabolism, which is known to inhibit polyclonal antibody secretion[45]. These C3a effects could be mimicked by C-terminal oligopeptides while C3a des Arg was inactive[46,47]. C3a was not able to suppress antigen- or mitogen-induced B and T cell proliferation, whereas C5a was capable of potentiating antigen-induced but not mitogen-induced T cell proliferative responses.

The stimulating effect of C5a involves helper T cells, demonstrated with soluble T cell-replacing factors (Fc)TRF, which rendered lymphocyte cultures refractory to the enhancing properties of C5a[48]. In contrast to C3a, the C-terminal arginine of C5a is not essential for the immune response. C5a des Arg was shown in a recent study to induce a similar level of IL-6 from peripheral blood-derived mononuclear cells as C5a[49]. IL-6 is thought to be in part responsible for the immunoregulatory activities of C5a.

FROM PHYSIOLOGICAL TO PATHOLOGICAL ACTION

The anaphylatoxins are mediators of inflammatory reactions and important messenger molecules between the humoral and cellular branch of the early immune response, shifting a localized or systemic humoral cascade reaction to the cellular level of phagocytic cells with their non-specific and specific immune functions. The genetic deficiencies of C3 and C5 are complicated by severe localized and systemic pyogenic infections (see Chapter 6) due to lack of opsonization (in the case of C3), assembly of the cytolytic membrane attack complex (for both C3 and C5) and lack of anaphylatoxins. Thus, one should be cautious before declaring that anaphylatoxin activities are unnecessary and undesirable. Inflammation is an important host–defence mechanism and not a disease. However, occasionally excessive production of anaphylatoxins produces pathological consequences, which will be discussed in detail below. In the remainder of this chapter, we will focus on the role of anaphylatoxins in the pathogenesis of the adult respiratory distress syndrome (ARDS) and other diseases. In addition, we will discuss possible implications of the therapeutic anaphylatoxin blockade.

THE ADULT RESPIRATORY DISTRESS SYNDROME (ARDS)

The anaphylatoxins play a major role in the pathogenesis of ARDS and measurement of their plasma concentrations has been used as a predictive marker for its development and severity.

The first clinical description of this acute pulmonary disorder more than twenty years ago led to an overwhelming interest in this disease. In the USA, 150 000 cases of ARDS occur each year with a mortality above 50%. Thus, understanding the pathogenesis of this disorder is one of the major goals of pulmonary research[50–52].

ARDS is a disease never 'sui generis' but the result of direct parenchymal lung injury or of an excessive inflammatory response of the whole body after polytrauma, septic shock, burns, etc. (Table 11.3). In the early stages, increased vascular permeability is the striking feature of the disease, followed by necrosis and remodelling of the lung architecture which leads to impaired oxygenation and decreased compliance, often with a lethal outcome. Interaction of humoral mediators with polymorphonuclear leukocytes, microvascular endothelial cells, alveolar macrophages and type II epithelial cells seems to be responsible for the vascular leakage. The anaphylatoxins, as potent humoral mediators, are thought to play an important role in initiating the inflammatory cascade reaction, although, alone, they are not sufficient to induce a complete ARDS. Based on data from different animal models and the finding of elevated levels of inflammatory mediators in plasma and bronchoalveolar fluid in man, it seems likely that mediators must act in concert to induce severe ARDS. Thus, blockade of inflammatory cascade at key points may have therapeutic potential. The main humoral and cellular mediators taking part in this inflammatory concert are listed in Figure 11.2. Subsequently, we will try to outline a pathogenetic concept focusing on the early events in ARDS based on *in vitro* and *in vivo* findings, mostly in animal models. Because of the mass of *in vitro* data we will discuss only those results which correlate with *in vivo* findings in animals or humans. We will discuss first the adherence of neutrophil polymorphonuclear leukocytes (neutrophils) to vascular endothelial cells as the initial step in ARDS and secondly the activation of neutrophils as a key event in the increase in vascular permeability which leads to pulmonary oedema. We will not focus on the later phenomena which are linked to the irreversible lung remodelling because they are only poorly understood and the role of anaphylatoxins, if any, is unknown.

Pathogenesis

Adherence of neutrophils

In the case of all events listed in Table 11.3, the plasma enzyme systems in inflammation, i.e. the clotting, kinin, fibrinolytic and the complement systems, are activated. One of the most potent inflammatory mediators released is C5a. As a neutrophil chemoattractant, it is able to induce neutrophil aggregation and adhesion to vascular endothelium, respectively. This was investigated in a guinea-pig *in vivo* model[53,54]. After intravenous injection of purified C5a or C3a,

Table 11.3 Risk factors for development of an ARDS

Direct	*Indirect*
Aspiration pneumonia	Shock
Pulmonary contusion	Sepsis
Inhalation of toxic gas	Multiple blood transfusions
Infection (pneumonia)	Polytrauma
	Acute pancreatitis

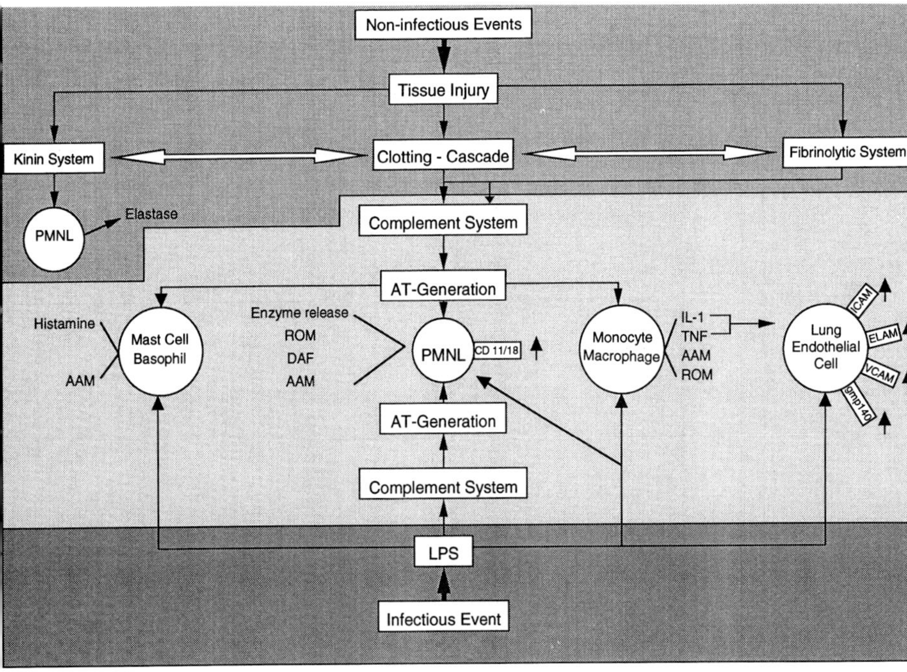

Figure 11.2 Network of main humoral and cellular mediators at the early stage of ARDS. At the top, the consequences of non-infectious (polytrauma, multiple blood transfusions, pancreatitis and other) events on the humoral enzyme and cellular system in inflammation are pictured. At the bottom, the pathway of LPS interaction in Gram-negative sepsis is shown. ROM, reactive oxygen metabolites; PAF, platelet activating factor; AAM, arachidonic acid metabolites; IL-1, interleukin 1; TNF, tumour necrosis factor; ICAM, intracellular adhesion molecule; ELAM, endothelial leucocyte adhesion molecule; VCAM, vascular cell adhesion molecule; GMP 140, granule membrane protein 140; < or > secretion.

granulocytes and platelets disappeared from circulating within a minute, returned to starting values after 2 min and increased to approximately double the normal level after 1–4 h (Figure 11.3). Simultaneously with the fall in the circulating neutrophils, the neutrophil content of the lung increased about three-fold (Figure 11.4), but gradually declined over the next 24 h. All the neutrophils were in the blood vessels with no evidence of migration towards the interstitial or the alveolar spaces. Recent *in vitro* data indicate that this adhesion process is mediated by members of the CD11/CD18 family of leukocyte integrins[55–58]. C5a as well as LTB_4 can induce a rapid increase (maximum in 2 min) of CD11/CD18 glycoproteins on neutrophils. In contrast, the adhesivity of endothelial cells, depending on upregulation of endothelial–leukocyte adhesion molecule-1 (ELAM-1) and intracellular adhesion molecule-1 (ICAM-1), increased after 4–6 h, requiring *de novo* RNA and protein synthesis. Thus, upregulation of CD11/CD18 on neutrophils appears to be responsible for the rapid margination of neutrophils in the pulmonary microcirculation following the intravenous injection of C3a or C5a. Furthermore, flow cytometric measurements with

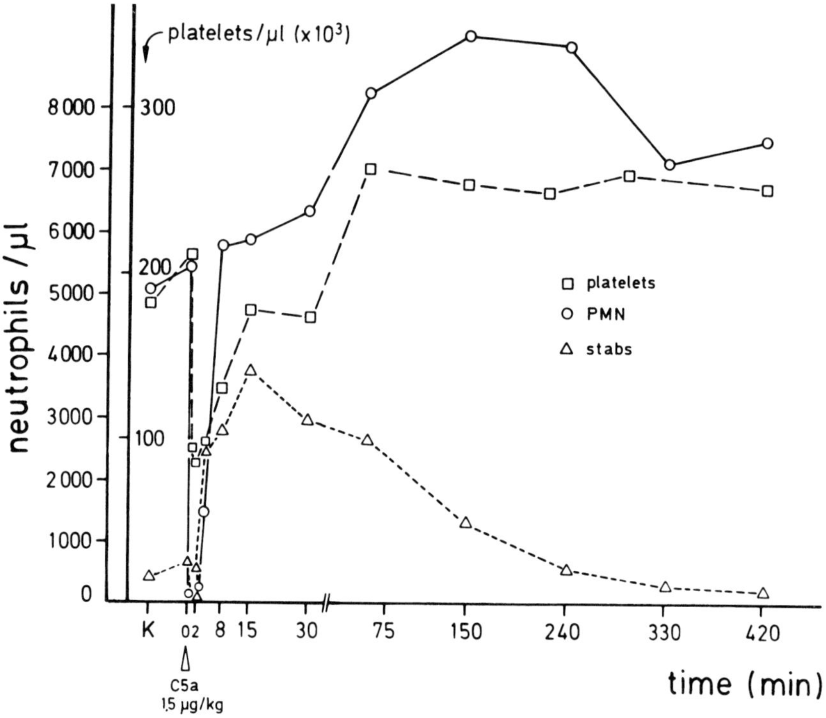

Figure 11.3 Reaction of circulation PMNS, stabs and platelets after injection of C5a. Dose of AT peptide: 1.5 μg kg^{-1}. At time −10 and 0 min, blood samples, serving as controls, were removed. All values are corrected for dilution. Data of representative animals are given (Taken from Hoffmann, T., Bottger, E. C., Baum, H. P., Dennebaumm, R., Hadding, U. and Bitter-Suermann, D. (1986). Evaluation of low dose anaphylatoxic peptides in the pathogenesis of the adult respiratory distress syndrome (ARDS). Monitoring of early C5a effects in a guinea-pig *in vivo* model after i.v. application. *Eur. J. Clin. Invest.* **16**, 500–8, with permission)

fluoresceinated C5a indicate that C5a does not bind specifically to human vein endothelial cells[59] showing that the anaphylatoxin C5a is not directly responsible for the upregulation of ELAM-1 or ICAM-1 on endothelial cells; this process involves other cell types, such as monocytes, which release IL-1 in response to C5a and C3a[60,12].

Although this animal model is a good example for the adhesion-promoting properties of the anaphylatoxins, it demonstrates that elevated plasma levels of anaphylatoxins alone are not sufficient to induce increased microvascular permeability in the lung. Only the administration of anaphylatoxins by unphysiological routes, like intratracheal instillation[62], the use of extremely high doses (double the maximal amount of C3a which could be generated in the animal) intravenously, combined with the administration of an inhibitor of serum carboxypeptidase-N to prevent degradation of C3a[63], produced histological evidence of lung injury. Although these models do not mimic clinical situations, they do show that, in circumscribed areas, high anaphylatoxin concentrations may produce tissue damage.

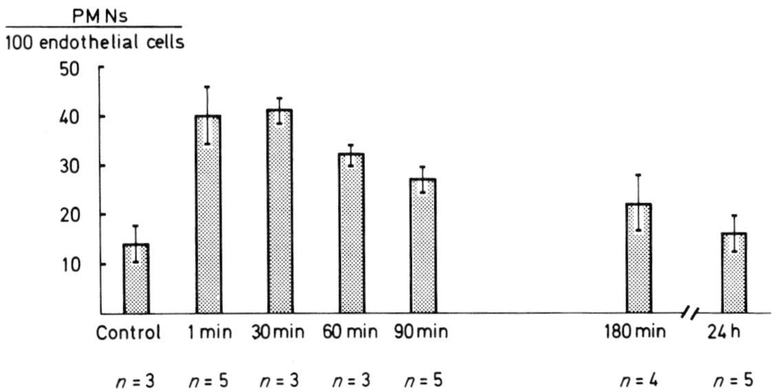

Figure 11.4 Number of PMNs per 100 endothelial cells in the lung at different times after C5a injection. Abscissa: time after C5a injection when the animal was sacrificed. (for details see Hoffmann, T., Bottger, E. C., Baum, H. P., Dennebaum, R., Hadding, U. and Bitter-Suermann, D. (1986). Evaluation of low dose anaphylatoxic peptides in the pathogenesis of the adult respiratory distress syndrome (ARDS). Monitoring of early C5a effects in a guinea-pig *in vivo* model after i.v. application. *Eur. J. Clin. Invest.*, **16**, 500–8, with permission)

Vascular leakage mediated by neutrophils

Because of the high frequency of ARDS following Gram-negative sepsis and of septic shock with lipopolysaccharide (LPS) as the causative agent, most animal models of ARDS depend on the administration of LPS.

As a result of these studies on animal models and humans with ARDS, it is evident that humoral mediators other than anaphylatoxins play a role in the development of ARDS (Figure 11.2). LPS stimulates monocytes to release cytokines, for example IL-1, IL-6 and TNFα, and to trigger neutrophils and endothelial cells to undergo an oxidative burst. However, as LPS can activate both the classical and alternative pathways of complement, the role of anaphylatoxins in LPS-induced ARDS has been investigated in different animal models. Primates[64–66] infused with *E. coli* showed an increase in C3a, C4a and C5a plasma levels associated with sequestration of neutrophils in the lung and an increase of extravascular fluid in the lungs. Thus, in addition to a neutrophil margination, increased vascular permeability occurred. LPS-primed adherent neutrophils are probably responsible for the plasma leakage, as neutrophil depletion by nitrogen mustard[67] or the use of oxygen radical scavengers reduced the lung injury.

Furthermore, it has been shown that adherent neutrophils produce more reactive oxygen species than non-adherent neutrophils[68]. The reactive oxygen-derived species include superoxide anion (O_2^-), hydrogen peroxide (H_2O_2) and hydroxyl radical (OH), which can be released from adherent granulocytes upon stimulation with C5a[68,69]. These reactive oxygen species are considered to be the major neutrophil products responsible for acute microvascular damage in the lung[70], which leads to enhanced permeability and pulmonary oedema.

Recently, however, the role of the neutrophil as the main effector cell in vascular leakage has been questioned as ARDS may also occur in patients with neutropenia[71–74]. It is therefore likely that other cells, such as alveolar macrophages or alveolar endothelial cells, may contribute to vascular leakage, an area requiring further investigation. Experimental and clinical studies have shown that activated neutrophils release proteases, such as elastase and collagenase[75–77]; their roles in the pathogenesis of ARDS are unclear.

Sequestration of neutrophils from blood vessels in the alveolar space

Anaphylatoxins are not involved in the events leading to neutrophil adherence and activation but are also thought to be responsible for the transalveolar traffic of granulocytes into the alveolar space. In principle, neutrophils have the ability to penetrate the endothelial/epithelial barrier by diapedesis, but migration is greatly enhanced by chemotaxis. Both C5a and C5a des Arg are chemotactic factors and have been detected in the bronchoalveolar lavage fluids of ARDS patients.[78] This C5a could be generated locally within the extravascular space or may have diffused from the plasma (as C5a des Arg), although most C5a generated intravenously binds rapidly to circulating neutrophils. Intact C5 could be present in the extravascular space as a result of diffusion from the microcirculation, secondary to increased vascular permeability, or may be synthesized locally. In this regard, it has been shown that human alveolar type II cells in culture *in vitro* synthesize C5, as well as C2, C4, C3 and factor B[79]. As the incubation of radio-labelled C5 with bronchoalveolar lavage fluid from ARDS patients results in the generation of C5a, enzymes capable of activating C5 must be present. Whether these enzymes are the C5 convertases of the complement system or the neutrophil proteases, or both, is unknown. However, the generation of C5a locally in the extravascular space will permit the establishment of a chemotactic gradient so that neutrophil migration from blood vessels into the alveolar space occurs. C5a will also stimulate secretion of neutrophil proteases so that more C5a is generated and a vicious circle has developed. In addition to C5a, transendothelial traffic of neutrophils is also stimulated by the actions of IL-1 or TNFα on endothelial cells, without any chemotactic gradient[80]. Thus, there are at least two mechanisms which contribute to the extravascular emigration of neutrophils in ARDS. Interestingly, it has been shown that C5a leads to shedding of soluble 20 kDa TNFα receptors by neutrophils[81,82]. As these receptors retain their ligand-binding capacity, it is possible that this process may limit neutrophil emigration as TNFα in the circulation and extravascular fluid would be bound by these receptors. Studies of the effects of C5a on TNF receptor expression by endothelial cells are required.

Therapeutic implications

According to the presented pathogenetic concept for the early events in ARDS, different therapeutic approaches are conceivable. There are at least two different neutrophil products which are able to induce the vascular leakage in ARDS: the proteinases and the reactive oxygen species. Although elastase is present at sites of inflammation[83] and increases vascular permeability *in vitro*, because of the presence of α_1 antiprotease *in vivo*[75], it is unlikely to increase vascular permeability in ARDS. Thus, therapeutic blockade of the neutrophil oxidative burst appears to be an attractive option. Free radical scavengers, such as dimethylurea, dimethylsulphoxide and N-acetylcysteine, have been used in animal models to try to prevent the toxic effects of reactive oxygen species and resulted in the extent of pulmonary oedema being reduced. Despite this apparent success, the use of free radical scavengers in patients must be tempered with the knowledge that the ability of phagocytes to kill bacteria depends principally on reactive oxygen species. This is best demonstrated in chronic granulomatous disease patients who suffer from recurrent bacterial infections as their neutrophils cannot undergo a normal respiratory burst.

Perhaps a better therapeutic approach would be to arrest the generation of ARDS at an earlier stage, perhaps inhibiting the generation or activity of anaphylatoxins or the cytokines IL-1 and TNFα. In a mouse model, prevention of death has been observed with an anti-TNFα antibody after LPS challenge[84]. Recently, a human IL-1 receptor antagonist was tested in a rabbit model of ARDS, and shown to prevent the massive transudation and cellular infiltration of alveolar spaces and to reduce mortality[85,86]. These *in vivo* experiments indicate that blocking of IL-1 and TNFα could effectively interrupt the inflammatory cascade after LPS challenge.

The earliest event in ARDS appears to be the adhesion of neutrophils to the pulmonary vascular endothelium. As the anaphylatoxins represent key mediators in this initial phase of ARDS, their blockade should result in a decreased neutrophil adhesion, activation and, in consequence, a reduced vascular permeability of the lung. The blockade of the most powerful anaphylatoxin, C5a, was achieved by administration of an anti-C5a antibody in a primate model prior to the infusion of *E. coli*. This reduced the increase in pulmonary vascular permeability, the decrease in blood oxygenation and mortality[65]. Similar results could be obtained[87] from a rat model after LPS challenge using $F(ab')_2$ fragments of rabbit anti-rat C5a. These data. suggest that blocking the C5a peptide at an early stage of the disease could be a practical approach of great benefit.

In summary, some early intervention strategies show great promise in the prevention of ARDS. Antagonists of mediators such as anaphylatoxins and cytokines could be given prophylactically to high-risk patients to prevent ARDS and to decrease mortality.

Anaphylatoxin levels in patients at risk from ARDS

As anaphylatoxins are involved in the pathogenesis of ARDS, measurement of C3a and C5a levels in plasma and bronchoalveolar fluid could be important in the management of these patients. However, although the results of studies performed over the past decade have been somewhat inconsistent, they show that anaphylatoxin levels are elevated during episodes of sepsis and that persistent elevation tends to be associated with the development of complications[85–95].

In a more recent study, C3a and C4a levels were shown to be elevated and a clear correlation between mortality and anaphylatoxin levels was documented[96].

However, there was no relationship between anaphylatoxin levels and the development of ARDS or deterioration in lung function. C3a/C4a plasma levels were elevated both in patients with ARDS and those without ARDS and the mean levels in each group did not differ significantly. Thus, these findings are surprising as the high mortality of septic shock correlates with anaphylatoxin plasma levels. In contrast, the results of a recent study of 48 patients with trauma and sepsis, in which plasma levels of phospholipase A_2, the macrophage stimulation marker neopterin, elastase and C3a des Arg were measured, showed that only elastase and C3a des Arg levels could be used to distinguish between patients with uncomplicated sepsis and those with ARDS[97]. In addition to these differences, patients who developed ARDS had circulating C5a-deactivated neutrophils, with impaired migratory responses and reduced degranulation following C5a exposure[98].

Apart from the differentiation of those sepsis patients with ARDS from those without ARDS, plasma anaphylatoxin levels have been used to detect pulmonary deterioration. High-risk patients, with worsening arterial blood gases, had significantly higher C3a and C5a levels than those with stable blood gases. The authors concluded that monitoring arterial blood gases and anaphylatoxin levels in ARDS-risk patients permitted earlier and more precise diagnosis of ARDS[99].

The results of a recent multicentre study have verified the importance of measurement of plasma anaphylatoxin levels for the early identification of ARDS in high-risk polytrauma patients at an early stage (within 6–12 h) of the

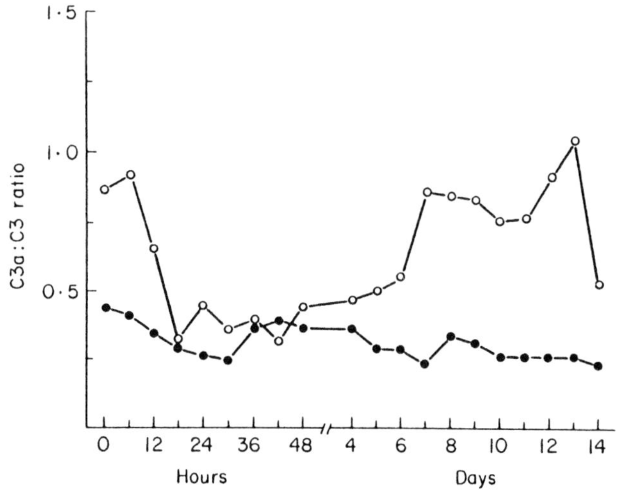

Figure 11.5 C3a:C3 ratio in 14 polytrauma patients with adult respiratory distress syndrome (ARDS) (open circles) and 17 patients without ARDS (closed circles). Differences in the first 12 h and from day 4 to 14 between the two groups are significant. (Taken from Zilow, G., Sturm, J. A., Rother, U. and Kirschfink, M. (1990). Complement activation and the prognostic value of C3a in patients at risk of adult respiratory distress syndrome. *Clin. Exp. Immunol.* **79**, 151–7, with permission).

disease. C3a and the C3a:C3 ratio proved to be important parameters in distinguishing between those patients who will develop ARDS and those who will not[100] (Figure 11.5). The ARDS group had significantly higher C3a levels 6 h after admission to the intensive care unit with a second rise on days 4–14. In contrast, the non-ARDS group showed only minor increases. The same was true for the C3a:C3 ratio. These data suggest that monitoring plasma anaphylatoxin levels with a minimum of two blood samples a day may serve as an early indicator for the development of ARDS in critically ill patients. Changes in anaphylatoxin levels can be confirmed by measurement of the C5b-9 terminal complement complex[101], plasma elastase[97] or IL-6[102].

Measurement of plasma anaphylatoxin concentrations by RIA or ELISA is time consuming with considerable delay between blood sampling and obtaining the final result. If anaphylatoxin assays are to be used in patient management, rapid on-line procedures must be developed.

ANAPHYLATOXIN GENERATION DURING HAEMODIALYSIS AND CARDIOPULMONARY BYPASS

Complement activation through the alternative pathway is an event which is independent of antigen–antibody complexes. A wide range of agents from LPS of Gram-negative bacteria, virus-infected cells and the cell wall of yeasts are able to activate this pathway. Besides these natural activators, iatrogenic activation occurs, most commonly during haemodialysis and during cardiopulmonary bypass using bubble oxygenation. Patients undergoing either of these procedures may develop complications associated with a systemic inflammatory reaction, either immediately at the onset of extracorporeal circulation or during the postoperative period. The symptoms range from urticaria and angio-oedema to life-threatening profound organ dysfunction, often manifest in the lung with neutrophil sequestration and increased microvascular permeability[103].

The striking similarities between the early events in ARDS and these observed clinical findings suggests a pathogenetic role for anaphylatoxins released during complement activation on the surface of the biomembranes. As a consequence, C3a, C4a and C5a plasma levels have been measured: C3a, but not C4a, was found to be elevated during both haemodialysis and cardioplumonary bypass[104]. These findings indicate that the alternative pathway is predominantly responsible for complement activation in these patients. When radio-immunoassays were used to quantitate plasma anaphylatoxin levels, C5a appeared to be normal whereas elevated C5a levels were demonstrated when the ELISA technique was used[16,105] (Figure 11.6).

In the recent literature, concentrations of the terminal complement complex have been used as a measure of bioincompatibility. With respect to the investigated biomembranes (Cuprophane, Hemophane and Polysulphone), the results seem to be analogous to those found using anaphylatoxin assays[106,107].

Since haemodialysis was first practised with Cellophane membranes, great progress has been made with regard to a better biocompatibility of the material. Today, at least three groups of dialyser membranes can be distinguished[108]: the first with high complement-activation potential, e.g. the classical regenerated

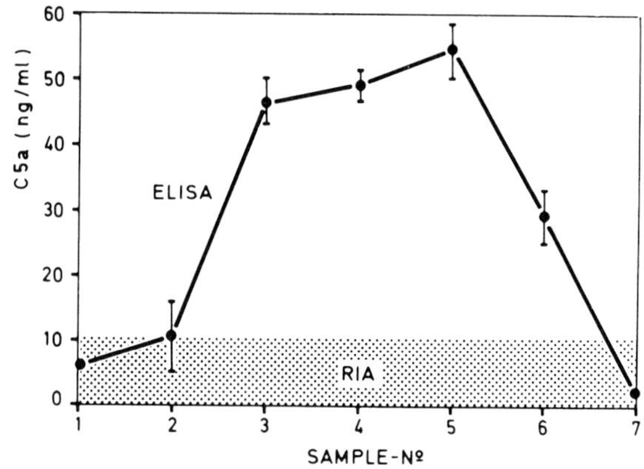

Figure 11.6 Time course of C5a plasma levels in patients with cardiopulmonary bypass. C5a plasma levels of two patients detected by ELISA (filled circles) and RIA. Threshold of detection of the C5a RIA for EDTA plasma samples is shown by the shaded area. 1: preoperative sample; 2: 5 min after partial bypass; 3: 5 min after complete bypass; 4: 30 min after complete bypass; 5: at the end of complete bypass; 6: 2 h postoperative; 7: first postoperative day. (Taken from Klos, A., Ihrig, V., Messner, M., Grabbe, J. and Bitter-Suermann, D. (1988). Detection of native human complement components C3 and C5 and their primary activation peptides C3a and C5a (anaphylatoxic peptides) by ELISA with monoclonal antibodies. *J. Immunol. Meth.*, **111**, 241–52, with permission).

cellulose (Cuprophane); the second with moderate activation potential, e.g. modified cellulose (cellulose acetate); and the third with a low activation potential, e.g. polycarbonate, polysulphone, polyacrylonitrile and modified cellulose (Hemophane)[109,110]. The polyacrylonitrile membranes which were characterized originally as weak activators of the complement system have recently been shown to produce marked complement activation but the majority of generated C3a binds to the membrane and evades fluid-phase detection[111,112]. Nevertheless, it is conceivable that specific interaction with neutrophils with membrane-bound anaphylatoxins may occur and lead to inflammation. In order to reduce complement activation, dialyser membranes have been reused as it has been shown that these membranes activate complement less effectively than new ones[113].

In addition to complement activation by the alternative pathway, there are reports of classical pathway complement activation occurring during extracorporeal circulation. Such activation does not depend on activation biomembranes but is due to C1 activation by protamine–heparin complexes.[114] Heparin is used routinely to prevent coagulation in the extracorporeal circulation (EC). On completion of the operation, protamine is used to reverse the anticoagulation action of heparin rapidly. The heparin–protamine complexes, which bind to red blood cells, activate the classical pathway of complement[115].

Protamine also inhibits plasma carboxypeptidase-N[116], which inactivates anaphylatoxins and kinins. Thus, by inhibiting the carboxypeptidase while simultaneously triggering complement activation and anaphylatoxin release, anaphylatoxins will not only be generated but remain active following protamine administration. As a result, some authors advise against the use of protamine to reverse heparin anticoagulation, particularly in patients with ischaemic heart disease[117].

Another problem is the increased risk of infection in patients with chronic renal failure undergoing either chronic haemodialysis or continuous ambulatory peritoneal dialysis (CAPD). This may be in part due to the recurrent C5a generation which has been shown to downregulate specific C5a receptors on phagocytes[118,119]. Neutrophils and monoctyes which have been deactivated by C5a have their bactericidal activity reduced markedly as both chemotactic responsiveness and the oxidative burst are reduced.

In summary, the anaphylatoxins play an important role in the clinical complications of extracorporeal circulation. At present, all known biomembranes activate complement, although Hemophane or Polysulphone membranes produce low levels of activation. Investigations to improve those membranes should be continued to minimize the occurrence of acute problems during extracorporeal circulation and to prevent impairment of antimicrobial defence mechanisms.

ANAPHYLATOXINS IN ATHEROMA AND MYOCARDIAL INFARCTION

Myocardial infarction is normally the result of severe coronary artery atheroma. The disease originates in early childhood when diffuse thickening of the musculo-elastic intima is seen. During adolescence and adulthood, the lesions progress through the formation of fatty intimal streaks, which contain smooth muscle cells surrounded by deposits of lipids (mainly cholesterol oleate), fibrous plaques, which contain lipid-laden (mainly cholesterol linoleate) macrophages and smooth muscle cells. This leads to a complicated lesion, in which the fibrous plaque has undergone calcification, cell necrosis, mural-thrombosis and possibly haemorrhage. Endothelial injury is thought to be the initiating event followed by the migration of smooth muscle cells and monocytes into the lesion. Complement activation occurs in atheromatous lesions and cholesterol-rich liposomes have been shown to activate complement activation in atheromatous lesions resulting in the formation of anaphylatoxins.

Anaphylatoxins and other chemotactic agents will stimulate the migration of phagocytes into the atheromatous lesions and amplify the inflammatory response. Thus, anaphylatoxins may play a significant role in the pathogenesis of atheroma. Anaphylatoxins also play a role in the pathogenesis of tissue injury occurring in response to myocardial ischaemia. *In vivo* studies have shown that cardiac muscle constituents are released from ischaemic and infarcted tissue. One of these, a mitochondrial constituent, will bind C1 and activate the classical pathway. The importance of C5a in the subsequent inflammatory process has been emphasized by the demonstration that, following the intracoronary perfusion of C5a, neutrophils accumulate rapidly in the coronary blood vessels, coronary blood flow decreases and myocardial contractility is reduced. The effects of C5a on myocardial ischaemia and myocardial contractility are likely to depend on members of the lipoxygenase (leukotriene D/E_4) and the cyclooxygenase (thromboxane A_2) pathways[120]. The use of antagonists to the arachidonic acid metabolites following C5a challenge has shown that both cyclooxygenase and lipoxygenase metabolites contribute to the negative inotropic effects and myocardial ischaemia, while they do not affect neutrophil accumulation. Thus, the pathophysiological findings after intracoronary C5a infusion depended mainly on release of arachidonic acid metabolites[121,122]. Neutrophil migration is probably the result of direct chemotactic response to C5a. These findings were confirmed for human C3a in a guinea-pig model[123].

In addition to the experimental evidence suggesting a role for anaphylatoxins in myocardial infarction, a recent study has shown that plasma levels of C3a are elevated for up to 10 days after acute myocardial infarction[124]. However, further evidence is required to confirm a pathogenetic role of anaphylatoxins in this disease.

OTHER DISORDERS

Psoriasis

Although the classification of this dermatosis as an immunological disease is still open to discussion, the inflammatory nature of psoriasis is well documented. There are two pathological features which characterize the clinical picture: the increased cell proliferation and the infiltration of the epidermis by neutrophils. These inflammatory responses are probably mediated through anaphylatoxins since large amounts of C3a, C4a and C5a were found in scale extracts of psoriatic patients[125,126]. Nevertheless, C5a is not the only chemotactic factor present in scale extracts[127] as LTB_4[128] as well as neutrophil-activating peptide[129] have been isolated. The latter mediator has properties which are similar to the cytokine IL-1. The finding of elevated C4a levels indicates the occurrence of classical pathway activation. Recent evidence suggests that this activation is due to complexes of psoriasis-associated antigen, pso p27, with IgG[130].

In addition to complement activation occurring locally in dermal lesions, systemic complement activation may occur, since plasma levels of C3a and C4a are increased in psoriatic patients compared with non-psoriatic controls[131,132]. Thus, the continuous local and systemic generation of anaphylatoxins could, at least in part, be responsible for the ongoing transepidermal migration of neutrophils in psoriatic disease.

Rheumatoid arthritis

The initial event of this autoimmune systemic disorder of connective tissue is still unknown but there is no doubt that significant complement activation occurs via both the classical and alternative pathways. Within the joints' immune complexes (IgG–IgG and IgG–IgM), complement activation products and a predominant neutrophil infiltration are found[133]. Neutrophils are thought to play an important role in the inflammatory process in the joint because of their great destructive potential. The levels of anaphylatoxins in synovial fluid are sevenfold higher in patients with rheumatoid arthritis than in patients with degenerative joint disease[134,135]. This suggests that anaphylatoxins have a role in the persistent neutrophil influx and activation[136]. However, because neutrophils will be deactivated after stimulation with anaphylatoxins[137], the role of other phlogistic mediators has to be considered, e.g. IL-1[138]. This cytokine has been found in high concentrations in knee-joint effusions of patients with rheumatoid arthritis.

Plasma anaphylatoxin levels, like C-reactive protein levels and erythrocyte sedimentation rate, correlate with disease activity and are therefore useful in patient management[134]. The best correlations were seen when two of these three parameters were compared with disease activity. Therefore, it is probably more useful to measure plasma anaphylatoxin levels in association with one other parameter in order to monitor disease activity in rheumatoid arthritis.

Systemic lupus erythematosus (SLE)

There is extensive evidence which shows that activation of complement by both the classical and alternative pathways occurs in SLE and that complement activation increases as the illness relapses and decreases as it remits. A number of single case reports have shown that measurement of plasma levels of both C3a and C5a were useful indicators for a flare of SLE. Moreover, it could be demonstrated that plasma C3a levels were elevated 1–2 months prior to a clinical exacerbation of the disease and therefore could serve as a predictive marker[139,140]. Interestingly, the plasma levels of C3a in patients with central nervous system involvement were significantly higher than in those without central nervous system involvement. The cerebral blood vessels of patients who died of acute central nervous system disease were occluded with aggregated neutrophils which may have been mediated by anaphylatoxins.

CONCLUDING REMARKS

The anaphylatoxins play an important role in the mediation of acute inflammation and can be generated by activation of any of the plasma enzyme systems. The variety of activation pathways, either by direct cleavage through proteases (e.g. factor XIIa, neutrophil elastase) or as a consequence of alternative or classical activation of the complement system, ensures that anaphylatoxins participate in any inflammatory process. In most instances, this is beneficial to the organism and provides a mechanism for interaction between the humoral and cellular components of inflammation. However, in chronic inflammation due to autoimmune phenomena (SLE or RA) or in conditions of excessive complement activation (e.g. due to plasma coming into contact with a foreign surface or in patients with polytrauma or septic shock), anaphylatoxins produce disease.

The diverse biological properties of anaphylatoxins are due to specific cellular receptor/ligand interactions. Until now, the list of receptor-bearing cells is somewhat longer for C5a than for C3a but awaits further expansion for both peptides. The interaction of the anaphylatoxins with their corresponding receptors is well characterized for C3a through C-terminal oligopeptides but is only poorly understood for C5a, where a minimum of three different binding sites may be involved. As the C5a receptor has been cloned recently, it is to be expected that genetic and immunological approaches will clarify the extra- and intracellular mechanisms leading to the release of the diverse cell-derived mediators which are ultimately responsible for the effects of anaphylatoxins *in vivo*. This information may permit the development of pharmacological agents which could block the release of mediators by interfering with ligand–receptor interactions or by blocking signal transduction.

References

1. Bitter-Suermann, D. (1987). The anaphylatoxins. In Rother, K. and Till, G. (eds.) *The Complement System*, pp. 367–95. (Heidelberg: Springer Verlag)
2. Johnson A. R., Hugli, T. E. and Müller-Eberhard, H. J. (1975). Release of histamine from mast cells by the complement peptides C3a and C5a. *Immunology*, **28**, 1067–87
3. Grossklaus, C., Damerau, B., Lemgo, E. and Vogt, W. (1976). Induction of platelet aggregation by the complement-derived peptides C3a and C5a. *Naunyn-Schmiedeberg's Arch. Pharmacol.*, **295**, 71–6
4. Meuer, S., Ecker, U., Hadding, U. and Bitter-Suermann, D.(1981). Platelet serotonin-release by C3a and C5a. Two independent pathways of activation. *J. Immunol.*, **126**, 1506–9
5. Zanker, B., Rasokat, H., Hadding, U. and Bitter-Suermann, D. (1982). C3a induced activation and stimulus specific desensitization of guinea pig platelets. *Agents Actions (Suppl.)*, **11**, 147–57
6. Hartung, H. P., Bitter-Suermann, D. and Hadding, U. (1983). Induction of thromboxane release from macrophages by anaphylatoxic peptide C3a of complement and synthetic hexapeptide C3a. *J. Immunol.*, **130**, 72–7
7. Dias da Silva, W. and Lepow, I. (1967). Complement as a mediator of inflammation. II. Biological properties of anaphylatoxin prepared with purified components of human complement. *J. Exp. Med.*, **125**, 921–46
8. Björk, J., Hugli, T. E. and Smedegard, G. (1985). Microvascular effects of anaphylatoxins C3a and C5a. *J. Immunol.*, **134**, 1115–19
9. Fernandez, H. N., Henson, P. M., Otani, A. and Hugli, T. E. (1978). Chemotactic response to human C3a and C5a anaphylatoxins. I. Evaluation of C3a and C5a leukotaxis in vitro under simulated in vivo conditions. *J. Immunol.*, **120**, 102–8
10. Goldstein, I. M. and Weissmann, G. (1974). Generation of C5-derived lysosomal enzyme-releasing activity (C5a) by lysates of leucocyte lysosomes. *J. Immunol.*, **113**, 1583–8
11. Goldstein, I. M., Ross, D., Kaplan, H. B. and Weissmann, G. (1975). Complement and immunoglobulins stimulate superoxide production by human leucocytes independently of phagocytosis. *J. Clin. Invest.*, **56**, 1155–63
12. Haeffner-Cavaillon, N., Cavaillon, J. M., Laude, M. and Kazatchkine, M. D. (1987). C3a (desarg) induces production and release of interleukin 1 by cultured human monocytes. *J. Immunol.* **139**, 794–9
13. Goodmann, M. G., Chenoweth, D. E. and Weigle, W. O. (1982). Induction of interleukin 1 secretion and enhancement of humoral immunity by binding of human C5a to macrophage surface C5a receptors. *J. Exp. Med.*, **1156**, 912–17
14. Bischoff, S. C., De Weck, A. L. and Dahinden, C. A. (1990). Interleukin 3 granulocyte/macrophage-colony-stimulating factor render human basophils responsive to low concentrations of complement component C3a. *Proc. Natl. Acad. Sci. USA*, **87**, 6813–17
15. Kurimoto, Y., De Weck, A. L. and Dahinden A. (1989). Interleukin 3 dependent mediator release in basophils triggered by C5a. *J. Exp. Med.*, **170**, 467–79
16. Klos, A., Ihrig, V., Messner, M., Grabbe, J. and Bitter-Suermann, D. (1988). Detection of native human complement components C3 and C5 and their primary activation peptides C3a and C5a(anaphylatoxic peptides) by ELISA's with monoclonal antibodies. *J. Immunol. Meth.*, **241**, 241–52
17. Burger, R., Zilow, G., Bader, A., Friedlein, A. and Naser, W. (1988). The C terminus of the anaphylatoxin C3a generated upon complement activation represents a neoantigenic determinant with diagnostic potential. *J. Immunol.*, **141**, 553–8

18. Hugli, T. E. and Chenoweth, D. E. (1980). Biologically active peptides of complement: Techniques and significance of C3a and C5a measurements. In *Immunoassays: Clinical Laboratory Technique for the 1980s*, pp. 443–60. (New York: A.R. Liss Inc.)
19. Nilsson, B., Svensson, K. E., Inganas, M., and Nilsson, U. R. (1988). A simplified assay for the detection of C3a in human plasma employing a monoclonal antibody raised against denatured C3. *J. Immunol. Meth.*, **107**, 281–7
20. Takeda, J., Kinoshita, T., Takata, Y., Kozono, H., Tanaka, E., Hong, K., and Inoue, K., (1987). Rapid and simple measurement of human C5a-des-Arg level in plasma or serum using monoclonal antibodies. *J. Immunol. Meth.*, **101**, 265–70
21. Oppermann, M., Schulze, M. and Gotze, O. (1991). A sensitive enzyme immunoassay for the quantitation of human C5a/C5a (desArg) anaphylatoxin using a monoclonal antibody with specificity for a neoepitope. *Complement Inflamm.*, **8**, 13–24
22. Meuer, S., Zanker, B., Hadding, U. and Bitter-Suermann, D. (1982). Low zone desensitization: a stimulus-specific control mechanism of cell-response. Investigations on anaphylatoxin-induced platelet-secretion. *J. Exp. Med.*, **155**, 698–710
23. Craddock, P. R., Fehr, J., Dalmasso, A. P., Brigham, K. L. and Jacob, H. S. (1977). Hemodialysis leucopenia: pulmonary vascular leucostasis resulting from complement activation by dialyzer cellophane membranes. *J. Clin. Invest.*, **59**, 879–88
24. Gerardy-Schahn, R., Ambrosius, D., Casaretto, M., Grötzinger, J., Saunders, D., Wollmer, A., Brandenburg, D. and Bitter-Suermann, D. (1988). Design and biological activity of a new generation of synthetic C3a analogues by combination of peptidic and non-peptidic elements. *Biochem. J.*, **255**, 209–16
25. Ember, J. A., Johansen, N. L. and Hugli, T. E. (1991). Designing synthetic superagonists of C3a anaphylatoxin. *Biochemistry*, **30**, 3603–12
26. Mandecki, W., Mollison, K. W., Bolling, T. J., Powell, B. S., Carter, G. W. and Fox, J. L. (1985). Chemical synthesis of a gene encoding the human complement fragment C5a and its expression in Escherichia coli. *Proc. Natl. Acad. Sci. USA*, **82**, 3542–7
27. Mollison, K. W., Mandecki, L.W.L., Zuiderweg, E. R. P., Fayer, L., Fey, T. A., Krause, R. A., Conway, R. G., Miller, L., Edalji, R. P., Shallcross, M. A., Lane, B., Fox, J. L., Greer, J. and Carter, G. W. (1989). Identification of receptor-binding residues in the inflammatory complement protein C5a by site-directed mutagenesis. *Proc. Natl. Acad. Sci. USA*, **86**, 292–6
28. Köhl, J., Casaretto, M., Gier, M., Karwath, G., Gietz, C., Bautsch, W., Saunders, D. and Bitter-Suermann, D. (1990). Reevaluation of the C3a active site using short synthetic C3a analogues. *Eur. J. Immunol.*, **20**, 1463–8
29. Hugli, T. E. (1986). Biochemistry and biology of anaphylatoxins. *Complement*, **3**, 111–27
30. Köhl, J., Kola, A., Bautsch, W. and Bitter-Suermann, D. (1991). Comparative analysis of synthetic anaphylatoxic peptides in ATP-release and ileum contraction assay. *Complement Inflamm.*, **8**, 175
31. Fukuoka, Y. and Hugli, T. E. (1988). Demonstration of a specific C3a receptor on guinea pig platelets. *J. Immunol.*, **140**, 3496–501
32. Gerardy-Schahn, R., Ambrosius, D., Saunders, D., Casaretto, M., Mittler, C., Karwath, G., Görgen, S. and Bitter-Suermann, D. (1989). Characterization of C3a receptor-proteins on guinea pig platelets and human polymorphonuclear leukocytes. *Eur. J. Immunol.*, **19**, 1095–102
33. Grötzinger, J., Engels, M., Jacoby, E. and Wollmer, A. (1991). A model for the C5a receptor and for its interaction with the ligand. *Protein Eng.*, **4**, 767–71
34. Bautsch, W., Stühmer, T., Emde, M., Kretzschmar, T., Köhl, J. and Bitter-Suermann, D. (1991). A recombinant hybrid anaphylatoxin with dual C3a/C5a activity. *Complement Inflamm.*, **8**, 127–8
35. Jacob, H. S., Craddock, P. R., Hammerschmidt, D. E. and Moldow, C. R. (1980). Complement-induced granulocyte aggregation. *N. Engl. J. Med.*, **302**, 789–94
36. Rollins, T. E. and Springer, M. S. (1985). Identification of the polymorphonuclear leukocyte C5a receptor. *J. Biol. Chem.*, **260**, 7157–60
37. Kretzschmar, T., Kahl, K., Rech, K., Bautsch, W., Köhl, J. and Bitter-Suermann, D. (1991). Characterization of the C5a receptor on guinea pig platelets. *Immunobiology*, **183**, 418–32
38. Gerard, N. P. and Gerard, C. (1991). The chemotactic receptor for human C5a and anaphylatoxin. *Nature*, **349**, 614–17
39. Boulay, F., Mery, L., Tardif, M., Brouchon, L. and Vignais, P. (1991). Expression cloning of a receptor for C5a anaphylatoxin on differential HL-60 cells. *Biochemistry*, **30**, 2993–9

40. Boulay, F., Tardiff, M., Brouchon, L. and Vignais, P. (1990). Synthesis and use of a novel N-formyl peptide derivative to isolate a human N-formyl peptide receptor cDNA. *Biochem. Biophys. Res. Commun.*, **168**, 1103–9
41. Dixon, R. A., Kobilka, B. K., Strader, D. J., Benovic, J. L., Dohlman, H. G., Frielle, T., Bolanowski, M. A., Bennett, C. D., Rands, E. and Diehl, R. E. (1986). Cloning of the gene and cDNA for mammalian beta-adrenergic receptor and homology with rhodopsin. *Nature*, **321**, 75–9
42. Gerard, N. P. and Gerard, C. (1990). Construction and expression of a novel recombinant anaphylatoxin, C5a–N19, as a probe for the human C5a receptor. *Biochemistry*, **29**, 9274–81
43. Morgan, E. L. (1986). Modulation of the immune response by anaphylatoxins. *Complement*, **3**, 128–36
44. Morgan, E. L., Thoman, M. L., Hobbs, M. V., Weigle, W. O. and Hugli, T. E. (1985). Human C3a-mediated suppression of the immune responses. II. Suppression of human in vitro polyclonal antibody responses occurs through the generation of nonspecific OKT8+ suppressor T cells. *Clin. Immunol. Immunopathol.*, **37**, 114–23
45. Morgan, E. L. (1987). The role of prostaglandins in C3a-mediated suppression of human in vitro polyclonal antibody responses. *Clin. Immunol. Immunopathol.*, **44**, 1–11
46. Morgan, E. L., Weigle, W. O., Erickson, B. W., Fok, K. F. and Hugli, T. E. (1983). Suppression of humoral immune responses by synthetic C3a peptides. *J. Immunol.*, **131**, 2258–61
47. Morgan, E. L., Weigle, W. O. and Hugli, T. E. (1984). Anaphylatoxin-mediated regulation of human and murine immune responses. *Fed. Proc.*, **43**, 2543–7
48. Morgan, E. L., Thoman, M. L., Weigle, W. O. and Hugli, T. E. (1983). Anaphylatoxin-mediated regulation of the immune response. II. C5a-mediated enhancement of human humoral and T cell-mediated immune responses. *J. Immunol.*, **130**, 1257–61
49. Scholz, W., McClurg, M. R., Cardenas, G. J., Smith, M., Noonan, D. J., Hugli, T. E. and Morgan, E. L. (1990). C5a-mediated release of interleukin 6 by human monocytes. *Clin. Immunol. Immunopathol.*, **57**, 297–307
50. Rinaldo, J. E. and Rogers, R. M. (1982). Adult respiratory distress syndrome – changing concepts of lung injury and repair. *N. Engl. J. Med.*, **306**, 900–9
51. Simon, R. H. and Ward, P. A. (1988). *Adult Respiratory Distress Syndrome Inflammation: Basic Principles and Clinical Correlates*, pp. 815–26. (New York: Raven Press, Ltd.)
52. Herndon, D. N. and Traber, D. L. (1990). Pulmonary failure and acute respiratory distress syndrome. Multiple organ failure. In: Deitch, E. A. (ed.), *Pathophysiology and Basic Concepts of Therapy*, pp. 192–214. (New York: Thieme)
53. Hoffman, T., Böttger, E. C., Baum, H. P., Dennebaum, R., Hadding, U. and Bitter-Suermann, D. (1986). Evaluation of low dose anaphylatoxin peptides in the pathogenesis of the adult respiratory distress syndrome (ARDS). Monitoring of early C5a effects in a guinea pig in vivo model after i.v. application. *Eur. J. Clin. Invest.*, **16**, 500–8
54. Hoffmann, T., Böttger, E. C., Baum, H. P., Messner, M., Hadding, U. and Bitter-Suermann, D. (1988). *In vivo* effects of C3a on neutrophils and its contribution to inflammatory lung processes in a guinea pig model. *Clin. Exp. Immunol.*, **71**, 486–92
55. Lo, S. K., van Seventer, G. A., Levin, S. M. and Wright, S. D. (1989). Two leukocyte receptors (CD11a/CD18 and CD11b/CD18) mediate transient adhesion to endothelium by binding to different ligands. *J. Immunol.*, **143**, 3325–9
56. Lo, S. K., Detmers, P. A., Levin, S. M. and Wright, S. D. (1989). Transient adhesion of neutrophils to endothelium. *J. Exp. Med.*, **169**, 1779–93
57. Tonnesen, M. G. (1989). Neutrophil–endothelial cell interaction mechanism of neutrophil adherence to vascular endothelium. *J. Invest. Dermatol.*, **93**, 53S–58S
58. Tonnesen, M. G., Anderson, D. C., Springer, T. A., Knedler, A., Avdi, N. and Henson, P. M. (1989). Adherence of neutrophils to cultured human microvascular endothelial cells. Stimulation by chemotactic peptides and lipid mediators and dependence upon the mac-1, lfa-1, p.150,95 glycoprotein family. *J. Clin. Invest.*, **83**, 637–46
59. Yancey, K. B., Lawley, T. J., Dersookian, M. and Harvath, L. (1989). Analysis of the interaction of human C5a and C5a desarg with human monocytes and neutrophils: flow cytometric and chemotaxis studies. *J. Invest. Dermatol.*, **92**, 184–9
60. Goodman, M. C., Chenoweth, D. E. and Weigle, W. O. (1982). Induction of interleukin-1 secretion and enhancement of humoral immunity by binding of human C5a to macrophage surface C5a receptors. *J. Exp. Med.*, **156**, 6652

61. Burger, R., Bader, A., Kirschtink, M., Rother, U., Schrod, L., Wörner, I., Zilow, G. (1987). Functional analysis and quantification of the complement C3 derived anaphylatoxin C3a with a monoclonal antibody. *Clin. Exp. Immunol.*, **68**, 703–11
62. Stimler, N. P., Hugli, T. E. and Bloor, C. M. (1980). Pulmonary injury induced by C3a and C5a anaphylatoxins. *Am. J. Pathol.*, **100**, 327–48
63. Huey, R., Bloor, C. M., Kawahara, M. S. and Hugli, T. E. (1983). Potentiation of the anaphylatoxins *in vivo* using an inhibitor of serum carboxypeptidase N (SCPN). I. Lethality and pathologic effects on pulmonary tissue. *Am. J. Pathol.*, **112**, 48–60
64. Hangen, D. H., Segall, G. M., Harney, E. W., Stevens, J. H., McDougall, I. R. and Raffin, T. A. (1990). Kinetics of leukocyte sequestration in the lungs of acutely septic primates. A study using 111IN-labelled autologuos leukocytes. *J. Surg. Res.*, **48**, 196–203
65. Hangen, D. H., Stevens, J. H., Satoh, P. S., Hall, E. W., O'Hanley, P. T. and Raffin, T. A. (1989). Complement levels in septic primates treated with anti-C5a antibodies. *J. Surg. Res.*, **46**, 195–9
66. Stevens, J. H., O'Hanley, P., Shapiro, J. M., Mihm, F. G., Satoh, P. S., Collins, J. A. and Raffin, T. A. (1986). Effects of anti-C5a antibodies in the adult respiratory distress syndrome in septic primates. *J. Clin. Invest.*, **77**, 1812–18
67. Worthen, G. S., Haslett, C., Rees, J., Irving, C. G., Gumbay, R. S., Henson, J. E. and Henson, P. M. (1987). Neutrophil-mediated pulmonary vascular injury: synergistic effect of trace amounts of lipopolysaccharide and neutrophil stimuli on vascular permeability and neutrophil sequestration in the lung. *Am. Rev. Respir. Dis.*, **136**, 19–28
68. Neumann, M. and Kownatzki, E. (1989). The effect of adherence on the generation of reactive oxygen species by human neutrophilic granulocytes. *Agents Actions*, **26**, 183–5
69. Craddock, P. R. (1984). Complement, granulocytes and shock lung. *Am. J. Emerg. Med.*, **2**, 78–81
70. Till, G. O. and Ward, P. A. (1985). Oxygen radicals in complement and neutrophil mediated acute lung injury. *J. Free Radical Biol. Med.*, **1**, 163–8
71. Braude, S., Krausz, T., Apperley, J., Goldman, J. M. and Royston, D. (1985). Adult respiratory distress syndrome after allogenic bone-marrow transplantation: evidence for a neutrophil independent mechanism. *Lancet*, **1**, 1239–42
72. Laufe, M. D., Simon, H., Flint, A. and Keller, J. B. (1986). Adult respiratory distress syndrome in neutropenic patients. *Am. J. Med.*, **80**, 1022–6
73. Maunder, R. J., Hackman, R. C., Riff, E., Albert, R. K. and Springmeyer, S. C. (1986). Occurrence of the adult respiratory distress syndrome in neutropenic patients. *Am. Rev. Respir. Dis.*, **133**, 313–16
74. Ognibene, F. P., Martin, S. E., Parker, M. M., Schlesinger, T., Roach, P., Burch, C. *et al.* (1986). Adult respiratory distress syndrome in patients with severe neutropenia. *N. Engl. J. Med.*, **315**, 547–51
75. Fowler, A. A., Walchak, S., Giclas, P. C., Henson, P. H. and Hyers, T. M. (1982). Characterization of antiproteinase activity in the adult respiratory distress syndrome. *Chest*, **81**, 50S–51S
76. Lee, C. T., Fein, A. M., Lippman, M., Holtzman, H., Kimbel, P. and Wienbaum, G. (1981). Elastolytic activity in pulmonary lavage fluid from patients with the adult respiratory distress syndrome. *N. Engl. J. Med.*, **304**, 192–6
77. McGuire, W. W., Spragg, R. G., Cohen, A. M. and Cochrane, C. G. (1982). Studies on the pathogenesis of the adult respiratory distress syndrome. *J. Clin. Invest.*, **69**, 543–53
78. Robbins, C. A., Russ, W. D., Rasmussen, J. K. and Clayton, M. M. (1987). Activation of the complement system in the adult respiratory distress syndrome. *Am. Rev. Respir. Dis.*, **135**, 651–8
79. Strunk, R. C., Eidlen, D. M. and Mason, R. J. (1988). Pulmonary alveolar type II epithelial cells synthesize and secrete proteins of the classical and alternative complement pathways. *J. Clin. Invest.*, **81**, 1419–26
80. Moser, R., Schleiffenbaum, B., Groscurth, P. and Fehr, J. (1989). Interleukin 1 and tumor necrosis factor stimulate human vascular endothelial cells to promote transendothelial neutrophil passage. *J. Clin. Invest.*, **83**, 444–55
81. Schleiffenbaum, B. and Fehr, J. (1990). The tumor necrosis factor receptor and human neutrophil function. *J. Clin. Invest.*, **86**, 184–95
82. Porteu, F. and Nathan, C. (1990). Shedding of tumor necrosis factor receptors by activated human neutrophils. *J. Exp. Med.*, **172**, 599–607

83. Grisham, M. B., Evers, J. and Janssen, H. F. (1988). Endotoxemia and neutrophil activation in vivo. *Am. J. Physiol.*, **254**, H1017–22
84. Beutler, B., Milsark, I. W. and Cerami, A. C. (1985). Passive immunization against cachectin/tumor necrosis factor protects mice from lethal effect of endotoxin. *Science*, **229**, 869–71
85. Ohlsson, K., Björk, P., Bergenfeldt, M., Hageman, R. and Thompson. R. C. (1990). Interleukin-1 receptor antagonist reduces mortality from endotoxin shock. *Nature*, **348**, 550–3
86. Wakabayashi, G., Gelfand, J. A., Durke, J. K., Thompson, R. C. and Dinarello, C. A. (1991). A specific receptor antagonist for interleukin-1 prevents Eschericha coli-induced shock in rabbits. *FASEB J.*, **5**, 338–43
87. Smedegard, G., Lianxian, C. and Hugli, T. E. (1989). Endotoxin-induced shock in the rat: A role for C5a. *Am. J. Pathol.*, **135**, 489–97
88. Bengtson, A. and Heideman, M. (1988). Anaphylatoxin formation in sepsis. *Arch. Surg.*, **123**, 645–9
89. Davis, J. M., Meyer, J. D., Barie, P. S., Yurt, R. W., Duhaney, R., Dineen, P. and Shires, G. T. (1990). Elevated production of neutrophil leukotriene B_4 precedes pulmonary failure in critically ill surgical patients. *Surg. Gynecol. Obstet.*, **170**, 495–500
90. Hallgren, R., Samuelsson, T. and Modig, J. (1987). Complement activation and increased alveolar-capillary permeability after major surgery and in adult respiratory distress syndrome. *Crit. Care Med.*, **15**, 189–93
91. Heidemann, M. and Hugli, T. E. (1984). Anaphylatoxin generation in multisystem organ failure. *J. Trauma*, **24**, 1038–43
92. Heidemann, M., Norder-Hanssen, B., Bengston, A. and Mollnes, T. E. (1988). Terminal complement complexes and anaphylatoxins in septic and ischemic patients. *Arch. Surg.*, **123**, 188–92
93. Lamy, M., Deby-Dupont, G., Pincemail, J., Braun, M., Dochateau, J., Deby, C., van Erck, J., Bodson, L., Damas, P. and Franchimont, P. (1985). Biochemical pathways of active lung injury. *Bull. Eur. Physiopathol. Respir.*, **21**, 221–9
94. Langlois, P. F., Gawryl, M. S., Zeller, J. and Lint, T. (1989). Accentuated complement activation in patient plasma during the adult respiratory distress syndrome: a potential mechanism for pulmonary inflammation. *Heart Lung*, **18**, 71–84
95. Tennenberg, S. D., Jacobs, M. P. and Solomkin, J. S. (1987). Complement-mediated neutrophil activation in sepsis- and trauma-related adult respiratory distress syndrome. Clarification with radioaerosol lung scans. *Arch. Surg.*, **122**, 26–32
96. Hack, C. E., Nuijens, J. H., Felt-Bersma, R. J. F., Schreuder, W. O., Eerenberg-Belmer, A. J. M., Paardekooper, J., Bronsveld, W. and Thijs, L. G. (1989). Elevated plasma levels of the anaphylatoxins C3a and C4a are associated with fatal outcome in sepsis. *Am. J. Med.*, **86**, 20–6
97. Kellermann, W., Frentzel-Beyme, R., Welte, M. and Jochum, M. (1989). Phospholipase a in acute lung injury after trauma and sepsis: its relation to the inflammatory mediators PMN-elastase, C3a and neopterin. *Klin. Wochenschr.*, **67**, 190–5
98. Solomkin, J. S., Cotta, L. A., Satoh, P. S., Hurst, J. M. and Nelson, R. D. (1985). Complement activation and clearance in acute illness and injury: evidence for c5a as a cell-directed mediator of the adult respiratory distress syndrome in man. *Surgery*, **97**, 668–78
99. Weigelt, J. A., Chenoweth, D. E., Borman, K. R. and Norcross, J. F. (1988). Complement and the severity of pulmonary failure. *J. Trauma*, **28**, 1013–19
100. Zilow, G., Sturm, J. A., Rother, U. and Kirschfink, M. (1990). Complement activation and the prognostic value of C3a in patients at risk of adult respiratory distress syndrome. *Clin. Exp. Immunol.*, **79**, 151–7
101. Langlois, P. F. and Gawryl, M. S. (1988). Accentuated formation of the terminal C5b–9 complement complex in patient plasma precedes development of the adult respiratory distress syndrome. *Am. Rev. Respir. Dis.*, **138**, 368–75
102. Hack, C. E., DeGroot, E. R., Felt-Bersma, R. J., Nuijens, J. H., Strack Van Schijndel, R. J., Eerenberg-Belmer, A. J., Thijs, L. G. and Aarden, L. A. (1989). Increased plasma levels of interleukin 6 in sepsis. *Blood*, **74**, 1704–10
103. Chenoweth, D. E. (1987). The properties of human C5a anaphylatoxin. The significance of C5a formation during hemodialysis. *Contrib. Nephrol.*, **59**, 51–71
104. Chenoweth, D. E. (1986). Anaphylatoxin formation in extracorporal circuits. *Complement*, **3**, 152–65

105. Bingel, M., Arndt, W., Schulze, M., Floege, J., Shaldon, S., Koch, K. M. and Goetze, O. (1989). Comparative studies of C5a plasma levels with different hemodialysis membranes using an enzyme-linked immunosorbent assay. *Nephron*, **51**, 320–4
106. Deppisch, R., Schmitt, V., Bommer, J., Hansch, G. M., Ritz, E. and Rauterberg, E. W. (1990). Fluid phase generation of terminal complement complex as a novel index of bioincompatibility. *Kidney Int.*, **37**, 669–706
107. Schaefer, R. M., Rauterberg, E. W., Deppisch, R. and Vienken, J. (1990). Assembly of SC5b–9 complement complex: A new index of blood–membrane interaction. *Miner. Electrolyte Metab.*, **16**, 73–6
108. Chenoweth, D. E. and Henderson, L. W. (1987). Complement activation during hemodialysis: Laboratory evaluation of hemodialyzers. *Artif. Organs*, **11**, 155–62
109. Falkenhagen, D., Bosch, T., Brown, G. S., Schmidt, B., Holtz, M., Baurmeister, U., Gurland, H. and Klinkmann, H. (1987). A clinical study on different cellulosic dialysis membranes. *Nephrol. Dial. Transplant.*, **2**, 537–45
110. Lucchi, L., Bonucchi, D., Acerbi, M. A., Cappelli, G., Spattini, A., Innocenti, M., Castellani, A. and Lusvarghi, E. (1989). Improved biocompatibility by modified cellulosic membranes: the case of hemophan. *Artif. Organs*, **13**, 417–21
111. Cheung, A. K. (1989). Adsorption of unactivated complement proteins by hemodialysis membranes. *Am. J. Kidney, Dis.*, **14**, 472–7
112. Cheung, A. K., Parker, J. F., Wilcox, L. A. and Janatova, J. (1990). Activation of complement by hemodialysis membranes: Polyacrylonitrile bind more C3a than Cuprophan. *Kidney Int.*, **37**, 1055–9
113. Horl, E. I., Wanner, C., Frischmuth, N., Gosele, A. and Masry, S. G. (1990). Plasma levels of main granulocyte components during hemodialysis. Comparison of new and reused dialyzers. *Am. J. Nephrol.*, **10**, 53–7
114. Cavarocci, N. C., Schaff, H. V., Orszulak, T. A., Homburger, H. A., Schnell, W. A. Jr and Pluth, J. R. (1985). Evidence for complement activation by protamine–heparin interaction after cardiopulmonary bypass. *Surgery*, **89**, 525–31
115. Shastri, K. A., Phillips, M. J., Raza, S., Logue, G. and Rustagi, P. K. (1988). Effects of RBCs on the activation of human complement by heparin–protamine complexes. *Blood*, **71**, 36–40
116. Tan, F., Jackman, K., Skidgel, R. A., Zsigmond, E. K. and Erdos, E. G. (1989). Protamine inhibits plasma carboxypeptidase N, the inactivator of anaphylatoxins and kinins. *Anaesthesiology*, **70**, 267–75
117. Click, R. L., Homburger, H. A. and Bove, A. A. (1989). Complement activation from protamine sulfate administration after coronary angiography. *Cathet. Cardiovasc. Diagn.*, **16**, 221–5
118. Lewis, S. L., Van Epps, D. E. and Chenoweth, D. E. (1987). Leukocyte C5a receptor modulation during hemodialysis. *Kidney Int.*, **31**, 112–20
119. Lewis, S. L. and Van Epps, D. E. (1987). Neutrophil and monocyte alternations in chronic dialysis patients. *Am. J. Kidney Dis.*, **9**, 381–95
120. Stahl, G. L., Amsterdam, E. A., Symons, J. D. and Longhurst, J. C. (1990). Role of thromboxane A_2 in the cardiovascular response to intracoronary C5a. *Circ. Res.*, **66**, 1103–11
121. Del Balzo, U., Sakuma, I. and Levi, R. (1990). Cardiac dysfunction caused by recombinant human C5a anaphylatoxin: mediation by histamine adenosine and cyclooxygenase arachidonate metabolites. *J. Pharmacol. Exp. Ther.*, **253**, 171–9
122. Ito, B. R., Roth, D. M. and Engler, R. L. (1990). Thromboxane A_2 and peptidoleukotrienes contribute to the myocardial ischemia and contractile dysfunction in response to intracoronary infusion of complement C5a in pigs. *Circ. Res.*, **66**, 596–607
123. Del Balzo, U. H., Levi, R. and Polley, M. J. (1985). Cardiac dysfunction caused by purified human C3a anaphylatoxin. *Proc. Natl. Acad. Sci. USA*, **82**, 886–90
124. Yasudam, M., Kawarabayashi, T., Akioka, K., Teragaki, M., Oku, H. and Kanayama, Y. (1989). The complement system in the acute phase of myocardial infarction. *Jpn. Circ. J.*, **53**, 1017–22
125. Christophers, E. and Henseler, T. (1989). Patient subgroups and the inflammatory pattern in psoriasis. *Acta Derm. Venereol. Suppl. Stockh.*, **151**, 88–92
126. Takematsu, H., Ohkohchi, K. and Tagami, H. (1986). Demonstration of anaphylatoxin C3a, C4a and c5a in the scales of psoriasis and inflammatory pustular dermatoses. *Br. J. Dermatol.*, **114**, 1–6

127. Takematsu, H., Terui, T., Ohkohchi, K., Tagami, H., Suzuki, R. and Kuhmagi, K. (1986). Presence of chemotactic peptides other than C5a anaphylatoxin in scales of psoriasis and sterile pustular dermatoses. *Acta Derm. Venereol. Suppl. Stockh.*, **66**, 93–7
128. Takematsu, H., Terui, T. and Tagami, H. (1986). Demonstration of leukotriene B_4 in the scale extracts of psoriasis and inflammatory pustular dermatoses. Correlation with leukocyte chemotactic activity and C5a anaphylatoxin. *Acta Derm. Venereol. Suppl. Stockh.*, **66**, 6–10
129. Schroder, J. M. and Christophers, E. (1986). Identification of C5a desarg and a neutrophil activating peptide (ANAP) in psoriatic scales. *J. Invest. Dermatol.*, **87**, 53–8
130. Asbakk, K., Bergh, K. and Iversen, O. J. (1990). The psoriasis associated antigen, pso p27, participates in the formation of complement activating immune complexes in psoriatic scale. *Acta Pathol. Microbiol. Immunol. Scand.*, **98**, 143–9
131. Kapp, A., Wokalek, H. and Schopf, E. (1985). Involvement of complement in psoriasis and atopic dermatitis measurement of C3a and C5a, C3, C4 and C1 inactivator. *Arch. Dermatol. Res.*, **277**, 359–61
132. Ohkochi, K., Takematsu, H. and Tagami, H. (1985). Increased anaphylatoxins (C3a and C4a) in psoriatic sera. *Br. J. Dermatol.*, **113**, 189–96
133. Weissmann, G. and Korchak, H. (1984). Rheumatoid arthritis. The role of neutrophil activation. *Inflammation*, **8**, S3–S14
134. Moxley, G. and Rudy, S. (1987). Elevated plasma C3 anaphylatoxin levels in rheumatoid arthritis patients. *Arthritis Rheum.*, **30**, 1097–104
135. Moxley, G. and Rudy, S. (1985). Elevated plasma C3 anaphylatoxin levels in synovial fluids from patients with rheumatoid arthritis. *Arthritis Rheum.*, **28**, 1089–95
136. Haslett, C., Jose, P. J., Giclas, P. C., William, T. J. and Henson, P. M. (1989). Cessation of neutrophil influx in C5a-induced acute experimental arthritis is associated with loss of chemoattractant activity from the joint space. *J. Immunol.*, **142**, 3510–17
137. Elmgreen, J. and Hansen, T. M. (1985). Subnormal sensitivity of neutrophils to complement split product C5a in rheumatoid arthritis: relation to complement catabolism and disease extent. *Ann. Rheum. Dis.*, **44**, 514–18
138. Hermann, E., Vogt, P., Hagemann, W., Dunky, A. and Muller, W. (1988). Synovial level of interleukin-1 and C3a in chronic polyarthritis, psoriatic arthritis and activated arthritis. *Z. Rheumatol.*, **47**, 20–5
139. Belmont, H. M., Hopkins, P., Edelson, H. S., Kaplan, H. B., Ludewig, R., Weissmann, G. and Abramson, S. (1986). Complement activation during systemic lupus erythematosus. C3a and C5a anaphylatoxins circulate during exacerbations of disease. *Arthritis Rheum.*, **29**, 1085–9
140. Hopkins, P., Belmont, H. M., Buyon, J., Phillips, M., Weissmann, G. and Abramson, S. B. (1988). Increased levels of plasma anaphylatoxins in systemic lupus erythematosus predict flares of the disease and may elicit vascular injury in lupus cerebritis. *Arthritis Rheum.* **31**, 632–41

12
Cellular responses to the membrane attack complex

B. P. MORGAN

INTRODUCTION

Complement was first identified over a century ago as a result of the observation that fresh serum caused lysis of bacteria and erythrocytes – activities we now recognize as being mediated by the membrane attack complex (MAC). It is not surprising that, until recently, the MAC was considered by the majority of immunologists, and even by complementologists, as a lytic entity whose only role was to kill target cells. The concept that the MAC might also cause more subtle (and often more pathologically relevant) changes in target cells has only recently gained widespread recognition. This is particularly relevant when targets are nucleated and metabolically active, although important non-lethal changes may also be induced in non-nucleated cells.

This chapter summarizes the current understanding of the non-lethal effects of the MAC on metabolically active eukaryotic cells. It details the types of non-lethal changes observed in diverse cell types and explains the intracellular signalling pathways by which the MAC brings about these changes. In order to set the scene, the first section of this chapter summarizes current ideas of MAC assembly and structure while the second section describes the protective factors – both inhibitory proteins and active cell responses – which enable a cell to resist lysis by the MAC. The final section of the chapter relates these non-lethal changes, most of which have been observed only *in vitro*, to diseases in which cell stimulation by the MAC may be of pathogenic importance.

ASSEMBLY AND STRUCTURE OF THE MEMBRANE ATTACK COMPLEX

The membrane attack pathway begins with the cleavage of C5 by the C5 convertase of either the classical (C4b2a3b) or the alternative (C3bBb3b) pathways on the target membrane. Cleavage of C5 is the final enzymatic step in the complement sequence and the first step in MAC assembly[1,2]. The large C5b fragment remains attached to the convertase where it transiently expresses a binding site for a single molecule of the next component in the series, C6. Binding of C6 creates a stable complex with the capacity to bind the next component C7. The C5b6 complex remains attached to the convertase until C7 is bound, whereupon the trimolecular C5b-7 complex may be released into the fluid phase. Unlike its hydrophilic precursor molecules, the C5b-7 complex is amphiphilic, thus possessing the capacity to bind and insert into the lipid bilayer. The membrane-binding capacity of the C5b-7 complex is short-lived because the complex has a marked propensity to self-aggregate and because of the presence in serum of several plasma proteins with the capacity to bind and inactivate the complex. Binding of C5b-7 complexes is therefore limited to the membrane immediately adjacent to the C5 convertase. Once bound, the C5b-7 complex is extremely stable, at least on metabolically inert targets, enabling cellular intermediates bearing C5b-7 sites to be made and stored for long periods with no loss of C8- and C9-binding activity.

Although the C5b-7 complex does insert into the lipid bilayer, it causes little or no disturbance of bilayer integrity. Upon binding to the complex, C8 undergoes a hydrophilic–amphiphilic transition, inserts deeply into the bilayer and forms small 'pores' through which water and ions can leak. This C5b-8 leak may be sufficient to cause the slow lysis of inert targets[3], but is insufficient to lyse metabolically active cells. Exceptions to this rule exist and some nucleated tumour cell lines have been shown to be susceptible to C5b-8-mediated lysis[4,5].

The final step in the assembly of the membrane attack complex is the binding and insertion of several C9 molecules, each of which must undergo a hydrophilic–amphiphilic transition prior to insertion[6]. Insertion of a single C9 molecule is sufficient to potentiate the lytic potential of the C5b-8 complex markedly, but incorporation of more C9 molecules enhances lysis further by increasing the size of the functional pore. Production of the well-recognized ring lesions seen by electron microscopy on complement-lysed membranes requires the incorporation of between twelve and eighteen C9 molecules per MAC which become arranged in a circular polymer. This ring lesion is not a requirement for MAC lysis; indeed, there is persuasive evidence that circular polymerization of C9 in the MAC serves to reduce the lytic potential of the lesion. Thrombin-cleaved C9 is more lytic for erythrocytes and bacteria than is native C9 yet is unable to form circular polymers in the MAC, forming instead elongated string-like membrane lesions[7,8]. The majority of MACs on these targets must contain very much fewer than twelve C9 molecules, as the measured ratio of C9:C8 on complement-lysed erythrocyte membranes is only about 3.5:1[9,10]. The membrane attack pathway and the structure of the MAC are illustrated in Figure 12.1.

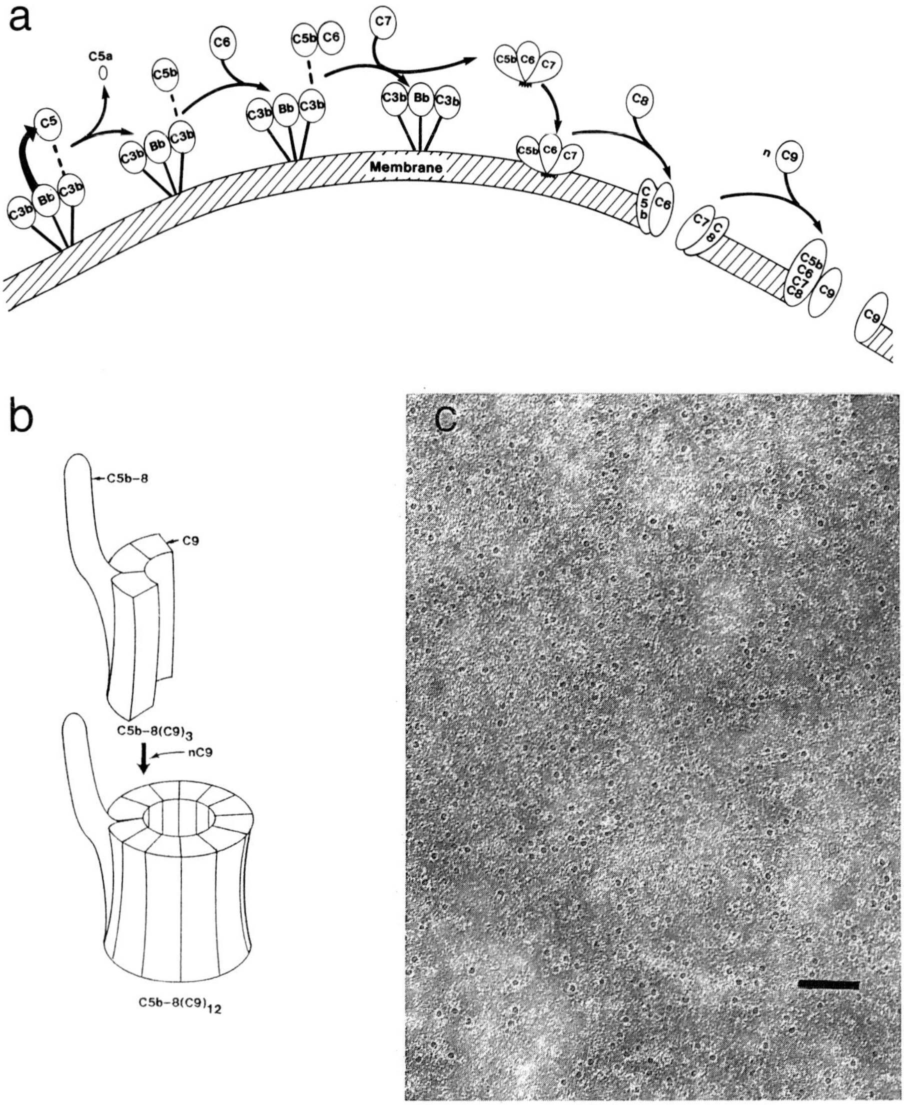

Figure 12.1 Formation and structure of the membrane attack complex (MAC). **a** Schematic of the assembly of the MAC. Cleavage of C5 is the final step in the activation pathways and initiates MAC formation. The large fragment, C5b, remains attached to the convertase and binds C6 and C7 from the fluid phase. The C5b-7 complex is released from the convertase and binds to adjacent membrane via a newly expressed hydrophobic domain. A single C8 and multiple C9 molecules subsequently bind to form the MAC. **b** Structure of the MAC. When only a few C9 molecules are present, incomplete rings are formed (top). Formation of complete ring lesions requires at least twelve C9 molecules per complex (bottom). **c** Electron micrograph of ring lesions on a complement-lysed sheep erythrocyte. Bar is 100 nm. Modified from Morgan, B. P. (1990). *Complement, Clinical Aspects and Relevance to Disease*, pp. 21–26. (London: Academic Press)

With the availability of complete sequence information on each of the terminal complement components[11–14], it has become possible to suggest mechanisms of component interaction during MAC assembly. The components, C6, C7, C8α, C8β and C9, all share sequence homology. In particular, they all contain highly conserved cysteine-rich sequences, which serve as intermolecular fasteners, locking each compartment in its correct configuration in the MAC[12]. This 'modular fusion hypothesis' provides an elegant model for MAC assembly, but some findings, particularly the demonstration that C8 binds to C5b in the C5b-7 complex and not to the homologous components, C6 and C7, appear not to fit the hypothesis[15].

CONTROL OF MEMBRANE ATTACK COMPLEX FORMATION

Complement membrane attack on cells is controlled by a number of fluid-phase and membrane-associated proteins. The fluid-phase inhibitors bind C5b-7, preventing its insertion into membranes. The major C5b-7-inhibiting factor in plasma is C8[16,17]. If C8 binds to the C5b-7 complex prior to its insertion into the bilayer, the resultant fluid-phase C5b-8 complex is unable to insert and is hence inactive. S protein, also known as vitronectin or serum spreading factor, is an acidic glycoprotein, present in plasma at a concentration of about 0.3 g/L, which efficiently inhibits MAC assembly[18,19]. Two or three molecules of S protein bind to the fluid-phase C5b-7 complex to form the inactive, hydrophilic SC5b-7 complex. SC5b-7 still binds C8 and two or three molecules of C9; the resultant SC5b-9 complex is present in plasma during episodes of complement activation and has a half-life *in vivo* of about 30 minutes.

Yet another C5b-7 inhibitor has recently been described. This protein, known as SP-40,40 or cytolysis inhibitor (CLI), is present in plasma at a concentration of about 0.1 g/L and combines with and inactivates the fluid-phase C5b-7 complex[20–22]. SC5b-9 complexes formed *in vivo* contain both S protein and SP-40,40 and it is likely that these two proteins act in similar ways to inactivate and solubilize C5b-7. Recently, it has become apparent that SP-40,40 has other functions. It is present in extremely high concentration in seminal plasma, where it may play a role in sperm adhesion[23], and is identical to apolipoprotein J, an apolipoprotein present in specific subclasses of high-density lipoproteins[24]. Very low-, low- and high-density lipoproteins have all previously been shown to inhibit C5b-7[25,26] but the inhibitory activity was assumed to reside within the lipid core rather than within constituent apoproteins. However, it is possible that these other apolipoproteins may also directly interact with the complex and cause inhibition.

Fluid-phase inhibition of MAC formation is therefore a rather non-specific process mediated by a diverse group of plasma proteins which interact with the C5b-7 complex. Each of these C5b-7 inhibitors has other specific functions and none appear to exist solely or mainly to inhibit complement. Nevertheless, they prevent bystander lysis by minimizing spread of MACs from the site of activation. Control of MAC formation on the membrane is a much more specific process. The proteins involved appear to have evolved for this role and exhibit homologous restriction in their inhibitory actions. The first membrane inhibitor of the MAC to be described was a 60 kDa protein purified from human erythrocyte membranes, named C8-binding protein (C8bp)[27], C9-binding protein (C9bp), homologous restriction factor (HRF)[28] or MAC-inhibitory protein (MIP)[29]. This protein has been shown to be present on leukocytes, platelets and a variety of other cell types and, at least on circulating cells, is linked to the membrane by a glycosyl phosphatidyl inositol (GPI) anchor[30,31]. The purified protein retains its GPI anchor and thus has the capacity to incorporate into a membrane bilayer. Incorporation of human C8bp into sheep, chicken or guinea-pig erythrocytes inhibits lysis of the cells by human C5b-9 but not by C5b-9 of other species, demonstrating that inhibition is homologously restricted. C8bp/HRF acts late in the assembly of the MAC and becomes incorporated into the forming MAC, but the details of its inhibitory action remain uncertain[32]. Fluid-phase forms of the protein have been identified in plasma[33] and in urine[34], and protein isolated from both these sources retains some inhibitory activity.

The presence of a second MAC-inhibiting protein on erythrocyte membranes was first reported in 1988 but, despite its recent discovery, a great deal is known about its structure and mode of action. In the original report[35], the isolated protein was found to have a molecular weight of 18 kDa and was thus named P-18. Within six months of the original report, at least three other groups, using diverse methods, reported independently the isolation of 18–20 kDa inhibitory proteins from human erythrocyte membranes, resulting in a profusion of names: membrane inhibitor of reactive lysis (MIRL)[36], MAC inhibitory factor (MACIF)[37], homologous restriction factor-20 (HRF-20)[38], H19[39], CD59 antigen[40] and protectin[41]. Most of these proteins have now been sequenced and shown to be identical and therefore, for the remainder of this chapter, the term protectin is used. Like the larger inhibitor, protectin is attached to the membrane by a GPI anchor and the purified protein is therefore able to incorporate efficiently into lipid bilayers. Neutralization of endogenous protectin on human erythrocytes using specific antibody renders the cells more susceptible to lysis by human C5b-9 and incorporation of protectin into foreign erythrocytes renders them less susceptible to lysis by human C5b-9. Thus, restriction of lysis by protectin has been reported to be homologously restricted, so that human protectin restricts lysis by human C5b-9. However, recent studies indicate incorporation of protectin into foreign cells also reduces lysis by C5b-9 from some, but not all, animal species. Protectin does not influence the number of complexes formed on the cell but binds to C8 in the forming MAC and limits subsequent incorporation of C9[41,42]. MACs formed on erythrocytes in the presence of protectin contain an average of only 1.5 C9 molecules, compared with 3.5 in the absence of the inhibitor, and are non-lytic.

Both MAC-inhibitory proteins are also present on many nucleated cells and evidence of their importance in control of complement activation on these cells *in vitro* and *in vivo* is now accumulating. Both proteins are deficient on defective erythrocytes in paroxysmal nocturnal haemoglobinuria (PNH), a disease previously ascribed to deficiency of decay-accelerating factor (DAF). The recent reports of individuals specifically deficient in DAF who do not have PNH[43], and of PNH patients specifically deficient in protectin (HRF-20)[44], demonstrate that PNH is primarily due to a defect in control of MAC formation.

RESISTANCE AND RECOVERY PROCESSES IN METABOLICALLY ACTIVE CELLS

Background

It has long been recognized that nucleated cells are far more difficult to lyse with complement than are erythrocytes, and, in the late 1950s, the mechanisms of this cell resistance to complement lysis attracted considerable research interest. Two distinct possibilities were suggested: firstly, that complement was not activated efficiently on the cell surface, resulting in the formation of only small numbers of MACs; and, secondly, that complement activation occurred and many MACs were formed, but active processes within the cell resisted lysis. Evidence in favour of this latter possibility was provided by an elegant series of studies of complement attack on a nucleated tumour cell line by Goldberg, Green and colleagues over thirty years ago[45–47]. Complement attack caused cell swelling and release of intracellular amino acids, nucleic acids and ions without completely disrupting the cell membrane, leading these workers to conclude that MAC-mediated complement injury could occur in nucleated cells in the absence of lysis. Others continued to pursue the first possibility, with inefficient activation being attributed to low antigen density or diminished binding of activated components to the cell surface[48,49]. This hypothesis was not supported by studies which examined the variation in susceptibility to complement lysis between different nucleated cell lines or between cells at different stages of the cell cycle[50–52]. These studies revealed no consistent relationship between antigen density or the amount of early or late complement component[53,54] bound on the membrane and the degree of lysis, but did indicate an association between cell metabolic activity and survival.

By the early 1970s, it was clear that nucleated cells had the capacity to survive limited complement membrane attack and that this capacity is, at least in part, dependent on the metabolic status of the cell. However, the nature of the metabolic responses which permitted cell survival was completely unknown. In an attempt to elucidate the important responses, Ohanian and coworkers performed a comprehensive series of studies using a wide variety of metabolic inhibitors. They found that treatment of guinea-pig hepatoma cells with the anti-tumour drugs, puromycin, adriamycin and actinomycin D, either alone or in combination, increases the susceptibility of the cells to lysis by complement[55], whereas treatment with anabolic hormones, such as insulin and hydrocortisone, diminish lytic susceptibility[56]. Surprisingly, inhibition of cellular energy production, using the respiratory chain poisons, sodium cyanide and sodium azide, caused only a small enhancement of complement-mediated cytolysis[57]. These studies suggest that changes in lipid metabolism are the central events in modulation of lytic susceptibility[58]. The mechanisms by which lipid modulation affects susceptibility are not clear from these studies although an effect on membrane repair mechanisms was postulated. Direct modulation of membrane lipid composition in liposomes, erythrocytes and nucleated cells was also shown to alter lytic susceptibility[59–61], primarily by influencing the efficiency of pore formation by the MAC.

A second group of agents which caused significant enhancement of lytic susceptibility in these studies are the enzymes, neuraminidase, trypsin, pepsin and pronase[62]. Although not proven, it is likely that these enzymes work by stripping non-specific or specific protective factors (cell surface inhibitors) from the cell surface.

Lability of the MAC on nucleated cells

Aged sheep erythrocytes, the popular target for assessing complement lytic activity, are little more than membrane bags containing proteinaceous fluid. Formation of transmembrane pores in these targets leads to influx of water, causing the cell to swell and burst. Kinetic analysis of the lytic process has demonstrated that only a single functional lesion (single hit) is required to cause cell lysis[63]. Although lysis requires only a single functional lesion, many hundreds of MACs are present on the cell at the minimum lytic dose, demonstrating that lesion formation is highly inefficient and that most of the MACs are ineffective. Functional pores formed by the MAC on erythrocyte ghosts or on liposomes are highly stable, remaining in the membrane for several days after formation[64,65].

In contrast, MAC pores on nucleated cells are labile. Pores which allow efflux of small markers, such as rubidium ions, or influx of calcium ions can be formed on nucleated cells without lysis ensuing[66,67], and nucleated cells can be 'rescued' from a potentially lytic dose of the MAC by incubating with cyclic AMP[68,69], suggesting that pores can be repaired or removed from the membrane. A direct demonstration of pore closure was first provided by patch-clamping studies on isolated nerve and muscle cells during complement attack[70,71]. The MAC induced transient changes in membrane potential in these cells, and opening and closing of individual pores could be observed. It was therefore not surprising that kinetic analysis of nucleated cell killing revealed that cytolysis obeyed multi-hit kinetics, indicating that multiple effective lesions were required on the membrane in order to bring about lysis[72]. The lifespan of MAC pores on the tumour cell line, U937, measured by release of rubidium ions, has been shown to be very brief, lasting only a few minutes before being closed or removed[73]. Inhibition of ion pumps had little effect on pore closure and lytic susceptibility in U937 cells[74], implying that, at least in this cell line, increased removal of ions and water from the cell was not a major factor in resisting lysis.

Routes of elimination of the MAC

Nucleated cells, therefore, appear to possess escape mechanisms not present on aged erythrocytes, which allow them to withstand limited complement membrane attack. Functional studies demonstrate pore closure but provide few clues to the mechanisms involved. The MAC could be functionally inactivated but remain on the cell surface or could be physically removed from the membrane, with or without prior inactivation. Unusual morphological changes in cells during complement attack, including the appearance of multiple protrusions[75] and the shedding of vesicles from the cell surface[45,76,77], have been noted in diverse cells, but involvement of these changes in the process of cell recovery was first demonstrated in neutrophils. These cells, which are highly resistant to lysis by homologous complement, shed numerous vesicles from their surfaces when subjected to membrane attack. Using monoclonal antibodies, it was shown that these vesicles stain strongly for C9, and so presumably contain MACs[78]. These antibodies were used to monitor the fate of the complex on neutrophils bearing a non-lethal MAC load. Complexes rapidly disappeared from the cell surface, 50% of the bound MACs being removed within 3.5 min at 37°C, and it was suggested that these complexes are removed on shed membrane vesicles (Figure 12.2). These findings were confirmed in later studies which showed that an average of 25 000 MACs per cell could be formed on human neutrophils

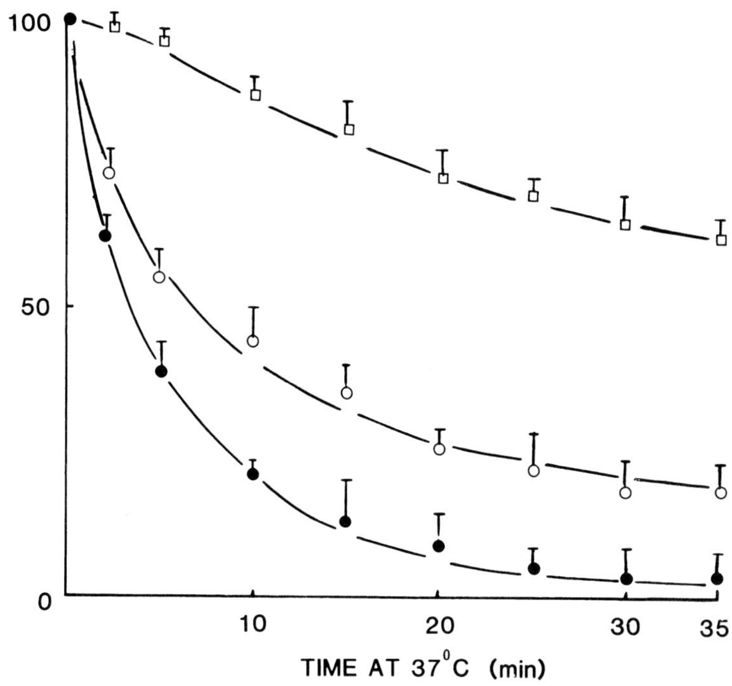

Figure 12.2 Removal of MACs from human neutrophils. Neutrophils were attacked with a non-lethal amount of the MAC by first making C5b-8 sites on the cell surface and then binding C9 on ice. The cells were then warmed to 37°C and portions removed at intervals and placed on ice. The quantity of MAC remaining on the cell surface at each time point was then assessed by measuring the binding of radio-labelled monoclonal anti-C9 antibodies to the cells (all on ice). The results are expressed as the percentage of binding at time zero and show a rapid loss of antibody-binding sites (MAC) from the cell surface in the presence of extracellular calcium (closed circles). The open circles show the effect on MAC removal of chelating extracellular calcium; and the open squares the effect of chelating both extra- and intracellular calcium. From Morgan and Campbell (1985). *Biochem. J.*, **231**: 205 (with permission)

without causing significant lysis[79]. Of these lesions, 65% are rapidly shed on membrane vesicles which constituted just 2% of the cell surface. The remainder of the cell-bound MACs are internalized and degraded by the cell. Shed vesicles isolated from the supernatant are densely covered with MACs, whereas MACs are not detected on the cell membrane within 5 minutes of attack (Figure 12.3).

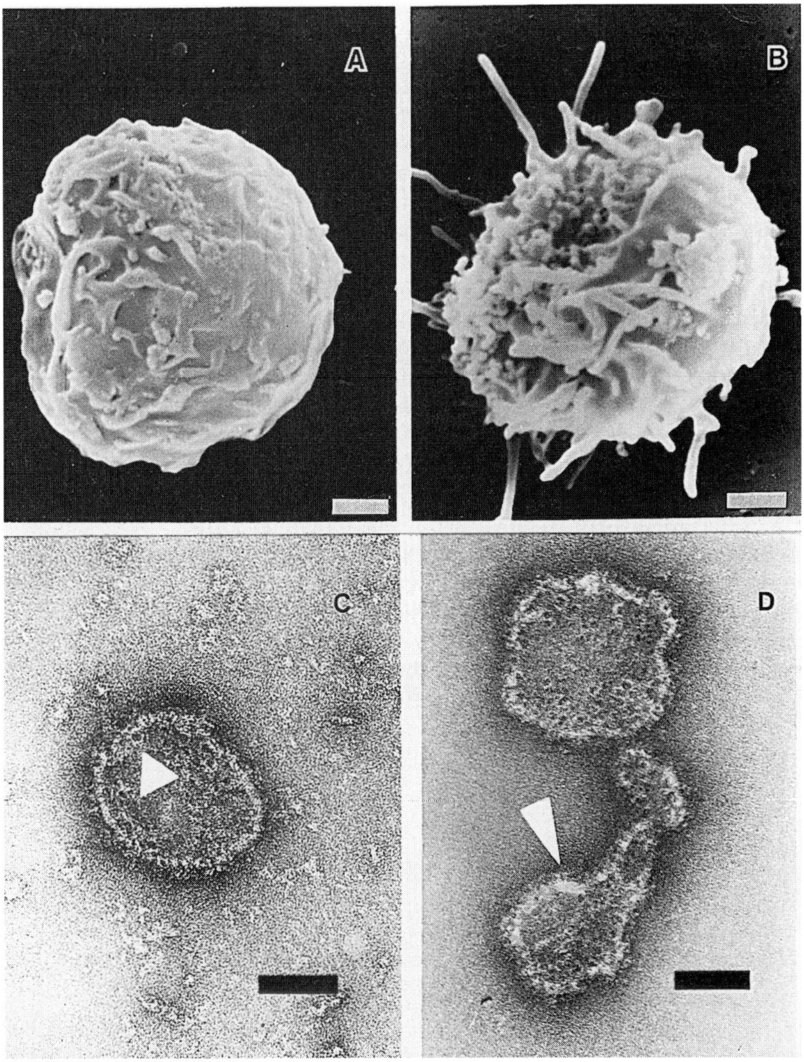

Figure 12.3 Recovery of neutrophils from membrane attack. **A**, **B** Scanning electron micrographs of neutrophils before (**A**) and 2 minutes after (**B**) attack with non-lethal amounts of the MAC. Bar represents 1 μm. **C**, **D** Transmission electron micrographs of vesicles shed from neutrophils during non-lethal complement membrane attack. The surfaces of the vesicles are covered with ring lesions. Bar represents 100 nm. Modified from Morgan *et al.* (1987). *J. Immunol.*, **138**: 246–53 (with permission)

Physical removal of MACs by vesiculation (ectocytosis) and/or endocytosis has now been demonstrated in a large number of cell types (see Table 12.1). In some cells (e.g. the Ehrlich murine carcinoma cell line), endocytosis appears to be the principal route of MAC elimination, removing MACs at rates comparable to those achieved by ectocytosis in the neutrophil[80]. C5b-8 sites on neutrophils are relatively stable, with a halflife for removal of over 60 min at 37°C. However, on Ehrlich cells, C5b-8 sites are rapidly removed, albeit at a slower rate than C5b-9 sites (halflife about 20 min), and even C5b-7 sites, which presumably cause little or no membrane perturbation, are efficiently cleared from the cell surface, suggesting that the events signalling lesion removal are different in this system. These experiments were performed using a heterologous system – murine cells and human complement – and it is possible that this species incompatibility could account for the differences observed.

Like the neutrophil, the human histiocytic cell line, U937, removes human C5b-9 efficiently, primarily via ectocytosis, but C5b-8 sites are stable and, if present on the membrane in sufficient numbers, can cause cell killing. Addition of trace amounts of C9 to U937 cells bearing C5b-8 markedly enhances removal and decreases killing[4]. The C5b-8 lesion thus appears to be an insufficient stimulus for recovery in cells attacked by homologous complement, but may be sufficient in heterologous systems because of the lack of other inhibitory factors. Cultured rat renal glomerular epithelial cells remove MACs by vesiculation[81] and, recently, a transcytotic route of MAC elimination by these cells *in vivo* has been described[82]. These workers used immunoelectron microscopy to monitor the fate of MACs formed in the kidney in experimental glomerulonephritis and showed that MACs are endocytosed at the abluminal surface of the epithelial cell, and, after traversing the cell, are exocytosed into the urinary space. MACs are detected in the urine of animals with glomerulonephritis, suggesting that transcytosis is a major route of MAC elimination from the kidney in this disease. Preliminary studies in our laboratory have detected MACs in the urine of patients with glomerulonephritis, indicating that similar processes may be occurring in human renal disease (unpublished observations).

Table 12.1 Routes of MAC elimination

Cell	*Route*	*Ca^{2+} dependence*	*Reference*
Neutrophil (rat and human)	Ecto⟫endo	Yes	78,79,86
EAT cell	Endocytosis	Yes	80,88
U937 cells	Ectocytosis	?	4
Glomerular epithelial cells (rat)	Ectocytosis	?	81
	Transcytosis	?	82
Oligodendrocytes (rat)	Ectocytosis	Yes	90
Rheumatoid synovial cells (human)	Ectocytosis	Yes	*
K562 cells	Ectocytosis	?	114
Platelets	Ectocytosis	Yes	89

* = unpublished observations

Intracellular signals for MAC elimination

An early clue to the intracellular signals responsible for mediating recovery was provided by the studies of Campbell *et al.* who showed that the first intracellular event detectable upon formation of the MAC on a cell was a rapid increase in intracellular free calcium concentration ($[Ca^{2+}]i$)[83,84]. The increase occurs within seconds of adding C9 to cells bearing C5b-8 sites and precedes cell lysis by several minutes[85]. These workers proposed that this rapid rise in $[Ca^{2+}]i$ could, under conditions of mild attack, signal MAC removal from the cell surface[84]. In the neutrophil, transient changes in $[Ca^{2+}]i$ are detectable even in the absence of lysis, rising from a resting level of about 0.2 μM to a peak of up to 5 μM within 1 min of MAC formation and then falling rapidly to the resting level[86]. In the absence of extracellular calcium, the MAC-induced increase in $[Ca^{2+}]i$ is inhibited, though not completely; MAC removal is concomitantly slowed, and cell death is enhanced. Chelation of intracellular calcium ablates MAC removal and further enhances lysis, firmly implicating calcium as a mediator of MAC removal and demonstrating that the increase in $[Ca^{2+}]i$ is due, not only to influx of calcium via the pore, but also to release from intracellular stores (Figure 12.2). Above a certain threshold level, which probably varies among cell types, $[Ca^{2+}]i$ is toxic and cell lysis ensues[87]. Calcium signals recovery of a variety of cells, including Ehrlich cells[88], platelets[89], oligodendrocytes[90], synovial cells[91] and glomerular epithelial cells[92] (Table 12.1). Interestingly, the higher the peak $[Ca^{2+}]i$ reached in Ehrlich cells during non-lethal attack, the faster intracellular levels subsequently fall, further showing that calcium is the major intracellular signal for recovery.

Most of the intracellular effects of raised $[Ca^{2+}]i$ are mediated by calmodulin and involve modulation of the activity of protein kinases which phosphorylate, and regulate, key enzymes in the cell[93]. MAC-induced protein kinase activation has been directly demonstrated in several cell types, and specific inhibitors of protein kinases or of calmodulin increase lytic susceptibility of these cells[92,94–97].

Evidence suggests that other intracellular signals might also influence recovery processes. A role of cyclic AMP (cAMP) is suggested by several studies: incubation of nucleated cells bearing potentially lytic amounts of the MAC with cAMP 'rescued' these cells from subsequent death; lysis was inversely related to the intracellular cAMP concentration[98]; and the non-metabolizable adenosine agonist, 2-chloroadenosine, which modulates intracellular cAMP levels, inhibits MAC removal in neutrophils and enhances cell lysis[99]. The mechanism by which the MAC brings about an increase in intracellular cAMP is unclear but Ca^{2+}–calmodulin complexes can modulate the enzymes responsible for cAMP production and breakdown. Increased $[Ca^{2+}]i$ may cause a secondary increase in cAMP which enhances recovery. It is also possible that the MAC directly influences membrane signalling systems. This possibility is supported by the observation that the MAC causes release of calcium from intracellular stores in neutrophils and in glomerular epithelial cells in the absence of extracellular calcium[86,92]. One candidate is the G protein system which couples diverse cell surface receptors with multiple intracellular effectors, including cyclic nucleotides and inositol phospholipids[100,101]. The increase in cAMP levels in response to the MAC in Erhlich cells is inhibited[102] and MAC-mediated lysis of synovial cells is enhanced[103] by specific inhibitors of G proteins. Direct interaction of the MAC with G proteins in the membrane has yet to be demonstrated.

It is clear that the signalling of recovery in nucleated cells is a complex process involving calcium, cyclic nucleotides and perhaps other intracellular effectors, such as the inositol phosphates. Influx of calcium via the MAC pore plays a central role but the MAC may also interact with and influence signalling systems within the membrane. The products of MAC-mediated cell activation, which include eicosanoids and cytokines (see below) may also contribute to recovery processes (see Figure 12.5).

Mechanisms of MAC elimination

The physical processes of removal of MACs by shedding (ectocytosis) or endocytosis have not yet been fully characterized. In Erhlich cells, endocytic elimination of MACs or incomplete complexes involves accumulation of the complexes in clathrin-coated pits on the cell surface followed by internalization and subsequent degradation in lysosomes[88]. Transcytotic elimination of MACs in glomerular cells may also utilize clathrin-coated or uncoated pits and intracellular vesicle transport systems[82]. Similarly ectocytic elimination of MACs similarly involves the accumulation of complexes in 'patches' on the cell surface but there is no evidence of association with specific surface structures and the intracellular processes causing this accumulation are unknown. Patching and vesiculation of MACs on the neutrophil surface is little affected by the presence of inhibitors of microfilament or microtubule function, or by the inclusion of metabolic poisons (cyanide or azide) (Morgan and Dankert, unpublished observations). Similarly, MAC-induced vesiculation in platelets is not influenced by disruption of the cytoskeleton or by depletion of cellular ATP[104], implying that the immediate response can occur independently of target-cell activity. MACs may accumulate in patches by adhering together when they meet during their random migrations in the cell membrane. It has been suggested that this aggregation of complexes disturbs the integrity of the surrounding bilayer and may be a sufficient stimulus to vesiculation[79]. However, the evidence implicating intracellular signalling in recovery does not support this attractive hypothesis.

Sorting of membrane proteins and lipids occurs during MAC-induced ectocytosis in neutrophils[105]. As shed vesicles contain higher proportions of cholesterol and diacylglycerol than the parent plasma membrane, preferential sorting of these two lipids may contribute to vesicle formation. Diacylglycerol may initiate localized membrane curvature and membrane fusion[106], and cholesterol has a condensing effect on membrane phospholipids[107], which would again favour increased membrane curvature. Furthermore, calcium destabilizes artificial lipid bilayers by interacting with cholesterol[108], and calcium flux through the MAC in glomerular epithelial cell membranes causes activation of phospholipases[109], which may also contribute to membrane destabilization around the lesion. The combination of increased [Ca^{2+}]i and membrane areas rich in cholesterol may represent a potent stimulus for vesiculation.

Calcium and cyclic nucleotides may also directly influence the MAC. C9, the major component of the MAC, has recently been shown to be a calcium-binding protein[15] and to be susceptible to phosphorylation *in vitro*[95]. Calcium uptake or phosphorylation of C9, brought about by increased intracellular calcium or cyclic nucleotide concentrations, might enhance elimination of MACs by increasing their aggregation in the membrane.

Although ectocytosis may not require an active response on the part of the cell, non-lethal membrane attack renders the target cell metabolically depleted and functionally impaired, implying a considerable energy cost in restoring cellular equilibria after attack[90,110]. Immediately after recovery, these metabolically depleted cells are more susceptible to lysis by a second attack but, in the presence of suitable substrates, energy stores and cell resistance are rapidly restored.

Role of MAC inhibitory proteins in recovery

Both of the membrane-associated MAC-inhibitory proteins described in a preceding section have been shown to incorporate into the forming MAC on erythrocytes[32,41]. These proteins have been identified on a variety of nucleated cells where recent evidence would suggest that they serve the same regulatory function as the erythrocyte protein[111–113]. It might therefore be expected that the bulk of MACs formed by homologous complement on nucleated cells would be rendered inactive by CD59/protectin and/or HRF/MIP prior to their removal from the cell surface. This would explain why vesicles released from neutrophils attacked by the MAC are not leaky despite being covered with ring lesions[79]. Preliminary evidence suggests that protectin is selectively removed from the cell surface in association with the MAC during recovery[114]. Surface expression of endogenous protectin, measured on the fluorescence-activated cell sorter, falls by 25% during non-lethal attack on K562 cells and reincorporated radio-labelled protectin is shed in a MAC-rich vesicle fraction (Figure 12.4). Thus, physical removal of MACs may be a secondary protective phenomenon – a highly efficient garbage disposal system clearing the membrane of large numbers of inactive MACs, perhaps together with the occasional active complex which has escaped the attentions of the inhibitory proteins.

NON-LETHAL EFFECTS OF THE MAC ON NUCLEATED CELLS

Background

Nucleated cells are highly resistant to lysis by homologous C5b-9 because of the array of protective and recovery mechanisms described above. However, complement membrane attack on these cells is not without consequence. Non-lethal stimulatory effects of complement on cells *in vitro* were first observed over twenty years ago and included release of lysosomal enzymes by cartilage cells[115], release of serotonin from platelets[116] and stimulation of prostaglandin synthesis and bone resorption in fetal long bone cultures[117,118]. Bone

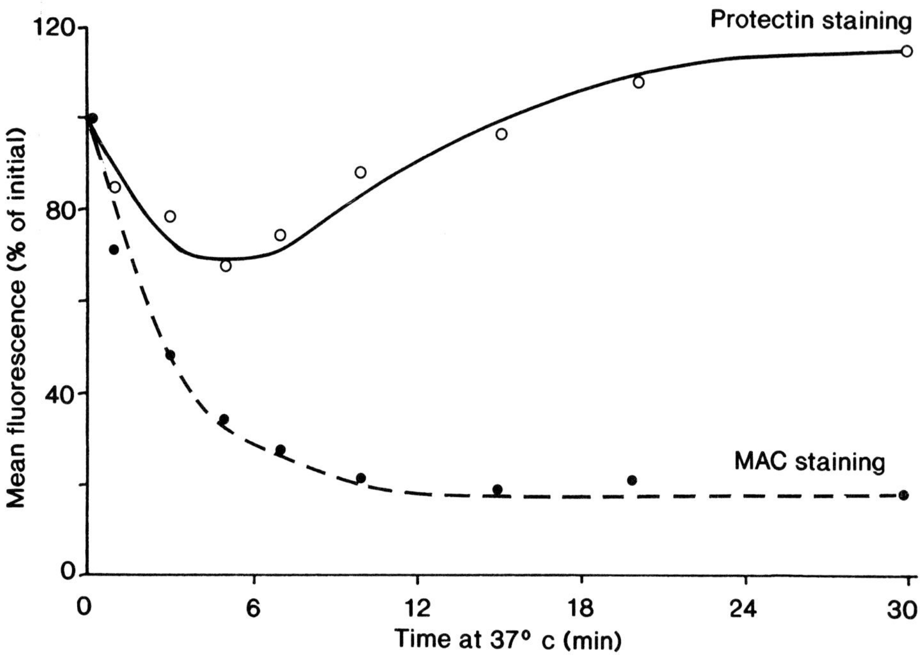

Figure 12.4 Removal of protectin (CD59) during non-lethal membrane attack. K562 cells, a protectin-positive human erythroleukaemia cell line, were subjected to non-lethal membrane attack by first forming C5b-7 sites and then adding C8 and C9 on ice. The cells were then warmed to 37°C, portions removed at intervals, placed on ice and fixed in 1% paraformaldehyde. Fixed cells at each time point were then stained with a monoclonal antiprotectin antibody or with a monoclonal anti-MAC antibody. After washing and incubating with fluorescent second antibody, the cells were analysed in a fluorescence-activated cell sorter. Mean protectin and MAC fluorescence was measured at each time point. Cell surface protectin initially falls in parallel with the loss of MACs from the cell, but pre-attack levels are rapidly restored

resorption in fetal long bone cultures was shown to be dependent on the formation of the MAC, C6-deficient serum causing no prostaglandin synthesis or bone resorption, the first evidence of a stimulatory effect of the MAC. With the recognition that nucleated cells usually survive attack by homologous C5b-9, research interest has focussed on the non-lethal effects of the complex. A wide range of human and non-human cells have been chosen as targets, attacked with homologous or heterologous complement and a host of parameters subsequently measured. The result is a complex and often contradictory literature from which it is difficult to extract a logical summary. *In vivo*, cells are exposed to homologous complement, thus the non-lethal effects of homologous attack are most relevant to pathogenesis. The consequences of non-lethal attack are predominantly proinflammatory. This section describes some of these effects, lists the cell types in which each effect has been observed *in vitro* and discusses the likely contribution of these non-lethal effects to disease pathogenesis.

Release of reactive oxygen metabolites

Reactive oxygen metabolites (ROMs), a term which encompasses the many reactive species of oxygen, including O_2^-, OH and H_2O_2, are highly toxic, causing a wide range of deleterious effects on membranes and molecules[119,120]. Phagocytic cells have the capacity to make ROMs for intracellular killing of microorganisms. ROMs are released in inflammatory diseases, such as rheumatoid arthritis. Since the original demonstration that ROMs are released when rat and human neutrophils are exposed to antibody and low lytic doses of human complement[67], it has been shown that complement attack will stimulate ROM release from several cell types (Table 12.2). Release of ROMs requires formation of the complete MAC and occurs with non-lethal MAC doses[86,99]. MAC-induced ROM released has subsequently been observed from human macrophages[121], rat glomerular mesangial cells[122] and human synovial cells[123,91]. In all these targets, ROM release has been shown to require the assembly of the complete MAC and the presence of extracellular calcium. The C5b-8 complex does not cause significant ROM release in the absence of C9 and calcium chelation after the formation of C5b-7 sites on the cell completely inhibits the release of these metabolites on subsequent addition of C8 and C9. Thus, MAC-induced increase in $[Ca^{2+}]i$, the primary signal for recovery mechanisms, is also responsible for signalling cell activation.

Table 12.2 Release of inflammatory mediators during non-lethal complement attack

Cell	*Mediators*	*References*
Neutrophil (rat and human)	ROM	67,86,99
	LT, TBX	130,131
Macrophages (human)	ROM	121
	PG	121
	CK	121
Glomerular mesangial cells (rat)	ROM	122
	PG	125
	CK	125
Rheumatoid synovial cells (human)	ROM	91,123
	PG	91,103,129
	LT	91
	CK	91
	Collagenase	142
Glomerular epithelial cells (rat)	PG	126
Pulmonary endothelial cells (human)	PG	127
Amniotic epithelial cells (human)	PG	128
Platelets (human)	TBX	132
	Prothrombinase	144
Oligodendrocytes (rat)	LT	133

ROM = reactive oxygen metabolites; PG = prostaglandins; LT = leukotrienes; TBX = thromboxanes; CK = cytokines

Release of eicosanoids

The eicosanoids are a group of biologically active molecules derived from arachidonic acid which have diverse effects, including the production of pain and inflammation, *in vivo*[124]. Complement-dependent prostaglandin synthesis and release from cells *in vitro* was first noted over 15 years ago[117] and is dependent on MAC formation[118]. The relationship of prostaglandin release to cell death was not investigated in these early studies. More recently, release of eicosanoids in response to non-lethal complement membrane attack has been observed in a variety of target cells (Table 12.2). Two distinct eicosanoid biosynthetic pathways exist in nucleated cells: the cyclooxygenase pathway which yields prostaglandins, prostacyclins and thromboxanes; and the lipoxygenase pathway which produces leukotrienes[124]. The cyclooxygenase pathway is widely distributed in mammalian cells and is constitutively active, requiring only a supply of substrate, arachidonic acid. The lipoxygenase pathway is restricted mainly to bone-marrow-derived nucleated cells and is activated by increased $[Ca^{2+}]i$. Stimulation of prostaglandin synthesis by non-lethal amounts of the MAC has been observed in macrophages[121], glomerular mesangial[125] and epithelial cells[126], pulmonary endothelial cells[127], amniotic epithelial cells[128] and synovial cells[91,103,129]. MAC-induced release of leukotrienes and/or thromboxanes has been demonstrated in rat and human neutrophils[130,131], human platelets[132], rat oligodendrocytes[133] and a variety of other cells (Table 12.2). The role of calcium has not been investigated for all the targets listed, but, in all cases where calcium has been examined, it appears to be important in signalling the response. Chelation of extracellular calcium abolishes eicosanoid release from most targets, and, even in the one reported case where removal of calcium did not completely block, release of calcium from intracellular stores was observed[132]. Inhibitors of calmodulin block MAC-induced eicosanoid production[127], suggesting that calcium effects are mediated via calmodulin. Unlike ROM release, which requires formation of the complete MAC, eicosanoid release from some targets is observed at the C5b-8 stage[91,127,131,133], with addition of C9 causing little or no enhancement of production. In other targets, an absolute requirement for the complete MAC has been found[130]. These inconsistencies are unexplained but may relate to different methods of cell preparation and formation of cell intermediates. In all these targets, C5b-8-mediated stimulation of eicosanoid release is dependent on extracellular calcium and it is likely that the slow calcium leak known to occur through the C5b-8 lesion[134,135] causes a sufficient increase in $[Ca^{2+}]i$ to initiate release of eicosanoids (but not of ROMs) from these targets. The release of leukotriene B_4 in response to non-lethal membrane attack by rat oligodendrocyte/glioma hybrid cells is calcium dependent and is also inhibited by protein kinase antagonists[136]. The sequence of events may be: increased $[Ca^{2+}]i$ activates protein kinases which activates membrane phospholipases, thereby releasing arachidonic acid, the substrate for the lipoxygenase enzymes. This proposed pathway bears many similarities to that outlined above for cell recovery.

Because MACs are rapidly cleared from the cell surface, non-lethal complement membrane attack *in vitro*, using reactive lysis or cell intermediates and purified components, is transient. Nevertheless, eicosanoid release is often observed over many hours following attack[91,103,126,129]. The mechanisms of this prolonged response have been studied in human rheumatoid synovial cells[91,103] which release PGE_2 in response to the MAC in a biphasic manner; an early phase peaks about 30 min post-attack and a second, larger phase persists for at least 24 hours. Both phases are inhibited by removal of extracellular calcium during the initial attack. Protein synthesis inhibitors abolish the second prolonged phase but not the early release, suggesting that the early phase results from increased activity (calcium-mediated) of pre-existing enzymes of PGE_2 synthesis, whereas the second phase is due to *de novo* synthesis of cyclooxygenase enzymes[91]. The second phase is also inhibited by pertussis toxin, an inhibitor of G protein-mediated signalling systems[103], implying that multiple messages are involved. Non-lethal doses of a variety of other pore-forming agents, including bacterial toxins[137], antibiotics[138], melittin, ionophores and T cell perforins[103] also stimulate the release of eicosanoids from cells. In all instances, eicosanoid release depends on extracellular calcium, demonstrating that the influx of calcium through membrane pores is the primary stimulus.

Release of cytokines

Cytokines are a group of secreted proteins which can act locally on the secreting cell (autocrine effect), on nearby cells (paracrine effect), or systemically (endocrine effect). Cytokine release in response to non-lethal MAC injury was first observed in glomerular mesangial cells[125]. These cells release an autocrine growth factor which resembles interleukin 1 (IL-1) and stimulates cell proliferation. Rheumatoid synovial cells release interleukin 6 (IL-6) in response to the MAC[91]. Release is not detectable until 5 hours after attack and then rises steadily over the ensuing 20 hours. Neutralization of the released protein with anti-IL-6 antibody inhibits the second phase of prostaglandin release described above[139], suggesting that released IL-6 acts as an autocrine stimulus, mediating eicosanoid synthesis. It is probable that the MAC mediates the release of cytokines from many cell types and this is likely to be a fruitful area of research.

Other non-lethal effects of the MAC

Non-lethal effects of the MAC on specialized functions in nucleated cells include: production of type IV collagen by glomerular epithelial cells[140], implicated in the genesis of glomerulosclerosis[141]; synthesis of collagenase by rheumatoid synovial cells, implicated in joint destruction[142], and inhibition of synthesis of myelin proteins by oligodendrocytes[143]. Although non-nucleated, the platelet is metabolically active and able to resist complement attack. Sims *et al.* have demonstrated that non-lethal complement membrane attack on platelets induces calcium-dependent prothrombinase activation[144], degranulation[94] and increased expression of surface receptor proteins[104,145]. Degranulation occurs without platelet aggregation[146]. Thus, non-lethal complement attack provides a potential mechanism for the persistence of activated platelets *in vivo*.

Signalling of non-lethal effects of the MAC

The preceding sections describe the diverse effects of non-lethal complement attack on different cell types. The intracellular signals initiating these effects may differ in detail from cell to cell but the basic pathways remain the same. Recovery and cell stimulation are both dependent on calcium. Influx of calcium via the MAC pore initiates a chain of events which result in the removal of MACs from the cell surface and in the activation of cellular enzyme systems. Products of activation depend on the synthetic pathways present in the cell and include pro-inflammatory molecules, growth factors and tissue-degrading enzymes. The signalling pathways which have been implicated in recovery from and cell activation by the MAC, and the complex interactions between the pathways, are summarized in Figure 12.5.

Non-lethal effects of the MAC *in vivo*

The MAC may play a role in the pathogenesis of numerous inflammatory and immune-mediated diseases as demonstrated by terminal complement complexes (TCCs) in the fluid phase and/or MACs in the tissues (reviewed in Ref. 147). Table 12.3 lists some of the diseases in which the MAC may play a role. Despite widespread deposition of the cytolytic MAC on tissues in these diseases, necrosis is not a dominant feature. Rather, these conditions are characterized by

Table 12.3 Examples of diseases in which the MAC is implicated

System	*Disease*	*Evidence*		
		TCC	*MAC*	*Model*
Renal	Lupus nephritis	+	+	+
	Post-strep. nephritis	?	+	+
	IgA nephropathy	?	+	+
	Membranous nephropathy	?	+	+
	MPGN type III	?	+	–
Rheumatological	Rheumatoid arthritis	+	+	+
	Sjogren's syndrome	+	?	–
	Psoriatic arthritis	+	+	–
	Behcet's disease	+	+	–
Dermatological	Pemphigus vulgaris	?	+	–
	Bullous pemphigoid	?	+	–
	Dermatitis herpetif.	?	+	–
Neurological	Multiple sclerosis	+	+	+
	Myasthenia gravis	?	+	+
	Cerebral lupus	+	?	–
Others	Atheroma/infarct	–	+	+
	Grave's disease	+	+	–
	Myositis	?	+	–

TCC, fluid-phase complexes detected; MAC, localization of MAC in tissue; Model, evidence for MAC dependence from animal studies. + = evidence obtained; – = no evidence; ? = untested.
The table is derived from data in Refs. 147–155

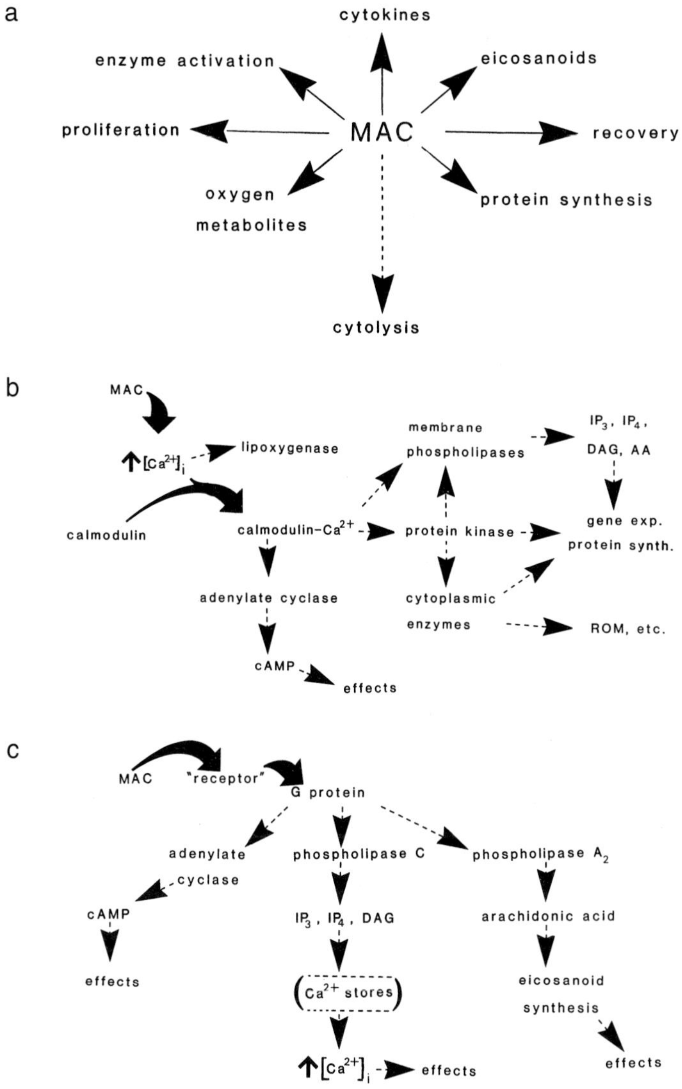

Figure 12.5 Non-lethal effects of the MAC. **a** A simplified summary of the important consequences of complement membrane attack on nucleated cells. The MAC activates diverse processes in the cell, initiates the release of potent mediators and stimulates its own removal. Cytolysis is, in comparison with these non-lethal events, a rare consequence. **b** Calcium flux through the MAC as an initiating stimulus. Increased intracellular free calcium concentration ($[Ca^{2+}]$i), operating primarily through calmodulin, activates protein kinase, adenylate cyclase and phospholipase, which in turn release secondary mediators and activate other cell systems. **c** MAC interaction with membrane signalling systems. The MAC binds an unidentified receptor molecule resulting in activation of G proteins within the membrane. G protein activation switches on cyclases and phospholipases in the membrane, resulting in the production of secondary mediators, which, in turn, modulate many intracellular events. These mediators cause a secondary increase in ($[Ca^{2+}]$i) by initiating release from stores. These schemes are 'best guess' models based on the available data. The realities in this complex signalling network may be quite different. Modified from Ref. 155

cell activation, including proliferation and release of inflammatory mediators, features which are typical of non-lethal complement attack *in vitro*. Although caution is essential when extrapolating results from a simple *in vitro* system to the intact organism, the similarities are persuasive.

The best evidence for a pathogenic role of non-lethal complement membrane attack has emerged from animal studies, where it is possible to block MAC formation specifically. Rat models of human nephritis have been particularly informative: in both antiglomerular basement membrane (GBM) nephritis and Heymann nephritis, glomerular injury is a consequence of complement activation[148,149]. Recently, the MAC has been implicated as the causative factor in both these model diseases. C6 deficiency protects rabbits against the development of anti-GBM nephritis[150], and in an isolated perfused kidney variant of Heymann nephritis, proteinuria, induced by perfusion of the antibody-sensitized kidney with serum, was dependent on the presence of C8[151]. The role of the MAC in experimental autoimmune myasthenia gravis is discussed in Chapter 13.

There is abundant evidence for complement activation and MAC formation in the rheumatoid joint. TCCs are present in the synovial fluid and the MAC is deposited in the synovial membrane[152,153]. Cells in the joint fluid and the synovial membrane, including infiltrating neutrophils, macrophages, lymphocytes and fibroblasts, are exposed to complement attack, yet necrosis is not a major histological feature. Instead, the synovial membrane is thickened as a result of cellular infiltration and proliferation, and the synovial fluid contains cytokines, eicosanoids and reactive oxygen species, products of resident and infiltrating cells. Synovial cells and phagocytic cells *in vitro* have been shown to produce all these inflammatory mediators in response to non-lethal complement membrane attack (Table 12.2) and it is reasonable to speculate that the MAC contributes to inflammation in the rheumatoid joint. Membrane fragments bearing MACs have also been found in the synovial fluid, providing further evidence that non-lethal attack and cell recovery occur *in vivo*[123]. Although other factors are also likely to be involved in pathogenesis, a role for the MAC in perpetuating inflammation in rheumatoid arthritis is probable. Specific therapies which inhibit MAC formation or its non-lethal effects might be of benefit in this disease and in numerous others where non-lethal membrane attack contributes to pathology.

Acknowledgements

I thank the Wellcome Trust for financial support through the award of a Wellcome Senior Research Fellowship, and Mrs Jeannie Burt for secretarial assistance.

References

1. Mayer, M. M., Imagawa, D. K., Ramm, L. E. and Whitlow, M. B. (1983). Membrane attack by complement and its consequences. *Prog. Immunol.*, **5**, 427–44
2. Hansch, G. M. (1989). The complement attack phase. In Rother, K and Till, G. O. (eds.) *The Complement System*, pp. 202–30. (Berlin: Springer Verlag)

3. Stolfi, R. L. (1968). Immune lytic transformation: a state of irreversible damage generated as a result of the reaction of the eighth component of complement in the guinea pig system. *J. Immunol.*, **100**, 46–54
4. Morgan, B. P., Imagawa, D. K., Dankert, J. R. and Ramm, L. E. (1986). Complement lysis of U937, a nucleated mammalian cell line, in the absence of C9: effect of C9 on C5b-8 mediated cell lysis. *J. Immunol.*, **136**, 3402–6
5. Martin, D. E., Chiu, F. J., Gigli, I. and Muller-Eberhard H. J. (1987). Killing of human melanoma cells by the membrane attack complex of human complement as a function of its molecular composition. *J. Clin. Invest.*, **80**, 226–33
6. Stanley, K. K. (1989). The molecular mechanism of complement C9 insertion and polymerisation in biological membranes. *Curr. Top. Microbiol. Immunol.*, **140**, 49–65
7. Dankert, J. R. and Esser, A. F. (1985). Proteolytic modification of human complement protein C9: loss of poly (C9) and circular lesion formation without impairment of function. *Proc. Natl. Acad. Sci. USA*, **82**, 2128–32
8. Esser, A. F. (1986). C9-mediated cytotoxicity and the function of poly (C9). *UCLA Symp. Mol. Cell. Biol.*, **45**, 411–22
9. Stewart, J. L. and Sodetz, J. M. (1985). Analysis of the specific association of the eighth and ninth components of human complement: identification of a direct role for the α subunit of C8. *Biochemistry*, **24**, 4598–602
10. Sims, P. J. (1983). Complement pores in erythrocyte membranes. Analysis of C8/C9 binding required for functional membrane damage. *Biochim. Biophys. Acta*, **732**, 541–52
11. Di Scipio, R. and Hugli, T. E. (1989). The molecular architecture of human complement component C6. *J. Biol. Chem.*, **264**, 16197–206
12. Di Scipio, R. G., Chakravarti, D. N., Muller-Eberhard, H. J. and Fey, G. H. (1988). The structure of human complement component C7 and the C5b-7 complex. *J. Biol. Chem.*, **263**, 549–60
13. Sodetz, J. M. (1989). Structure and function of C8 in the membrane attack sequence of complement. *Curr. Top. Microbiol.*, **140**, 19–31
14. Stanley, K. K., Kocher, H. P., Luzio, J. P., Jackson, P. and Tschopp, J. (1985). The sequence and topology of human complement C9. *EMBO J.*, **4**, 375–82
15. Esser, A. F. (1990). The membrane attack pathway of complement. *Year Immunol.*, **6**, 229–44
16. Nemerov, G. R., Yamamoto, K. and Lint, T. F. (1979). Restriction of complement-mediated membrane damage by the eighth component of complement: a dual role for C8 in the complement attack sequence. *J. Immunol.*, **123**, 1245–52
17. Zeitz, H. J., Zeff, R. A., Gewurz, H. and Lint, T. F. (1983). Decreased C5b67-inhibitor activity in two families with hereditary functional deficiency of the eighth component of complement. *J. Immunol.*, **130**, 2809–13
18. Kolb, W. P. and Muller-Eberhard, H. J. (1975). The membrane attack mechanism of complement: verification of a stable C5b-9 complex in free solution. *J. Exp. Med.*, **141**, 724–32
19. Podack, E. R. and Muller-Eberhard, H. J. (1978). Binding of deoxycholate, phosphatidyl choline vesicles, lipoprotein and of the S-protein to complexes of terminal complement components. *J. Immunol.*, **121**, 1025–30
20. Murphy B. F., Kirszbaum, L., Walker, I. D. and d'Apice, A. J. F. (1988). SP-40,40, a newly identified normal human serum protein found in the SC5b-9 complex of complement and in the immune deposits in glomerulonephritis. *J. Clin. Invest.*, **81**, 1858–64
21. Murphy, B. F., Saunders, J. R., O'Bryan, M. K., Kirszbaum, L., Walker, I. D. and d'Apice, A. J. F. (1989). SP40,40 is an inhibitor of C5b-6 initiated haemolysis. *Int. Immunol.*, **1**, 551–4
22. Jenne, D. E. and Tschopp, J. (1989). Molecular structure and functional characterisation of a human complement cytolysis inhibitor found in blood and seminal plasma: identity to sulfated glycoprotein 2, a constituent of rat testis fluid. *Proc. Natl. Acad. Sci. USA*, **86**, 7123–7
23. Kirszbaum, L., Sharpe, J. A., Murphy, B., Hudson, P. and Walker, I. D. (1989). Molecular cloning and characterisation of the novel, human complement-associated protein, SP40,40: a link between the complement and reproductive systems. *EMBO J.*, **8**, 711–18
24. de Silva, H. V., Harmony, J. A. K., Stuart, W. D., Gil, C. M. and Robbins, J. (1990). Apolipoprotein J: Structure and tissue distribution. *Biochemistry*, **29**, 5380–9
25. Lint, T. F., Behrends, C. L. and Gewurz, H. (1977). Serum lipoproteins and C5b7-inhibitor activity. *J. Immunol.*, **119**, 883–8
26. Rosenfeld, S. I., Packman, C. H. and Leddy, J. P. (1983). Inhibition of the lytic action of cell-bound terminal complement components by human high density lipoproteins and apoproteins. *J. Clin. Invest.*, **71**, 795–808

27. Schonermark, S., Rauterberg, E. W., Shin, M. L., Loke, S., Roelcke, D. and Hansch, G. M. (1986). Homologous species restriction in lysis of human erythrocytes: a membrane-derived protein with C8-binding capacity functions as an inhibitor. *J. Immunol.*, **136**, 1772–6
28. Zalman, L. S., Wood., L. M. and Muller-Eberhard, H. J. (1986). Isolation of a human erythrocyte membrane protein capable of inhibiting expression of homologous complement transmembrane channels. *Proc. Natl. Acad. Sci. USA*, **83**, 6975–9
29. Watts, M. J., Patel, A. K. and Morgan, B. P. (1987). C9-binding protein: purification, characterization and re-incorporation into lipid vesicles. *Complement*, **4**, 236 (Abstr.)
30. Low, M. G. (1989). Glycosyl-phosphatidylinositol: a versatile membrane anchor for cell surface proteins. *FASEB J.*, **3**, 1600–8
31. Hansch, G. M., Weller, P. and Nicholson-Weller A. (1988). Release of C8bp from the cell membrane by phosphatidylinositol specific phospholipase C. *Blood*, **72**, 1089–92
32. Hansch, G. M. (1988). The homologous species restriction of complement attack: Structure and function of the C8 binding protein. *Curr. Top. Microbiol. Immunol.*, **140**, 109–18
33. Watts, M. J., Dankert, J. R. and Morgan, B. P. (1990). Isolation and characterisation of membrane attack complex inhibitory protein present in human serum and other biological fluids. *Biochem. J.*, **265**, 471–7
34. Zalman, L. S., Brothers, M. A. and Muller-Eberhard, H. J. (1989). Isolation of homologous restriction factor from human urine: Immunochemical properties and biological activity. *J. Immunol.*, **143**, 1943–7
35. Sugita, Y., Nakano, Y. and Tomita, M. (1988). Isolation from human erythrocytes of a new membrane protein which inhibits the formation of complement transmembrane channels. *J. Biochem. (Tokyo)*, **104**, 633–7
36. Holguin, M. H., Frederick, L. R., Bernshaw, N. J., Wilcox, L. A. and Parker, C. J. (1989). Isolation and characterisation of a membrane protein from normal human erythrocytes that inhibits reactive lysis of the erythrocytes of paroxysmal nocturnal haemoglobinuria. *J. Clin. Invest.*, **84**, 7–17
37. Sugita, Y., Tobe, T., Oda, E., Tomita, M., Yasukawa, K., Yamaji, N., Takemoto, T., Furichichi, K., Takayana, M. and Yano, S. (1989). Molecular cloning and characterisation of MACIF, an inhibitor of membrane channel formation of complement. *J. Biochem. (Tokyo)*, **106**, 555–7
38. Okada, N., Harada, R., Fujita, I. and Okada, H. (1989). A novel membrane glycoprotein capable of inhibiting membrane attack by homologous complement. *Int. Immunol.*, **1**, 205–9
39. Whitlow, M. B., Iida, K., Stefanova, I., Bernard, A. and Nussenzweig, V. (1990). H19, a surface membrane molecule involved in T-cell activation, inhibits channel formation by human complement. *Cell. Immunol.*, **162**, 176–84
40. Davies, A., Simmons, D. L., Hale, G., Harrison, R. A., Tighe, H., Lachmann, P. J. and Waldmann, H. (1989). CD59, an LY-6-like protein expressed in human lymphoid cells, regulates the action of the complement membrane attack complex on homologous cells. *J. Exp. Med.*, **170**, 637–54
41. Meri, S., Morgan, B. P., Davies, A., Daniels, R. H., Olavesen, M. G., Waldmann, H. and Lachman, P. J. (1990). Human protectin (CD59), an 18 000–20 000 MW complement lysis restricting factor, inhibits C5b-8 catalysed insertion of C9 into bilayers. *Immunology*, **71**, 1–9
42. Rollins, S. A. and Sims, P. J. (1990). The complement inhibitory activity of CD59 resides in its capacity to block incorporation of C9 into membrane C5b-9. *J. Immunol.*, **144**, 3478–83
43. Merry, A. H., Rawlinson, V. I., Uchikawa, M., Daha, M. R. and Sim, R. B. (1989). Studies of the sensitivity to complement mediated lysis of erythrocytes (Inab phenotype) with a deficiency of DAF (decay accelerating factor). *Br. J. Haematol.*, **73**, 248–53
44. Yamashina, M., Ueda, E., Kinoshita, T., Takami, T., Ojina, A., Ono, H. *et al.* (1990). Inherited complete deficiency of 20-kilodalton homologous restriction factor (CD59) as a cause of paroxysmal noctural haemoglobinuria. *N. Engl. J. Med.*, **323**, 1184–9
45. Goldberg B. and Green, H. (1959). The cytotoxic action of immune gamma globulin and complement on Krebs ascites tumor cells. I. Ultrastructural studies. *J. Exp. Med.*, **109**, 505–10
46. Green, H., Barrow P. and Goldberg, B. (1959). Effect of antibody and complement on permeability control in ascites tumor cells and erythrocytes. *J. Exp. Med.*, **110**, 689–713
47. Green, H. and Goldberg, B. (1960). The action of antibody and complement on mammalian cells. *Ann. NY Acad. Sci.*, **87**, 352–61
48. Moller, E. and Moller, G. (1962). Quantitative studies of sensitivity of normal and neoplastic cells to the cytotoxic action of isoantibodies. *J. Exp. Med.*, **115**, 527–34

49. Linscott, W. D. (1970). An antigen density effect on the hemolytic efficiency of complement. *J. Immunol.*, **104**, 1307–9
50. Cikes, M. (1970). Antigenic expression of an immune lymphoma during growth in vitro. *Nature (London)*, **225**, 645–6
51. Ferrone, S., Cooper, N. R., Pellegrino, M. A. and Reisfeld, R. A. (1973). Interaction of histocompatibility (HLA) antibodies and complement with synochronized human lymphoid cells in continuous culture. *J. Exp. Med.*, **137**, 55–68
52. Pellegrino, M. A., Ferrone, S., Cooper, N. R., Dierich, M. P. and Reisenfeld, R. A. (1974). Variation in susceptibility of a human lymphoid cell line to immune lysis during the cell cycle: lack of correlation with antigen density and complement binding. *J. Exp. Med.*, **140**, 578–90
53. Ohanian, S. H. and Borsos, T. (1975). Lysis of tumor cells by antibody and complement. II. Lack of correlation between amount of C4 and C3 fixed and cell lysis. *J. Immunol.*, **114**, 1292–5
54. Cooper, N. R., Polley, M. J. and Oldstone, M. B. A. (1974). Failure of terminal complement components to induce lysis of moloney virus transformed lymphocytes. *J. Immunol.*, **112**, 866–8
55. Segerling, M. S., Ohanian, S. H. and Borsos, T. (1975). Chemotherapeutic drugs increase killing of tumor cells by antibody and complement. *Science*, **188**, 55–7
56. Schlager, S. I., Ohanian, S. H. and Borsos, T. (1976). Inhibition of antibody-complement mediated killing of tumor cells by hormones. *Cancer Res.*, **36**, 3672–7
57. Segerling, M. S., Ohanian, S. H. and Borsos, T. (1975). Enhancing effect by metabolic inhibitors on the killing of tumour cells by antibody and complement. *Cancer Res.*, **35**, 3195–203
58. Ohanian, S. H. and Schlager, S. I. (1981). Humoral immune killing of nucleated cells: mechanisms of complement-mediated attack and target cell defense. *CRC Crit. Rev. Immunol.*, **1**, 165–209
59. Shin, M. L., Paznekas, W. A. and Mayer, M. M. (1978). On the mechanism of membrane damage by complement: the effect of length and saturation of the acyl chains in liposomal bilayers and the effect of cholesterol concentration in sheep erythrocytes and liposomal membranes. *J. Immunol.*, **120**, 1996–2002
60. Yoo, T. J., Chin, H. C., Spector, A. A., Whitaker, R. J., Denning, C. M. and Lee, N. F. (1980). Effect of fatty acid modifications of cultured hepatoma cells on susceptibility to complement-mediated cytolysis. *Cancer Res.*, **40**, 1084–90
61. Ohanian, S. H., Schlager, S. I. and Saha, S. (1982). Effect of lipids, structural precursors of lipids and fatty acids on complement-mediated killing of antibody-sensitized nucleated cells. *Mol. Immunol.*, **19**, 535–42
62. Boyle, M. D. P., Ohanian, S. and Borsos, T. (1978). Effect of protease treatment on the sensitivity of tumor cells to antibody-GPC killing. *Clin. Immunol. Immunopathol.*, **10**, 84–94
63. Mayer, M. M. (1972). Mechanisms of cytolysis by complement. *Proc. Natl. Acad. Sci. USA*, **69**, 2954–8
64. Ramm, L. E. and Mayer, M. M. (1980). Life span and size of the transmembrane channels formed by large doses of complement. *J. Immunol.*, **124**, 2281–7
65. Ramm, L. E., Whitlow, M. B. and Mayer, M. M. (1983). Size distribution and stability of the transmembrane channels formed by complement complex C5b-9. *Mol. Immunol.*, **20**, 155–60
66. Boyle, M. D. P., Ohanian, S. and Borsos, T. (1976). Lysis of tumor cells by antibody and complement VII. Complement-dependent ^{86}Rb release – a non-lethal event. *J. Immunol.*, **117**, 1346–50
67. Hallett, M. B., Luzio, J. P. and Campbell, A. K. (1981). Stimulation of Ca^{2+}-dependent chemiluminescence in rat polymorphonuclear leucocytes by polystyrene beads, and the non-lytic action of complement. *Immunology*, **44**, 569–77
68. Kaliner, M. and Austen, K. F. (1974). Adenosine 3′5-monophosphate: inhibition of complement mediated cell lysis. *Science*, **183**, 659–61
69. Boyle, M. D. P., Ohanian, S. and Borsos, T. (1976). Studies on the terminal stages of antibody-complement-mediated killing of a tumor cell. II. Inhibition of transformation of T^* to dead cells by 3′5′ cAMP. *J. Immunol.*, **116**, 1276–9
70. Stephens, C. L. and Henkart, P. A. (1979). Electrical measurements of complement-mediated membrane damage in cultured nerve and muscle cells. *J. Immunol.*, **122**, 455–8
71. Jackson, M. B., Stephens, C. L. and Lecar, H. (1981). Single channel currents induced by complement in antibody-coated cell membranes. *Proc. Natl. Acad. Sci. USA*, **79**, 6421–5

72. Koski, C. L., Ramm, L. E., Hammer, C. H., Mayer, M. M. and Shin, M. L. (1983). Cytolysis of nucleated cells by complement: cell death displays multi-hit characteristics. *Proc. Natl. Acad. Sci. USA*, **80**, 3816–20
73. Ramm, L. E., Whitlow, M. B., Koski, C. L., Shin, M. L. and Mayer, M. M. (1983). Elimination of complement channels from the plasma membranes of U937, a nucleated mammalian cell line: temperature dependence of the elimination rate. *J. Immunol.*, **131**, 1411–15
74. Ramm, L. E., Whitlow, M. B. and Mayer, M. M. (1984). Complement lysis of nucleated cells: effect of temperature and puromycin on the number of channels required for cytolysis. *Mol. Immunol.*, **21**, 1015–19
75. Ohanian, S. H., Schlager, S. I. and Borsos, T. (1977). Molecular interactions of cells with antibody and complement. *Contemp. Top. Mol. Immunol.*, **7**, 153–75
76. Richardson, P. J. and Luzio, J. P. (1980). Complement-mediated production of plasma membrane vesicles from rat fat cells. *Biochem. J.*, **186**, 897–906
77. Podack, E. R. and Muller-Eberhard, H. J. (1981). Complement-mediated membrane injury of tumor cells: release of membrane vesicles. *Fed. Proc.*, **40**, 359 (abstract)
78. Campbell, A. K. and Morgan, B. P. (1985). Monoclonal antibodies demonstrate protection of polymorphonunclear leukocytes against complement attack. *Nature* (*London*), **317**, 164–6
79. Morgan, B. P., Dankert, J. R. and Esser, A. F. (1987). Recovery of human neutrophils from complement attack removal of the membrane attack complex by endocytosis and exocytosis. *J. Immunol.*, **138**, 246–53
80. Carney, D. F., Koski, C. L. and Shin, M. L. (1985). Elimination of terminal complement intermediates from the plasma membrane of nucleated cells: The rate of disappearance differs for cells carrying C5b-7 or C5b-8 or a mixture of C5b-8 with a limited number of C5b-9. *J. Immunol.*, **134**, 1804–9
81. Camussi, G., Salvidio, G., Biesecker, G., Brentjens, J. and Andres, G. (1987). Heymann antibodies induce complement-dependent injury of rat glomerular visceral epithelial cells. *J. Immunol.*, **139**, 2906–14
82. Kerjaschki, D., Schulze, M., Binder, S., Kain, R., Ojha, P. P., Susani, M., Horvat, R., Baker, P. J. and Couser, W. G. (1989). Transcellular transport and membrane insertion of the C5b-9 membrane attack complex of complement by glomerular epithelial cells in experimental membranous nephropathy. *J. Immunol.*, **143**, 546–52
83. Campbell, A. K., Daw, R. A. and Luzio, J. P. (1979). Rapid increase in intracellular free Ca^{2+} induced by antibody plus complement. *FEBS Lett.*, **107**, 55–60
84. Campbell, A. K. and Luzio, J. P. (1981). Intracellular calcium as a pathogen in cell damage initiated by the immune system. *Experientia*, **37**, 110–12
85. Campbell, A. K., Daw, R. A., Hallett, M. B. and Luzio, J. P. (1981). Direct measurement of the increase in intracellular free Ca^{2+} concentration in response to the action of complement. *Biochem. J.*, **194**, 551–60
86. Morgan, B. P. and Campbell, A. K. (1985). The recovery of human polymorphonuclear leucocytes from sublytic complement attack is mediated by changes in intracellular free calcium. *Biochem. J.*, **231**, 205–8
87. Morgan, B. P., Luzio, J. P. and Campbell, A. K. (1986). Intracellular Ca^{2+} and cell injury: a paradoxical role of Ca^{2+} in complement membrane attack. *Cell Calcium*, **7**, 399–411
88. Carney, D. F., Hammer, C. H. and Shin, M. L. (1986). Elimination of terminal complement complexes in the plasma membrane of nucleated cells: influence of extracellular Ca^{2+}. *J. Immunol.*, **137**, 263–70
89. Sims, P. J. and Wiedmer, T. (1986). Repolarization of the membrane potential of blood platelets after complement damage: evidence for a Ca^{2+}-dependent exocytic elimination of C5b-9 pores. *Blood*, **68**, 556–61
90. Scolding, N. J., Houston, W. A. J., Morgan, B. P., Campbell, A. K. and Compston, D. A. S. (1989). Reversible injury of cultured rat oligodendrocytes by complement. *Immunology*, **67**, 441–6
91. Daniels, R. H., Houston, W. A., Petersen, M. M., Williams, J. D., Williams, B. D. and Morgan, B. P. (1990). Stimulation of rheumatoid synovial cells by non-lethal complement membrane attack. *Immunology*, **69**, 237–42
92. Cybulsky, A. V., Bonventre, J. V., Quigg, R. J., Lieberthal, W. and Salant, D. J. (1990). Cytosolic calcium and protein kinase C reduce complement-mediated glomerular epithelial injury. *Kidney Int.*, **38**, 803–11

93. Campbell, A. K. (1982). In *Intracellular Calcium: Its Universal Role as Regulator*, pp. 257–304. (Chichester: Wiley)
94. Weidmer, T., Ando, B. and Sims P. J. (1987). Complement C5b-9-stimulated platelet secretion is associated with a Ca^{2+}-initiated activation of cellular protein kinases. *J. Biol. Chem.*, **272**, 13674–81
95. Fischelson, Z., Kopf, E., Paas, Y., Ross, L. and Reiter, Y. (1989). Protcin phosphorylation as a mechanism of resistance against complement damage. *Prog. Immunol.*, **7**, 205–10
96. Carney, D. F., Lang, T. I. and Shin, M. L. (1990). Multiple signal messengers generated by terminal complement complexes and their role in terminal complex elimination. *J. Immunol.*, **145**, 623–9
97. Scolding, N. J., Morgan, B. P., Frith, S., Campbell, A. K. and Compston, D. A. S. (1990). Intracellular calcium and oligodendrocyte injury. *J. Neurol. Neurosurg. Psych.*, **53**, 811 (abstract)
98. Lo, T. N. and Boyle, M. D. P. (1979). Relationship between the intracellular cyclic adenosine 3′:5′-monophosphate level of tumor cells and their sensitivity to killing by antibody and complement. *Cancer Res.*, **39**, 3156–62
99. Roberts, P. A., Morgan, B. P. and Campbell, A. K. (1985). 2-Chloroadenosine inhibits complement-induced reactive oxygen metabolite production and recovery of human polymorphonuclear leucocytes attacked by complement. *Biochem. Biophys. Res. Commun.*, **126**, 692–7
100. Casey, P. J. and Gilman, A. G. (1988). G protein involvement in receptor-effector coupling. *J. Biol. Chem.*, **263**, 2577–80
101. Taylor, C. W. (1990). The role of G proteins in transmembrane signalling. *Biochem. J.*, **272**, 1–13
102. Carney, D. F. and Shin, M. L. (1987). Multiple signals are generated by terminal complement complexes (TCCs) to stimulate the elimination of TCC from the surface of nucleated cells (NC). *Complement*, **4**, 140 (abstract)
103. Daniels, R. H., Williams, B. D. and Morgan, B. P. (1990). Human rheumatoid synovial cell stimulation by the membrane attack complex and other pore-forming toxins in vitro; the role of calcium in cell activation. *Immunology*, **71**, 312–16
104. Weidmer, T., Shattil, S. J., Cunningham, M. and Sims, P. J. (1990). Role of calcium and calpain in complement-induced vesiculation of the platelet plasma membrane and in the exposure of the platelet factor Va receptor. *Biochemistry*, **29**, 623–32
105. Stein, J. M. and Luzio, J. P. (1990). Ectocytosis caused by sublytic autologous complement attack on human neutrophils: the sorting of endogenous plasma membrane proteins and lipids into shed vesicles. *Biochem. J.*, **274**, 381–6
106. Allan, D. and Michell R. H. (1979). The possible role of lipids in control of membrane fusion during secretion. *Symp. Soc. Exp. Biol.*, **33**, 323–36
107. Levine, Y. K. (1972). Physical studies of membrane structure. *Prog. Biophys. Mol. Biol.*, **24**, 1–74
108. Cheetham, J. J., Chen, R. J. B. and Epand, R. M. (1990). Interaction of calcium and cholesterol sulphate induces membrane destabilization and fusion: implications for the acrosome reaction. *Biochim. Biophys. Acta*, **1024**, 367–72
109. Cybulsky, A. V., Salant, D., Quigg, R. J., Badalamenti, J. and Bonventre, J. V. (1989). Complement C5b-9 complex activates phospholipases in glomerular epithelial cells. *Am. J. Physiol.*, **257**, F826–36
110. Morgan, B. P. (1988). Non-lethal complement membrane attack on human neutrophils: transient cell swelling and metabolic depletion. *Immunology*, **63**, 71–7
111. Nose, M., Katoh, M., Okada, N., Kyogoku, M. and Okada, H. (1990). Tissue distribution of HRF20, a novel factor preventing the membrane attack of homologous complement, and its predominant expression on endothelial cells in vivo. *Immunology*, **70**, 145–9
112. Rooney, I. A. and Morgan, B. P. (1990). Protection of human amniotic epithelial cells (HAEC) from complement-mediated killing: expression of three complement inhibitory membrane proteins. *Immunology*, **71**, 308–11.
113. Rooney, I. A., Davies, A., Griffiths, D., Williams, J. D., Davies, M., Meri, S., Lachmann, P. J. and Morgan, B. P. (1991). The complement inhibiting protein, protectin (CD59 antigen) is present and functionally active on glomerular epithelial cells. *Clin. Exp. Immunol.*, **83**, 251–6
114. Morgan, B. P. (1992). Effects of the membrane attack complex of complement on nucleated cells. *Curr. Top. Microbiol. Immunol.*, **178**, 115–40

115. Lachmann, P. J., Coombs, R. R. and Fell, H. B. (1969). The breakdown of embryonic (chick) cartilage and bone cultivated in the presence of complement–sufficient antiserum. 3. Immunological analysis. *Int. Arch. Allergy Appl. Immunol.*, **36**, 469-85
116. Cines, D. B. and Schreiber, A. D. (1979). Effect of anti-P1A1 antibody on human platelets. The role of complement. *Blood*, **53**, 567–77
117. Raisz, L. G., Sandberg, A. L., Goodson, J. M., Simmons, H. A. and Mergenhagen, S. E. (1974). Complement-dependent stimulation of prostaglandin synthesis and bone resorption. *Science*, **185**, 787–91
118. Sandberg, A. L., Raisz, L. G., Goodson, M. J., Simmons, H. A. and Mergenhagen, S. E. (1977). Limitation of bone resorption by the classical and alternative pathways and its mediation by prostaglandin. *J. Immunol.*, **119**, 1378–81
119. Halliwell, B. and Gutteridge, J. M. C. (1984). Oxygen toxicity, oxygen radicals, transition metals and disease. *Biochem. J.*, **219**, 1–14
120. Slater, T. F. (1984). Free-radical mechanisms in tissue injury. *Biochem. J.*, **222**, 1–15
121. Hansch, G. M., Seitz, M. and Betz, M. (1987). Effect of the late complement components C5b-9 on human monocytes: release of prostanoids, oxygen radicals and of a factor inducing cell proliferation. *Int. Arch. Allergy Appl. Immunol.*, **82**, 317–20
122. Adler, S., Baker, P., Johnson, R. J., Ochi, R., Pritzl, P. and Couser, W. G. (1986). Complement membrane attack complex stimulates production of reactive oxygen metabolites by cultured rat mesangial cells. *J. Clin. Invest.*, **77**, 762–7
123. Morgan, B. P., Daniels, R. H., Watts, M. J. and Williams, B. D. (1988). In vivo and in vitro evidence of cell recovery from complement attack in rheumatoid synovium. *Clin. Exp. Immunol.*, **73**, 467–72
124. Salmon, J. A. and Higgs, G. A. (1987). Prostaglandins and leukotrienes as inflammatory mediators. *Br. Med. Bull.*, **43**, 285–96
125. Lovett, D. H., Haensch, G. M., Goppelt, M., Resch, K. and Gemsa, F. (1987). Activation of glomerular mesangial cells by the terminal membrane attack complex of complement. *J. Immunol.*, **138**, 2473–80
126. Hansch, G. M., Betz, M., Gunther, J., Rother, K. O. and Sterzel, B. (1988). The complement membrane attack complex stimulates the prostanoid production of cultured glomerular mesangial cells. *Int. Arch. Allergy Appl. Immunol.*, **85**, 87–93
127. Suttorp, N., Seeger, W., Zinsky, S. and Bhakdi, S. (1987). Complement complex C5b-8 induces PGI_2 formation in cultured endothelial cells. *Am. J. Physiol.*, **253**, C13–21
128. Rooney, I. A. and Morgan, B. P. (1990). Non-lethal doses of antibody and complement stimulate release of prostaglandin E_2 from human amniotic cells *in vitro*. *Biochem. Soc. Trans.*, **18**, 617
129. Von Kempis, J., Torbohm, I., Schonermark, M., Jahn, B., Seitz, M. and Hansch, G. M. (1989). Effect of the late complement components C5b-9 and of platelet-derived growth factor on the prostaglandin release of human synovial fibroblast-like cells. *Int. Arch. Allergy Appl. Immunol.*, **90**, 248–55
130. Imagawa, D. K., Barbour, S. E., Morgan, B. P., Wright, T. M., Shin, H. S. and Ramm, L. E. (1987). Role of complement C9 and calcium in the generation of arachidonic acid metabolites from rat polymorphonuclear leukocytes. *Mol. Immunol.*, **24**, 1263–71
131. Segger, W., Suttorp, N., Helliwig, A. and Bhakdi, S. (1986). Non-cytolytic complement complexes may serve as calcium gates to elicit leukotriene B4 generation in human polymorphonuclear leukocytes. *J. Immunol.*, **137**, 1286–93
132. Betz, M., Seitz., M. and Hansch, G. M. (1987). Thromboxane B2 synthesis in human platelets induced by the late complement components C5b-9. *Int. Arch. Allergy Appl. Immunol.*, **82**, 323–6
133. Shirazi, Y., Imagawa, D. K. and Shin, M. L. (1987). Release of leukotriene B4 from sublethally injured oligodendrocytes by terminal complement complexes. *J. Neurochem.*, **48**, 271–8
134. Ramm, L. E., Whitlow, M. B. and Mayer, M. M. (1982). Size of the transmembrane channels produced by complement proteins C5b-8. *J. Immunol.*, **129**, 1143–6
135. Morgan, B. P. (1984). The biochemistry and pathology of complement component C9. *PhD Thesis*, pp. 235–74. University of Wales
136. Shirazi, Y., McMorris, F. A. and Shin, M. L. (1989). Arachidonic acid mobilization and phosphoinositide turnover by the terminal complement complex, C5b-9, in rat oligodendrocyte $\times$ C6 glioma cell hybrids. *J. Immunol.*, **142**, 4385–91

137. Suttorp, N., Seeger, W., Zucker-Reimann, J., Roka, L. and Bhakdi, S. (1987). Mechanism of leukotriene generation in polymorphonuclear leukocytes by staphylococcal alpha-toxin. *Infect. Immun.*, **55**, 104–10
138. Wiegard, R., Betz, M. and Hansch, G. M. (1988). Nystatin stimulates prostaglandin E synthesis and formation of diacylglycerol in human monocytes. *Agents Actions*, **24**, 243–50
139. Daniels, R. H., Williams, B. D. and Morgan, B. P. (1990). Non-lethal complement membrane attack on cultured synovial cell induces G-protein and calcium-dependent PGE_2 release and release of IL-6. *Complement Inflamm.*, **7**, 137 (abstract)
140. Hansch, G. M., Torbohm, I. and Rother, K. (1989). Chronic glomerulonephritis: inflammatory mediators stimulate the collagen synthesis in glomerular epithelial cells. *Int. Arch. Allergy Appl. Immunol.*, **88**, 139–43
141. Torbohm, I., Schonermark, M., Wingen, A. M., Berger, B., Rother, K. and Hansch, G. M. (1990). C5b-8 and C5b-9 modulate the collagen release of human glomerular epithelial cells. *Kindney Int.*, **37**, 1098–104
142. Jahn, B., von Kempis, J. and Hansch, G. M. (1990). Induction of prostaglandin E2 (PGE2) and collagenase synthesis in human synovial fibroblast-like cells (SFC) by terminal complement components C5b-9. *Complement Inflamm.*, **7**, 138 (abstract)
143. Shirazi, Y., Macklin, W. B. and Shin, M. L. (1990). Terminal complement complexes (TCC) inhibit myelin protein mRNA expression in oligodendrocytes (OLG). *FASEB J.*, **4**, A2017 (abstract)
144. Wiedmer, T., Esmon, C. T. and Sims, P. J. (1986). On the mechanism by which complement proteins C5b-9 increase platelet prothrombinase activity. *J. Biol. Chem.*, **261**, 14587–92
145. Ando, B., Wiedmer, T., Hamilton, K. K. and Sims, P. J. (1988). Complement proteins C5b-9 initiate secretion of platelet storage granules without increased binding of fibrinogen or von Willebrand factor to newly expressed cell surface GPIIb-IIIa. *J. Biol. Chem.*, **263**, 11907–14
146. Ando, B., Wiedmer, T. and Sims, P. J. (1989). The secretory release reaction initiated by complement proteins C5b-9 occurs without platelet aggregation through glycoproteins IIb-IIIa. *Blood*, **73**, 462–7
147. Morgan, B. P. (1989). Mechanisms of tissue damage by the membrane attack complex of complement. *Complement Inflamm.*, **6**, 104–11
148. Couser, W. G., Baker, P. J. and Adler, S. (1985). Complement and the direct mediation of immune glomerular injury: a new perspective. *Kidney Int.*, **28**, 879–90
149. Salant, D. J., Quigg, R. J. and Cybulsky, A. V. (1989). Heymann nephritis: mechanisms of renal injury. *Kidney Int.*, **35**, 976–90
150. Groggel, G. C., Salant, D. J., Darby, C., Rennke, H. G. and Couser, W. G. (1985). Role of terminal complement pathway in the heterologous phase of antiglomerular basement membrane nephritis. *Kidney Int.*, **27**, 643–51
151. Cybulsky, A. V., Rennke, H. G., Feintzeig, I. D. and Salant, D. J. (1986). Complement-induced glomerular epithelial cell injury. Role of the membrane attack complex in rat membranous nephropathy. *J. Clin. Invest.*, **77**, 1096–107
152. Morgan, B. P., Daniels, R. H. and Williams, B. D. (1988). Measurement of terminal complement complexes in rheumatoid arthritis. *Clin. Exp. Immunol.*, **73**, 473–8
153. Sanders, M. E., Kopicky, J. A., Wigley, F. M., Shin, M. L., Frank, M. M. and Joner, K. A. (1986). Membrane attack complex of complement in rheumatoid synovial tissue demonstrated by immunofluorescent microscopy. *J. Rheumatol.*, **13**, 1028–34
154. Rauterberg, E. W. (1987). Demonstration of complement deposits in tissues. In Rother, K. and Till, G. O. (eds.) *The Complement System*, pp. 287–326. (Berlin: Springer-Verlag)
155. Morgan, B. P. (1990). *Complement, Clinical Aspects and Relevance to Disease.* (London: Academic Press)

13 Complement in diseases of the nervous system

B. P. MORGAN

INTRODUCTION

Tissue damage in many neurological diseases is mediated, at least in part, by components of the immune system. Both cellular and humoral elements have been implicated and immune complex deposition demonstrated. This chapter focusses on the evidence implicating complement in these diseases. Excellent reviews of the role of the immune system in the pathogenesis of several neurological diseases exist, and the interested reader is urged to consult these to obtain a less focussed overview.

The potential role of complement in pathogenesis has been investigated in only a small number of conditions. These include diseases in which activation of complement may be directly responsible for tissue damage (for example, multiple sclerosis), and conditions where a defective complement system contributes to pathogenesis (for example, meningococcal meningitis). Evidence of complement involvement has been obtained from *in vitro* observations, from animal models and from observations in human diseases. For the sake of clarity, each of these diseases will be discussed separately.

COMPLEMENT IN MULTIPLE SCLEROSIS

Multiple sclerosis is a chronic inflammatory disease of the central nervous system characterized histologically by localized areas of tissue damage and demyelination scattered throughout the white matter. It is one of the commonest neurological diseases, particularly in temperate climates where its prevalence may exceed 1 in 1000. There is a slight female preponderance and associations with HLA antigens DR2, DR4 and DRw6 have been reported. The clinical presentation and progress of the disease are extremely variable, but the majority of cases present in the third or fourth decades of life with evidence of disease at a single site. The subsequent course is usually one of remissions and relapses, each attack leaving some residual disability, the cumulative effect being a gradual deterioration over the course of 10–20 years[1,2].

Despite intensive research efforts, the cause of multiple sclerosis remains unknown. Evidence suggesting a genetic susceptibility (HLA associations, increased incidence in first-degree relatives), an infective agent ('epidemics' of disease, increased antiviral antibody titres) and autoimmunity has been produced and theories of pathogenesis combining some or all of these factors abound[3,4]. Involvement of the immune system is suggested by the demonstration of increased amounts of immunoglobulin[5,6], immune complexes[7,8] and T and B lymphocytes[9,10] in the brain and cerebrospinal fluid in multiple sclerosis.

The presence of increased levels of immunoglobulin in cerebrospinal fluid from multiple sclerosis patients was first noted over 40 years ago[11]. Subsequently, it was shown that this increase is due to intrathecal synthesis of immunoglobulin by a small number of B cell clones – an oligoclonal response[12]. A small proportion of these immunoglobulin species appear to be directed against CNS proteins, antibodies against myelin and cellular elements being present in some but not all patients[13]. The possibility that these antibodies alone or in concert with complement might be responsible for the pathology of multiple sclerosis has been intensively investigated. Evidence has emerged from studies of demyelination of myelinated tissue *in vitro*, from the principal animal model of multiple sclerosis, experimental allergic encephalomyelitis, and directly from studies of the human disease. This evidence is summarized in the following sections.

Depolarization and demyelination *in vitro*

A variety of *in vitro* systems have been developed to examine the effects of serum and CSF from multiple sclerosis patients on the function and morphology of neural tissue. Initially it was shown that sera from patients with multiple sclerosis (or from animals with experimental allergic encephalomyelitis, see below) blocked neural conduction in spinal cord and cerebral explants from rodents and frogs[14,15], whereas serum from normal individuals or patients with other neurological diseases does not cause blocking. Furthermore, in multiple sclerosis patients, the degree of blocking activity correlates with disease severity. Blocking activity is lost upon heating of the serum to 56°C but is restored upon adding fresh normal serum, suggesting a requirement for active complement. The specific factor in multiple sclerosis serum and cerebrospinal fluid resides within the immunoglobulin fractions, thus implying that activation of complement by antibody is responsible for the effect. Blockade is rapid (onset within a few minutes) and partially reversible, suggesting that it is due to a transient depolarization of the conducting elements and not to their destruction.

Sera and cerebrospinal fluid from multiple sclerosis patients (and from animals with experimental allergic encephalomyelitis) also cause demyelination of myelinated cultures of rat neural tissue[16–18]. The patterns of demyelination observed in these culture systems closely resemble the changes seen in multiple sclerosis brain lesions. As with the effects on conduction, the demyelinating activity is heat labile, but restorable by fresh normal serum, and the disease-specific heat-stable factor is an immunoglobulin, implicating complement and antibody respectively. It has recently been suggested that demyelination of myelinated cultures by multiple sclerosis serum is not entirely complement dependent but is mediated, at least in part, by an as yet unidentified heat-labile non-complement factor[19]. This report awaits clarification. Nevertheless, complement is certainly capable of causing demyelination *in vitro*. Shin and co-workers examined the role of complement in demyelination of myelinated mouse cerebellum cultures by antispinal cord antibody and serum. They found that serum deficient in C8 does not cause demyelination, and restoration of C8 to the serum restores its demyelinating capacity. As the only known function of C8 is to participate in the formation of the membrane attack complex (MAC), these studies implicate the MAC directly as the cause of myelin damage in this system[20,21]. The vesicular disruption of myelin caused by the MAC *in vitro* closely resembles that seen upon exposure of myelin to the calcium ionophore A23187[22], suggesting that damage is the result of calcium flux through the MAC[23]. It has recently been shown that calcium influx through the MAC activates endogenous calcium-dependent neutral proteases in myelin, thereby causing hydrolysis of myelin basic protein and myelin degradation[24]. Isolated myelin activates the classical pathway of complement even in the absence of antibody[25–27]. Areas of damaged myelin may therefore provide foci for complement activation *in vivo*, enabling complement-mediated demyelination to proceed even in the absence of antibrain antibodies.

Complement effect on glial cells *in vitro*

The oligodendrocyte is the cell responsible for synthesizing myelin within the central nervous system and for maintaining it in lamellar sheaths around exons. Damage to or destruction of oligodendrocytes will therefore have profound effects on the ability of axons to conduct. Recent studies have shown that rat oligodendrocytes activate homologous complement via the classical pathway in the absence of antibody and are highly susceptible to killing by the MAC[28,29]. This property is shared by adult oligodendrocyte/type-2 astrocyte precursor cells but not by other cells of the central nervous system. It has been suggested that a selective complement-induced loss of these susceptible cell types might explain the failure of remyelination which is a central feature of multiple sclerosis[30,31]. Oligodendrocytes are not killed upon exposure to rat serum specifically depleted of C1 or of C9, but adding back the missing component restores killing, confirming that activation occurs via the classical pathway and that lysis is caused by the MAC. The specific features of the oligodendrocyte which allow C1 binding and activation in the absence of antibody are as yet unidentified. Susceptibility of oligodendrocytes to complement killing is not merely a reflection of their capacity to activate, the cells also appear to be highly vulnerable to killing by amounts of the MAC which are not lethal for other nucleated cells. One possible explanation for this phenomenon is that these cells lack surface MAC inhibitory proteins (HRF, CD59 – see Chapter 12) present on other cell types, a hypothesis which has yet to be tested.

Sublytic complement activation and MAC formation on oligodendrocytes cause a number of non-lethal changes. These include the release of arachidonic acid metabolites[32,33], changes in intracellular calcium and ATP concentrations and vesiculation[34]. The MAC-induced increase in intracellular calcium concentration is an essential signal in the induction of these non-lethal effects and removal of extracellular calcium prevents their occurrence. Vesiculation, which is also calcium dependent, appears to be a recovery mechanism, limiting cell lysis by removing MACs from the cell surface (see Chapter 12). It has recently been shown that non-lethal amounts of the MAC cause decreased expression of myelin basic protein message in cultured oligodendrocytes, suggesting a direct effect of the MAC on myelin synthesis[35]. Thus, formation of MACs on oligodendrocytes may cause cell death or initiate a number of non-lethal effects, including metabolic depletion, release of inflammatory mediators and decreased synthesis of myelin proteins. Both non-lethal and lethal events may occur *in vivo* and contribute to oligodendrocyte damage following their exposure to levels of complement which do not damage other cells in the central nervous system.

Complement in animal models of multiple sclerosis

Experimental allergic encephalomyelitis is induced in experimental animals by immunization with tissue or specific purified proteins of the central nervous system in Freund's complete adjuvant. In the classical acute disease signs develop about ten days after immunization and follow a predictable course of weight loss and ascending paralysis, terminating in death or recovery. In survivors, recovery is complete and relapse is rare. Acute experimental allergic encephalomyelitis is an autoimmune reaction against central nervous system antigens and is characterized histologically by perivascular infiltrates of inflammatory cells. The clinical signs are attributable to oedema of the central nervous system, and demyelination is sparse or absent. Despite these obvious differences from multiple sclerosis, which is a chronic demyelinating disease, experimental allergic encephalomyelitis has been widely used as an experimental model. Several strategies have been employed to produce variants which more closely resemble the human disease. Chronic, demyelinating forms have been induced in a variety of species[36], and immunization with a demyelinating antibody during the induction of acute experimental allergic encephalomyelitis in rats produces a severe demyelinating form of the disease[37].

Evidence for a primary role of T cells in the pathogenesis of experimental allergic encephalomyelitis is compelling. Disease can be transferred from affected animals to naive recipients by transfusion of T cells, and encephalitogenic clones of T cells have been generated *in vitro*[38]. Nevertheless, there is also substantial evidence that complement contributes to pathogenesis. Decomplementation of animals prior to the onset of clinical disease, using cobra venom factor, delays or suppresses the development of symptoms in acute experimental allergic encephalomyelitis and, to a lesser extent, in the antibody-enhanced and T cell transfer variants of the disease[39–42] (Figure 13.1). Although in the initial studies of acute experimental allergic encephalomyelitis[42], decomplementation had little effect on central nervous system inflammation despite the marked

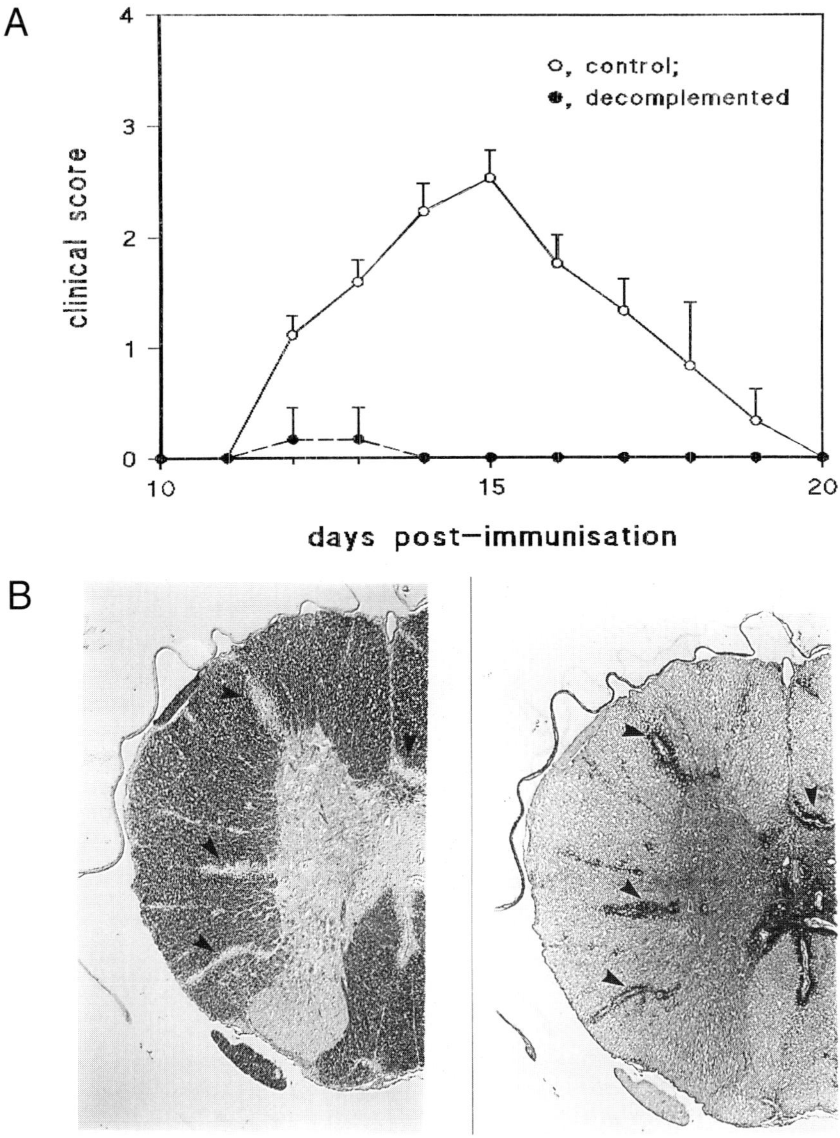

Figure 13.1 Complement in experimental allergic encephalomyelitis (EAE). **A** Effect of decomplementation on clinical disease in acute EAE. Ten Lewis rats were inoculated with myelin basic protein in adjuvant on day 0. Ten days later, half the animals were decomplemented using cobra venom factor, the other half receiving a sham injection. Clinical disease was assessed daily in all animals and scored on a scale of 0 (no disease) to 4 (moribund or dead). The points represent the average clinical scores for the animals in the decomplemented group (closed circles) and the control group (open circles) on each day and vertical bars represent standard deviations. Modified from Ref. 42. **B** MAC deposition in the CNS in EAE. Serial sections of spinal cord from rat with EAE showing co-localization of extensive demyelination (left: pale areas, arrowed) and heavy deposits of C9 (right: dark staining, arrowed). Magnification ×42. Courtesy of Dr H. Lassmann, Austrian Academy of Sciences, Vienna, Austria

inhibition of clinical disease, it has recently been shown that the maintenance of complete decomplementation can only be achieved by giving multiple doses of cobra venom factor during the experimental period: under these circumstances, inflammation in the central nervous system is markedly diminished[43]. It is therefore likely that complement activation in the central nervous system is an important stimulus for the infiltration of inflammatory cells in acute experimental allergic encephalomyelitis. An acute demyelinating form of experimental allergic encephalomyelitis can be induced by the intravenous infusion of an antibody against myelin-oligodendrocyte glycoprotein during the induction of disease, and chronic demyelinating forms can be induced in susceptible rat strains by immunization with a homogenate of central nervous system tissue. Although there is no direct evidence that complement is involved in demyelination in these forms of experimental allergic encephalomyelitis, a role for the MAC is suggested by the demonstration of granular deposits of C9 (indicative of MAC formation) around inflamed vessels and in areas of active demyelination in both models[44] (Figure 13.1). Macrophages also contribute to demyelination in these models and the roles and interactions between these effectors in bringing about demyelination remain uncertain.

Evidence for complement in multiple sclerosis (Table 13.1)

Early studies of complement activation in multiple sclerosis involved the measurement of the levels of native components (C3, C4, factor B) or haemolytic

Table 13.1 Evidence implicating complement in demyelination

Source	*Evidence*	*References*
In vitro	MS/EAE sera and CSF cause DM in CNS culture	14,15
	DM *in vitro* requires assembly of complete MAC	20,21
	Isolated myelin activates complement	25–27
	Oligodendrocytes activate and are readily damaged by complement	28–31
Animal model (EAE)	Decomplementation with CVF ameliorates	39–42
	MAC deposition in areas of active disease in CNS	43,44
Human disease	Alterations in haemolytic complement and individual components in CSF	45–49
	Presence of TCCs in CSF	54,55
	Oligodendrocyte-derived MAC-positive fragments in CSF	29
	MAC deposition in and around plaques in brain	56

DM, demyelination; MS, multiple sclerosis; EAE, experimental allergic encephalomyelitis; CNS, central nervous system; CSF, cerebrospinal fluid; MAC, membrane attack complex; TCC, terminal complement complex; CVF, cobra venom factor

complement activity in cerebrospinal fluid and/or plasma of patients and controls[45–49]. The results of these studies were contradictory and confusing. Measurement of the terminal complement component C9 in the cerebrospinal fluid of patients with neurological disease demonstrated significantly lower levels of C9 in multiple sclerosis and this was interpreted as evidence for complement activation and MAC formation within the central nervous system[50,51]. Two subsequent studies have found only small and insignificant decreases in C9 levels in cerebrospinal fluid of patients with multiple sclerosis[52,53]. In retrospect, it seems likely that the choice of control group in the initial report, which included several individuals with pathologically elevated C9 levels, served to magnify small differences. Nevertheless, the report focussed attention on the possibility of complement involvement in multiple sclerosis and led to the investigation of other indices of activation.

Measurement of activation products provides a superior index of complement activation as it is much less influenced by parameters such as the acute-phase response or blood–brain barrier leakage. The fluid-phase terminal complement complex (TCC) has been shown to be present in increased amounts in the cerebrospinal fluid in up to 70% of patients with multiple sclerosis[54,55], providing strong evidence that complement activation occurs to completion in the central nervous system (Figure 13.2). The TCC has also been localized immunocytochemically within the brain in autopsy tissue from 5 out of 7 multiple sclerosis patients but is absent in control tissue[56] (Figure 13.2). MACs are present in and around the walls of blood vessels of the plaques of the brains of patients with multiple sclerosis, but are not present in central nervous system tissue which is remote from the plaques[56]. This distribution is similar to that occurring in the central nervous system of animals with experimental allergic encephalomyelitis. The granular nature of the deposits in and around the blood vessels suggests that they are derived from myelin or cellular elements within the central nervous system. In support of this, examination of cerebrospinal fluid samples from patients with multiple sclerosis revealed the presence of membrane fragments in eleven of nineteen cases. These fragments stained strongly for the oligodendrocyte/myelin marker, galactocerebroside, and also for the MAC[29]. Their staining characteristics and close physical similarity to the vesicles shed from oligodendrocytes *in vitro* prompted the suggestion that these fragments represent vesicles shed from oligodendrocytes and/or myelin during non-lethal complement attack *in vivo*.

A hypothesis for complement involvement in multiple sclerosis

The experimental evidence obtained *in vitro*, from animal studies and from examination of the human disease, supports an involvement of complement in the pathogenesis of multiple sclerosis. It is possible that opening of the blood–brain barrier by T cells or other initiating effectors allows entry of complement components into the central nervous system.

Complement activation could then occur spontaneously on damaged myelin or on cells, releasing inflammatory mediators, further damaging myelin and selectively killing the highly sensitive oligodendrocytes. The anaphylatoxin C5a

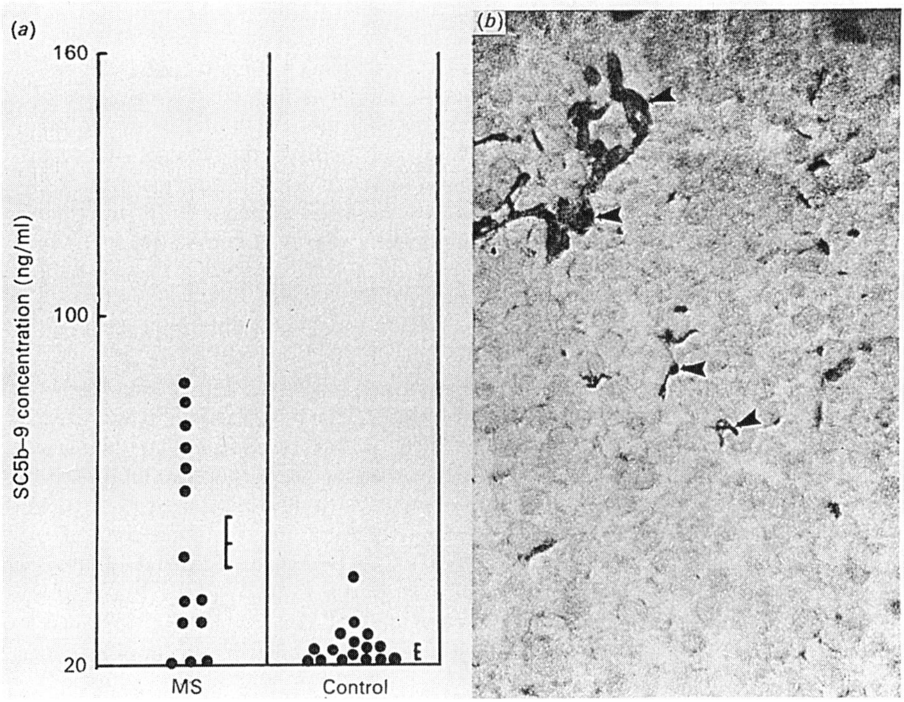

Figure 13.2 Cerebrospinal fluid and tissue terminal complement complexes (TCCs) in multiple sclerosis. (***a***) Concentrations of TCCs (SC5b-9) in the cerebrospinal fluid of multiple sclerosis patients compared with those in control individuals. Bars represent mean plus or minus standard error for each group. (***b***) A plaque from the brain of a patient with multiple sclerosis stained with TCC-specific (antineoantigenic) antibodies. Granular staining is present in and around capillaries (arrowed). (From Morgan, *Biochem. J.*, **264**, 1–14 (1989), with permission)

which is formed during complement activation, together with mediators released from attacked oligodendrocytes, will attract phagocytic cells into the forming lesion and activate them, further exacerbating inflammation. A variety of agents and insults which raise intracellular calcium levels have been observed to cause disruption of myelin *in vitro*[22,57–59], and non-lethal complement membrane attack on oligodendrocytes and myelin may damage myelin by this mechanism. Complement could therefore be involved in inflammation, demyelination and failure to remyelinate, all of which are characteristic of the disease (Figure 13.3). This hypothesis envisages complement as a secondary factor, acting only after the initiating agent has breached the blood–brain barrier, but then playing a major role in the evolution of the lesion.

Why then does not blood–brain barrier breakdown in other diseases of the central nervous system or following trauma initiate a chronic demyelinating disease akin to multiple sclerosis? It is possible that demyelination occurs in multiple sclerosis because blood–brain barrier leakage is widespread and occurs

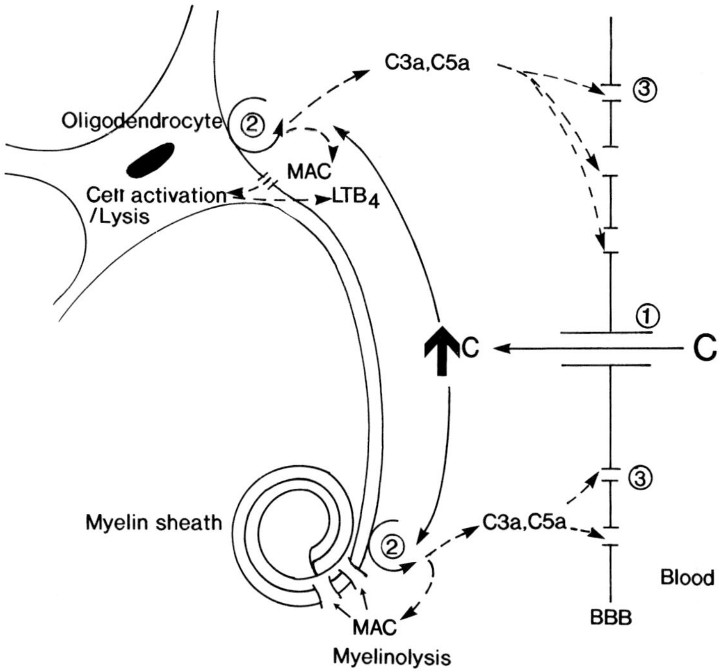

Figure 13.3 Role of complement in demyelination. A schematic representation of the potential role of complement in demyelination. ① The initial insult causing blood–brain barrier (BBB) damage allows influx of complement components into the CNS, exposing tissues to abnormally high concentrations of complement. ② Activation of complement and MAC formation on oligodendrocytes causes lethal or non-lethal changes, disturbing the capacity of the cell to maintain myelin. Direct complement attack on myelin initiates myelin breakdown. ③ Anaphylatoxins C3a and C5a released during intrathecal complement activation further disturb BBB integrity and allow entry of yet more complement.

The important contributions of cellular effectors, some of which may be recruited by complement activation products, are omitted from this simplified scheme

frequently or because some additional abnormality of the glial cells is present. This important area is now a major focus of investigation.

COMPLEMENT AND THE GUILLAIN–BARRÉ SYNDROME

Guillain–Barré syndrome is an acute or subacute generalized polyneuropathy which may occur spontaneously, may follow a viral infection or, occasionally, vaccination[60]. The annual incidence rate in the USA is about 1.7 per 100 000 and the incidence in women is twice that in men[61]. In most cases, the disease is self-limiting and at least 75% of patients make a complete recovery. Involved nerves are infiltrated with mononuclear cells and phagocytes, and segmental demyelination occurs[62].

Many aetiological factors have been implicated. It has long been suspected that an infectious agent is involved. Although increased viral antibody titres are often present, extensive investigation has failed to reveal a consistent association with any one organism. However, the possibility remains that viral infection of cells within the peripheral nervous system is the initiating factor.

The pathological appearances of the lesions in Guillain–Barré syndrome are highly suggestive of an immune reaction, and a role of the immune system in the disease process is supported by several lines of evidence. The animal model for Guillain–Barré syndrome, experimental allergic neuritis, appears to be mediated primarily by T cells, and the target antigen has been identified in peripheral nerve myelin[63,64]. However, in the human disease, evidence for cellular immunity is tenuous and contradictory[65,66]. Humoral immunity was first implicated in the pathogenesis with the demonstration that sera from some patients with the Guillain–Barré syndrome caused demyelination of peripheral nerve in culture and *in vivo*[67,68]. It was subsequently shown that the great majority of patients have complement-fixing serum antibodies reactive with Schwann cells and/or peripheral nerve myelin[69,70]. These antibodies are predominantly IgM and react with several peripheral nerve myelin antigens, including a neutral glycolipid which resembles the Forssman antigen[71]. The titre of antibodies in the serum closely correlates with disease activity[72], and plasmapheresis, which markedly reduces antibody titres, shortens the course of the disease[73], suggesting a causative role for antibody in pathogenesis.

Direct evidence of complement activation in Guillain–Barré syndrome has been provided by the demonstration of high levels of the anaphylatoxins, C3a and C5a, in cerebrospinal fluid[74], and of the TCC in both cerebrospinal fluid and serum[54,75]. The TCC has also been localized in peripheral nerves of patients with the disease[72]. It is therefore possible that the MAC is directly responsible for the observed demyelination. This concept is supported by the observation that sera of patients with Guillain–Barré syndrome are able to demyelinate peripheral nerve *in vitro*[67,68]. These sera cause demyelination in a tissue culture model prior to, but not following, heat treatment to destroy complement. Addition of fresh

Table 13.2 Antibody and complement in peripheral neuropathies

Evidence	*References*	
	GBS	*PN*
Sera from some patients causes demyelination *in vitro*	67,68	79
Complement-fixing IgM antibodies against peripheral nerve myelin in serum	69,70	76–78
Antibody titre proportional to disease activity	72	—
Plasmapheresis ameliorates disease	73	80
Complement activation products in serum and/or CSF	54,74,75	75
Complement activation products and MAC in peripheral nerve	72	81,82
MAC-dependence of demyelination *in vitro*	72	83

GBS, Guillain–Barré syndrome; PN, paraprotein neuropathy; CSF, cerebrospinal fluid; MAC, membrane attack complex

normal serum as a source of complement restores the demyelinating capacity of heat-inactivated Guillain–Barré syndrome serum whereas serum depleted of C7 does not. Thus, at least in this model system, formation of the MAC is a requirement for demyelination[72].

Complement and the MAC, activated by specific antimyelin antibodies, are therefore strong candidates as major demyelinating factors in Guillain–Barré syndrome. As with multiple sclerosis, the events which breach the blood–nerve or blood–brain barriers, allowing these agents access to myelin antigens, remain unknown. Cell-mediated mechanisms, already implicated in multiple sclerosis, are likely to be responsible for this vital stage in pathogenesis. The evidence implicating antibody and complement in the pathogenesis of Guillain–Barré syndrome is summarized in Table 13.2.

COMPLEMENT AND PARAPROTEIN NEUROPATHY

A minority of patients with malignant or benign paraproteinaemia develop a slowly progressive demyelinating peripheral neuropathy. Most of these individuals have a complement-fixing IgM paraprotein which recognizes myelin-associated glycoprotein and a specific ganglioside in peripheral nerve myelin[76–78]. The histological picture is one of patchy demyelination and remyelination and the IgM antibody is deposited on myelin sheaths in areas of demyelination. Evidence that this antibody is causally related to pathogenesis is provided by the demonstration that serum from these patients causes demyelination *in vitro*[79], and by the therapeutic efficacy of plasmapheresis[80].

Recently, direct evidence of a causative role of complement in demyelination associated with the neuropathy has accumulated. Ongoing complement activation in patients with this syndrome is indicated by the demonstration of increased levels of TCC in serum[75] and the co-localization of complement components, C1q, C3b, C5 and MAC, with the IgM antibody in myelin sheaths of affected nerve[81,82]. IgM-mediated complement-dependent demyelination has also been demonstrated in a model system and the MAC implicated in bringing about the typical myelin changes observed in the human disease[83].

The frequent association of IgM antibodies, but not IgG antibodies, against myelin antigens with peripheral neuropathy is noteworthy. Because a single IgM molecule can bind and activate C1, IgM antibodies are far more efficient than IgG antibodies at fixing complement, particularly when the target antigen is sparse and evenly distributed on the surface[84–86]. Thus IgG antibodies against the minor myelin surface antigens are unlikely to fix complement and cause disease. The use of IgG antibodies against specific myelin antigens as ‘blocking antibodies’ to prevent binding of IgM antibodies to myelin might be efficacious in the treatment of paraprotein neuropathy and Guillain–Barré syndrome.

COMPLEMENT AND MYASTHENIA GRAVIS

Myasthenia gravis is a chronic disease characterized by abnormal muscle fatiguability which may be localized or generalized. Ocular and facial muscles are most commonly affected and diplopia and ptosis are common presenting complaints. In severe cases, involvement of respiratory muscles can lead to shortness of breath or even respiratory failure. The disease may occur at any age, but there are marked sex differences, females most commonly having an early age of onset (10–30 years) whereas in males onset is more often late (50–70 years). Hyperplastic changes are commonly seen in the thymus in myasthenia gravis and thymic tumours are present in a minority of patients[87].

It was suggested over 90 years ago that myasthenia gravis is caused by a circulating curare-like toxin which caused blockage or destruction of the motor end plate[88]. The concept of a circulating toxin is supported by the demonstration that some myasthenic sera cause neuromuscular blockade[89], and by the observation that a proportion of infants born to myasthenic mothers had a transient form of the disease during the first two months of life[90]. The active factor was subsequently shown to be immunoglobulin directed against muscle fibres[91,92], which is also reactive with thymic epithelium[93].

A major advance in the understanding of myasthenia gravis came from studies examining the binding in myasthenic muscle of neurotoxins specific for the acetylcholine receptor (AChR)[94]. These studies demonstrated that AChR numbers are decreased markedly in myasthenia gravis, implying that the central defect is receptor loss, and suggest that the circulating antibody in myasthenic serum is directed against the receptor. These concepts are supported by the results of animal studies. Immunization of a wide range of species with purified AChR induced disease, experimental autoimmune myasthenia gravis, which closely resembled human myasthenia gravis[95,96]. The disease can be passively transferred to naive animals by serum or immunoglobulin, confirming that it is antibody mediated.

There is abundant evidence for a role of complement in the pathogenesis of both the naturally-occurring and experimentally-induced disease. Complement-fixing anti-AChR antibodies are present; thus, the potential for complement activation at the end-plate exists. Hypocomplementaemia[97] and decreased levels of C2 and C4[98] have been observed during exacerbations of myasthenia gravis, and complement components, C3 and C9, and the MAC have all been localized at the motor end-plate in association with IgG[99–101]. Complement components are also found at the end-plate in experimental autoimmune myasthenia gravis[102], and animals depleted of complement by treatment with cobra venom factor are refractory to active (immunization with AChR) or passive (transfusion of antibody) induction of disease[103], suggesting a central role for complement in pathogenesis of this disease.

Definitive evidence for a direct role for complement in mediating AChR loss in experimental autoimmune myasthenia gravis has recently emerged from studies in rats which were specifically depleted of C6 by injection of the Fab′ fragment of an anti-C6 antibody[104]. Animals rendered C6-deficient in this way failed to develop signs when transfused with immunoglobulin from diseased animals, whereas their C6-sufficient litter mates developed classical features of the disease (Figure 13.4). The early parts of the pathway and all the inflammatory-cell-recruiting elements are intact in the C6-depleted animals, suggesting that formation of MACs is directly responsible for receptor loss in this disease.

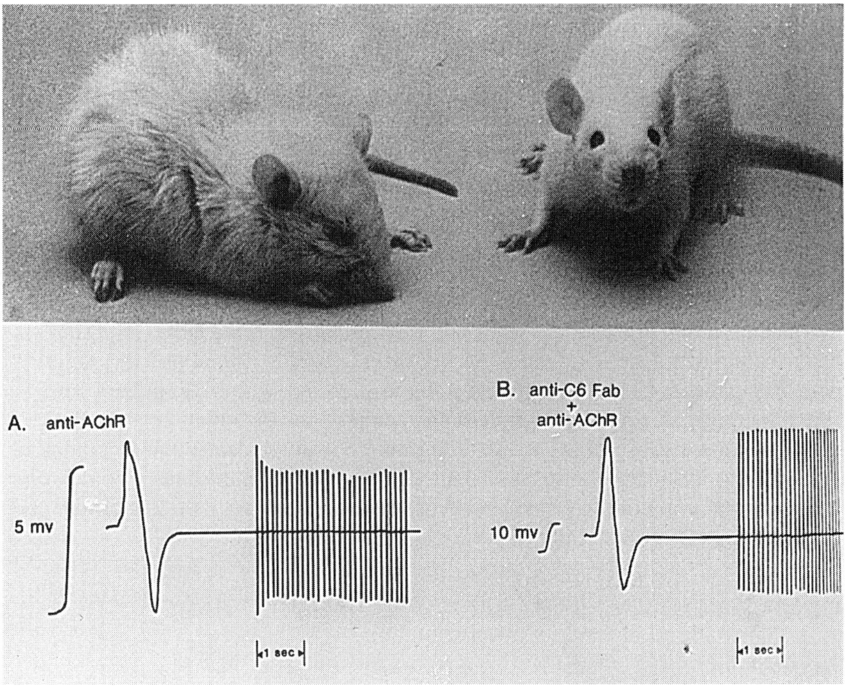

Figure 13.4 Effect of C6 depletion on experimental myasthenia gravis (EAMG). EAMG induced in rats by injection of anti-acetylcholine receptor antibody (anti-AChR) with or without the Fab fragment of an anti-C6 monoclonal antibody to produce C6 depletion *in vivo*. **Top**: animal on left, anti-AChR alone; on right, anti-AChR plus anti-C6. **Bottom**: markedly reduced electromyographic response in the anti-AChR-treated animal (left) compared with relatively normal response in the animal treated with anti-AChR plus anti-C6. (From Biesecker and Gomez, *J. Immunol.*, **142**, 2654–9 (1989), with permission)

The mechanism by which the MAC brings about AChR loss in both the naturally-occurring and experimentally-induced form of the disease remains uncertain. It has been suggested that receptor loss occurs subsequent to 'microlysis' at the end-plate, focal destruction by the MAC resulting in loss of membrane together with receptors[101,105]. In the light of our current knowledge of nucleated cell resistance to MAC killing (Chapter 12), it is more likely that receptors are lost by endocytosis or vesiculation together with MACs during cell recovery processes. The C9-rich 'fragments' identified in the synaptic cleft would then represent membrane vesicles shed during recovery.

COMPLEMENT AND DEMENTIA

Alzheimer's disease is a chronic degenerative disease of the central nervous system characterized clinically by progressive dementia. Pathological changes include diffuse cerebral atrophy and the presence of characteristic lesions in the brain (senile plaques, neurofibrillary tangles, amyloid). Many factors have been implicated but the cause of the disease remains unknown. Evidence of an underlying immunological defect has accumulated in recent years[106]. An acute-phase response is detectable in the plasma of the majority of individuals with Alzheimer's disease, and the plasma levels of the complement proteins, C3, C4, properdin and factor B, are elevated[107]. Complement components, including C1, C3 and C4, are also present in the senile plaques and amyloid[108–110], and the MAC has recently been localized in association with neurofibrillary tangles and dystrophic neurones in Alzheimer brain[111]. Alternative pathway components are not found in these regions, suggesting that complement activation occurs via the classical pathway. Clusters of oligodendrocytes and myelin sheaths coated with the complement breakdown products, C3d and C4d, have been identified in brain tissue from patients with Alzheimer's disease and other degenerative neurological disorders[112], reinforcing the impression that the exquisite sensitivity of oligodendrocytes to complement-mediated damage may be an important factor in diverse CNS disorders. Although there is no evidence that complement activation is a primary factor in Alzheimer's disease, its contribution to neurone loss and inflammation in the central nervous system may be important and certainly merits further study.

COMPLEMENT AND SUBARACHNOID HAEMORRHAGE

Subarachnoid haemorrhage occurs as a result of rupture of a blood vessel in a site which allows the blood access to the subarachnoid space. It is usually due either to rupture of an intracranial aneurysm or to bleeding from a cerebral angioma but may occur occasionally in the absence of an anatomical defect secondary to severe hypertension. The blood spreads from the site of leakage through the subarachnoid space of the brain and spinal cord, causing compression of underlying structures. Treatment involves detection and surgical ligation of the source of bleeding. Even after successful treatment of the acute bleed, a proportion of patients develop severe delayed cerebral vasospasm. The aetiology of this potentially fatal complication is still uncertain but several studies have suggested a role for complement. Activation of complement is detectable in plasma and cerebrospinal fluid of most patients following subarachnoid haemorrhage, and the extent of activation is much greater in those who develop cerebral vasospasm[113,114]. In experimental animals, intracisternal or intraventricular injection of C3adesArg causes breakdown of the blood–brain barrier and influx of cells[115,116]. Thus, complement activation in subarachnoid haemorrhage may be responsible for cerebral vasospasm by causing disruption of the blood–brain barrier or by initiating other inflammatory reactions within the central nervous system.

COMPLEMENT AND NEUROLOGICAL MANIFESTATIONS OF SYSTEMIC AUTOIMMUNE DISEASES

Central nervous system involvement is a feature of several multisystem autoimmune diseases. Neurological disease is present in about one third of individuals with systemic lupus erythematosus (SLE), the prototype human autoimmune disease, and is second only to renal disease as a cause of morbidity and death[117]. Symptoms are extremely varied, ranging from behavioural disturbances or psychosis to organic brain disease with convulsions or paralysis[118,119]. The first indication that complement activation might be occurring within the central nervous system in this disease came from a study of complement levels in the cerebrospinal fluid[120]. SLE patients with central nervous system involvement have markedly lowered cerebrospinal fluid C4 levels which are not merely a reflection of the serum level. Subsequent studies found C4 depletion in the central nervous system only during acute attacks of disease[121], supporting the notion that complement activation might be relevant to pathogenesis. It has recently been reported that elevated levels of TCCs are present in the cerebrospinal fluid of only those SLE patients with central nervous system involvement[122]. In some of the patients, TCCs were detectable in cerebrospinal fluid but not in serum, confirming that activation was occurring within the central nervous system. The mechanisms by which complement is activated in the central nervous system in SLE are uncertain but antineuronal antibodies[123] and immune complexes[124] are present and may be involved.

Sjogren's syndrome is a common rheumatic disease in which joint symptoms are accompanied by diminished lacrimal and salivary gland secretions. Central nervous system complications, which approach in diversity those seen in SLE, occur in a proportion of patients and can cause significant morbidity[125]. An immunological cause of the central nervous system disease is suggested by the demonstration of intrathecal IgG synthesis and the presence of inflammatory cells in the cerebrospinal fluid[126]. The cerebrospinal fluid also contains markedly elevated levels of TCCs, indicating a high level of intrathecal complement activation[122].

Although intrathecal complement activation clearly occurs in these autoimmune disorders, its contribution to the pathogenesis of central nervous system complications remains uncertain. It is also unclear why a proportion of individuals develop central nervous system disease while, despite having similar systemic immune disturbances, the remainder do not.

COMPLEMENT AND BACTERIAL MENINGITIS

Deficiencies of early complement components predispose to infection by a wide range of organisms. These aspects are discussed elsewhere (Chapter 6) and will not be reiterated here. Inherited deficiencies of a terminal component (C5, C6, C7, C8 or C9) or of properdin renders the individual specifically susceptible to systemic Neisserial infections, the commonest manifestation of which is meningococcal meningitis. Deficiencies of terminal components render the individual unable to form lytic MACs, indicating that the MAC is particularly important in neutralizing *Neisseria* species[127]. Several features distinguish meningococcal infection in individuals deficient in terminal components from that in non-deficient individuals – meningitis is commonly accompanied by meningococcaemia, relapse and recurrence of infections are common, severe disease is rare, the first episode of infection occurs at an older age and the causative organism is often of a serogroup not normally associated with disease[128–130]. Deficiency of C5 carries the highest risk of infection, perhaps because of the added loss of the ability to make the active C5a fragment. Deficiencies of C6, C7, or either of the subunits of C8 carry similar risks, at least 50% of the reported cases having had systemic Neisserial infections, although the problems associated with ascertainment bias mean that the true prevalence among deficient individuals is probably much lower than this[131]. The consequences of C9 deficiency are more controversial. Only a minority of the reported cases have had infections, and early reports from Japan, where C9 deficiency is one of the commonest inherited defects[132], implied that the deficiency is not associated with any increase in disease susceptibility[133]. However, a recent study of complement deficiencies in Japanese patients with meningococcal meningitis showed a highly significant association between C9 deficiency and disease, 25% of the patients being C9 deficient compared with a population incidence of 0.036%[134].

Properdin deficiency is inherited in an X-linked manner, and thus predominantly affects males. Deficiency is associated with fulminant and often rapidly fatal meningococcal infections[135]. Until recently, properdin deficiency was considered to be very rare but a recent spate of case reports, particularly from Scandinavia and Holland, suggests that it may not be uncommon[136,137]. Properdin-deficient individuals have a normal classical pathway and, on the second encounter with an organism, can mount a normal response. Recurrent infection is not a feature and screening of male relatives of the index case, followed by immunization of deficient individuals, will reduce the risk. A recent case report describing an individual deficient in factor D suggests that this deficiency may also render individuals particularly susceptible to Neisserial infections and meningitis[138].

Meningococcal meningitis is therefore not infrequently associated with deficiencies of terminal or alternative pathway complement components. Screening of patients with meningococcal meningitis, particularly when the clinical features are unusual, is simple to perform and would identify individuals and families at risk. The features suggestive of an underlying complement deficiency are summarized in Table 13.3.

Table 13.3 Features of meningococcal meningitis suggestive of complement deficiency

Features suggestive of terminal component deficiency
Age at first attack >10 years
Mild recurrent infections
Family history of recurrent meningitis
Infection with unusual serogroups
Accompanying systemic meningococcal infection
Features suggestive of properdin deficiency
Male
Age at first attack >10 years
Family history restricted to males
Severe fulminant non-recurrent infection
Infection with unusual serogroups
Systemic meningococcal infection

CONCLUDING REMARKS

This chapter gives a highly focussed view of the potential relevance of the complement system in a variety of neurological diseases. It is, by design, an unbalanced account, providing abundant evidence for an involvement of complement but little or no information on the potential role of other effector systems. All the diseases discussed are likely to be multifactorial and several effectors will contribute to pathogenesis. It is hoped that this chapter will persuade the reader that the potential role of complement in the initiation and/or perpetuation of tissue damage in neurological disease is worthy of investigation. Even if complement is only secondarily involved, measurement of complement activation may be helpful in diagnosis and management, and manipulation of the complement system may prove therapeutically useful.

References

1. Matthews, B. (1987). Multiple sclerosis. *Med. Int.*, **47**, 1961–6
2. Rodriguez, M. (1989). Multiple sclerosis: Basic concepts and hypothesis. *Mayo Clin. Proc.*, **64**, 570–6
3. Sayetta, R. B. (1986). Theories of the etiology of multiple sclerosis. *J. Clin. Lab. Immunol.*, **21**, 55–70
4. Tourtellotte, W. V. (1989). Current concepts about multiple sclerosis. *Mayo Clin. Proc.*, **64**, 592–7
5. Lowenthal, A., Van Sande, M. and Karcher, D. (1960). The differential diagnosis of neurological diseases by fractionating electrophoretically the CSF gamma globulins. *J. Neurochem.*, **6**, 51–6
6. Tourtellotte, W. W. and Parker, J. A. (1966). Multiple sclerosis: Correlation between immunoglobulin G in cerebrospinal fluid and brain. *Science*, **154**, 1044–6
7. Dasgupta, M. K., Warren, K. G., Johny, K. V. and Dassetor, J. B. (1982). Circulating immune complexes in multiple sclerosis: relation with disease activity. *Neurology*, **32**, 1000–4
8. Salmi, A., Ziola, B., Reunaanen, M., Julkinen, I. and Wager, O. (1982). Immune complexes in serum and cerebrospinal fluid of multiple sclerosis patients and patients with other neurological disorders. *Acta Neurol. Scand.*, **66**, 1–15
9. Prineas, J. W. and Wright, R. G. (1978). Macrophages, lymphocytes and plasma cells in the perivascular compartment in chronic multiple sclerosis. *Lab. Invest.*, **38**, 409–21
10. Traugott, U. (1985). Characterization and distribution of lymphocyte subpopulations in multiple sclerosis plaques versus autoimmune demyelinating lesions. *Springer Semin. Immunopathol.*, **8**, 71–95
11. Kabat, E. A., Glusman, M. and Knaub, V. (1948). Quantitative estimation of the albumin and gamma globulin in normal and pathologic cerebrospinal fluid by immunochemical methods. *Am. J. Med.*, **4**, 653–62
12. Vandvick, B. (1977). Oligoclonal IgG and free light chains in the cerebrospinal fluid of patients with multiple sclerosis and infectious diseases of the central nervous system. *Scand. J. Immunol.*, **6**, 913–22
13. Ryberg, B. (1982). Antibrain antibodies in multiple sclerosis: relation to clinical variables. *J. Neurol. Sci.*, **54**, 239–61
14. Cerf, G. A. and Carels, G. (1966). Multiple sclerosis: serum factor producing reversible alteration in bioelectric responses. *Science*, **152**, 1066–8
15. Schauf, C. L. and Davis, F. A. (1978). The occurrence, specificity and role of neuroelectric blocking factors in multiple sclerosis. *Neurology*, **28**, 34–9
16. Bornstein, M. D. and Crain, S. M. (1965). Functional studies of cultured brain tissues as related to demyelinative disorders. *Science*, **148**, 1242–4
17. Raine, C. S., Hummelglard, A., Swanson, E. and Bornstein, M. B. (1973). Multiple sclerosis serum induced demyelination *in vitro*. A light and electron microscopic study. *J. Neurol. Sci.*, **20**, 127–39

18. Tabira, T., Wolfgran, F. J., Webster, H., Wray, S. H. and McFarlin, D. E. (1977). Myelintoxicity of CSF fractions from multiple sclerosis patients tested in an *in vivo* model. *Neurology*, **27**, 374–83
19. Grundke-Iqbal, I. and Bornstein, M. B. (1980). Multiple sclerosis – serum gamma globulins and demyelination in organ culture. *Neurology*, **30**, 749–54
20. Liu, W. T., Vanguri, P. and Shin, M. L. (1983). Studies on demyelination *in vitro*: the requirements of membrane attack components of the complement system. *J. Immunol.*, **131**, 778–82
21. Silverman, B. A., Carney, D. F., Johnston, C. A., Vanguri, P. and Shin, M. L. (1984). Isolation of membrane attack complex of complement from myelin membranes treated with serum complement. *J. Neurochem.*, **42**, 1024–9
22. Schlaepfer, W. W. (1977). Vesicular disruption of myelin stimulated by exposure of nerve to calcium ionophore. *Nature*, **265**, 734–6
23. Morgan, B. P. and Campbell, A. K. (1985). The recovery of human polymorphonuclear leucoytes from sublytic complement attack is mediated by changes in intracellular free calcium. *Biochem. J.*, **231**, 205–8
24. Vanguri, P. and Shin, M. L. (1988). Hydrolysis of myelin basic protein in human myelin by terminal complement complexes. *J. Biol. Chem.*, **263**, 7228–34
25. Cyong, J. C., Witkin, S. S., Reiger, B., Barbarese, E., Good, R. A. and Day, N. K. (1982). Antibody-independent complement activation by myelin via the classical complement pathway. *J. Exp. Med.*, **155**, 587–98
26. Vanguri, P., Koski, C. L., Silverman, B. and Shin, M. L. (1982). Complement activation by isolated myelin: activation of the classical pathway in the absence of myelin-specific antibodies. *Proc. Natl. Acad. Sci. USA*, **79**, 3920–34
27. Tanaka, M. and Cyong, J. C. (1985). The development of complement-activating ability as an age-related factor in murine brains. *Microbiol. Immunol.*, **29**, 1219–27
28. Scolding, N. J., Morgan, B. P., Houston, W. A. J., Campbell, A. K., Linington, C. and Compston, D. A. S. (1989). Normal rat serum cytotoxicity against syngenic oligodendrocytes: complement activation and attack in the absence of antimyelin antibodies. *J. Neurol. Sci.*, **89**, 289–300
29. Scolding, N. J., Morgan, B. P., Houston, W. A. J., Linington, C., Campbell, A. K. and Compston, D. A. S. (1989) Vesicular removal by oligodendrocytes of membrane attack complexes formed by activated complement. *Nature (London)*, **339**, 620–2
30. Wren, D. R. and Noble, M. (1989). Oligodendrocyte/type-2 astrocyte progenitor cells of adult rats are specifically susceptible to the lytic effects of complement in absence of antibody. *Proc. Natl. Acad. Sci. USA*, **86**, 9025–9
31. Scolding, N. J., Morgan, B. P., Campbell, A. K. and Compston, D. A. S. (1990). Complement-mediated serum cytotoxicity against oligodendrocytes: a comparison with other cells of the oligodendrocyte-type II astrocyte lineage. *J. Neurol. Sci.*, **97**, 155–62
32. Shirazi, Y., Imagawa, D. K. and Shin, M. L. (1987). Release of leukotriene B4 from sublethally injured oligodendrocytes by terminal complement complexes. *J. Neurochem.*, **48**, 171–8
33. Shirazi, Y., McMorris, F. A. and Shin, M. L. (1989). Arachidonic acid mobilization and phosphoinositide turnover by the terminal complement complex, C5b-9, in rat oligodendrocyte × C6 glioma cell hybrids. *J. Immunol.*, **142**, 4285–91
34. Scolding, N. J., Houston, W. A. J., Morgan, B. P., Campbell, A. K. and Compston, D. A. S. (1989). Reversible injury of cultured rat oligodendrocytes by complement. *Immunology*, **67**, 441–6
35. Shirazi, Y., Macklin, W. B. and Shin, M. L. (1989). Terminal complement complexes (TCC) inhibit myelin protein mRNA expression in oligodendrocytes. *FASEB J.*, **3**, A2017 (abstract)
36. Lublin, F. D. (1985). Relapsing experimental allergic encephalomyelitis a autoimmune model of multiple sclerosis. *Springer Semin. Immunopathol.*, **8**, 197–208
37. Linington, C., Bradl, M., Lassmann, H., Brunner, C. and Vass, K. (1988). Augmentation of demyelination in rat acute allergic encephalomyelitis by circulating mouse monoclonal antibodies directed against a myelin/oligodendrocyte glycoprotein (MOG). *Am. J. Pathol.*, **130**, 443–54
38. Ben-Nun, A., Wekerle, H. and Cohen, I. R. (1981). The rapid isolation of clonable antigen-specific T lymphocyte lines capable of mediating autoimmune encephalomyelitis. *Eur. J. Immunol.*, **11**, 195–9
39. Pabst, H., Day, N. K., Gewurz, H. and Good, R. A. (1971). Prevention of experimental allergic encephalomyelitis with cobra venom factor. *Proc. Soc. Exp. Biol. Med.*, **136**, 555–60

40. Levine, S., Cochran, C. G. and Carpenter, C. B. (1977). Allergic encephalomyelitis: effect of complement depletion with cobra venom. *Proc. Soc. Exp. Biol. Med.*, **138**, 285–9
41. Morariau, M. A. and Dalmasso, A. P. (1978). Experimental allergic encephalomyelitis in cobra venom factor-treated and C4-deficient guinea pigs. *Ann. Neurol.*, **4**, 427–30
42. Linington, C., Morgan, B. P., Scolding, N. J., Piddlesden, S., Wilkins, P. and Compston, D. A. S. (1989). The role of complement in the pathogenesis of experimental allergic encephalomyelitis. *Brain*, **112**, 895–911.
43. Piddlesden, S., Lassmann, H., Laffafian, I., Morgan, B. P. and Linington, C. (1990). Antibody-mediated demyelination in experimental allergic encephalomyelitis is independent of complement membrane complex formation. *Clin. Exp. Immunol.*, **83**, 245–50
44. Linington, C., Lassmann, H., Morgan, B. P. and Compston, D. A. S. (1989). Immuno-histochemical localisation of complement component C9 in experimental allergic encephalomyelitis. *Acta Neuropathol.*, **79**, 78–85
45. Kuwert, E., Pette, E., Firnhaber, W. and Mai, K. (1965). Demonstration of complement in spinal fluid in multiple sclerosis. *Ann. NY Acad. Sci.*, **122**, 429–35
46. Link, H. (1972). Complement factors in multiple sclerosis. *Acta Neurol. Scand.*, **48**, 521–8
47. Trouillas, P., Moindrot, J., Betuel, H., Quinay, C1., Aimard, G. and Devic, M. (1976). Scleroses en plaques avec hypocomplementemie et scleroses en plaques normocomplementaires correlation cliniques et genetiques. *Rev. Neurol.* (*Paris*), **132**, 681–704
48. Caspary, E. A. (1977). Humoral factors involved in immune processes in multiple sclerosis and allergic encephalomyelitis. *Br. Med. Bull.*, **33**, 50–3
49. Yam, P., Petz., L. D., Tourellote, W. W. and Ma, B. I. (1980). Measurement of complement components in cerebral spinal fluid by radioimmunoassay in patients with multiple sclerosis. *Clin. Immunol. Immunopathol.*, **17**, 492–505
50. Morgan, B. P., Campbell, A. K. and Compston, D. A. S. (1984). Terminal component of complement (C9) in cerebrospinal fluid of patients with multiple sclerosis. *Lancet*, **2**, 251–4
51. Compston, D. A. S., Morgan, B. P., Oleesky, D., Fifield, R. and Campbell, A. K. (1986). Cerebrospinal fluid C9 in demyelinating disease. *Neurology*, **36**, 1503–6
52. Halawa, I., Lolli, F. and Link, H. (1989). Terminal component of complement C9 in CSF and plasma of patients with MS and aseptic meningitis. *Acta Neurol. Scand.*, **80**, 130–5
53. Rodriguez, M., Wynn, D. R., Kimlinger, T. K. and Katzmann, J. A. (1990). Terminal component of complement (C9) in the cerebrospinal fluid of patients with multiple sclerosis and neurological controls. *Neurology*, **40**, 855–7
54. Sanders, M. E., Koski, C. L., Robbins, D., Shin, M. L., Frank, M. M. and Joiner, K. A. (1986). Activated terminal complement in cerebrospinal fluid in Guillain–Barre syndrome and multiple sclerosis. *J. Immunol.*, **135**, 4456–9
55. Mollnes, T. E., Vandvick, B., Lea, T. and Vartdal, F. (1987). Intrathecal complement activation in neurological diseases evaluated by analysis of the terminal complement complex. *J. Neurol. Sci.*, **78**, 17–28
56. Compston, D. A. S., Morgan, B. P., Campbell, A. K., Wilkins, P., Cole, G., Thomas, N. D. and Jasani, B. (1989). Immunocytochemical localization of the terminal complement complex in multiple sclerosis. *Neuropathol. Appl. Neurobiol.*, **15**, 307–16
57. Smith, K. J., Hall, S. M. and Schauf, C. L. (1985). Vesicular demyelination induced by raised intracellular calcium. *J. Neurol. Sci.*, **71**, 19–37
58. Smith, K. J. and Hall, S. M. (1988). Peripheral demyelination and remeylination initiated by the calcium-selective ionophore ionomycin: in vivo observations. *J. Neurol. Sci.*, **83**, 37–53
59. Waxman, S. G., Davis, P. K., Black, J. A. and Ransom, B. R. (1990). Anoxic injury of mammalian central white matter: decreased susceptibility in myelin-deficient optic nerve. *Ann. Neurol.*, **28**, 335–40
60. Asbury, A. K. (1990). Guillain–Barre syndrome: Historical aspects. *Ann. Neurol.*, **27** (suppl.), S2–6
61. Alter, M. (1990). The epidemiology of Guillain–Barre syndrome. *Ann. Neurol.*, **27** (suppl.), S7–12
62. Prineas, J. W. (1981). Pathology of the Guillain–Barre syndrome. *Ann. Neurol.*, **9** (suppl.), S6–19
63. Astrom, K. E. and Waksman, B. H. (1962). The passive transfer of experimental encephalomyelitis and neuritis with living lymphoid cells. *J. Pathol. Bacteriol.*, **83**, 39–106
64. Carlo, D. J., Karkhanis, Y. D. and Bailey, P. J. (1975). Experimental neuritis: evidence for the involvement of the P0 and P2 proteins. *Brain Res.*, **88**, 580–4

65. Cook, S. D., Dowling, P. C. and Whitaker, J. N. (1970). The Guillain–Barre syndrome: relationship of circulating immunocytes to disease activity. *Arch. Neurol.*, **22**, 470–4
66. Iquabal, A., Oger, J. J-F. and Arnason, B. G. W. (1981). Cell-mediated immunity in idiopathic polyneuritis. *Ann. Neurol.*, **9** (suppl.), S65–9
67. Cook, S., Dowling, P. C., Murray, M. R. and Whitaker, J. N. (1971). Circulating demyelinating factors in acute idiopathic polyneuropathy: myelinotoxic antibody in the Guillain-Barre syndrome. *Arch. Neurol.*, **24**, 136–44
68. Saida, T., Saida, K. and Lisak, R. P. (1982). In vivo demyelinating activity of sera from patients with Guillain–Barre syndrome. *Ann. Neurol.*, **11**, 69–75
69. Nyland, H. and Aarli, J. A. (1978). Guillain–Barre syndrome: demonstration of antibodies to peripheral nerve tissue. *Acta Neurol. Scand.*, **58**, 35–43
70. Koski, C. L., Gratz., E., Sutherland, J. and Mayer, R. F. (1986). Clinical correlation with anti-peripheral nerve myelin antibodies in Guillain-Barre syndrome. *Ann. Neurol.*, **19**, 573–7
71. Koski, C. L., Chou, D. K. H. and Jungalwala, F. B. (1989). Antiperipheral nerve myelin antibodies in Guillain–Barre syndrome bind a neutral glycolipid of peripheral myelin and cross-react with Forssman antigen. *J. Clin. Invest.*, **84**, 280–7
72. Koski, C. L. (1990). Characterisation of complement-fixing antibodies to peripheral nerve myelin in Guillain–Barre syndrome. *Ann. Neurol.*, **27** (suppl.), S44–7
73. McKhann, G. M., Griffin, J. W., Cornblath, D. R., Mellits, E. D., Fisher, R. S. and Quaskey, S. A. (1988). Plasmapheresis and Guillain–Barre syndrome: analysis of prognostic factors and the effect of plasmapheresis. *Ann. Neurol.*, **23**, 347–53
74. Hartung, H-P., Schwenke, C., Bitter-Suermann, D. and Toyka, K. V. (1987). Guillain–Barre syndrome: activated complement components C3a and C5a in CSF. *Neurology*, **37**, 1006–9
75. Koski, C. L., Sanders, M. E., Swoveland, P. T., Lawley, T. J., Shin, M. L., Frank, M. M. and Joiner, K. A. (1987). Activation of terminal components of complement in patients with Guillain–Barre syndrome and other demyelinating neuropathies. *J. Clin. Invest.*, **80**, 1492–7
76. Latov., N., Sherman, W. H., Nemni, R., Galasi, G., Shyong, J. S., Penn, A. S., Chess, L., Orlate, M. R., Rowland, L. P. and Osserman, E. F. (1980). Plasma cell dyscrasia and peripheral neuropathy with a monoclonal antibody to peripheral nerve myelin. *N. Engl. J. Med.*, **303**, 618–21
77. Latov, N., Gross, R. B., Kastelman, J., Flanagan, T., Lamme, S., Alkaitis, D. A., Olarte, M. R., Sherman, W. H., Chess, L. and Penn, A. S. (1981). Complement-fixing anti-peripheral nerve myelin antibodies in patients with inflammatory polyneuritis and polyneuropathy and paraproteinaemia. *Neurology*, **31**, 1530–4
78. Ilyas, A. A., Quarles, R. H., MacIntosh, I. D., Dobersen, M. J., Trapp, B. D., Dalakas, M. C. and Brady, R. O. (1984). IgM in a human neuropathy related to paraproteinaemia binds to a carbohydrate determinant in the myelin-associated glycoprotein and to a ganglioside. *Proc. Natl. Acad. Sci. USA*, **81**, 1225–9
79. Hays, A. P., Latov, N., Takasu, M. and Sherman, W. H. (1987). Experimental demyelination of nerve induced by serum of patients with neuropathy and an anti-MAG IgM M-protein. *Neurology*, **37**, 242–56
80. Haas, D. C. and Tatum, A. H. (1988). Plasmapheresis alleviates neuropathy accompanying IgM anti-myelin-associated glycoprotein paraproteinaemia. *Ann. Neurol.*, **23**, 394–6
81. Hays, A. P., Lee, S. and Latov, N. (1988). Immune reactive C3d on the surface of myelin sheaths in neuropathy. *J. Neuroimmunol.*, **18**, 231–44
82. Monaco, S., Bonetti, B., Ferrari, S., Moretto, G., Nardelli, E., Tedesco., F., Mollnes, T. E., Nobile-Orazio, E., Manfredini, E., Bonazzi, L. and Rizzuto, N. (1990). Complement-mediated demyelination in patients with IgM monoclonal gammopathy and peripheral neuropathy. *N. Engl. J. Med.*, **322**, 649–52
83. Monaco, S., Ferrari, S., Nardelli, E., Bonetti, B., Rizzuto, N. and Tedesco, F. (1990). Experimental models for complement-mediated demyelination. *Complement Inflamm.*, **7**, 138 (abstract)
84. Borsos, T. and Rapp, H. J. (1965). Complement fixation on cell surfaces by 19S and 7S antibodies. *Science*, **150**, 505–6
85. Borsos, T., Chapuis, M. and Langone, J. J. (1981). Distinction between fixation of C1 and the activation of complement by natural IgM anti-hapten antibody: Effect of cell surface hapten density. *Mol. Immunol.*, **18**, 863–8
86. Borsos, T. and Circolo, A. (1983). Binding and activation of C1 by cell bound IgG: Activation depends on cell surface hapten density. *Mol. Immunol.*, **20**, 433–8

87. Newsome-Davis, J. and Vincent, A. (1982). Myasthenia gravis. In Lachmann, P. J. and Peters, D. K. (eds.) *Clinical Aspects of Immunology*, pp. 1011–68. (Oxford: Blackwell)
88. Campbell, H. and Bramwell, E. (1990). Myasthenia gravis. *Brain*, **23**, 277–336
89. Wilson, A. and Stoner, H. B. (1944). Myasthenia gravis. A consideration of its causation in fourteen cases. *Q. J. Med.*, **13**, 1–18
90. Teng, P. and Osserman, K. E. (1956). Studies in myasthenia gravis, neonatal and juvenile types. *J. Mt. Sinai Hosp.*, **23**, 711–20
91. Strauss, A. J. L., Deitch, A. and Hsu, K. C. (1961). Further observations on the localization of a muscle-binding complement-fixing serum globulin fraction in myasthenia gravis. *Fed. Proc.*, **20**, 38 (abstract)
92. Parkes, J. D. and McKinna, J. A. (1966). Neuromuscular blocking activity in the blood of patients with myasthenia gravis. *Lancet*, **1**, 338–91
93. Van der Geld, H., Feltkamp, T. E. W. and Oosterhuis, H. J. G. H. (1964). Reactivity of myasthenia gravis serum γ-globulin with skeletal muscle and thymus demonstrated by immunofluorescence. *Proc. Soc. Exp. Biol. Med.*, **115**, 782–5
94. Fambrough, D. M., Drachman, D. B. and Satyamurti, S. (1973) Neuromuscular junction in myasthenia gravis: decreased acetylcholine receptors. *Science*, **182**, 293–5
95. Patrick, J. and Lindstrom, J. (1973). Autoimmune response to acetylcholine receptor. *Science*, **189**, 871–2
96. Tarab-Hazdai, R., Aharanov, A., Silbman, I., Fuchs, S. and Abramsky, O. (1975). Experimental autoimmune myasthenia induced in monkeys by purified acetylcholine receptor. *Nature*, **256**, 128–30
97. Nastuk, W. L., Plescia, O. and Osserman, K. E. (1960). Changes in serum complement levels in patients with myasthenia gravis. *Proc. Soc. Exp. Med.*, **105**, 177–84
98. Plescia, O. J., Segovia, J. M. and Strampp, A. (1966). An assessment of changes in the complement level of myasthenic sera. *Ann. N. Y. Acad. Sci.*, **135**, 580–7
99. Engel, A. G., Lambert, E. H. and Howard, F. M. (1977). Immune complexes (IgG and C3) at the motor end-plate in myasthenia gravis. Ultra-structural and light microscopical localization and electrophysiological correlations. *Mayo Clin. Proc.*, **52**, 267–80
100. Sahashi, K., Engel, A. G., Lambert, E. H. and Howard, F. M. (1980). Ultrastructural localization of the terminal and lytic 9th complement component (C9) at the motor end-plate in myasthenia gravis. *J. Neurol. Exp. Neuropathol.*, **39**, 160–72
101. Engel, A. G. and Arahata, K. (1987). The membrane attack complex of complement at the motor end-plate in myasthenia gravis. *Ann. NY Acad. Sci.*, **505**, 326–32
102. Engel, A. G., Sakakibara, H., Sahashi, K., Lindstrom, J. M., Lambert, E. H. and Lennon, V. A. (1979). Passively transferred experimental autoimmune myasthenia gravis: sequential and quantitative studies of the motor end-plate fine structure and ultrastructural localization of immune complexes (IgG and C3), and of the acetylcholine receptor. *Neurology*, **29**, 179–88
103. Lennon, V. A., Seybold, M. E., Lindstrom, J. M., Cochrane, C. and Ulevitch, R. (1978). Role of complement in the pathogenesis of experimental autoimmune myasthenia gravis. *J. Exp. Med.*, **147**, 973–83
104. Biesecker, G. and Gomez, C. M. (1989). Inhibition of acute passive transfer experimental autoimmune myasthenia gravis with Fab antibody to complement C6. *J. Immunol.*, **142**, 2654–9
105. Engel, A. G. and Fumagalli, G. (1982). Mechanisms of acetylcholine receptor loss from the neuromuscular junction. In *Receptors, Antibodies and Disease. CIBA Foundation Symposium 90*, pp. 197–224. (London: Pitman)
106. Hulette, C. M. and Walford, R. L. (1987). Immunological aspects of Alzheimer disease: a review. *Alzheimer Dis. Assoc. Discord.*, **1**, 72–82
107. Giometto, B., Argentiero, V., Sanson, F., Ongaro, G. and Tavolato, B. (1988). Acute phase proteins in Alzheimer's disease. *Eur. Neurol.*, **28**, 30–3
108. Eikelenboom, P. and Stam, F. C. (1982). Immunoglobulins and complement factors in senile plaques: an immunohistoperoxidase study. *Acta Neuropathol.*, **57**, 239–42
109. Ishii, T., Haga, S. and Akiyama, H. (1988). Presence of immunoglobulins and complement in the amyloid plaques in the brain of patients with Alzheimer's disease. In Pouplard-Barthelaix, Emile and Christen (eds.) *Immunology and Alzheimer's Disease*, pp. 17–29. (Berlin: Springer)
110. Eikelenboom, P., Hack, C. E., Rozemuller, J. M. and Stam, F. C. (1989). Complement activation in amyloid plaques in Alzheimer's dementia. *Virchow's Arch.* (*Cell Pathol.*), **56**, 259–62

111. McGeer, P. L., Akinyama, H., Iltagaki, S. and McGeer, E. G. (1989). Activation of the classical complement pathway in brain tissue of Alzheimer patients. *Neurosci. Lett.*, **107**, 341–6
112. Yamada, T., Akiyama, H. and McGeer, P. L. (1990). Complement-activated oligodendrocytes: a new pathogenic entity identified by immunostaining with antibodies to human complement proteins C3d and C4d. *Neurosci. Lett.*, **112**, 161–6
113. Ostergard, J. R., Kristensen, B. O., Svehag, S. E., Teisner, B. and Miletic, T. (1987). Immune complexes and complement activation following rupture of intracranial saccular aneurysms. *J. Neurosurg.*, **66**, 891–7
114. Kasuya, H. and Shimizu, T. (1989). Activated complement components C3a and C4a in cerebrospinal fluid and plasma following subarachnoid haemorrhage. *J. Neurosurg.*, **71**, 741–6
115. Hollerhage, H. G., Wilgand, H. and Stolke, D. (1986). The effect of the cleavage peptide C3adesArg of the third complement component on the accumulation of leukocytes in cerebrospinal fluid (CSF) and on the permeability of the blood–CSF barrier. In Wenker, H., Klinger, M. and Brock, M. (eds.) *Advances in Neurosurgery*, 14, pp. 252–6. (Berlin: Springer)
116. Hollerhage, H. G. (1988). Possible role of complement peptides in SAH. *J. Neurosurg.*, **69**, 802–3
117. Small, P., Mass, M. F., Kohler, P. F. and Harbeck, R. J. (1977). Central nervous system involvement in SLE. Diagnostic profile and clinical features. *Arthritis Rheum.*, **20**, 869–978
118. Johnson, R. T. and Richardson, E. P. (1968). The neurological manifestations of systemic lupus erythematosus. *Medicine*, **47**, 337–69
119. Ellis, S. G. and Verity, M. A. (1979). Central nervous system involvement in systemic lupus erythematosus: a review of neuropathologic findings in 57 cases, 1975–1977. *Semin. Arthritis Rheum.*, **8**, 212–21
120. Petz, L. D., Sharp, G. C., Cooper, N. R. and Irvin, W. S. (1971). Serum and cerebral spinal fluid complement and serum autoantibodies in systemic lupus erythematosus. *Medicine*, **50**, 259–75
121. Hadler, N. M., Gerwin, R. D., Frank, M. M., Whitaker, J. N., Baker, M. and Decker, J. L. (1973). The fourth component of complement in the cerebrospinal fluid in systemic lupus erythematosus. *Arthritis Rheum.*, **16**, 507–21
122. Sanders, M. E., Alexander, E. L., Koski, C. L., Frank, M. M. and Joiner, K. A. (1987). Detection of activated terminal complement (C5b-9) in cerebrospinal fluid from patients with central nervous system involvement of primary Sjogren's syndrome or systemic lupus erythematosus. *J. Immunol.*, **138**, 2095–9
123. Bluestein, H. G., Williams, G. W. and Steinberg, A. D. (1981). Cerebrospinal fluid antibodies to neuronal cells: association with neuropsychiatric manifestations of systemic lupus erythematosus. *Am. J. Med.*, **70**, 240–6
124. Seibold, J. R., Buckingham, R. B., Medsger T. A. Jr. and Kelly, R. H. (1982). Cerebrospinal fluid immune complexes in systemic lupus erythematosus involving the central nervous system. *Semin. Arthritis Rheum.*, **12**, 68–76
125. Alexander, G. E., Provost, T. T., Stevens, M. B. and Alexander, E. L. (1982). Sjogren's syndrome: central nervous system manifestations. *Neurology*, **31**, 1391–6
126. Alexander, E. L., Lijewski, J. E., Jordan, M. S. and Alexander, G. E. (1986). Evidence of an immunopathogenic basis for central nervous system disease in primary Sjogren's syndrome. *Arthritis Rheum.*, **29**, 1223–31
127. Harriman, G. R., Esser, A. F., Podack, E. R., Wunderlich, A. C., Braude, A. I., Lint, T. F. and Curd, J. G. (1980). The role of C9 in complement-mediated killing of Neisseria. *J. Immunol.*, **125**, 2252–7
128. Ross, S. C. and Densen, P. (1984). Complement deficiency states and infection: Epidemiology, pathogenesis and consequences of Neisserial and other infections in an immune deficiency. *Medicine*, **63**, 243–73
129. Fries, L. F., O'Shea, J. J. and Frank, M. M. (1986). Inherited deficiencies of complement and complement-related proteins. *Clin. Immunol. Immunopathol.*, **40**, 37–49
130. Fijen, C. A. P., Kuijper, E. J., Hannema, A. J., Sjoholm, A. G. and van Putten, J. P. M. (1989). Complement deficiencies in patients over ten years old with meningococcal disease due to uncommon serogroups. *Lancet*, **2**, 585–8
131. Inai, S. H., Kitamura, S., Hiramatsu, S. and Nagaki, K. (1979). Deficiency of the ninth component of complement in man. *J. Clin. Invest.*, **71**, 183–91

132. Inaba, S., Okochi, K., Fukada, K., Kinoshita, S., Maeda, Y. and Yoshinari, M. (1987). The occurrence of precipitating antibodies in transfused Japanese patients with hereditary ninth component of complement deficiency and frequency of C9 deficiency. *Transfusion*, **27**, 475–7
133. Fukumori, Y., Yoshimuro, K. and Ohnoki, S. (1989). A high incidence of C9 deficiency among healthy blood donors in Osaka, Japan. *Int. Immunol.*, **1**, 85–9
134. Nagata, M., Hara, T., Aoki, T., Mizuno, Y., Akeda, H., Inaba, S., Tsumoto, K. and Ueda, K. (1989). Inherited deficiency of ninth component of complement: An increased risk of meningococcal meningitis. *J. Paediatr.*, **114**, 260–4
135. Sjoholm, A. G., Braconier, J-H. and Soderstrom, C. (1982). Properdin deficiency in a family with fulminant meningococcal infections. *Clin. Exp. Immunol.*, **50**, 291–7
136. Sjoholm, A. G., Kuijper, E. J., Tijssen, C. C., Jansz, A., Bol, P., Spanjaard, L. and Zanen, H. C. (1988). Dysfunctional properdin in a Dutch family with meningococcal disease. *N. Engl. J. Med.*, **319**, 33–7
137. Sjoholm, A. G., Soderstrom, C. and Nilsson, L.-A. (1988). A second variant of properdin deficiency: The detection of properdin at low concentrations in affected males. *Complement*, **5**, 130–40
138. Hiemstra, P. S., Langeler, E., Compier, B., Keepers, Y., Leijh, P. C. J., van den Barselaar, M. T., Overbosch, D. and Daha, M. R. (1989). Complete and partial deficiencies of complement factor D in a Dutch family. *J. Clin. Invest.*, **84**, 1957–61

Index